Pediatric
Radiology

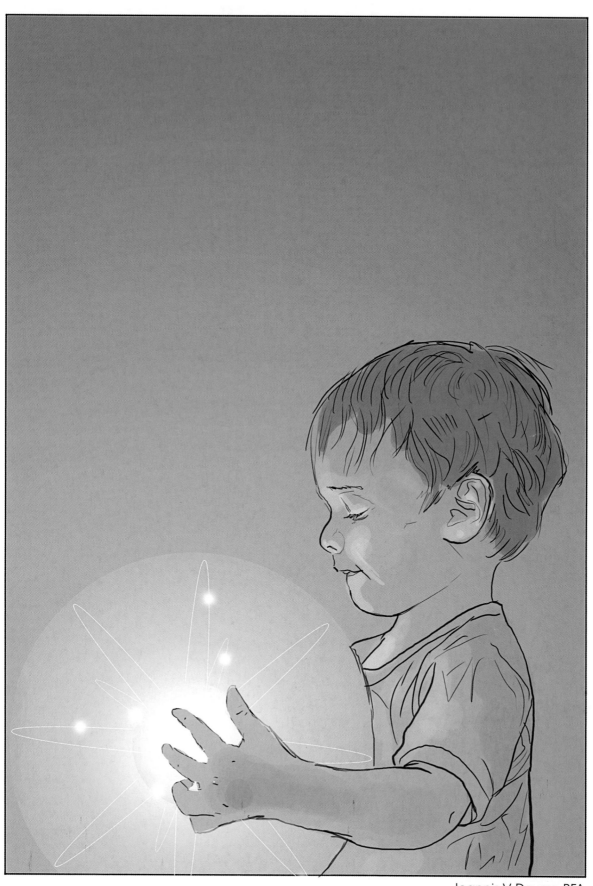

Ioannis V. Davros, BFA.
Savannah College of Art and Design

Future Books in the **Rotations in Radiology** Series

Cardiac Imaging

Charles White, Linda Haramati, Joseph J.S. Chen,
and Jeffrey Levky

Chest Imaging

Melissa Rosado de Christensen, SanjeevBhalla, Gerald Abbott,
and Santiago Martinez-Jiminez

Gastrointestinal Imaging

Angela Levy, Koenraad Mortele, and Benjamin Yeh

Rotations in Radiology

Pediatric Radiology

Edited by

Janet R. Reid, MD, FRCPC

Associate Professor of Radiology
The University of Pennsylvania
The Children's Hospital of Philadelphia
Philadelphia, PA

Angelisa Paladin, MD

Associate Professor of Radiology
University of Washington School of Medicine
Seattle Children's Hospital
Seattle, WA

William J. Davros, PhD, ABMP(D)

Senior Member, Section of Medical Physics
Cleveland Clinic
Cleveland, OH

Edward Y. Lee, MD, MPH

Associate Professor of Radiology
Harvard Medical School
Children's Hospital Boston
Boston, MA

Caroline W. T. Carrico, MD

Associate Professor of Radiology
Duke University School of Medicine
Duke Children's Hospital and Health Center
Durham, NC

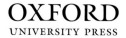

OXFORD
UNIVERSITY PRESS

OXFORD
UNIVERSITY PRESS

Oxford University Press is a department of the University of Oxford.
It furthers the University's objective of excellence in research, scholarship,
and education by publishing worldwide.

Oxford   New York
Auckland   Cape Town   Dar es Salaam   Hong Kong   Karachi
Kuala Lumpur   Madrid   Melbourne   Mexico City   Nairobi
New Delhi   Shanghai   Taipei   Toronto

With offices in
Argentina   Austria   Brazil   Chile   Czech Republic   France   Greece
Guatemala   Hungary   Italy   Japan   Poland   Portugal   Singapore
South Korea   Switzerland   Thailand   Turkey   Ukraine   Vietnam

Oxford is a registered trademark of Oxford University Press in the UK
and certain other countries.

Published in the United States of America by
Oxford University Press
198 Madison Avenue, New York, NY 10016

© Oxford University Press 2014

Library of Congress Cataloging-in-Publication Data
Pediatric radiology / edited by Janet R. Reid…[et al.].
      p. ; cm. — (Rotations in radiology)
Includes bibliographical references and index.
Summary: "Presented in a concise and readable format, Pediatric Radiology provides a
comprehensive review of 120 pathologies commonly encountered by practicing radiologists
and residents. As part of the Rotations in Radiology series, this volume offers a guided
approach to imaging diagnosis with a constant depth of coverage, a structured template, and
incorporation of applied physics, distinguishing it from other texts in the field. A definition
is given for each pathology in this volume, followed by: demographics, clinical presentation,
imaging modalities and features, imaging algorithm, applied physics, differential diagnoses
and pitfalls, and a bulleted summary of key points. Designed for point-of-care use while
training on a specific rotation, as well as for exam review and ongoing reference, Pediatric
Radiology is the perfect tool to impart to residents, as well as to refresh for practitioners,
the essential facts of common pathologies and the various modalities used to interpret
them"—Provided by publisher.
ISBN 978–0–19–975532–5 (alk. paper) — ISBN 978–0–19–998575–3 (alk. paper)
I. Reid, Janet.   II. Series: Rotations in radiology.
[DNLM: 1. Radiography.   2. Child.   3. Infant. WN 240]
LCClassification not assigned
618.92′00757—dc23
2013000987

9 8 7 6 5 4 3 2 1
Printed in China
on acid-free paper

Contents

Preface

There are many excellent resources for pediatric radiology now available as textbooks, online textbooks, online courses, etc. Why create yet another book about pediatric radiology? Our thoughts were this: let's set out to create the most comprehensive resource for the radiology resident, an adult student of radiology who may not know his or her future career path, but who is curious about pediatric radiology and who must also pass a test at the end of training. And let's cast a wide net to gather content from experts from around the country to eliminate regional bias. Using adult learning principles, we chose to present the most relevant and current information within context of the resident experience- first to give the granular facts and illustrate the findings in a templated succinct style, but to then suggest an "imaging strategy" to provide guidance while navigating the waters of a pediatric rotation; to give a soundbite summary in "key points" but to go beyond this in presenting "imaging pitfalls" and "common variants" so that they could be prepared to think of pediatric disease on a grayscale rather than black and white. Where necessary, original illustrations were created by a team of 8 medical illustrators from the Department of Medical Illustration and Photography at the Cleveland Clinic, where a common style was adopted to ensure uniformity. Lastly, embracing the philosophy of the new certification process, our medical physicist and I carefully crafted individualized "related physics" sections for each of the 120 topics offered in this book. This is the book I needed when I was a resident. And this will hopefully serve as the foundation for a future enduring electronic resource.

Janet R. Reid MD, FRCPC
Patricia Borns Chair for Radiology Education
Associate Professor of Radiology
University of Pennsylvania
The Children's Hospital of Philadelphia
Philadelphia, PA

Foreword

Pediatric imaging has grown tremendously in scope and practice since I began my own career in 1985. At that time, MRI was in its infancy, producing blurred, artifact-filled images needing hours to acquire, usually requiring sedation or general anesthesia. Although radiation dose reduction has always been a part of the pediatric radiologists' mantra, the use of lower kVp and girth-based mA settings for CT scanning, as well as pulsed fluoroscopy were not in our armamentarium. Current practice requires the integrated use of multiple modalities to reach a diagnosis in an efficient, cost-effective, non-invasive and safe manner, with particular attention paid to minimizing radiation dose. This current paradigm results in a strong need for a readable, introductory text for trainees beginning their exploration of pediatric imaging. There are few high quality review texts for residents and fellows that have been properly peer reviewed and checked for accuracy and error. *Pediatric Radiology* fits this bill quite well. Dr. Janet Reid, the editor of this work is no stranger to pediatric radiology education. She has taken many of the concepts she developed for the widely recognized and used "Children's Hospital Cleveland Clinic Pediatric Radiology" educational website* and applied them to the current textbook.

The resulting book presents high quality, state of the art imaging with current information that will serve as a very useful review of the specialty of pediatric imaging. Every chapter has been reviewed and carefully edited for authenticity, currency and quality. *Pediatric Radiology* is authored by a cross-section of practicing pediatric radiologists from around the United States, and reflects the broad diversity of our specialty. *Pediatric Radiology* is logically organized into 8 main anatomic sections including a section on systemic disease encompassing important multi-system diseases such as cystic fibrosis, sickle cell disease, child abuse, and others. Each section is divided into concise chapters on specific disease entities, organized around the concepts of clinical presentation, anatomic considerations, imaging findings, strategies, and variants. Each chapter also provides topical insights into the physical principles of the appropriate imaging techniques to help with dose and image optimization. By doing so, the curriculum of the American Association of Physicists in Medicine is effectively embedded into each chapter by matching relevant topics with each of the 120 chapters. Many chapters contain anatomic drawings that further explain the basis of imaging findings. These are excellent, original illustrations that help to clarify complex imaging concepts. The style is well suited for trainees. It is streamlined, up to date and quite readable.

Pediatric Radiology fills an important niche as an accessible introduction to pediatric imaging, and will serve as an excellent reference for medical students, for fellows and residents in radiology, and for the general radiologist who practices pediatrics.

George A. Taylor, M.D.
John A. Kirkpatrick Professor of Radiology (Pediatrics)
Harvard Medical School
Radiologist-in-Chief Emeritus, Boston Children's Hospital
Boston, MA

*https://www.cchs.net/pediatricradiology/

Foreword

This book serves as a general introduction to Pediatric Radiology that is sure to be useful as an introductory textbook, a source for review, and a reference text for people with limited exposure to imaging children. In a field where there are already excellent textbooks, what makes Dr. Reid's book unique?

The first distinguishing feature is the book's format. There is a healthy emphasis on key points and imaging strategies, making concepts easier to retain and their applicability easier to understand. The text has also been configured with plans for an electronic version, and I strongly believe that in this day and age an electronic textbook has the greatest appeal to trainees.

The volume contains valuable imaging insights combined with concepts of physics. One hundred and twenty AAPM curriculum offerings are paired with topics. Pertinent physical concepts are very nicely integrated into the discussion of the imaging findings, such as in the chapter of Adult Polycystic Kidney Disease, which includes a discussion of harmonic ultrasound imaging.

Dr. Reid is a passionate teacher. She has demonstrated an amazing talent for integrating a large body of knowledge into an easily understandable format. The web-based Pediatric Radiology Curriculum she has contributed to has become one of the most widely used references in the field and is a teaching tool in almost 60 countries. Moreover, this coauthored text has been written by many outstanding authors. Since the authors come from many institutions, the text is representative of the pediatric radiology community rather than reflecting the bias of a single institution.

This is an excellent pediatric radiology textbook which will be useful for trainees and for those interested in reviewing current concepts in the subspecialty. Dr. Reid and her coauthors should feel very proud of having produced a superb compilation of pediatric imaging knowledge.

Diego Jaramillo, MD, MPH
Professor of Radiology
The University of Pennsylvania
The Children's Hospital of Philadelphia
Philadelphia, PA

Acknowledgements

Sincere appreciation and thanks to Christina Rasi, MA, for her tireless work as Editorial Assistant for this text. I could not have done this without her organizational skills, interactions within the team and meticulous combing of everything that went into this book.

Special thanks to assistant editors Angelisa Paladin MD, Caroline Caricco MD, Edward Lee MD and William Davros PhD who did more work than they originally signed up for!

Thank you to Ann Paladino, Jeff Loerch, Joseph Pangrace, Dave R. Schumick, Beth Halasz, Joseph Kanasz, Ross Papalardo, Bill Garriott, and Mark Sabo with their summer students from the Department of Medical Illustration and Photography at the Cleveland Clinic for their beautiful medical illustrations and the rights to license their use in this book. Thank you also to Andria Powers, MD for reviewing image proofs.

We appreciate the tireless work of every contributing author.

To my loving husband, Andrew, and our three children for all of their endless patience and support.

Janet Reid MD, FRCPC

Contributors

Adebunmi O. Adeyiga, MD
Assistant Professor of Radiology and Pediatrics
The George Washington University School of
Medicine & Health Sciences
Children's National Medical Center
Washington D.C.

Michael E. Arch, MD
Department of Pediatric Radiology
Chris Evert Children's Hospital
Broward Health Medical Center
Fort Lauderdale, Florida

Joao Amaral, MD
Assistant Professor of Medical Imaging
University of Toronto
The Hospital for Sick Children
Toronto, Ontario, Canada

Paul Babyn, MDCM, FRCPC
Department of Medical Imaging
University of Saskatchewan
Saskatoon Health Region Royal University Hospital
Saskatoon, Saskatchewan

Zachary D. Bailey, MD
Department of Radiology
University of Missouri-Kansas City School
of Medicine
Kansas City, Missouri

Gerald Behr, MD
Assistant Professor of Clinical Radiology
Columbia University
Morgan Stanley Children's Hospital
New York, New York

Linda Bloom, MD
Department of Pediatrics
Stony Brook University School of Medicine
Stony Brook University Hospital
Stony Brook, New York

Lorna Browne, MB, FFRRCSI
Assistant Professor of Pediatric Radiology
Children's Hospital Colorado
Aurora, Colorado

Christopher Cassady, MD, FRANZCR
Associate Professor of Radiology
Baylor College of Medicine
Texas Children's Hospital
Houston, Texas

Varghese P. Cherian, MD, MS
Assistant Professor of Radiology and Emergency Medicine
Stony Brook University School of Medicine
Stony Brook University Hospital
Stony Brook, New York

Eric Chong, MD
Department of Radiology
Hospital del Niño
Republic of Panama

Jamie L. Coleman, MD
Assistant Member
Department of Radiological Sciences
St. Jude Children's Research Hospital
Memphis, Tennessee

Gabriella L. Crane, MD
Assistant Professor of Radiology and Pediatrics
Monroe Carell Jr. Children's Hospital at Vanderbilt
Vanderbilt University Medical Center
Nashville, Tennessee

Amy N. Dahl, MD
Assistant Professor of Radiology
University of Missouri – Kansas City School
of Medicine
Children's Mercy Hospital
Kansas City, Missouri

Kassa Darge, MD, PhD
Professor of Radiology
University of Pennsylvania
The Children's Hospital of Philadelphia
Philadelphia, Pennsylvania

Christopher A. Daub, MD
Department of Radiology
University of Missouri-Kansas City School of Medicine
Children's Mercy Hospital
Kansas City, Missouri

Melissa A. Daubert, MD
Department of Cardiology
Stony Brook University School of Medicine
Stony Brook University Hospital
Stony Brook, New York

Julianne Dean, DO
Department of Radiology
University of Missouri-Kansas City School of Medicine
Children's Mercy Hospital
Kansas City, Missouri

Adam Delavan
Department of Radiology
University of Colorado School of Medicine
Children's Hospital Colorado
Aurora, Colorado

Stephen L. Done, MD
Clinical Associate Professor of Radiology and Pediatrics
University of Washington School of Medicine
Seattle, Washington

Scott R. Dorfman, MD
Associate Professor of Radiology
Baylor College of Medicine
Texas Children's Hospital
Houston, Texas

L. Todd Dudley, MD
Radiological Associates of Sacramento
Sacramento, California

Alexia M. Egloff, MD
Department of Diagnostic Imaging and Radiology
Children's National Medical Center
Washington, D.C.

Monica Epelman, MD
Associate Professor of Radiology
Florida State University
Nemours Children's Clinic
Orlando, Florida

Eric James Feldmann, MD
Assistant Clinical Professor of Radiology
Stony Brook University School of Medicine
Stony Brook University Hospital
Stony Brook, New York

Laura Z. Fenton, MD
Associate Professor of Radiology
University of Colorado School of Medicine
Children's Hospital Colorado
Aurora, Colorado

Mark R. Ferguson, MD
Assistant Professor of Radiology
University of Washington School of Medicine
Seattle Children's Hospital
Seattle, Washington

Kristin Fickenscher, MD
Assistant Professor of Radiology
University of Missouri – Kansas City School of Medicine
Children's Mercy Hospital
Kansas City, Missouri

Lynn Ansley Fordham, MD, FACR
Associate Professor of Radiology
University of North Carolina School of Medicine
North Carolina Children's Hospital
Chapel Hill, North Carolina

Raul Galvez-Trevino, MD, MPH
Valley Radiologists, LTD
Banner Thunderbird Medical Center
Banner Estrella Medical Center
Phoenix, Arizona

John P. Gearhart, MD
Professor of Pediatric Urology
Johns Hopkins University School of Medicine
James Buchanan Brady Urological Institute
Baltimore, Maryland

Rachelle Goldfisher, MD
Assistant Professor of Pediatric Radiology
SUNY Downstate Medical Center
Brooklyn, New York

Mark Goldman, MD
Department of Cardiovascular Medicine
Stony Brook University School of Medicine
Stony Brook University Medical Center
Stony Brook, New York

R. Paul Guillerman, MD
Associate Professor of Radiology
Baylor College of Medicine
Texas Children's Hospital
Houston, Texas

Julie H. Harreld, MD
Assistant Member
Department of Radiological Sciences
St. Jude Children's Research Hospital
Memphis, Tennessee

Jeffrey C. Hellinger, MD, FACC
Associate Professor of Radiology and Pediatrics
Stony Brook University School of Medicine
Stony Brook University Medical Center
Stony Brook, New York

Kailyn Kwong Hing
Department of Medical Imaging
University of Saskatchewan
Saskatoon Health Region Royal University
Hospital Saskatoon
Saskatchewan

Terence Hong, MD
Clinical Research Associate
Department of Diagnostic Imaging
The Hospital for Sick Children
Toronto, Ontario, Canada

Anna Illner, MD
Assistant Professor of Radiology
Baylor College of Medicine
Department of Pediatric Radiology
Texas Children's Hospital
Houston, Texas

Gisele E. Ishak, MD
Assistant Professor of Radiology
University of Washington School of Medicine
Seattle Children's Hospital
Seattle, Washington

Ramesh S. Iyer, MD
Assistant Professor of Radiology
University of Washington School of Medicine
Seattle Children's Hospital
Seattle, Washington

Philip John, MBChB, DCH, FRCR, FRCP(C)
Associate Professor of Diagnostic Imaging
The University of Toronto
The Hospital for Sick Children
Toronto, Ontario, Canada

Nadja Kadom, MD
Assistant Professor of Radiology and Pediatrics
The George Washington University School of Medicine
and Health Sciences
Children's National Medical Center
Washington, D.C.

S. Pinar Karakas-Rothey, MD
Department of Radiology
Oakland Children's Hospital & Research Center
Oakland, California

Geetika Khanna, MD, MS
Associate Professor of Radiology
Washington University School of Medicine
Mallinckrodt Institute of Radiology
St. Louis, Missouri

Paritosh C. Khanna, MD
Assistant Professor of Pediatric Radiology
University of Washington School of Medicine
Seattle Children's Hospital
Seattle, Washington

Catherine Kier, MD
Associate Professor of Pediatrics
AStony Brook University School of Medicine
Stony Brook University Medical Center
Stony Brook, New York

Korgün Koral, MD
Associate Professor of Radiology
University of Texas Southwestern Medical Center
Children's Medical Center
Dallas, Texas

Neha S. Kwatra, MBBS, MD
Department of Diagnostic Imaging and Radiology
Children's National Medical Center
Washington, D.C.

Lisa H. Lowe, MD, FAAP
Professor of Radiology
University of Missouri-Kansas City
Children's Mercy Hospitals and Clinics
Kansas City, Missouri

Cheng Ting Lin
Department of Radiology
Stony Brook University School of Medicine Stony
Brook University
Medical Center Stony Brook, New York

Emily Maduro, MD
Department of Radiology
Hospital del Niño
Republic of Panama

Ihsan Mamoun, MD
Department of Diagnostic Radiology
Cleveland Clinic
Cleveland, Ohio

Neil Mardis, DO
Assistant Professor of Pediatrics
University of Missouri-Kansas City School of Medicine
Children's Mercy Hospitals and Clinics
Kansas City, Missouri

Charles Mason Maxfield, MD
Associate Professor of Radiology and Pediatrics
Duke University School of Medicine
Duke University Medical Center
Durham, North Carolina

Heather N. McCaffrey, MD
Department of Urology
Stony Brook University School of Medicine
Stony Brook University Medical Center
Stony Brook, New York

Siobhan McGrane, MD
Department of Diagnostic Imaging & Radiology
Children's National Medical Center
Washington, D.C.

Tracey R. Mehlman, MD
Department of Pediatric Radiology
Cleveland Clinic
Imaging Institute
Cleveland, Ohio

Amy R. Mehollin-Ray, MD, FAAP
Assistant Professor of Radiology
Baylor College of Medicine
Texas Children's Hospital
Houston, Texas

Himabindu Mikkilineni, MD
Department of Diagnostic Radiology
Cleveland Clinic
Cleveland, Ohio

Stuart Morrison, MB, ChB, FRCP
Department of Diagnostic Radiology
Cleveland Clinic
Cleveland, Ohio

Edrise Lobo Mueller, MD
Department of Diagnostic Imaging
The Hospital for Sick Children
Toronto, Ontario, Canada

Loren A. Murphy, MD
Department of Pediatrics
Stony Brook University School of Medicine
Stony Brook Long Island Children's Hospital
Stony Brook, New York

Kay L. North, DO
Assistant Professor of Pediatrics
University of Missouri-Kansas City School of Medicine
Kansas City, Missouri

Robert C. Orth, MD, PhD
Assistant Professor of Radiology
Baylor College of Medicine
Texas Children's Hospital
Houston, Texas

Randolph K. Otto, MD
Assistant Professor of Pediatric Radiology
University of Washington School of Medicine
Seattle Children's Hospital
University of Washington Medical Center
Seattle, Washington

Kamaldine Oudjhane, MD, MSc
Associate Professor of Radiology
University of Toronto
The Hospital for Sick Children
Toronto, Ontario, Canada

Marguerite T. Parisi, MD, MS Ed.
Professor of Radiology
Adjunct Professor of Pediatrics
University of Washington School of Medicine
Seattle Children's Hospital
Seattle, Washington

Shawn E. Parnell, MD
Assistant Professor of Radiology
University of Washington School of Medicine
Seattle Children's Hospital
University of Washington Medical Center
Seattle, Washington

Bhairav N. Patel, MD
Austin Radiological Associates
Dell Children's Medical Center
Austin, Texas

Jon Phelan, MD
Department of Radiology
University of Missouri-Kansas City School of Medicine
Kansas City, Missouri

Grace S. Phillips, MD
Associate Professor of Radiology
University of Washington School of Medicine
Seattle Children's Hospital
Seattle, Washington

Avrum N. Pollock, MD, FRCPC
Associate Professor of Clinical Radiology
University of Pennsylvania, Perelman School
of Medicine
Children's Hospital of Philadelphia
Philadelphia, Pennsylvania

Michael Poon, MD, FACC, FSCCT
Professor of Radiology, Emergency Medicine, and
Medicine
Stony Brook University School of Medicine
Stony Brook University Medical Center
Stony Brook, New York

Sumit Pruthi, MB,BS
Assistant Professor of Radiology and Pediatrics
Monroe Carell Jr. Children's Hospital at Vanderbilt
Vanderbilt University Medical Center
Nashville, Tennessee

Monther S. Qandeel, MD
Department of Pediatric Radiology
University of Colorado School of Medicine
The Children's Hospital Colorado
Aurora, Colorado

Ronald A. Rauch, MD
Assistant Professor of Radiology
Baylor College of Medicine
Texas Children's Hospital
Houston, Texas

Alexis B. Rothenberg, MD
Department of Radiology
Stony Brook University School of Medicine
Stony Brook University Medical Center
Stony Brook, New York

Noah D. Sabin, MD, JD
Assistant Member
Department of Radiological Sciences
St. Jude Children's Research Hospital
Memphis, Tennessee

Crystal Sachdeva, MD
Department of Internal Medicine – Pediatrics
Stony Brook University School of Medicine
Stony Brook University Medical Center
Stony Brook, New York

Nabile M. Safdar, MD
Department of Musculoskeletal Imaging
Children's National Medical Center
Washington, D.C.

Russell P. Saneto, MD
Associate Professor of Neurology
Adjunct Associate Professor of Pediatrics
University of Washington School of Medicine
Seattle Children's Hospital
Seattle, Washington

Alan E. Schlesinger, MD
Professor of Radiology
Baylor College of Medicine
Texas Children's Hospital
Houston, Texas

Victor J. Seghers, MD, PhD
Assistant Professor of Radiology
Baylor College of Medicine
Texas Children's Hospital
Houston, Texas

Laureen M. Sena, MD
Assistant Professor of Radiology
Harvard Medical School
Boston Children's Hospital
Boston, Massachusetts

Mohammed B. Shaikh, MD
Department of Radiology
New York University Langone Medical Center
New York, New York

Erjola Shehu, MD
Department of Radiology
Stony Brook University School of Medicine
Stony Brook University Medical Center
Stony Brook, New York

Sudha P. Singh, MBBS, MD
Assistant Professor of Radiology
Monroe Carell Jr. Children's Hospital
at Vanderbilt
Vanderbilt University Medical Center
Nashville, Tennessee

Lok Yun Sung, MD
Department of Radiology
Stony Brook University School of Medicine
Stony Brook University Medical Center
Stony Brook, New York

Jonathan O. Swanson, MD
Acting Assistant Professor of Radiology
University of Washington School of Medicine
Seattle Children's Hospital
Seattle, Washington

Mathew Swerdlow, MD
Department of Radiology
University of Colorado School of Medicine
Children's Hospital Colorado
Aurora, Colorado

Mahesh M. Thapa, MD
Associate Professor of Radiology
Seattle Children's Hospital
University of Washington
Seattle, Washington

Jason Tsai, MD
Department of Diagnostic Imaging and Radiology
Children's National Medical Center
Washington, D.C.

Unni Udayasankar, MD
Assistant Professor of Pediatric Neuroradiology
Cleveland Clinic Children's Hospital
Cleveland, Ohio

Alan F. Vainrib, MD
Department of Radiology
Stony Brook University School of Medicine
Stony Brook University Medical Center
Stony Brook, New York

Daniel N. Vinocur, MD
Department of Radiology
Boston Children's Hospital
Harvard Medical School
Boston, Massachusetts

C. Anne Waugh Moore, MD
Assistant Professor of Pediatrics
University of Missouri-Kansas City School of Medicine
Children's Mercy Hospital
Kansas City, Missouri

Sjirk J. Westra, MD
Associate Professor of Radiology
Harvard Medical School
Pediatric Radiologist
Massachusetts General Hospital
Boston, Massachusetts

Beverly P. Wood, MD, PhD
Professor Emerita of Radiology and Pediatrics
Keck School of Medicine
University of Southern California
Los Angeles, California

Jennifer L. Williams, MD
Assistant Professor of Radiology
Baylor College of Medicine
Texas Children's Hospital
Houston, Texas

Adam Zarchan, MD
Clinical Assistant Professor of Diagnostic Radiology
Kansas University School of Medicine – Wichita
Kansas City, Kansas

Evan J. Zucker, MD
Department of Radiology
Tufts University School of Medicine
Tufts Medical Center
Floating Hospital for Children
Boston, Massachusetts

Pediatric Radiology

Airway

CHAPTER 1

Epiglottitis

Jason Tsai, MD and Edward Y. Lee, MD, MPH

Definition

Epiglottitis is a life-threatening bacterial cellulitis of the epiglottis and surrounding supraglottic structures. The term supraglottitis is often preferred, as there is acute inflammatory involvement of tissues adjacent to the epiglottis, including the aryepiglottic folds and posterior base of the tongue. Progressive supraglottic edema may rapidly lead to complete upper airway obstruction and respiratory arrest, making prompt recognition and treatment of epiglottitis potentially life-saving.

Clinical Features

Historically, the most common cause of pediatric epiglottitis was *Haemophilus influenzae* type B (Hib), classically affecting children between the ages of 2 and 7 years. Following the introduction of widespread vaccination against Hib in the late 1980s, the incidence of pediatric epiglottitis has markedly declined, from 41 cases per 100,000 children less than 5 years of age in 1987 to an incidence of 1.3 cases per 100,000 children in 1997. This has led to a dramatic change in the epidemiological characteristics of the disease. In the post-Hib vaccine era, there has been a significant shift in the spectrum of disease toward older patients. The mean age of presentation has increased from an estimated 36 months during the time period from 1980 to 1986, to a mean age of 14.6 years from 1999 to 2002. In addition, although Hib remains the most common cause of epiglottitis, most cases are now caused by other microorganisms, including streptococcus, staphylococcus, other types of *H. influenzae*, *Klebsiella*, *Pseudomonas*, and *Candida*. Bacterial superinfection atop existing viral infection may also cause epiglottitis. Despite the decreasing incidence and changing epidemiology of the disease, epiglottitis remains a serious cause of pediatric upper airway obstruction.

Children with epiglottitis present with acute-onset fever, irritability, sore throat, and respiratory distress. Because of odynophagia, these patients often have difficulty controlling oral secretions. Classically, they adopt a tripod position, bracing themselves upright and forward on both arms, with uplifted chin and open mouth in an effort to maximize airway opening. Increasing anxiety, retractions, and stridor (a late finding) are indicative of substantial upper airway obstruction. Symptoms can progress rapidly if left untreated, culminating in complete airway obstruction and respiratory arrest.

Anatomy and Physiology

The epiglottis is a mucosa-covered flap of elastic cartilage projecting posteriorly and obliquely from the root of the tongue. Anteriorly, reflections of epiglottic mucosa attach laterally and midline at the posterior base of the tongue, bordering depressions known as the epiglottic vallecula. Posteriorly, the epiglottis is joined to the apices of the arytenoid cartilages on either side by mucosal folds, appropriately named the aryepiglottic folds, which define the opening into the lumen of the larynx. During deglutition, upward movement of the larynx flattens the leaf-shaped epiglottis against the tongue base, causing it to fold over the laryngeal inlet. This diverts the flow of a swallowed bolus and assists in protection of the airway.

In epiglottitis, there is acute infectious inflammation of the epiglottis and adjacent supraglottic structures. With increased edema, there is marked thickening of the aryepiglottic folds and enlargement of the epiglottis, resulting in rapidly progressive upper airway obstruction. There is often (although not always) sparing of the subglottic airway, as airway epithelium at the level of the vocal cords is more tightly bound, limiting swelling past this level.

Imaging Findings

Classic radiographic findings of epiglottitis mirror the underlying pathologic changes in the disease process. Epiglottic edema causes an enlarged and rounded appearance of the epiglottis on the lateral radiograph, termed the "thumb sign" (Fig. 1.1). There is partial obliteration of the vallecular air space resulting from epiglottic enlargement. Inflammation of the aryepiglottic folds manifests as thickening of the folds on the lateral radiograph. Width assessment is best made in the upper half of the folds. Distension of the hypopharynx can be seen resulting from supraglottic obstruction.

On the frontal radiograph, one may see symmetric subglottic narrowing of the tracheal air column, a nonspecific finding that is classically associated with croup. However, patients with epiglottitis commonly have subglottic sparing of inflammation and frontal radiographs

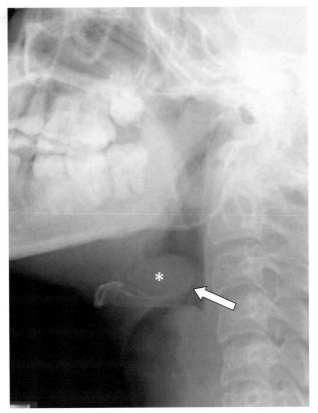

Figure 1.1. Lateral radiograph of the neck in a 5-year-old boy with fever, irritability, sore throat, and respiratory distress demonstrates enlargement of the epiglottis with the "thumb sign" (asterisk) and partial obliteration of the vallecular air space. There is also thickening (arrow) of the aryepiglottic folds.

may appear normal. Frontal views of the neck will not demonstrate thickening of the epiglottis or aryepiglottic folds and should not be obtained if there is high clinical suspicion for epiglottitis.

Imaging Strategy

Imaging is not advised if there is high clinical suspicion for epiglottitis, in which case patients should proceed to direct endoscopic visualization, with intubation once the diagnosis is confirmed.

If the clinical presentation is less clear, and if the patient is stable, a lateral radiograph of the neck is the single most useful imaging study to rule out epiglottitis. In all cases the child should be accompanied by personnel capable of obtaining a patent airway, with the necessary equipment readily available, as complete upper airway obstruction can occur at any time. Blood work generally reveals an elevated white count. However, as anxiety-provoking maneuvers may worsen airway obstruction, phlebotomy should not be performed in a child suspected to have epiglottitis until the airway has been secured. During the examination, the patient should be upright and kept as calm as possible.

Related Physics

For lateral neck radiography, soft tissue technique will help to optimize tissue contrast and identify the abnormal epiglottis. There are three types of inherent contrast to consider in planar imaging: subject, object, and detector contrast. Subject contrast is the inherent difference between two structures in a patient and can be described as differences in thickness, density, and atomic number. In the neck, air serves as subject contrast in that it is 1/1000 the density of soft tissue. Vertebral bodies are higher in density and have a higher atomic number than the epiglottis and surrounding tissues. These differences can be recorded on an image receptor medium that may or may not amplify the physical differences. Detectors are designed at a minimum to maintain subject contrast and ideally to augment it. This can be most effectively achieved with computed radiography (CR) and direct radiography (DR) plates. After the subject has been exposed to radiation and the image receptor has recorded the primary photons from the subject, the signals are rendered as an object on an image. The image display and its associated software controls can also augment subtle differences in subject contrast. An example of this would be the window width and level or brightness and contrast, settings available at the console or reading station.

Differential Diagnosis

- Omega epiglottis: As an imaging differential, the omega epiglottis represents a normal variant that can mimic epiglottitis. If the epiglottis is imaged obliquely on the lateral view, it may appear artificially thickened. However, thickening of the aryepiglottic folds is absent in cases of omega epiglottis, allowing for differentiation from epiglottitis.

- Croup: The most common cause of stridor in the pediatric patient, croup is typically a mild and self-limited viral-induced inflammation of the subglottic airway. Characterized by a barking cough, croup is a clinical diagnosis with a radiographic appearance of symmetric subglottic narrowing (steeple sign) on frontal radiographs. Bacterial tracheitis: Also called exudative tracheitis or membranous croup, this bacterial infection of the subglottic trachea affects young children, typically between 3 months to 3 years of age. Bacterial infection can be primary or superimposed on a viral respiratory infection, with the most common agent being *Staphylococcus aureus*. Resultant purulent exudative plaques can be seen as tracheal wall irregularities and airway filling defects on plain radiographs.

- Retropharyngeal abscess: These children often present with fever, stridor, neck pain, drooling, and dysphagia. Affected pediatric patients do not appear as sick as those with acute epiglottitis. On lateral radiographs, there is marked thickening of the retropharyngeal soft tissues. A CT scan can provide further characterization.Aspirated foreign body: These patients typically present with a history of sudden-onset airway obstruction or choking symptoms, without fever. Most tracheal foreign bodies are radiolucent, and the most common radiographic finding is asymmetric pulmonary aeration on chest radiographs if the aspirated foreign body is located in the bronchus.

Common Variants

Noninfectious epiglottitis, characterized by epiglottic and supraglottic swelling, may develop secondary to noninfectious causes, with similar presenting symptoms of upper airway obstruction. Traumatic injury from foreign body ingestion and burn injury from hot liquid or corrosive substances have been reported as causes of epiglottitis. Patient history generally allows for differentiation from infectious epiglottitis.

Clinical Issues

Epiglottitis is an airway emergency for which prompt recognition and treatment is critical. Although diagnosis is confirmed by direct observation of an erythematous and swollen epiglottis, visualization should not be attempted in the setting of impending airway obstruction. Control of the airway must take priority. Radiologic imaging is not obtained in many cases in which there is clinical suspicion for epiglottitis, as patients often proceed directly to endoscopic examination in the operating suite. In such a controlled setting, blood samples and specimens for culture may be obtained. For cases in which epiglottitis remains in the differential, but other conditions are felt more likely, radiographic examination may prove helpful.

Patients with epiglottitis are intubated and monitored in the intensive care unit. Broad-spectrum antibiotics are started, with adjustments made following the return of culture results. Extubation is performed once there is resolution of the supraglottic edema, evidenced by air leak about the endotracheal tube or confirmed with direct visualization of the epiglottis.

Key Points

- Epiglottitis is a life-threatening infectious inflammation of the epiglottis and supraepiglottic structures that can rapidly progress to complete upper airway obstruction and respiratory arrest if not recognized and treated promptly with aggressive airway control and antibiotics.
- Most commonly caused by *Haemophilus influenzae* type B, epiglottitis is now seen in older children in the post-Hib vaccine era, with a majority of cases caused by agents other than Hib.
- Diagnosis can be made by detecting enlarged epiglottis (thumb sign) and thickened aryepiglottic folds on lateral radiographs, but imaging should not be obtained at the expense of airway management.
- Patients with suspected epiglottitis should be accompanied at all times by medical personnel and equipment capable of securing airway patency if needed.

Further Reading

John SD, Swischuk LE. Stridor and upper airway obstruction in infants and children. *RadioGraphics*. 1992;*12*:625–643.

John SD, Swischuk LE, Hayden CK Jr, Freeman DH Jr. Aryepiglottic fold width in patients with epiglottitis: where should measurements be obtained? *Radiology*. 1994;*190*: 123–125.

Loftis L. Acute infectious upper airway obstructions in children. *Semin Pediatr Infect Dis*. 2005;*17*:5–10.

Shah RK, Roberson DW, Jones DT. Epiglottitis in the *Hemophilus influenza* type B vaccine era: changing trends. *Laryngoscope*. 2004;*114*:557–560.

Stroud RH, Friedman NR. An update on inflammatory disorders of the pediatric airway: epiglottitis, croup, and tracheitis. *Am J Otolaryngo*. 2001;*22*:268–275.

Wheeler DS, Dauplaise DJ, Giuliano JS Jr. An infant with fever and stridor. *Pediatr Emerg Care*. 2008;*24*:46–49.

CHAPTER 2

Croup

Jason Tsai, MD and Edward Y. Lee, MD, MPH

Definition

Croup (also known as laryngotracheobronchitis), is a respiratory illness of infants and young children, characterized by inspiratory stridor and a barking cough. Typically a result of viral-induced airway inflammation with subglottic and laryngeal narrowing, it is the most common cause of infectious upper airway obstruction in children.

Clinical Features

Croup predominantly affects infants and children under 6 years of age, with a peak incidence in the 1- to 2-year age range. Boys are affected approximately 1.4 times more frequently than girls. The most common cause of croup is the parainfluenza virus type 1. Other causative viral agents include parainfluenza types 2 and 3, respiratory syncytial virus, adenovirus, rhinovirus, and influenza A and B. Less commonly, croup may be caused by bacteria such as Mycoplasma pneumoniae. Most cases occur in the fall and early winter, coinciding with times of increased viral activity. A seasonal pattern of croup hospitalization has been observed, with biennial mid-autumn peaks and summer troughs.

Croup is a clinical diagnosis. Affected patients typically present with a several-day history of coryza, gradually progressing to hoarseness, inspiratory stridor, and the characteristic barking cough. Low-grade fever is a common finding. Laboratory studies are generally not useful in the evaluation of routine cases of croup, although blood work may show mild leukocytosis.

Most cases are mild and self-limited, with resolution of symptoms within several days to a week. More severe cases will show greater airway obstruction, including audible stridor at rest, biphasic stridor, suprasternal and intercostal retractions, increased patient agitation, and cyanosis. If symptoms appear more suddenly or progress more rapidly than expected, other conditions should be considered.

Anatomy and Physiology

The subglottic space is the narrowest part of the upper airway. Because of its small size and association with the complete cartilaginous ring of the cricoid, even mild airway inflammation can translate into clinically significant obstruction. In croup, the walls of the proximal trachea become edematous, typically resulting from viral infection. Soft tissues are infiltrated with lymphocytes, histiocytes, and neutrophils and they become swollen and erythematous. The resultant narrowing of the subglottic airway is responsible for the symptoms of croup.

Several predisposing factors may lead to respiratory compromise in infants and young children. According to Poiseuille's Law, resistance of flow through a tube is inversely proportional to the fourth power of the radius. Even a small degree of luminal narrowing can cause a marked increase in airflow resistance and work of breathing. Because of their smaller airways, young children are significantly more vulnerable to any degree of tracheal narrowing than older children and adults. In addition, the subglottic submucosa in children is nonfibrous and the overlying mucosa is more loosely attached than in adults, making it easier for fluid to accumulate in this region. Finally, cartilaginous support is not as well-developed in the airways of infants and young children, making them prone to collapse during inspiration. This can result in dynamic obstruction, superimposed on the subglottic obstruction already present in cases of croup.

Imaging Findings

Radiographic imaging can be useful in confirming a clinical diagnosis of croup and, more important, excluding other potentially more serious conditions in pediatric patients.

On frontal radiographs, the inferior margin of the pyriform sinuses represents the level of the true vocal cords, which is where the subglottic airway begins. From the undersurface of the true cords, the subglottic airway has a shouldered appearance. With croup, there is loss of these normal lateral convexities. Elevation of tracheal mucosa secondary to edema causes symmetric subglottic airway narrowing, manifested radiographically as an inverted V appearance to the tracheal air column, with the tip of the V at the level of the inferior margin of the true vocal cords (Fig. 2.1). Known as the steeple sign, this appearance is classically associated with croup, although it is nonspecific and can be seen with other conditions, such as epiglottitis, bacterial tracheitis, and angioneurotic edema.

On lateral radiographs, imaging findings of croup include distension of the hypopharynx and narrowing of the cervical trachea resulting from subglottic airway obstruction

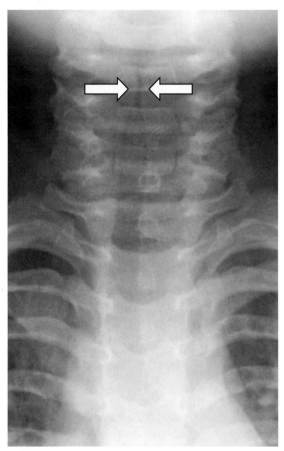

Figure 2.1. A 3-year-old boy who presented with a 3-day history of coryza, progressively worsening hoarseness, inspiratory stridor, and barking cough. Frontal radiograph of the neck shows symmetric subglottic narrowing (arrows) of the airway that creates an inverted V appearance to the tracheal air column (steeple sign).

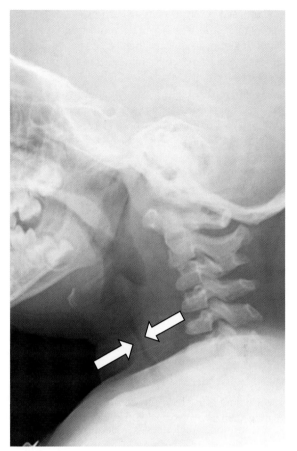

Figure 2.2. Lateral radiograph of the neck demonstrates narrowing (arrows) of the subglottic airway.

Although most aspirated foreign bodies are radiolucent, a radioopaque foreign body should not be missed.

(Fig. 2.2). If lateral expiratory views are obtained, one may see reversal of this pattern, with distension of the cervical trachea and collapse of the hypopharynx, findings also consistent with laryngeal obstruction. However, the extent of these findings in patients with croup is variable and has not been found to correlate with disease severity. The primary purpose of radiographic examination is the exclusion of other causes of airway obstruction.

Imaging Strategy

Croup is most often a self-limited illness that is managed conservatively without the need for radiographic imaging. However, plain radiographs may be helpful if the clinical course is atypical and the diagnosis is in doubt. On the lateral radiographs, enlargement of the epiglottis and thickening of the aryepiglottic folds should raise serious concern for epiglottitis, an airway emergency. Tracheal wall irregularities or airway filling defects could suggest bacterial tracheitis (membranous croup). Widening of the retropharyngeal soft tissues may represent an abscess.

Related Physics

One must be familiar with the many possible artifacts associated with pediatric airway and chest radiography. These may be caused by patient factors, equipment and operator error. Patient factors include distortion (elongation and foreshortening) as well as motion blurring. Equipment-related artifacts include bright pixels, dead pixels, no image, and light leaks. Operator error could induce scratches, insufficient cleaning of equipment, incomplete erasure, and double exposure. Elongation occurs when a curvilinear structure is imaged directly at 90 degrees, displaying it at maximum length. An example of this is the Towne's versus the Caldwell view of the skull. Foreshortening is a phenomenon whereby an object's true length is apparently decreased because the object does not lie parallel to the imaging plane. In both cases, care must be taken to orient the patient flat on the image receptor to minimize this effect and eliminate blurring. 'Bright pixels and dead pixels relate to over-amplification of the signal or nonexistent signal, respectively. With over-amplification, the system can be reinitialized or recalibrated by a service engineer. Dead pixels in marginal areas of the image may be acceptable; otherwise it will be necessary to replace the receptor. If no image appears, there are two possible causes: either there were no X-rays emitted from the tube, or the receptor reader failed. Both conditions require a service engineer for repair. Light leaks will appear on the image as dark shadows near the edges of the image and are most often caused by an improper seal or a crack in the cassette. This will require replacement of the cassette. It is important to maintain equipment through proper cleaning, which will minimize scratches to the receptor and residual dirt and dust. The cassettes must be organized and managed to avoid exposing the cassette twice before processing (double exposure), or imaging before all digital information from the prior study is fully erased from the cassette, leading to "ghosting" on the image.

Differential Diagnosis

- Epiglottitis: This is a life-threatening infectious inflammation of the epiglottis and the surrounding supraglottic structures. It is seen more often than croup in older children. Affected individuals have a more toxic presentation, but do not possess a barking cough. Lateral radiographs demonstrate an enlarged epiglottis and thickened aryepiglottic folds. Although uncommon, epiglottitis is a serious condition that must be excluded in every pediatric patient presenting with airway obstruction.
- Bacterial tracheitis: Also called exudative tracheitis or membranous croup, this is a bacterial infection of the subglottic trachea that affects young children, typically between 3 months to 3 years of age. Bacterial infection can be primary or superimposed on a viral respiratory infection, with the most common agent being *Staphylococcus aureus*. Resultant purulent exudative plaques can manifest as tracheal wall irregularities and airway filling defects on radiographs.
- Aspirated foreign body: These patients typically present with a history of sudden-onset airway obstruction or choking symptoms. Most foreign bodies lodged within the airway are radiolucent so that the most common finding is asymmetric pulmonary aeration on chest radiographs if the object is located within the bronchus.
- Retropharyngeal abscess: Presenting symptoms may include fever, stridor, neck pain, drooling, and dysphagia. On lateral radiographs, there is thickening of the retropharyngeal soft tissues. A CT scan can provide confirmation and further characterization.
- Subglottic hemangioma: Generally becoming clinically evident during the first year of life with croup-like symptoms, subglottic hemangiomas do not present acutely. On radiographs, they cause asymmetric subglottic narrowing.

Common Variants

Affecting the same age group as viral croup, spasmodic croup is characterized by recurrent night-time onset of inspiratory stridor and mild upper respiratory symptoms. Symptoms often improve within hours with minimal or no therapy. Unlike classic croup, which presents with a continuous course of symptoms, patients with spasmodic croup are clinically well between episodes. Imaging findings may be similar. Treatment for more severe cases is the same as for viral croup.

Clinical Issues

Most cases of croup are self-limited and treated conservatively with supportive measures. Traditional therapy has involved the use of humidified air, although its clinical effectiveness has not been scientifically substantiated. Corticosteroid treatment is now routinely recommended for all pediatric patients with croup. For more severe cases, nebulized epinephrine has been shown to be beneficial. Patients who fail these therapies are hospitalized for further work-up and supportive care. There is little role for additional imaging, unless another condition is suspected.

Key Points

- Croup is the most common cause of stridor in the pediatric patient, with peak age of 1 year.
- Generally croup is a mild and self-limited viral inflammation of the airway, with a characteristic barking cough.
- Croup is a clinical diagnosis, but with a classic radiographic appearance of symmetric subglottic narrowing (inverted V or steeple sign).
- The primary purpose of radiographic imaging is the exclusion of other causes of airway obstruction, such as epiglottitis.

Further Reading

Cherry JD. Clinical practice. Croup. *New Engl J of Med.* 2008;*358*:384–391.

Currarino G, Williams B. Lateral inspiration and expiration radiographs of the neck in children with laryngotracheitis (croup). *Radiology.* 1982;*145*:365–366.

Denny FW, Murphy TF, Clyde WA Jr, Collier AM, Henderson FW. Croup: an 11-year study in a pediatric practice. *Pediatric.* 1983;*71*:871–876.

Rotta AT, Wiryawan B. Respiratory emergencies in children. *Respir Care.* 2003;*48*:248–258.

Salour M. The steeple sign. *Radiology.* 2000;*216*:428–429.

Segal AO, Crighton EJ, Moineddin R, Mamdani M, Upshur RE. Croup hospitalizations in Ontario: a 14-year time-series analysis. *Pediatrics.* 2005;*116*:51–55.

CHAPTER 3

Exudative Tracheitis

Jason Tsai, MD and Edward Y. Lee, MD, MPH

Definition

Bacterial tracheitis is an infectious inflammation of the larynx and trachea characterized by subglottic edema and purulent membranous exudates. Also called exudative tracheitis or membranous croup, this entity is an uncommon but important cause of acute upper airway obstruction in children. Affected individuals require aggressive airway management and prompt antibiotic therapy.

Clinical Features

Bacterial tracheitis predominantly affects children between the ages of 1 month to 8 years, with the majority under 3 years of age. Bacterial infection can be primary or superimposed on a viral respiratory illness, with the most common bacterial agent being *Staphylococcus aureus*. Other microorganisms commonly recovered from infected individuals include alpha-hemolytic streptococcus, *Haemophilus influenzae*, *Pseudomonas*, and *Moraxella*. Most cases occur in the fall and winter months, mimicking the incidence pattern of croup, although bacterial tracheitis is a much less common illness, with an estimated incidence of 0.1 per 100,000 children per year based on the recent multi-center study performed in the United Kingdom and Australia.

Pediatric patients with bacterial tracheitis typically present with a hoarse cough, low-grade fever, and inspiratory stridor, preceded by several days of gradually progressive upper-respiratory-type symptoms, similar to that seen in viral croup. Affected children are generally more toxic in appearance, although the degree of respiratory distress is variable. As with other bacterial infections, patients will have an elevated white blood cell count, with a predominance of neutrophils.

If left untreated, patients with bacterial tracheitis can rapidly deteriorate, developing high fever and worsening upper airway obstruction. Conventional therapies for viral croup will be ineffectual, which should raise the concern for bacterial tracheitis. Definitive diagnosis of bacterial tracheitis is made endoscopically, by direct visualization of an edematous subglottic airway and membranous secretions in the trachea, along with positive culture.

Anatomy and Physiology

The subglottis is located in the region of the larynx bound by the cricoid cartilage. Extending from just below the level of the true vocal cords to the inferior margin of the cricoid ring, the subglottic area is the narrowest portion of the upper airway. Owing to this small size and association with the unyielding complete ring of the cricoid, the subglottic airway is especially susceptible to obstruction secondary to edema.

In bacterial tracheitis, infection of the upper airway results in subglottic inflammation and accumulation of thick mucopurulent secretions and sloughed epithelium into pseudomembranes. Detachment of these membranous exudates in a segment of airway already narrowed by edema can result in acute airway obstruction. In cases of bacterial superinfection, preceding viral infection may predispose the airway mucosa to injury.

Imaging Findings

On frontal radiographs, the upper portion of the subglottic airway normally has a shouldered appearance, tracing the undersurface of the true vocal cords. In patients with bacterial tracheitis, subglottic edema effaces these lateral convexities, and resultant symmetric subglottic narrowing creates an inverted V appearance to the proximal most tracheal air column (steeple sign), indistinguishable from that seen in viral croup.

On lateral radiographs, detached pseudomembranes manifest as tracheal wall irregularities or intraluminal filling defects (Fig. 3.1. More subtle cases may be visible only as an indistinct haziness to the tracheal wall. Cervical tracheal narrowing may also be present.

Imaging Strategy

Frontal and lateral radiographs of the neck are the initial imaging evaluation of choice for assessing children with clinically suspected bacterial tracheitis. Fluoroscopy can provide dynamic information of airway caliber and is used in many centers. However, if the radiographic imaging findings are atypical and the diagnosis is in doubt, definitive diagnosis can be made endoscopically, by direct visualization of an edematous subglottic airway and membranous secretions in the trachea, along with a positive culture.

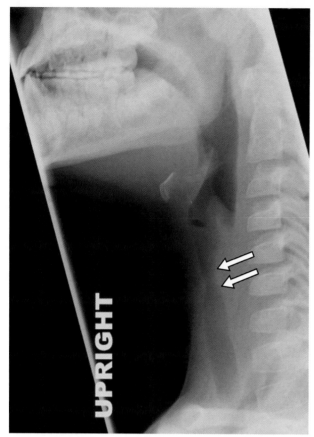

Figure 3.1. Lateral radiograph of the neck in a 9-year-old boy with a hoarse cough, low-grade fever, and inspiratory stridor demonstrates tracheal wall irregularity and narrowing (arrows) in a patient with bacterial tracheitis.

Related Physics

Airway fluoroscopy can confirm exudative tracheitis; however, caution must be used when performing airway fluoroscopy as this delivers a direct dose to sensitive organs such as the thyroid, breast, and esophagus. Anyone using fluoroscopy must be aware of the federal and state regulations, some of which include dose rate limits, audible alarms, metrics concerning exposure, and minimum source-to-skin distance. Dose rate limits are set by the Food and Drug Administration (FDA) and are constrained to 10 Roentgens per minute (R/minute) under normal conditions and 20 R/minute for high-exposure rate output. All equipment must emit an audible alarm for each 5-minute period of beam "on-time" and when in high-exposure dose rate mode. Most modern units now record total beam "on-time" that is storable and searchable in Digital Imaging and Communications in Medicine (DICOM) format. All units must have a minimum source-to-skin distance of 45 centimeters and all cases where peak skin exposure exceeds 15 Gy must be reported to the Joint Commission.

Differential Diagnosis

- Croup: The most common cause of stridor in the pediatric patient, croup is typically a mild and self-limited viral-induced inflammation of the subglottic airway. Characterized by a barking cough, croup is a clinical diagnosis. Bacterial superinfection in patients with viral croup can result in 0 tracheitis. Bacterial tracheitis can mimic croup radiographically. However, tracheal irregularities or linear plaques are not seen in croup and the presence of such findings should lead one to suspect bacterial tracheitis.

- Epiglottitis: A life-threatening infectious inflammation of the epiglottis and surrounding supraglottic structures, epiglottitis is usually seen in older children in comparison to bacterial tracheitis. Affected individuals are less able to control their oral secretions or to tolerate lying flat, as compared with bacterial tracheitis patients, but do not possess a substantial cough. Lateral radiographs demonstrate an enlarged epiglottis and thickened aryepiglottic folds.

- Retropharyngeal abscess: Presenting symptoms may include fever, stridor, neck pain, drooling, and dysphagia. On lateral radiographs, there is marked thickening of the retropharyngeal soft tissues. A CT scan can provide confirmation and further characterization of retropharyngeal abscess in pediatric patients.

- Aspirated foreign body: Affected pediatric patients typically present with a history of sudden-onset airway obstruction or choking symptoms, without fever. Intraluminal accumulation of membranous secretions in bacterial tracheitis may on occasion resemble a foreign body, but clinical history generally allows for distinction between the two entities.

- Laryngeal diphtheria: Rarely seen in the industrialized world because of widespread immunization, diphtheria is characterized by necrotic mucosal exudates secondary to *Corynebacterium diphtheria* toxin. Primary sites of infection include the tonsils and pharynx, and isolated laryngeal involvement is exceedingly rare. Diphtheria pseudomembranes are typically more adherent than those in bacterial tracheitis. Diagnosis is made by culture and testing for toxins.

Common Variants—None
Clinical Issues

Bacterial tracheitis is treated in the intensive care unit with airway intubation and broad-spectrum antibiotics. In addition to its role in diagnosis, endoscopy can serve a therapeutic function, by stripping purulent membranes and removing dead tissues from the airway. With appropriate therapy, clinical improvement generally occurs within 1 week.

Key Points

- Bacterial tracheitis is an infectious inflammation of the larynx and trachea, most commonly caused by *Staphylococcus aureus*, characterized by subglottic edema and mucopurulent membranous exudates in the airway.
- Radiographically, bacterial tracheitis manifests as symmetric subglottic narrowing on the frontal view and as tracheal irregularity, narrowing, and linear filling defects on the lateral view.
- Bacterial tracheitis is generally more toxic in clinical presentation than viral croup.
- Although bacterial tracheitis is a rare entity, it should be suspected in a pediatric patient who does not respond to treatment for croup.

Further Reading

Brook I. Aerobic and anaerobic microbiology of bacterial tracheitis in children. *Pediatr Emerg Care.* 1997;*13*:16–18.

Graf J, Stein F. Tracheitis in pediatric patients. *Semin Pediatr Infect Dis.* 2006;*17*:11–13.

Hopkins A, Lahiri T, Salerno R, Heath B. Changing epidemiology of life-threatening upper airway infections: the reemergence of bacterial tracheitis. *Pediatrics.* 2006;*118*:1418–1421.

Huang YL, Peng CC, Chiu NC, Lee KS, Hung HY, Kao HA, Hsu CH, Chang JH, Huang FY. Bacterial tracheitis in pediatrics: 12 year experience at a medical center in Taiwan. *Pediatr Int.* 2009;*51*:110–113.

Kasian GF, Bingham WT, Steinberg J, Ninan A, Sankaran K, Oman-Ganes L, Houston CS. Bacterial tracheitis in children. *CMAJ.* 1989;*140*:46–50.

Salamone FN, Bobbitt DB, Myer CM, Rutter MJ, Greinwald JH Jr. Bacterial tracheitis reexamined: is there a less severe manifestation? *Otolaryngol Head Neck Surg.* 2004;*131*:871–876.

CHAPTER 4

Retropharyngeal Abscess

Jason Tsai, MD and Edward Y. Lee, MD, MPH

Definition

Retropharyngeal abscess is a loculated infection of the posterior pharynx secondary to suppuration of retropharyngeal lymph nodes following upper respiratory tract infection. In older children and adults, retropharyngeal abscesses more commonly result from pharyngeal trauma.

Clinical Features

Retropharyngeal abscesses occur less frequently than peritonsillar or superficial neck infections and affect a younger age group. Most cases are seen in children under the age of 6 years, with a mean age of 2 to 3 years. There is a male predominance of approximately 1.5:1. Incidence increases in the winter months, coinciding with seasonality of upper respiratory tract disease. Common causative agents include group A streptococcus, *Staphylococcus aureus*, and anaerobic organisms such as *Bacteroides*, *Fusobacterium*, and *Peptostreptococcus*. Other organisms that have been implicated include *Haemophilus influenza*, *Neisseria*, and other streptococcus species. Polymicrobial involvement with aerobes and anaerobes is frequent, as is involvement of penicillin-resistant organisms.

Pediatric patients with retropharyngeal abscess classically present with fever, sore throat, and localizing neck symptoms such as swelling and pain. Other common symptoms include muffled voice, trismus, odynophagia, and dysphagia. Diagnosis of retropharyngeal abscess can be difficult in infants, who may present with irritability and neck stiffness, often mimicking meningitis. On physical examination, a neck mass is often palpable, representing lymphadenopathy or abscess extension. With progression of retropharyngeal swelling, affected patients can develop stridor and difficulty controlling oral secretions. Increased respiratory difficulty may be a sign of impending upper airway obstruction.

As with other infectious processes, patients generally have an elevated white blood cell count with a predominance of neutrophils. Blood cultures are rarely positive, although throat culture for group A streptococcus may be helpful. Radiologic evaluation may include lateral neck radiographs if clinical suspicion is low and other entities are suspected and/or CT of neck if suspicion is high and further delineation of disease extent is needed.

Anatomy and Physiology

Definition of the retropharyngeal space requires an understanding of the fascial anatomy of the neck. There are three layers of deep cervical fascia: superficial, middle, and deep. The superficial layer of the deep fascia encloses the neck and envelops the sternocleidomastoid muscles. The middle layer encloses the viscera of the neck. The deep layer surrounds the paraspinal muscles and vertebrae and consists of two components, a more anteriorly located alar fascia and a more posteriorly positioned prevertebral fascia.

The retropharyngeal space lies anterior to the alar layer of the deep cervical fascia and posterior to the middle cervical fascia, extending from the skull base to approximately T1, where these fascial layers fuse. Posterior to this, between the alar and prevertebral layers of the deep cervical fascia, there is a potential "danger space" that provides access inferiorly to the posterior mediastinum.

The retropharyngeal space normally contains fibrofatty tissue and paramedial lymph node chains that drain the nasopharynx, adenoids, and posterior sinuses. Retropharyngeal lymph nodes are more prominent in early childhood, and atrophy by 5 years of age, which likely explains the preponderance of retropharyngeal abscess formation in younger children. Disease typically begins as an upper respiratory tract infection with spread to these retropharyngeal lymph nodes. Infected lymph nodes undergo liquefactive necrosis and suppuration with extension of purulent material into surrounding tissues leads to abscess formation.

Imaging Findings

On a lateral radiograph, the normal preverterbal measurement at the level of C2, from the anterior border of C2 to the posterior border of the pharyngeal air space, ranges from 3 to 6 millimeters, although this figure may be somewhat higher in infants and very young children. As a general rule, the ratio of prevertebral soft tissue thickness at the C2 level to the anteroposterior dimension of the C2 vertebral body should be no more than 1:1 at 0 to 1 years of age and 1:2 by 6 to 10 years of age. Thickening of the retropharyngeal soft tissues is generally not subtle in pediatric patients with retropharyngeal abscess (Fig. 4.1). Other helpful signs include

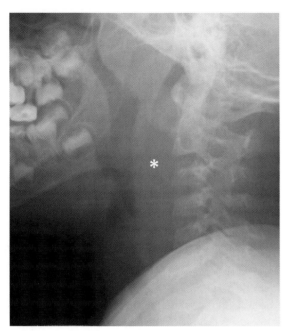

Figure 4.1. A 3-year-old boy with fever, sore throat, and neck pain. Lateral radiograph of the neck shows marked widening (asterisk) of the retropharyngeal soft tissues and straightening of the cervical lordosis.

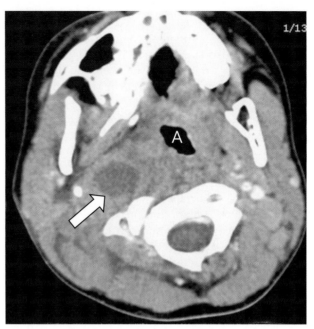

Figure 4.2. Axial contrast-enhanced CT through the level of C2 demonstrates a rim-enhancing low-attenuation collection (arrow) in the right retropharyngeal space, suspicious for abscess. There is mass effect on the airway (A) and effacement of fat planes.

anterior bowing of the airway resulting from mass effect, loss of the normal cervical lordosis from muscle spasm, or gas or fluid level in an abscess cavity.

On CT, a retropharyngeal abscess typically presents as a well-defined low-attenuation fluid collection with rim enhancement (Fig. 4.2). Mass effect and obliteration of fat planes would favor abscess over cellulitis. Although specific characteristics of a fluid collection on CT have not been found to be highly predictive for a purulent collection, evaluation of the location, size, and extent of any visualized collection is nevertheless important for treatment planning. One should also assess the relationship to nearby major vascular structures and evidence of vascular involvement. Special attention should be paid to any extension to the lateral neck spaces or superior mediastinum. Descending mediastinitis, in particular, has substantial associated morbidity and mortality.

Imaging Strategy

Lateral radiographs of the neck are sensitive in the detection of retropharyngeal abscess, manifested as abnormal widening of the prevertebral soft tissues. Radiographs should be obtained if possible at inspiration with the neck in extension, in order to avoid artifactual widening of the retropharyngeal soft tissues. If there is clinical suspicion for retropharyngeal abscess, a CT scan of the neck with intravenous contrast is the imaging test of choice because of its higher sensitivity and ability to better anatomically define the disease process.

Related Physics

When imaging the neck with CT, it is important to balance adequate dose with the potential for radiation damage to thyroid, lenses, breast and lung tissue. It has become increasingly evident that highly specialized techniques are required for pediatric CT imaging beyond age and weight to include patient girth and the presence of sensitive organs within the scan volume. One way to track technique optimization and development is to record a dose metric as well as an image quality metric. For dose metrics one has the choice of computed tomography dose index (CTDI) or dose-length product (DLP). The CTDI, given in milligray (mGy), was developed by the Food and Drug Administration to permit comparison of radiation output across vendors using a mathematical standard, which is the dose delivered in one 10-millimeter slice plus the scatter tails from 70 millimeters on either side of the slice using a 32-centimeter acrylic phantom. The weighted CTDI (CTDI-w) is a variant that preferentially weights peripheral dose by two-thirds and central dose by one-third. The CTDI-volume equals CTDI-w divided by the pitch factor. The DLP, given in milligray-centimeters (mGycm) is equal to the product of the CTDI-volume and scan length or the total distance that the table travels during the scan. One useful measurement of image quality is the noise content, measured in Hounsfield units, in a region of interest placed on a soft-tissue organ such as the liver. When noise is unacceptably high, low-contrast lesion detection becomes challenging, indicating that scan techniques are producing insufficient radiation for diagnosis.

Differential Diagnosis

- Croup: This is the most common cause of stridor in the pediatric patient and is typically a mild and self-limited viral-induced inflammation of the subglottic airway. Characterized by a barking cough, croup is a clinical diagnosis.
- Bacterial tracheitis: This affects young children, typically under 3 years of age. Bacterial infection can be primary or superimposed on a viral respiratory infection. Resultant purulent exudative plaques can be seen as tracheal wall irregularities and airway filling defects on radiographs.
- Epiglottitis: A life-threatening infectious inflammation of the epiglottis and surrounding supraglottic structures, epiglottitis is usually seen in older children. Lateral radiographs demonstrate an enlarged epiglottis and thickened aryepiglottic folds.
- Lymphatic malformation: This may involve the retropharyngeal space, but components are generally evident elsewhere. Although this entity is another potential cause of upper airway obstruction, infectious symptoms are absent.

Common Variants—None
Clinical Issues

Diagnosis of a retropharyngeal abscess is confirmed when there is expression of pus during surgical drainage. Although CT has very high sensitivity in the detection of a fluid collection, it is not as specific in predicting a purulent collection. Imaging must be utilized in conjunction with clinical evaluation. As with any disease process that may cause upper airway obstruction, security of the airway patency is paramount. Classic treatment of retropharyngeal abscess involves surgical drainage and intravenous antibiotics, including initial coverage for anaerobes and penicillin-resistant organisms. More recently, medical management alone has been advocated for treatment in uncomplicated cases, with performance of surgical drainage only when there has been no clinical improvement after several days of conservative therapy. Image-guided needle aspiration is another alternative to surgery in some centers.

Key Points

- Retropharyngeal abscess is a deep-space neck infection that occurs in young children as a complication of upper respiratory infection, with spread to and suppuration of retropharyngeal lymph nodes.
- Most commonly caused by *Staphylococcus aureus* and group A streptococcus, infections are commonly polymicrobial, with frequent involvement of anaerobes.
- Lateral radiograph shows thickening of retropharyngeal soft tissues.
- Contrast-enhanced CT is the preferred imaging study for differentiating retropharyngeal cellulitis and abscess and for defining extent of disease.

Further Reading

Brook I. Microbiology and management of peritonsillar, retropharyngeal, and parapharyngeal abscesses. *J Oral Maxillofac Surg.* 2004;*62*:1545–1550.

Craig FW, Schunk JE. Retropharyngeal abscess in children: clinical presentation, utility of imaging, and current management. *Pediatrics.* 2003;*111*:1394–1398.

Haug RH, Wible RT, Lieberman J. Measurement standards for the prevertebral region in the lateral soft-tissue radiograph of the neck. *J Oral Maxillofac Surg.* 1991;*49*:1149–1151.

Lee SS, Schwartz RH, Bahadori RS. Retropharyngeal abscess: epiglottitis of the new millennium. *J Pediatr.* 2001;*138*:435–437.

Nagy M, Backstrom J. Comparison of the sensitivity of lateral neck radiographs and computed tomography scanning in pediatric deep-neck infections. *Laryngoscope.* 1999;*109*:775–779.

Page NC, Bauer EM, Mieu JE. Clinical features and treatment of retropharyngeal abscess in children. *Otolaryngol Head Neck Surg.* 2008;*138*:300–306.

CHAPTER 5

Vascular Ring

Gabriella L. Crane, MD

Definition

The term "vascular ring" refers to a congenital anomaly of the thoracic aorta and its branches in which anomalous vessels encircle and compress the trachea and esophagus. The two classic subtypes of complete anatomic vascular rings are the double aortic arch and the right aortic arch with aberrant left subclavian artery (LSCA) and left ligamentum arteriosum. These rings encircle both the trachea and esophagus. The pulmonary artery (PA) sling, or anomalous pulmonary artery, is also considered a vascular ring but encircles the trachea only. The PA sling is formed when the left PA originates from the right PA.

Clinical Features

Infants with a complete vascular ring present more often with respiratory than swallowing difficulties secondary to compression on the trachea and esophagus. The most common symptoms include stridor, recurrent respiratory infections, choking with feeds, and the older child might describe pain with swallowing or "dysphagia lusoria." The double aortic arch is the most common of the vascular rings and the most symptomatic. Patients with a right arch with aberrant LSCA and left ligamentum arteriosum may also be symptomatic, especially if the ligamentum is tight or they have a large diverticulum of Kommerell (a dilated origin of the aberrant LSCA). There is an increased association with congenital heart disease in both subtypes. The PA sling presents with similar respiratory symptoms and is often associated with congenital tracheal stenosis.

Anatomy and Physiology

The embryonic development of vascular rings was described by Edwards in 1948. Edwards' hypothetical model consists of ventral and dorsal aortae that are connected by six primitive aortic arches. Early on, the first, second, and fifth arches regress. The third arches become the carotid arteries and the left sixth arch becomes the ductus arteriosus. The right sixth arch usually regresses. The fourth primitive arches will form the aortic arch depending on their pattern of regression. Normally, the right fourth arch involutes, leaving the left fourth arch as the aortic arch. If the left fourth arch involutes

instead of the right, a right aortic arch results. With persistence of a segment of the left dorsal arch, the aberrant LSCA is present and the ductus completes the ring. If both fourth arches persist, a double arch results (Fig. 5.1).

A PA sling is created when the left PA arises from the right PA, thus passing between the trachea and esophagus in order to reach the left hemithorax. The left PA can therefore compress the trachea posteriorly and the esophagus anteriorly. Sometimes, the right main stem bronchus may also be compressed laterally. The ductus travels from the origin of the right PA to the aorta, thereby completing the ring around the trachea.

Imaging Findings

A vascular ring will create abnormal impressions on the tracheal air column that can be detected by plain radiographs of the chest or airway. Extrinsic compression of the esophagus can be detected by esophagography. The detailed anatomy is clearly seen by MRI/MRA or CTA.

Double Aortic Arch

Plain radiography shows anterior and bilateral impressions on the trachea, causing concentric tracheal narrowing. The trachea may be midline or more commonly deviated to the side of the smaller arch. On the lateral view, the trachea may be bowed anteriorly. The descending aorta may be seen on either side. A barium esophagram will confirm posterior and bilateral compression of the esophagus (Fig. 5.2A, B). On MRA or CTA the double arch wraps around both the trachea and esophagus with both arches arising from a single ascending aorta anteriorly and joining to form a single descending aorta posteriorly (Fig. 5.3). The right arch is usually dominant.

Right Arch with Aberrant LSCA and Left Ligamentum

Radiographs show right lateral impression on the trachea, with tracheal deviation or buckling to the left, away from the arch. On the lateral view the trachea may be bowed anteriorly and in most cases, the proximal descending aorta will be on the right. The barium esophagram confirms posterior compression of the esophagus at the level of the arch. MRA or CTA shows the right arch with four branches, the last of which is the aberrant LSCA. There may be a diverticulum of Kommerell and the left ligamentum completes the ring (Fig. 5.4).

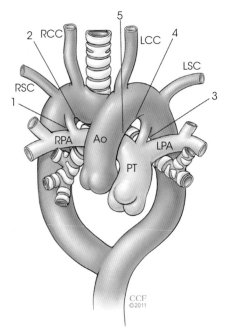

Figure 5.1. Illustration of Edwards' hypothetical double arch with bilateral ducti, after regression of first, second, and fifth primitive arches. Normal left arch anatomy results with involution at 1 and resorption of the right ductus. Involution at 2 results in left arch with aberrant right subclavian; typically the right ductus resorbs. Involution at 3 results in right arch with mirror-image branching. Involution at 4 results in right arch with aberrant left subclavian; typically the left ductus persists and completes the ring. Involution at 5 is similar to 4, but the aberrant vessel in this case is the left innominate.

Pulmonary Sling

Radiography shows posterior impression on the trachea with anterior bowing and an esophagram confirms anterior compression of the esophagus by the aberrant artery. An MRA or CTA shows the left PA originating from the right PA, then coursing between the trachea and esophagus to reach the left lung (Fig. 5.5). There may be associated congenital tracheal stenosis related to absence of the pars membranacea, which is best confirmed with CT with multiplanar reconstruction or three-dimensional volume rendering.

Imaging Strategy

Pulmonary artery and lateral chest radiography is the best screening study. Radiographs are used to determine the side of the arch, but may also offer an alternative explanation for a patient's symptoms, such as croup, aspirated foreign body, or a mediastinal mass giving the patient stridor. If a right arch or double arch is suspected, an esophagram can be performed to assess for a vascular ring and to determine the subtype based on the compressive effects on the esophagus. Both types of vascular rings will create a posterior impression on the esophagus, but only the double arch will create up to three impressions. In patients with a suspected vascular ring, CTA or MRI/MRA often replaces the esophagram as a preferred method for fully delineating the anatomy prior to surgery. Dynamic airway CT and virtual bronchoscopy may also demonstrate the degree and extent of tracheal narrowing and concomitant tracheomalacia, complete tracheal rings or congenital stenosis in greater detail.

Related Physics

Computed tomography angiography (CTA) is a special class of scanning whereby the efficient use of iodinated contrast is of utmost importance. This demands use of kVp that will maximize photoelectric absorption—a value as close to 80 is optimal. At each kVp, X-ray output can be finely tuned by adjusting mAs. The second most important parameter is bolus timing, which can be optimized through bolus tracking or empirical scan delay. If bolus tracking methods are used, it is important to carefully select the most appropriate

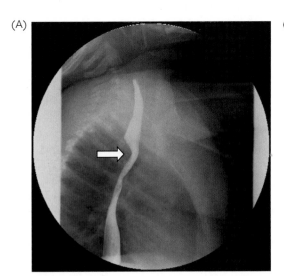

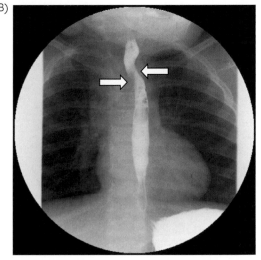

Figure 5.2. Lateral view (A) from a barium esophagram in an 18-month-old child with systolic murmur demonstrates posterior compression of the esophagus (arrow) and frontal view (B) shows bilateral lateral compression of the esophagus (arrows) suggestive of a double arch.

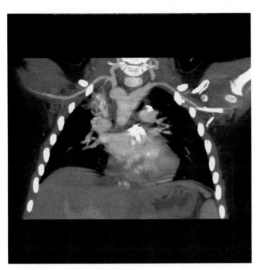

Figure 5.3. Coronal image from CT angiogram confirms the diagnosis of a double aortic arch. In this case, the right (red) and left (blue) arches are at the same level and are similar in size.

region of interest (ROI) (the descending aorta for vascular ring or main pulmonary artery for pulmonary sling). By applying extrinsic iodinated contrast, mAs may be decreased below values used for noncontrast scans. To detect smaller vessels, one chooses the smallest detector width and reconstructs at 1- to 2-millimeter image thickness offering excellent multiplanar and 3-D reconstructions.

Differential Diagnosis

If a right arch is diagnosed on plain radiography, the differential diagnosis includes a double aortic arch, right arch with aberrant LSCA, and right arch with mirror-image branching. If posterior compression of the esophagus is demonstrated by esophagography, the differential diagnosis would also include an aberrant right subclavian artery if the patient has a left aortic arch. An aberrant right subclavian artery arising from an otherwise normal left arch is the most common aortic arch anomaly, occurring in nearly 1 percent of the population. However, because it is almost never associated with an intact right ligamentum arteriosum, it is considered a normal variant, not a true vascular ring, and is rarely symptomatic. This aberrant artery creates an oblique impression on the posterior esophagus. A variety of posterior mediastinal masses could also cause extrinsic compression of the esophagus.

Common Variants

Innominate artery compression syndrome (IACS) is often classified under the heading "vascular ring" although it is not a true anatomic vascular ring. It occurs when the innominate artery takeoff from a left arch is abnormally distal and posterior, resulting in compression of the trachea anteriorly as it travels from the left hemithorax toward the right hemithorax.

In most cases of a right arch, the arch continues with the proximal descending aorta on the same side. A rare variant is the circumflex retroesophageal right arch, in which case the distal portion of the arch crosses the midline posterior to the esophagus and then continues as a left-sided descending aorta. On chest radiographs, the tracheal impression will be seen on the right while the entire descending aorta is seen on the left.

A cervical aortic arch extends above the clavicles and most commonly occurs in patients with a right arch. This type of arch is often tortuous and can be associated with aneurysmal dilatations and areas of narrowing.

(A)

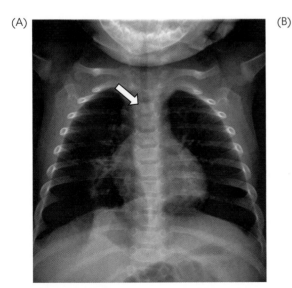

(B)

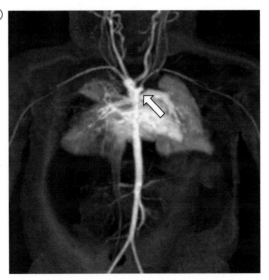

Figure 5.4. Frontal chest radiograph (A) in an 8-month-old child with trisomy 21, severe reflux, and vascular ring suggested by upper GI reveals buckling of the tracheal air column to the left (arrow), consistent with a right arch. Coronal MRA (B) demonstrates a right arch with aberrant left subclavian artery arising from a diverticulum of Kommerell (arrow).

(A) 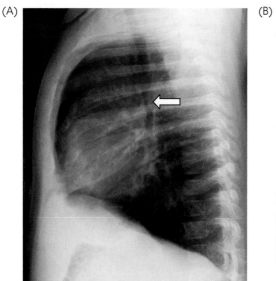   (B)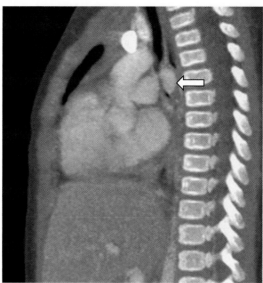

Figure 5.5. Lateral radiograph of the chest (A) in a 6-month-old child with stridor demonstrates posterior indentation of the trachea (arrow) and overinflation. Sagittal CTA (B) demonstrates the left PA (arrow) coursing between the trachea and esophagus, consistent with PA sling.

Clinical Issues

Treatment of symptomatic vascular rings is surgical division. Early treatment can prevent complications of long-standing extrinsic airway compression resulting in tracheomalacia or even sudden death. Asymptomatic patients do not require intervention.

Key Points

- Vascular rings are congenital anomalies that encircle the trachea and esophagus, most commonly causing stridor and respiratory symptoms.
- Older patients may complain of dysphagia lusoria.
- Pulmonary artery sling encircles the trachea and sometimes right main stem bronchus only.
- Left ligamentum arteriosum completes the ring with right arch and aberrant LSCA as well as pulmonary sling.
- Location of arch on chest radiograph can narrow differential diagnostic considerations.
- Treatment is surgical division of the ring.

Further Reading

Backer C, Mavroudis C. Congenital heart surgery nomenclature and database project: vascular rings, tracheal stenosis, pectus excavatum. *Ann Thorac Surg.* 2000:69(3)Suppl 1;308–318.

Berdon W. Rings, slings, and other things: vascular compression of the infant trachea updated from the midcentury to the millenium—the legacy of Robert E. Gross, MD, and Edward B. D. Neuhauser, MD. *Radiology.* 2000;*216*(3):624–632.

Hernanz-Schulman M. Vascular rings: a practical approach to imaging diagnosis. *Pediatr Radiol.* 2005;*35*(10):961–979.

Kimura-Hayama ET, Melendez G, Mendizabal AL, Meave-Gonzalez A, Zambrana GFB, Corona-Villalobos CP. Uncommon congenital and acquired aortic disease: role of multidetector CT angiography. *Radiographics.* 2010;*30*(1): 79–98.

Turner A, Gavel G, Coutts J. Vascular rings—presentation, investigation, and outcome. *Eur J Pediatr.* 2005;*164*:266–270.

CHAPTER 6

Airway Foreign Body

Daniel Vinocur, MD and Edward Y. Lee, MD, PhD

Definition

Foreign body (FB) aspiration refers the inhalation of exogenous material including food particles and broken fragments of teeth into the main or lobar bronchus. Peanuts are the most common aspirated particles in North America.

Clinical Features

The typical age group is 6 months to 4 years. Patients may present with the classic triad of choking, cough, and wheezing. When the presentation is classic, some practitioners proceed directly to bronchoscopy. In many cases, the aspiration is not witnessed and the diagnosis may be delayed and many children may present with recurrent pneumonia, hemoptysis, or atelectasis. In patients with nonspecific findings, the radiologist may be the first one to raise the possibility of an FB.

Anatomy and Physiology

Tracheal FBs are less common than bronchial FBs, constituting approximately 4 to 13 percent of cases and usually presenting with abrupt stridor or respiratory distress.

For tracheal FB, imaging is usually not performed but if obtained, foreign bodies usually lodge in the sagittal plane. Chest radiographs are usually normal. Laryngeal and subglottic FBs make up about 5 percent of the airway foreign bodies. Bronchial FBs are the most common, encompassing approximately 70 to 80 percent of the cases. The right main bronchus is a more common location of FBs than left main bronchi.

Imaging Findings

In the most common scenario, airway FBs tend to lodge in the main bronchi, leading to partial obstruction with the "one-way valve" mechanism and producing lobar or unilateral air trapping with a hyperlucent lung and mediastinal shift to the opposite site (Fig. 6.1). Expiratory or, in younger patients, lateral decubitus radiographs render air trapping more apparent. Atelectasis can be seen but is uncommon.

In approximately 10 percent of cases, the actual FBs are radio-opaque and can be seen by radiography (Fig. 6.2). More subtle secondary signs can sometimes be appreciated, such as soft-tissue density within the airways, and loss of visualization of the airway wall contour.

(A)

(B)

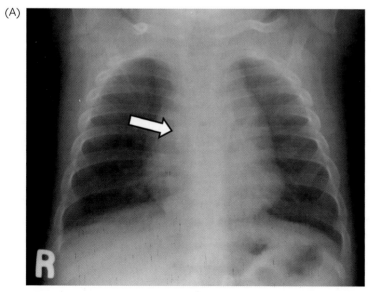
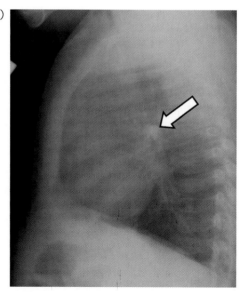

Figure 6.1. Frontal (A) and lateral (B) radiographs of the chest in an infant presenting with cough and a history of an aspirated foreign body show a rounded nonmetallic foreign body (arrows) lodged within the right mainstem bronchus with overinflation of the right lung.

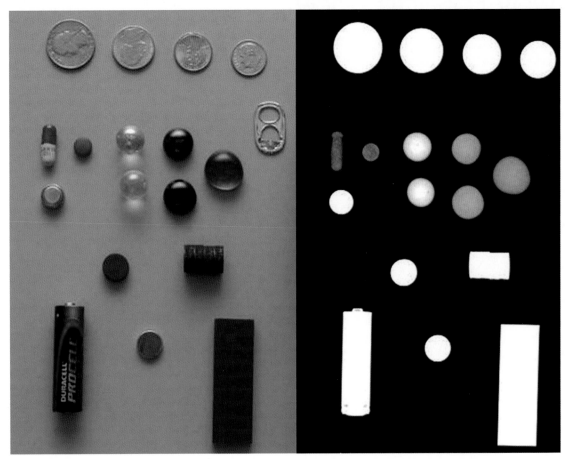

Figure 6.2. Photograph and specimen radiograph of commonly aspirated radio-opaque and radiolucent FBs. *(Courtesy Dr. Restrepo, Miami Children's Hospital)*

On CT, the presence of lobar collapse with localized pneumothorax should suggest the diagnosis of acute bronchial obstruction of any etiology. In addition, CT examination depicts complications more accurately including, necrotizing/cavitating pneumonia, pleural effusions, and signs of bronchopleural fistulae.

Imaging Strategy

Chest radiography remains the initial study of choice. Opaque FBs are easy to identify, however most are radiolucent. Laryngeal and tracheal foreign bodies constitute an acute emergency and radiography is frequently omitted. Chest fluoroscopy or CT can be performed if chest radiographic findings are equivocal.

Computed tomography is more sensitive than chest radiography, especially for radiolucent FB. Occasionally, CT may demonstrate subtle low-attenuation intrabronchial material, suggesting the diagnosis of radiolucent FB.

Related Physics

Before the introduction of computed radiography (CR) and direct radiography (DR), the mainstay of imaging for a radiographic foreign body in young children has been projection radiography. In traditional projection radiography, a two-dimensional image of a three-dimensional object is created and therefore geometric relationships are distorted. On a posteroanterior (PA) projection there is no information about the depth of a structure within the patient and a second projection is necessary. In addition, there are situations where laterality can be confused. There is also the problem of differential magnification dependent on depth

Table 6.1 – Radio-opacity of commonly aspirated foreign bodies.	
Opaque	• Glass (always) • Most metallic objects (except aluminum) • Sand and mineral fragments • Some pills, poisons/lead
Nonopaque	• Most fish bones • Wood/thorns • Plastics • Most foods • Aluminum including soda cans and pull tabs

of the structure so that true size measurements cannot be determined. Inhaled foreign bodies are often not well seen on radiography because of their similar density to adjacent soft tissue. More often we suspect an airway foreign body from secondary signs such as air trapping leading to hyperinflation and airway obstruction leading to atelectasis. Some foreign bodies such as plastic toys with sharp edges may be better visualized using image optimization measures such as edge enhancement and wide window settings. Scatter is the major impediment to the detection of low-contrast objects such as nonmetallic foreign bodies and can be decreased through the use of antiscatter grids, air gap or lowering the kVp (reducing the Compton scattering).

Differential Diagnosis

When the aspiration is not witnessed, acute airway obstruction would have a wider clinical differential diagnosis that includes upper airway obstruction (such as epiglottis, croup) and lower airway obstruction (such as bronchospasm, bronchiolitis). Rarely, an aspirated foreign body may mimic a congenital malformation or neoplasm.

Common Variants

Foreign bodies lodged within the proximal esophagus may also present with airway compression. In these cases, the symptoms are typically subacute or chronic because an inflammatory response to the foreign body needs to develop for the airway to be compressed. On frontal radiographs, foreign bodies typically lodge in the trachea in profile and in the esophagus en face. In misleading cases, lateral radiographs usually clarify the clinical dilemma.

Clinical Issues

The definitive treatment for airway foreign body is endoscopic removal. Some authors have suggested that all patients with suspected FB aspiration should undergo endoscopy, regardless of the chest radiographic findings. Others have advocated CT for elusive cases. If a CT examination is completely normal, the possibility of an airway FB is virtually excluded.

Key Points

- Most aspirated FBs lodge in the main bronchi (right > left).
- Tracheal foreign bodies are less common and imaging is usually not performed.
- Only 10 percent of foreign bodies are radio-opaque.
- Hyperlucent lung and mediastinal shift to the opposite site are the main radiographic findings.
- Airway FBs are usually better seen with expiratory or lateral decubitus films.

Further Reading

Franquet T, Giménez A, Rosón N, Torrubia S, Sabaté JM, Pérez C. Aspiration diseases: findings, pitfalls, and differential diagnosis. *Radiographics*. 2000;*20*:673–685.

Hunter TB, Taljanovic MS. Foreign Bodies. *Radiographics*. 2003;*23*:731–757.

John SD, Swischuk LE. Stridor and upper airway obstruction in infants and children. *Radiographics*. 1992;*12*:625–643.

Donnelly, L (Ed). *Fundamentals of Pediatric Radiology*. Chapter 2., Philadelphia, PA: Saunders; 2001.

Lucaya J (Ed). *Pediatric Chest Imaging*., Koplewitz BZ, Bar-Ziv J. Chapter 9 Foreign body aspiration: Imaging aspects. New York: Springer; 2008, pp. 195–286.

Chest

CHAPTER 7

Aspiration Pneumonia

Evan J. Zucker, MD and Edward Y. Lee, MD, MPH

Definition

Aspiration refers to a spectrum of clinical entities involving inhalation of liquids, solids, or vapors into the lungs and airways. Aspiration pneumonia generally denotes an infectious process caused by aspiration of bacteria-colonized oropharyngeal secretions. Aspiration pneumonia is different from aspiration pneumonitis, the latter of which results from a direct chemical insult caused by aspirated particles.

Clinical Features

Predisposing factors for aspiration pneumonia in children include neuromuscular disorders (muscular dystrophy, impaired swallowing), anatomic structural abnormalities (tracheoesophageal fistula, gastroesophageal reflux), and altered levels of consciousness (resulting from trauma, general anesthesia, metabolic disturbances). Clinical symptoms in children with aspiration pneumonia are variable and patients may be asymptomatic. Symptomatic patients may present with recurrent pneumonia, hoarseness and chronic cough, recurrent wheezing/asthma, or apnea. Clinical history should be carefully reviewed in children with suspected aspiration pneumonia because it may reveal the underlying material aspirated (e.g., foreign body, barium, mineral oil, etc.). Pertinent laboratory tests in patients with suspected aspiration pneumonia include complete blood count (CBC) with differential, sputum gram stain and culture, and arterial blood gas.

Anatomy and Physiology

Aspiration of colonized oropharyngeal secretions results in an acute pulmonary inflammatory response to the bacteria and their byproducts, leading to pneumonia. Such pneumonia may subsequently progress to cavitation and abscess without treatment. In children who aspirate while supine, the dependent portions of the lungs such as posterior segments of the upper lobes and the superior segment of the lower lobes are most commonly affected. In contrast, the basal segments of the lower lobes are typically affected in upright or semi-recumbent aspirators. Aspirated foreign materials may cause local obstruction within the tracheobronchial tree, hindering normal mucosal clearance of seeded pathogens. Factors that lead to recurrent aspiration events (e.g., stroke, impaired swallowing) increase bacterial colonization of oropharyngeal secretions. Impaired aspiration defense mechanisms (coughing, ciliary transport, immune mechanisms) further increase the risk of developing aspiration pneumonia.

Imaging Findings

> IMAGING PITFALLS: Imaging findings of aspiration pneumonia in children may vary with the time since the initial aspiration event.

Chest radiographs 1 to 3 days after aspiration of infectious material may be normal. Subsequently, heterogenous opacities will typically develop in the dependent portions of the lungs (Fig. 7.1). Within a couple of weeks, untreated aspiration pneumonia may progress to a more homogeneous opacity with air-fluid levels resulting from underlying lung necrosis and cavitation. Late-term sequelae of aspiration pneumonia after several months without treatment typically include: (1) focal lung abscess, often manifesting as a well-marginated lung mass, possibly with cavitation; (2) empyema; (3) bronchopleural fistula, which often appears as a large, loculated pleural effusion with air-fluid levels; and (4) bronchiectasis (Fig. 7.2). Hospitalized patients colonized with more virulent organisms tend to develop more severe disease with multifocal pneumonia that may progress to adult respiratory distress syndrome (ARDS).

Imaging Strategy

Chest radiography is the initial imaging modality of choice for evaluating aspiration pneumonia in pediatric patients. Chest CT is helpful in demonstrating late-term complications of aspiration pneumonia such as abscess, necrosis, cavitation, and bronchiectasis. Ultrasound can be useful for localizing and characterizing a complex pleural effusion resulting from complicated aspiration pneumonia. Fluoroscopic exams (barium esophagram, upper GI series, modified barium swallow) can be helpful for identifying underlying anatomic or physiologic abnormalities predisposing the patient to aspiration (e.g., swallowing dysfunction, tracheoesophageal fistula). Gastroesophageal scintigraphy ("milk scan") and radionuclide salivagram may detect gastroesophageal reflux and salivary aspiration, respectively.

(A)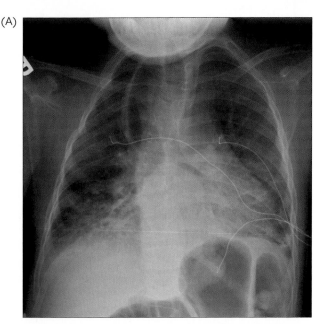

(B)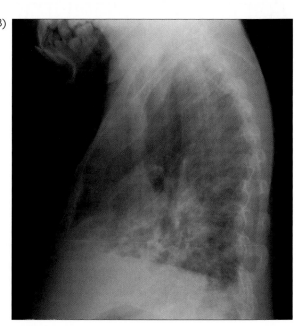

Figure 7.1. Frontal (A) and lateral (B) upright chest radiographs in a 12-year-old boy with history of vertebral, anorectal, cardiac, trachea-esophageal atresia, renal and limb anomalies (VACTERL association) status post-repair of esophageal atresia with tracheoesophageal fistula show bibasilar consolidation in a classical distribution for aspiration pneumonia. The esophagus is dilated and air-filled, compatible with prior esophageal atresia repair.

Related Physics

The modified barium swallow is often performed to detect aspiration and laryngeal penetration. There are four ways to acquire still images during a fluoroscopic examination. From lowest to highest patient dose, these include "frame grab," "last image hold," overhead radiographs, and digital spot films. The choice will affect the total dose to the patient and must be undertaken with great care. In general, last image hold and frame grab images are created with much lower radiation exposure than are overhead or digital

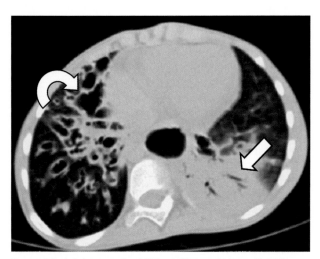

Figure 7.2. Axial noncontrast CT in a 13-year-old boy with history of VACTERL association and repaired esophageal atresia shows dense consolidation (arrow) with air bronchograms in the left lower lobe resulting from active aspiration pneumonia. There is severe bronchiectasis (curved arrow) at the right lung base as a result of chronic aspiration. The esophagus is also markedly dilated.

spot films. Magnification radiography will further increase patient dose for all of these modes. It is best to use last image hold whenever possible to document disease. This is at the expense of contrast and spatial resolution.

Differential Diagnosis

- Infectious pneumonia
- Pulmonary edema
- Primary neoplasm
- Secondary neoplasm
- Aspiration pneumonia from inhaled foreign body
- Chemical pneumonitis from aspiration of gastric acid, mineral oil, water-soluble contrast

Common Variants

In patients with recurrent aspiration pneumonia, underlying anatomic structural and/or physiologic anomalies may be responsible, such as tracheoesophageal reflux, gastroesophageal reflux disease, hiatal hernia, stroke, esophageal stricture, or mediastinal malignancy.

Clinical Issues

The main treatment for aspiration pneumonia is antibiotics, which can be tailored according to results from culture. If left untreated, patients may develop complications requiring invasive intervention such as tube drainage of empyema or surgical resection of severely damaged lung such as marked bronchiectasis. In antibiotic nonresponders, other entities such as tuberculosis, fungal infection, or malignancy should be considered. If the primary cause is foreign body obstruction, therapeutic efforts should focus on retrieving the object, typically by bronchoscopy. In recurrent aspirators, measures should be taken to identify and correct any underlying predisposing factors, which in turn may be associated with a myriad of multisystem anomalies.

Key Points

- Aspiration pneumonia has a predilection for dependent portions of lung.
- Late complications include empyema, abscess, bronchopleural fistula, and bronchiectasis.
- It is important to distinguish from foreign body obstruction and aspiration pneumonitis.
- Be wary of underlying anatomic or physiologic abnormalities, especially in recurrent aspirators.

Further Reading

Franquet T, Giménez A, Rosón N, Torrubia S, Sabaté JM, Pérez C. Aspiration diseases: findings, pitfalls, and differential diagnosis. *RadioGraphics.* 2000;*20*(3):673–685.

Lee KH, Kim WS, Cheon JE, Seo JB, Kim IO, Yeon KM. Squalene aspiration pneumonia in children: radiographic and CT findings as the first clue to diagnosis. *Pediatr Radiol.* 2005;*35*(6):619–623.

Marik PE. Aspiration pneumonitis and aspiration pneumonia. *N Engl J Med.* 2001;*344*(9):665–671.

Marom EM, McAdams HP, Erasmus JJ, Goodman PC. The many faces of pulmonary aspiration. *AJR Am J Roentgenol.* 1999;*172*(1):121–128.

Pikus L, Levine MS, Yang YX, Rubesin SE, Katzka DA, Laufer I, Gefter WB. Videofluoroscopic studies of swallowing dysfunction and the relative risk of pneumonia. *AJR Am J Roentgenol.* 2003;*180*(6):1613–1616.

CHAPTER 8

Bronchopulmonary Foregut Malformations

Mathew Swerdlow, MD and Laura Z. Fenton, MD

Definition

The bronchopulmonary foregut malformations (BPFM) are a subset of pulmonary developmental anomalies that result from abnormal budding of the foregut and tracheo-bronchial tree including congenital pulmonary airway malformation (CPAM), congenital lobar hyperinflation (CLH), pulmonary sequestration, bronchial atresia, and broncho-genic cyst.

Congenital pulmonary airway malformation (CPAM) is a hamartomatous malformation with proliferation of bronchi at the expense of alveoli. Formerly known as con-genital cystic adenomatoid malformation (CCAM), the new preferred term more accurately reflects the embryol-ogy and pathology, as not all lesions are cystic or adenom-atoid. Pathologically, there are five types with both cystic and solid components: type 0 (least common) involves the trachea or main bronchi; type I (60 to 70 percent) involves the bronchi or the proximal bronchioles; type II (15 to 20 percent) involves the bronchioles; type III (5 to 10 percent) involves the terminal bronchioles and/or the alveolar ducts; and type IV involves the distal acinus or alveolar sacs. Three types are utilized in clinical practice, based on imaging.

Congenital lobar hyperinflation (CLH), formerly known as congenital lobar emphysema (CLE), is overdis-tention of a lobe(s) resulting from bronchial obstruction without lung destruction (therefore no emphysematous component).

Pulmonary sequestration is lung tissue "sequestered from" the airway and pulmonary artery, supplied by a sys-temic artery from the aorta. There are two types: intralo-bar pulmonary sequestration (75 percent) and extralobar pulmonary sequestration (25 percent). Intralobar pulmo-nary sequestration is located within the lung and usually has pulmonary venous drainage, whereas extralobar pul-monary sequestration has a separate pleural covering and systemic venous drainage.

Bronchial atresia is obstruction of a bronchus whereby distal parenchyma is aerated (usually hyperaerated) by col-lateral air drift.

Bronchogenic cysts are congenital fluid-filled thin-walled masses located in the mediastinum (85 percent), resulting from error early in the embryologic sequence of airway branching, or pulmonary parenchyma (25 percent), from a later branching error.

Clinical Features

Clinical presentation of BPFM varies depending on size of the lesion, mass effect on the airway and adjacent lung, and superimposed infection. CPAM, extralobar sequestration and CLH often present in infancy with respiratory distress. Bronchogenic cyst, intralobar sequestration, and bronchial atresia have variable later presentations, most often with recurrent upper respiratory infection, but may be asymp-tomatic. Many are now being detected on prenatal ultra-sound and MRI.

Anatomy and Physiology

Bronchopulmonary foregut malformations are a spectrum of anomalies resulting from pulmonary obstruction and parenchymal dysplasia during gestational weeks 4 through 7. Development of the various malformations is determined by the timing of obstruction in utero. Bronchogenic cyst and CPAM are related to earlier obstruction; sequestra-tion and CLH form after later bronchial obstruction. Most foregut malformations have a component of bronchial atre-sia on pathological examination.

Imaging Findings

Radiographic manifestations include diffuse or focal asym-metric hyperaeration, air- or fluid-filled cysts, airspace consolidation, and pulmonary or mediastinal mass. In the neonatal period CPAM and CLH may be fluid-filled with progressive aeration. Mixed or "hybrid" lesions are com-mon at pathology (>50 percent) and imaging distinction between lesions may not be possible.

Congenital pulmonary airway malformation (Fig. 8.1): CPAM appears as a multilocular or unilocular cystic mass or solid mass, no lobar predilection; cysts may contain fluid if infected. The five pathological types discussed previously are classified into three imaging types based on size of cysts: type I (most common, 50 percent) has largest cyst (> 2cm); type II (40 percent) has smaller cysts (<2cm); and type III is solid with microscopic cysts.

Congenital lobar hyperinflation (Fig. 8.2): CLH is a hyperinflated, hyperlucent lobe with compression of adja-cent lobes and shift of the mediastinum away from the lesion. Left upper lobe is the most common location (50 percent),

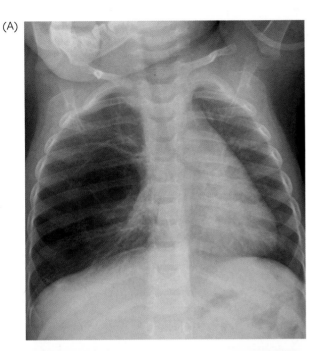

(A)

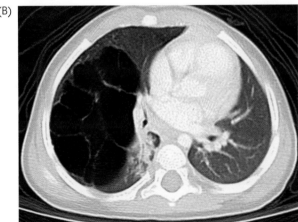

(B)

Figure 8.1. Frontal chest radiograph (A) in a 15-month-old boy shows a multilocular air-filled cystic mass in the right lower lobe causing shift of the heart and mediastinum to the left. Noncontrast CT (B) shows a multilocular air-filled cystic mass with multiple large (> 2 cm) thin-walled cysts consistent with congenital pulmonary airway malformation type I.

followed by the right middle lobe (30 percent) and right lower lobe (20 percent).

Pulmonary sequestration (PS; Fig. 8.3): PS appears as increased opacity (consolidation and/or cysts) in a basilar segment, most often the left lower lobe. Systemic vascular supply from the aorta is the key to diagnosis. Extralobar sequestration does not contain air unless infected, whereas intralobar sequestration may contain air via collateral air drift.

Bronchial atresia (BA; Fig. 8.4): BA appears as a perihilar tubular mass with adjacent hyperinflated lung and diminished vascularity, most common in the left upper lobe. Bronchogenic cyst (BC; Fig. 8.5): A BC appears as a round or oval mediastinal (fluid-filled) or pulmonary (air-filled) thin-walled mass. A mediastinal bronchogenic cyst may

be paratracheal, subcarinal, or hilar in location, does not contain air unless infected and density varies from simple to complex (proteinaceous or hemorrhagic). A pulmonary bronchogenic cyst is typically air-filled (communication with the airway), located in the medial third of the lung.

Imaging Strategy

The initial imaging modality of choice for assessing suspected BPFM begins with frontal and lateral chest radiographs. Chest CT distinguishes hyperaerated lung (CLH, bronchial atresia) from lung cysts (CPAM, intrapulmonary bronchogenic cyst). A CT scan or MRI can diagnose mediastinal bronchogenic cysts, which may be obscured by the thymus on chest radiograph when subcarinal. MRI can also confirm the cystic nature of proteinaceous bronchogenic cysts that are indeterminate on CT. Intravenous contrast is essential to visualize the systemic arterial supply in pulmonary sequestration on CT, however MRI or ultrasound with Doppler are radiation-free alternatives. Increased cost, sedation, propensity for artifact, and decreased spatial resolution are some drawbacks to MRI.

Related Physics

One limitation of MRI over CT is imaging time. Fetal MRI offers distinct advantages over CT in providing superior contrast-to-noise ratio without ionizing radiation, but fetal motion precludes conventional spin echo techniques that can take upward of 4 minutes per sequence. Ultrafast MRI has been developed to enable imaging of mobile structures in shorter time with two root origins; one is spin echo and the other gradient echo. Conventional spin echo applies a 90-degree pulse followed by a rephasing 180-degree pulse within one repetition time (TR). Fast or turbo spin echo applies a 90-degree pulse followed by a series of 180-degree pulses in a single TR given by the pulse "echo train length." The ultrafast sequence, HASTE (half-Fourier acquisition singleshot turbo spin-echo), is a fast spin echo technique that applies a very rapid train of 180-degree pulses in a "single shot" until half of k-space is filled; the other half is mirrored using the mathematical rules of fourier transforms. With this technique, a complete image set is obtained in seconds (as opposed to minutes with conventional spin echo). Gradient echo applies a flip angle of less than 90 degrees and rapid repetition of the sequence, affording imaging times of less than 1 minute per sequence. One of the most commonly employed techniques is FLASH (fast low angle shot), which utilizes low flip angle and very short TR; a fetal brain can be imaged in under 20 seconds with this technique.

Differential Diagnosis

CPAM:

- Congenital diaphragmatic hernia
- Pulmonary sequestration
- Pneumonia

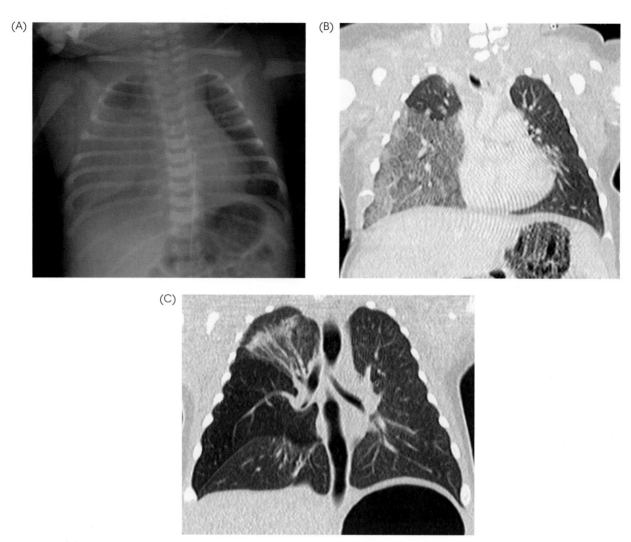

Figure 8.2. Frontal chest radiograph (A) and noncontrast CT (B) of a newborn with respiratory distress show fluid opacification of the right middle lobe (retained fetal lung fluid). Noncontrast CT (C) at day 24 shows a hyperlucent and hyperexpanded right middle lobe with mass effect on the right upper and lower lobes consistent with congenital lobar hyperinflation.

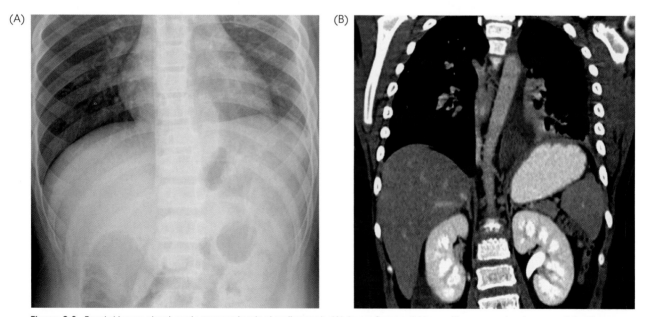

Figure 8.3. Frontal lower chest and upper adominal radiograph (A) in an 8-year-old boy with recurrent pulmonary infections shows a left lower thoracic paraspinal opacity (black arrow). Contrast-enhanced CT (B) shows a hypodense left lower lobe mass with arterial supply (white arrow) from the descending aorta consistent with intralobar pulmonary sequestration.

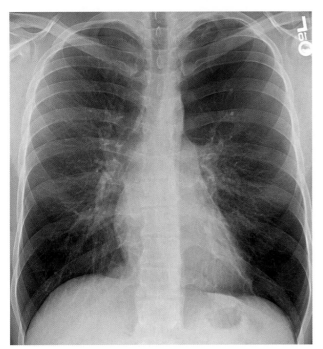

Figure 8.4. Frontal chest radiograph in a 17-year-old boy with intermittent respiratory distress shows a hyperlucent left upper lobe with attenuated vasculature and left suprahilar tubular opacity (arrow) consistent with bronchial atresia.

Pulmonary sequestration:
- CPAM
- Pneumonia
- Neurogenic tumor
- Pulmonary vascular anomaly

CLH:
- CPAM
- Pulmonary sequestration
- Pneumonia

Bronchial atresia:
- Airway foreign body
- Allergic bronchopulmonary aspergillosis

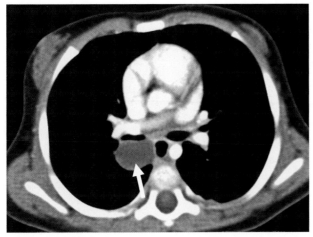

Figure 8.5. Contrast-enhanced CT in a 13-month-old boy with respiratory distress shows a thin-walled fluid-filled cyst posterior to and narrowing the right main bronchus (arrow) consistent with a mediastinal bronchogenic cyst.

Bronchogenic cyst:
- Esophageal duplication cyst
- Neuroenteric cyst
- Necrotic lymphadenopathy
- Pneumatocele
- Unilocular CPAM

Common Variants

Hybrid or mixed lesions are present at pathology in greater than 50 percent, most often comprised of CPAM and extralobar pulmonary sequestration. Pulmonary sequestration may rarely be extrathoracic, located in the left upper abdomen. Communication with the esophagus may occur with malformation involving one of the lower lobes. Fluid-filled cysts can occur with infected CPAM.

Clinical Issues

Because of risk for coexistent or future development of Pleuropulmonary blastoma or rhabdomyosarcoma, CPAMs are surgically removed. Some CPAMs will spontaneously involute, being identified on prenatal ultrasound and subsequently absent on postnatal imaging. Type II CPAM and extralobar sequestration may coexist with other congenital anomalies (congenital diaphragmatic hernia, cardiovascular anomalies, renal agenesis). Both intralobar and extralobar sequestrations are surgically removed because of compression of normal lung and risk of infection.

Key Points
- BPFMs are a spectrum and mixed "hybrid" lesions are common (>50 percent by pathology); imaging distinction is not always possible.
- CPAM and CLH most often present in infancy with respiratory distress because of mass effect and are best evaluated by CT (air-filled cysts in CPAM, hyperaerated lung in CLH).
- Pulmonary sequestration, both extralobar and intralobar, most often occurs in the left lower lobe; identification of systemic artery supply from the aorta is a key to diagnosis.

Further Reading
Berrocal T, Madrid C, Novo S, Gutierres J, Arjonilla A, Gomes-Leon N. Congenital anomalies of the tracheobronchial tree, lung, and mediastinum: embryology, radiology and pathology. *Radiographics*. 2004; *24*:e 17 (online only).

Daltro P, Fricke B, Kurocki I, Domingues R, Donnelly L. CT of congenital lung lesions in pediatric patients. *AJR*. 2004;*183*: 1497–1506.

Donnelly LF, Jones BV, O'hara SM. *Diagnostic Imaging: Pediatrics.* First Edition. Salt Lake City, UT: Amirsys; 2005.

Effmann E. Congenital lung malformations. In: Slovis T, ed. *Caffey's Pediatric Diagnostic Imaging.* Eleventh edition. Philadelphia, PA. Mosby Elsevier; 2008: 1086–1120.

Lee EY. Imaging evaluation of mediastinal masses in infants and children. In: Santiago ML, Applegate KE, Blackmore C, eds. *Evidence Based Imaging in Pediatrics.* First edition. New York, NY: Springer; 2009: 381–400.

Lee EY, Boiselle PM, Cleveland RH. Multidetector CT evaluation of congenital lung anomalies. *Radiology.* 2008;247(3): 632–648.

Newman, B. Congenital bronchopulmonary foregut malformations: concepts and controversies. *Pediatr Radiol.* 2006;36: 773–791.

CHAPTER 9

Congenital Diaphragmatic Hernia

Gerald Behr, MD

Definition

Congenital diaphragmatic hernia (CDH) is a developmental diaphragmatic defect that causes abdominal structures to herniate into the thoracic cavity. Congenital diaphragmatic hernias are typically classified into two types depending on the location of the diaphragmatic defect: Bochdaleck type and Morgagni type. There is a rare congenital form of hiatal hernia.

Clinical Features

The incidence of CDH is 1 in 2,000 to 3,000 live births. Pediatric patients with CDH present with varying clinical severity. Most cases of Bochdaleck hernia are sporadic. Overall, and in the absence of other findings, CDH has a mortality of approximately 20 percent although reported numbers vary widely. Major determinants for survival in patients with CDH include degree of underlying pulmonary hypoplasia and pulmonary hypertension. Lung hypoplasia results from compression of fetal lungs caused by mass effect from the herniated viscera. Such lung hypoplasia is characterized by decrease in total arteriolar cross-sectional area and distal arterial wall thickening. Both are thought to contribute to the often refractory pulmonary hypertension in patients with CDH.

The Morgagni (retrosternal or parasternal) hernia accounts for between 9 and 12 percent of infantile diaphragmatic hernias. These hernias frequently come to attention later in life, often in adulthood, either incidentally or as a cause of bowel obstruction or pneumonia. Because of the risk of bowel strangulation or incarceration, surgical repair is currently recommended for Morgagni hernias. An additional form of retrosternal hernia occurs as one feature of pentalogy of Cantrell, which is believed to result from failure of development of the septum transversum. This entity consists of the pentad of omphalocele, complex cardiac anomalies (including ectopia cordis), pericardial defects, inferior sternal cleft, and the retrosternal congenital diaphragmatic hernia.

Anatomy and Physiology

The diaphragm begins development during the fourth gestational week with structural contributions from the musculature of the lateral body wall, mediastinum, transverse septum and pleuroperitoneal folds (Fig. 9.1). Myoblasts migrate to muscularize these tissues. A remnant of the fibrous pleuroperitoneal folds persists as the lumbocostal trigone. Although it is often stated that the Bochdalek hernia arises from failure of the pleuroperitoneal folds to close or to fuse with the lateral musculature, several lines of evidence suggest an intrinsic defect within the pleuroperitoneal folds themselves that actually *predates* fold closure. The diaphragmatic defect is located within the posterolateral aspect of the diaphragm in cases of Bochdalek type. This is typically a left-sided defect but right-sided defects of this type may also occur.

The most common form of the restrosternal hernia is the Morgagni hernia. The foramen of Morgagni is thought to arise from failure of transverse septum fusion with the lateral muscular wall. It is situated between the sternum and eighth rib at the point of crossing of the internal mammary artery through the diaphragm. Interestingly, the Morgagni type congenital diaphragmatic hernia defect often occurs in patients with Trisomy 21 (1:1,000 incidence).

The rare congenital sliding hiatal hernia has been hypothesized to occur from late descent of the stomach below the diaphragm leaving an abnormally wide esophageal hiatus. Hiatal hernias, compromising less than 9 percent of infantile diaphragmatic hernias, are of three types: congenital short esophagus, sliding hiatus hernia, and paraesophageal hernia. The congenital short esophagus is characterized by a stomach that is fixed in position above the diaphragm. The sliding hiatus hernia and the paraesophogeal hernia comprise the other two, both of which are typically acquired in late childhood or adulthood although they also rarely may present at birth.

Imaging Findings

Chest radiography reflects the underlying abnormalities of CDH (Figs. 9.2 to 9.4). Specifically, the tip of a nasogastric tube overlies the left hemi-thorax while its esophageal course is deviated contralaterally. The mediastinum is shifted to the contralateral side. There is decreased or complete absence of intraabdominal bowel gas. Finally, air-filled bowel loops are seen in the chest. The initial chest radiographs, however, often show ipsilateral opacification as no air has yet reached the bowel.

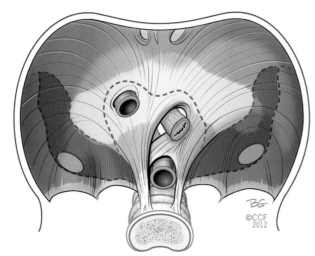

Figure 9.1. Illustration of fetal diaphragm in development and potential location of CDH. Transverse septum (yellow), Mediastinum (white), Pleuroperitoneal membrane (red), Lateral body wall (blue), Bochdalek hernia (pink).

No contralateral mediastinal shift will occur in a rare entity known as hepatopulmonary fusion whereby the right lung and liver are fused across a right-sided diaphragmatic defect. Rather than contralateral shift, the hepatopulmonary fusion causes an ipsilateral shift of the mediastinum that may be interpreted merely as atelectasis or right lung agenesis/hypoplasia.

Although the number of herniated bowel loops on chest radiographs correlates poorly with outcome, findings such as liver herniation are associated with a worse prognosis in patients with CDH. In fact, some have proposed a grading system for degree of liver herniation to estimate prognosis of patients with CDH. Another important prognostic factor is degree of underlying lung hypoplasia. Traditionally, fetal ultrasound measurements are expressed in terms of lung:head ratios. More recently, however, some have used more direct lung measurements calculated using three-dimensional ultrasound or fetal MRI compared with expected standards from age-matched controls.

In the postoperative setting, an ipsilateral pneumothorax is an expected finding (Fig. 9.5). The pneumothorax is gradually replaced by fluid. The lung demonstrates varying degrees of underlying pulmonary hypoplasia manifested by smaller size and decreased density of vessels. Evacuation of the pneumothorax by chest tube is generally avoided because the hypermobile neonatal mediastinum may undergo torsion, which can lead to compromise of the inferior vena cava.

Imaging Strategy

Often CDH is diagnosed prenatally by ultrasound, generally around gestational age of 24 weeks but may be seen as early as 18 weeks. Fetal MRI is often obtained to confirm the diagnosis, determine position of the liver, and search for additional associated congenital abnormalities.

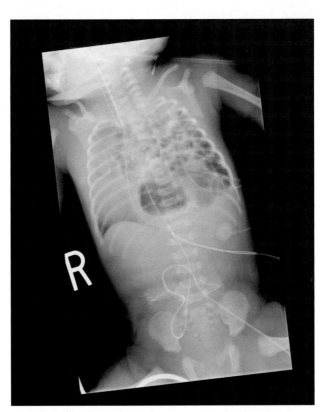

Figure 9.2. Frontal radiograph of a newborn with known left CDH shows multiple dilated bowel loops in the left hemithorax, supradiaphragmatic positioning of the nasogastric tube, and mediastinal shift to the right.

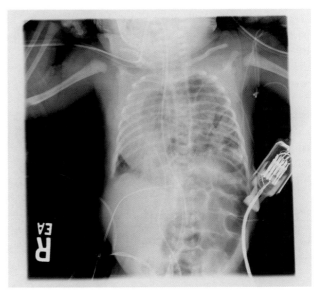

Figure 9.3. Frontal radiograph of a 1-day-old baby boy with known left CDH shows bowel loops located both above and below the left hemidiaphragm. Exact relationship of the umbilical venous catheter to right atrium is difficult to determine. There is rightward mediastinal (and NG tube) shift.

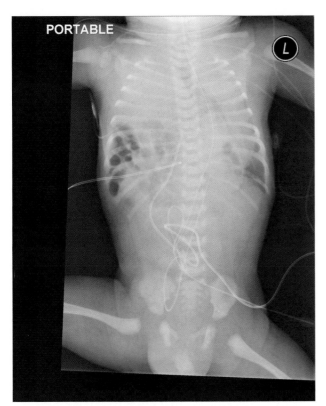

Figure 9.4. Frontal radiograph of a 1-day-old baby boy with known right CDH demonstrates multiple gas-filled bowel loops in the right hemithorax with a gasless abdomen. Leftward deviation of the NG tube is also seen.

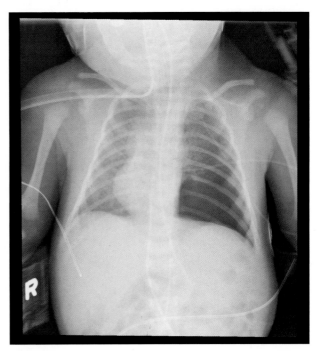

Figure 9.5. Frontal radiograph in a 3-day-old baby boy following surgical repair of left CDH shows left pneumothorax, an expected postoperative finding that does not require chest tube placement. This space will eventually fill with fluid and expanded left lung over time.

When the diagnosis is straightforward, only chest radiographs are obtained in the newborn undergoing surgical repair. If there is suspicion for an associated mass or the diagnosis is in doubt, a CT scan with coronal reconstruction images may be of benefit. Such reconstructed CT images are helpful to clearly display the complex anatomic relationships between the herniated organs or bowel and diaphragmatic defect. Intravenous contrast should be administered and CT angiography considered, particularly if an underlying sequestration or hepatopulmonary fusion is considered. Upper GI may reveal the stomach in the thorax although preoperative studies of this kind are currently rarely necessary. Midgut malrotation is an expected finding in patients with CDH because the bowel does not return to the abdomen to complete its normal counterclockwise turns in utero.

Complications from the underlying lung hypoplasia or the supportive therapy may occur such as contralateral pneumothorax. The course of umbilical vessel catheters on the plain film is often altered, particularly when the liver is herniated. Lateral views may help depict the course of the lines although, often, assessment of their precise localization is not possible.

Related Physics

Although it is safer than CT for fetal imaging because of lack of ionizing radiation, MRI is not without risk. Safety issues are related to tissue heating caused by radiofrequency energy, heat absorbed within metallic objects either within or on the patient, and mechanical torque of implanted devices. All equipment within the imaging area must be MRI-compatible to avoid objects acting as missiles when placed within the extremely strong magnetic field. The specific absorption rate expressed in units of Watts/kilogram (W/kg) is SAR. The FDA limit is 3 W/kg for brain and 4 W/Kg for whole body average in 15 minutes. The SAR will increase with static field strength; increasing from a 1.5 to 3 Tesla field will quadruple the SAR. Great care should be taken in imaging fetuses at 3T. The SAR also increases with radiofrequency and duty cycle and with the use of transmit-receive over receive-only coils. The SAR can be lowered by reducing the frequency of pulses applied (increasing echo train length or increasing the interecho spacing), increasing repetition time (TR), eliminating or reducing the spatial saturation pulses or applying parallel imaging techniques.

Differential Diagnosis

- Diaphragmatic eventration
- Congenital pulmonary airway malformation
- Bronchopulmonary foregut malformations
- Sequestrations
- Primary pulmonary hypoplasia or agenesis (direction of mediastinal shift is toward the small lung)

Common Variants

Most commonly, CDH presents as a Bochdaleck hernia; however, the Morgagni hernia and esophageal hernia are variants. Acquired diaphragmatic hernias in the first few months of life are not common; however, do tend to be right-sided. Of interest, these often arise in the setting of a history of Group B Streptococcal pneumonia.

Clinical Issues

Although most cases of CDH are sporadic, 15 to 45 percent of patients are born with associated congenital anomalies and 10 to 20 percent demonstrate chromosomal abnormalities such as Trisomy 13, 18, 21 and tetrasomy 12p (Pallister-Killian syndrome). Additionally, there are familial case reports of CDH. The more common associations include cleft palate, neural tube defects, esophageal atresia, and cardiac anomalies. Those with associated anomalies generally have a poorer prognosis. In fact, associated anomalies are reported in 95 percent of cases of stillborn infants with CDH. One lethal syndrome that features CDH is Fryns syndrome (coarse facies, micrognathia, distal limb and nail hypoplasia).

Apart from surgical repair of the underlying defect, treatment is directed toward the resultant pulmonary hypertension. No consensus has been established, but extracorporeal membrane oxygenation (ECMO), vasodilators such as nitric oxide and calcium channel blockers, high-frequency oscillation ventilation and surfactant have all been used with varying degrees of success for managing pulmonary hypertension associated with CDH. Over the past two decades there has been a trend away from immediate surgical management and toward elective repair after medical management. In addition, the past 15 years has seen a trend toward less aggressive ventilation, while tolerating some degree of hypercapnia, previously thought to be detrimental. These advances have led to decreased need for ECMO and have resulted in improved survival in patients with CDH.

Key Points

- Diagnosis of CDH is usually made prenatally.
- The most common form of CDH is a left-sided Bochdaleck hernia.
- Degree of bowel herniation depicted on radiograph carries little prognostic information.
- A herniated liver spells a worse prognosis.
- Survival is largely dependent on degree of underlying pulmonary hypoplasia and hypertension.
- Postoperative pneumothoraces should not routinely be evacuated.

Further Reading

Bosenberg AT, Brown RA. Management of congenital diaphragmatic hernia. *Curr Opin Anaesthesiol.* 2008;*21*(3):323–331.

Chavhan GB, Babyn PS, Cohen RA, Langer JC. Multimodality imaging of the pediatric diaphragm: anatomy and pathologic conditions. *Radiographics.* 2010;*30*(7):1797–1817.

Clugston RD, Klattig J, Englert C, Clagett-Dame M, Martinovic J, Benachi A, Greer JJ. Teratogen-induced dietary and genetic models of congenital diaphragmatic hernia share a common mechanism of pathogenesis. *Am J Pathol.* 2006;*169*(5): 1541–1549.

Gander JW, Kadenhe-Chiweshe A, Fisher JC, Lampl BS, Berdon WE, Stolar CJ, Zitsman JL. Hepatic pulmonary fusion in an infant with a right-sided congenital diaphragmatic hernia and contralateral mediastinal shift. *J Pediatr Surg.* 2010;*45*(1): 265–268.

Holt PD, Arkovitz MS, Berdon WE, Stolar CJ. Newborns with diaphragmatic hernia: initial chest radiography does not have a role in predicting clinical outcome. *Pediatr Radiol.* 2004;*34*(6):462–464.

Taylor GA, Atalabi OM, Estroff JA. Imaging of congenital diaphragmatic hernias. *Pediatr Radiol.* 2009; *39*(1):1–16.

CHAPTER 10

Surfactant Deficiency Disease

Emily Maduro, MD and Eric Chong, MD

Definition

Surfactant deficiency disease (SDD) is a condition characterized by the insufficient production of surfactant in the preterm neonate, resulting in alveolar collapse and eventually respiratory failure.

Clinical Features

Infants born after 34 weeks gestation have a less than 5 percent risk of developing SDD, although infants born before 28 weeks gestation have a 60 percent risk. Other risk factors for developing SDD include perinatal asphyxia, maternal diabetes, and multiple gestations. The deficiency of surfactant leads to increased breathing effort and diffuse atelectasis thus diminishing the functional residual capacity of the lungs, resulting in alveolar injury. Hypoxia and acidosis contribute to pulmonary vasoconstriction. Consequently, the threat of right-to-left shunting through the ductus arteriosus is greater and ventilation-perfusion mismatch is worsened. Additionally, alveolar injury produces edema, proteinaceous exudates, and hemorrhage that together inactivate the surfactant.

Nonspecific respiratory distress typically develops shortly after birth, worsens over time, and peaks at 24 to 48 hours. These symptoms include tachypnea, nasal flaring, expiratory grunting, substernal and intercostal retractions, central cyanosis, and apnea. Since 1990, endotracheal administration of surfactant has been the mainstay of therapy for SDD.

Babies who suffered prenatal stress, including prolonged ruptured membranes, have been observed to have fewer incidence of SDD. This is histologically associated with more mature lungs. Glucocorticoids have been shown to stimulate lung and surfactant maturation and reduce the risk of intracranial intraventricular hemorrhage and neonatal mortality. Therefore, in an attempt to prevent SDD, current recommendations include maternal administration of betamethasone 1 to 7 days before delivery in women at risk of preterm labor between 24 and 34 weeks of gestation.

Anatomy and Physiology

Fetal lung development is divided into five stages. The last three stages of lung development (canalicular, saccular, and alveolar) take place within the window of potential viability. The alveolar phase begins at about 36 weeks gestation. Mature alveoli create a larger surface area lined mostly by type I pneumocytes responsible for gas exchange, scattered with type II pneumocytes, which secrete surfactant. Surfactant is composed of phospholipids and proteins, which lower the surface tension within the alveoli preventing collapse during expiration. Cell debris, fibrin, and transudate come together to form thin membranes that line the inner alveolar wall, further inhibiting gas exchange. Although they are not part of the primary pathologic process in this disease, these characteristic hyaline membranes initially gave the disease its name.

Imaging Findings

The lack of abnormal radiographic findings at 6 hours after birth generally excludes SDD. The classic appearance of SDD is symmetric reticulogranular opacities of the lungs, which coalesce and worsen, effacing vascular markings and in the severe cases, resulting in "white out," obliterating cardiac and diaphragmatic contours. Low lung volumes create a characteristic bell-shaped appearance to the thorax (Fig. 10.1). Air bronchograms are caused by distended bronchioles overlying diffuse alveolar atelectasis.

The radiographic appearance of SDD changes drastically after the administration of surfactant (Fig. 10.2). Improved aeration is visible on the chest radiograph within an hour. The uneven distribution of endotracheally administered surfactant can lead to asymmetric improvement of aeration that may favor the right lung or present as focal over-aeration of acini seen as cystic lucencies or even a hyperlucent right lung mimicking barotrauma.

Imaging Strategy

Because these newborns are usually placed in the neonatal intensive care unit, portable frontal radiographs within the incubator are the standard method of examination. If barotrauma such as pneumothorax and pneumomediastinum are suspected on the frontal radiograph, a cross-table lateral view can be obtained.

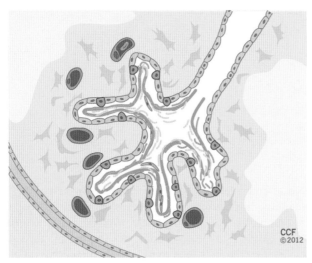

Figure 10.1. Illustration of pathophysiology in surfactant deficiency disease. Lack of surfactant production leads to poor alveolar compliance with multiple low volume acini containing 'hyaline membranes' (green).

Related Physics

Imaging using projection radiographic technology requires a balance between optimum image quality and radiation absorbed dose. It is fair to say that there is less room for error when using film-screen radiography, as an over- or under-exposed film cannot be postprocessed and must be taken again. On the other hand, computed radiography (CR) and direct radiography (DR) are more forgiving to underexposure where the underexposed imaging may be lesser in quality but still readable. The true danger lies in CR/DR overexposure, as this leads to a great reduction in noise and an apparently superior image, but one with an unacceptably high radiation dose. This latter phenomenon has been coined "radiation creep" as the radiologist becomes accustomed to the nice images and requests that technique be established as the routine. Film-screen imaging in the NICU requires attention to detail, as adequate preparation of the patient and equipment will lead to the lowest radiation dose. First, one should apply labels to identify side and patient information. If possible, one must remove equipment and linen lying between the X-ray source and the image receptor that may include the cassette, CR or DR plate. By positioning the patient flat on the receptor, oblique X-ray paths are avoided. Collimation should be employed to restrict the exposure to the region of interest and lead shielding may be placed under the gonads in males. The technologist must choose the technique manually (kVp and mAs) and this should be based on a technique chart for age and weight developed by a committee within one's department. The committee should include a board-certified radiologist, qualified medical physicist, and a pediatric technologist. In general, one should choose short exposure time with higher mA to limit effects from patient motion. When imaging infants in the NICU, it is advisable not to use an antiscatter grid, which will increase exposure techniques and patient dose by a factor of 3 to 5 when compared to the same imaging study without the use of a grid.

Differential Diagnosis

■ Meconium aspiration syndrome (MAS): This typically occurs in postmature infants who present with respiratory distress and meconium stain during delivery. Lungs are usually hyperinflated in MAS. Spontaneous pneumothorax is also frequently seen.

■ Neonatal pneumonia (NP): NP is often associated with premature rupture of membranes and chorioamnionitis. Respiratory distress is delayed by 3 or 4 days after birth. There is no specific radiographic pattern of lung opacifications, but the presence of a pleural effusion should raise the possibility of NP.

■ Transient tachypnea of the newborn (TTN): Respiratory distress is delayed by about 6 hours from birth. There is normal or increased lung volume, prominence of vascular markings and often a small pleural effusion with spontaneous clearing within 48 to 72 hours.

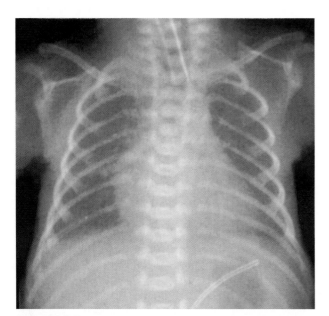

Figure 10.2. Frontal chest radiograph in a newborn male with respiratory distress shows bell-shaped thorax with diffuse hazy granular opacity of the lungs and air bronchograms.

Common Variants

The radiographic presentation of SDD is usually straightforward. When there is a variation in the imaging findings or clinical course, it is usually caused by one of the many complications that can arise, as discussed more fully in the following section.

Clinical Issues

The major clinical issues for SDD are associated with early complications, including air leak phenomena, hemodynamic shunting, pulmonary hemorrhage, and late complications such as bronchopulmonary dysplasia.

Air Leak

Infants with SDD often require mechanical ventilation with positive end-expiratory pressure, which aims to maintain the distention of the collapsed alveoli. High airway pressure and overdistention of alveoli are the main risk factors for rupture at the bronchiolo-alveolar junction. The air then dissects through the peribronchovascular interstitium, causing linear lucencies in tortuous patterns that radiate outward, not conforming to the branching pattern of air bronchograms and extending to the periphery. This is known as pulmonary interstitial emphysema (PIE) and it is the initial radiographic sign of barotrauma. Thin-walled pseudocysts may also be formed as a result of PIE (Fig. 10.3. Peripherally, subpleural blebs may rupture into the pleural space creating pneumothorax, whereas centrally, it may produce pneumomediastinum or pneumopericardium. In neonates, pneumothorax may be difficult to discern on chest radiographs. Radiologic findings of pneumothorax include a generalized increase in radiolucency of one hemithorax, increase in volume of a hemithorax with contralateral shift of the heart and mediastinum, depression of the ipsilateral diaphragm, and separation of the intercostal spaces. A pleural line may not be seen in the case of pneumothorax. A cross-table lateral view will demonstrate an anterior lucency that delineates the anterior margin of the collapsed lung. With pneumomediastinum, up to half of cases may go undetected without a lateral radiograph. The air may outline the inferior aspect of the heart producing the "continuous diaphragm" sign, elevate the lobes of the thymus in an "angel wing" sign, dissect into the soft tissues of the neck or outline the contour of the heart. It may be difficult to differentiate pneumomediastinum from pneumopericardium, and they may coexist. With pneumopericardium, the air is limited to the pericardial space, unable to extend past the roots of the great vessels, and it completely surrounds the heart on both frontal and lateral radiographs, without displacing the thymus.

Hemodynamic Shunting

Initially, severe hypoxia and acidosis cause pulmonary vasoconstriction that may serve to maintain a patent ductus arteriosus (PDA) with right-to-left shunting. As lung compliance and pulmonary artery pressure improve from approximately the third day to the end of the first week after birth, the direction of flow within the patent ductus changes from left to right. There is an increase in pulmonary flow with left heart failure, interstitial edema and a slight increase in heart size on the chest radiograph. These findings may be the earliest signs of PDA.

Hemorrhage

Parenchymal hemorrhage is a rare yet potentially serious complication of SDD. It can appear early (in the first or second day of life) as a complication of surfactant treatment, or after 1 week of age, in relation with barotrauma or hemorrhagic pulmonary edema resulting from left-to-right shunting through a PDA. Affected infants usually present with acute respiratory worsening accompanied by new airspace opacifications.

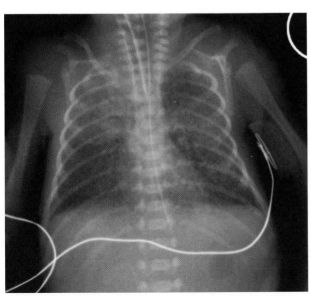

Figure 10.3. Frontal chest radiograph in the same patient following endotracheal surfactant administration shows greater expansion of the lungs with the reticulogranular opacities still apparent in a patchy uneven distribution.

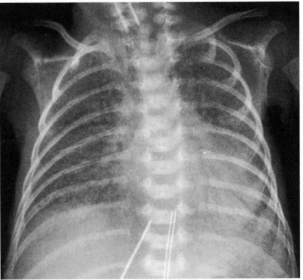

Figure 10.4. Frontal chest radiograph of an 8-day-old baby girl with respiratory distress shows a coarse appearance of the lungs with the characteristic tortuous lucencies of pulmonary interstitial emphysema.

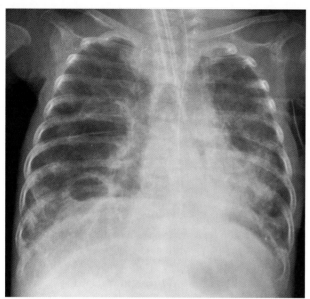

Figure 10.5. Frontal chest radiograph of a 5-week-old baby girl who has developed bronchopulmonary dysplasia shows hyperinflated lungs with lucent areas and some patchy opacities. There is a pseudocyst projected just above the right hemidiaphragm and a pneumomediastinum shown by right paravertebral lucency.

Bronchopulmonary Dysplasia

Bronchopulmonary dysplasia (BPD), also known as chronic lung disease of infancy, is a frequent chronic complication of SDD and is a form of chronic lung disease that develops in preterm neonates treated with oxygen and positive-pressure ventilation. Histologically, necrotizing alveolitis and diffuse alveolar-septal fibrosis are usually present. Radiographically, BPD is characterized by patchy and coarse opacities and small cystic lucencies that evolve to hyperinflation and larger lucent areas, often referred to as "bubbly lung"(Fig. 10.4).

Key Points

- SDD is a disease of prematurity mostly seen in infants born before 34 weeks of gestation, caused by lack of surfactant.
- In SDD, clinical respiratory distress and radiologic changes develop shortly after birth.
- The classic imaging features of SDD include low lung volume, homogeneous granular opacity, and air bronchograms.
- Air leaks are a common complication of SDD and include pulmonary interstitial emphysema, pneumothorax, pneumomediastinum, and pneumopericardium.
- In presumed SDD, if there is no improvement after 3 days of treatment with administration of surfactant, additional underlying conditions such as left-to-right shunt through PDA, hemorrhage, fluid overload, and infection should be considered.

Further Reading

Agrons GA, Courtney SE, Stocker JT, Markowitz RI. Lung disease in premature neonates: radiologic-pathologic correlation. *Radiographics.* 2005;*25*(July):1047–1073.

Hedlund GL, Griscom NT, Cleveland RH, Kirks D. Respiratory system. In: Kirks D, ed. *Griscom NT Practical Pediatric Imaging: Diagnostic Radiology of Infants and Children.* Philadelphia, PA: Lippincott-Williams & Wilkins;1998: 693–700.

Slovis TL, Bulas DI. Congenital and aquired lesions (most causing respiratory distress) of the neonatal lung and thorax. In: Slovis TL, Adler BH, Bloom DA, et al., eds. *Caffey's Pediatric Diagnostic Imaging.* Philadelphia, PA:Mosby; 2008: 104–122.

WarrenJB, Anderson JM. Core concepts: respiratory distress syndrome. *NeoReviews.* 2009;*10*(7):e351–e361.

CHAPTER 11

Neonatal Pneumonia

Jonathan O. Swanson, MD

Definition

Neonatal pneumonia (NP) is defined as pulmonary infection within the first 28 days of life. The inoculation responsible for NP can occur in utero, during labor and delivery, as well as after birth.

Clinical Features

Neonatal pneumonia represents a great medical burden in the developing world (estimated mortality as high as 29 in 1,000 live births), yet also remains a substantial source of morbidity and mortality in the developed world with an incidence is 0.5 to 1.0 percent of live births. Premature infants are at greater risk of infection, with the incidence reaching an estimated 10 percent of preterm infants. The major risk factor for intrauterine development of pneumonia is prolonged rupture of the membranes, particularly if labor is active during this period. Importantly, NP is often associated with sepsis. At the onset of neonatal pneumonia, there are no dependable clinical markers. Septic neonates cannot always mount a febrile response; therefore fever cannot reliably be used as a clinical marker for infection. A neonate with pneumonia may initially look well or demonstrate only mild respiratory distress. However, over the course of days, the clinical picture often worsens as NP becomes complicated by sepsis with multi-organ involvement. Although the diagnosis may remain elusive initially, early clinical suspicions may be raised if a neonate has a birth history of prolonged rupture of membranes, is premature, or if there is maternal fever.

Anatomy and Physiology

The transmission of infection for NP can occur in utero, during delivery, or after birth (often nosocomially). Congenital infections causing NP include rubella, congenital syphilis, cytomegalovirus (CMV), and listeriosis. Conversely, perinatal pneumonia is most often caused by group B beta-hemolytic streptococcus (GBS). Neonates who acquire the infection in the perinatal setting may have early respiratory distress, but it can often be delayed by as many as 3 to 4 days. The most frequent cause of post-amnionitis pneumonia is GBS, with Escherichia coli and Enterococcus as the next most common agents.

Imaging Findings

The radiographic findings of NP mimic many of the other major respiratory ailments of the neonate. Two common radiographic patterns suggestive of NP are the diffuse granular opacification throughout both lungs (mimics surfactant deficiency disease, SDD; Fig. 11.1) and the coarse reticular pattern (mimics meconium aspiration or partially treated SDD; Fig. 11.2). In a smaller subset of patients, NP can have bilateral fine reticular opacities like those seen in the setting of transient tachypnea of the newborn (TTN; Fig. 11.3). Although these look-alikes make a pure radiographic diagnosis difficult, the following chest radiographic findings can support the diagnosis of NP: pleural effusions, hyperinflation, and worsening or persistent bilateral fine reticular opacities. Effusions are much more likely in NP than in SDD or meconium aspiration. Hyperinflation can help distinguish NP from the typical low lung volumes of SDD. Finally, the worsening or persistent bilateral fine reticular opacities of NP are in stark contrast to the TTN pattern of lung clearing over 1 to 3 days.

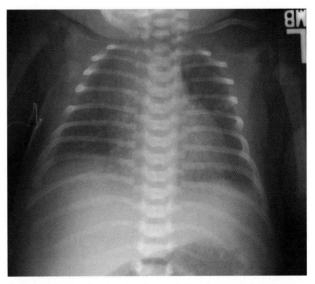

Figure 11.1. Frontal chest radiograph in a 1-day-old boy born at 34 weeks gestation with respiratory distress shows diffuse granular opacities bilaterally with a small right-sided pleural effusion.

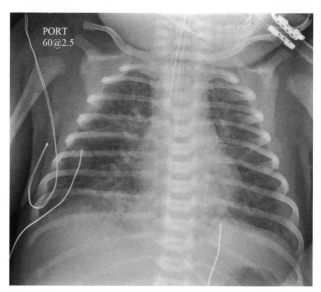

IMAGING PITFALLS: The pleural effusions are often subtle, seen as mild thickening of the costophrenic angle on the frontal view.

Imaging Strategy

Chest radiography is the imaging modality of choice. Repeat chest radiographs can be used to distinguish TTN (which improves) from NP. As mentioned above, special attention should be paid to the costophrenic angles to identify a subtle pleural effusion. Because of the subtleties, the diagnosis must be made in conjunction with the patient's history and clinical presentation.

Related Physics

The use of computed radiography systems (CR) or digital radiography systems (DR) has several distinct advantages over film-based systems. The CR and DR systems permit the use of image-enhancement techniques such as low-contrast object detectability, noise reduction, edge enhancement, window and level capabilities. The end result is the improved ability to characterize chest

Figure 11.3. Frontal chest XR in a 4-day-old full-term boy with respiratory distress shows central reticular opacities and pleural effusion.

disease in newborns that, in the case of NP, can be quite subtle.

Differential Diagnosis

- Surfactant deficiency disease: SDD (also known as hyaline membrane disease and respiratory distress syndrome[RDS] of the newborn) typically affects premature infants ranging from 26 weeks through 33 weeks gestational age. The radiographic appearance is typically a fine granular opacity throughout both lungs in the setting of low lung volumes and pleural effusions are rare.
- Meconium aspiration syndrome (MDS): MDS refers to neonatal respiratory distress that occurs secondary to intrapartum/intrauterine aspiration of meconium, the thick material found in the neonatal bowel. The coarse reticular, rope-like pattern on the newborn chest is most frequently seen in the setting of meconium aspiration and NP. The presence of pleural effusion is more often seen in the setting of NP.
- Transient tachypnea of the newborn (TTN): TTN represents prolongation of the normal physiologic clearing of fluid from the lungs. The infant with TTN may present with mild or moderate respiratory distress but this benign, self-limited condition, resolves with supportive measures.
- Congestive heart failure (CHF): Pulmonary edema in the setting of congenital heart disease can have a similar appearance as TTN, without the spontaneous clearing after 1 to 3 days. Suspected congenital heart disease is best evaluated with an echocardiogram.

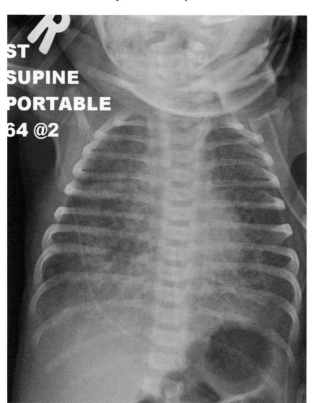

Figure 11.2. Frontal chest radiograph in a 2-day-old boy with persistent respiratory distress and mother who was GBS-positive at the time of delivery shows bilateral coarse parenchymal opacities and possible bilateral small pleural effusions.

Common Variants

Although *Chlamydia* is a less common cause of NP, timing may suggest this diagnosis. Neonates with chlamydia NP can present several weeks after birth. These patients may present with a concomitant conjunctivitis and may have diffuse reticular nodular opacities in the setting of large lung volumes. *Candida*, herpes simplex, and syphilis are also potential NP pathogens.

Of note, delayed right-sided diaphragmatic hernia is associated with a prior GBS neonatal pneumonia. The pathophysiology remains unknown.

Clinical Issues

The diagnosis of NP is complicated by the fact that neither the clinical nor radiographic findings are sensitive or specific. The radiographic evaluation must be taken in context with the clinical findings. As an example, when a radiologist evaluates a chest radiograph with diffuse granular opacities, distinguishing between RDS and NP may be extremely difficult. However, when the chest radiograph is presented with concurrent clinical information (e.g., a 36-week-old newborn), it may lead to closer inspection of the radiograph. On inspection, when a small right pleural effusion is seen, NP would be the far more likely diagnosis. In this example, RDS is less likely because of both gestational age and the presence of an effusion.

Key Points

- NP mimics the radiographic appearance of SDD, meconium aspiration, and TTN.
- Pleural effusion, persistent abnormality over time, and hyperinflation support NP.
- Risk factors include prolonged rupture of membranes, maternal fever, and prematurity.
- Knowledge of the clinical presentation (gestational age, presence/absence of meconium at birth, patient's clinical trajectory) sharpens the radiographic diagnosis.

Further Reading

Ablow RC, Gross I, Effmann EL, Uauy R, Driscoll S. The radiographic features of early onset Group B streptococcal neonatal sepsis. *Radiology.* 1977;*124*(3):771–777.

Bang AT, Bang RA, Morankar VP, Sontakke PG, Solanki JM. Pneumonia in neonates: can it be managed in the community? *Arch Dis Child.* 1993; 68:550–556.

Cleveland RH. A radiologic update on medical diseases of the newborn chest. *Pediatr Radiol.* 1995;*25*(8):631–637.

Haney PJ, Bohlman M, Sun CC. Radiographic findings in neonatal pneumonia. *AJR Am J Roentgenol.* 1984;*143*(1):23–26.

McCarten KM, Rosenberg HK, Borden S, Mandell GA. Delayed appearance of right diaphragmatic hernia associated with group B streptococcal infection in newborns. *Radiology.* 1981; *139*(2):385–389.

Slovis SL, Bulas DI. Congenital and acquired lesions (most causing respiratory distress) of the neonatal lung and thorax. In. Slovis TL, ed. *Caffey's Pediatric Diagnostic Imaging.* Philadelphia, PA: Mosby Elsevier; 2008.120–122.

CHAPTER 12

Meconium Aspiration Syndrome

Raul Galvez-Trevino, MD, MPH

Definition

Meconium aspiration syndrome (MAS) is defined as respiratory distress in an infant born through meconium-stained amniotic fluid (MSAF) whose symptoms cannot be explained otherwise. Hallmarks include early onset of respiratory distress, poor lung compliance, hypoxemia, and characteristic radiographic features.

Clinical Features

Infants are born through MSAF in approximately 10 to 15 percent of live births beyond 34 weeks gestation, but only 1 to 5 percent of newborns develop MAS, affecting males and females equally. Risk factors for MAS include post-term pregnancy, placental insufficiency, maternal hypertension and preeclampsia, oligohydramnios, and maternal drug use, among others.

The clinical presentation of an infant with MAS is variable. Signs depend on the severity of the hypoxic insult and the amount and viscosity of the meconium aspirated. Infants with MAS often exhibit signs of postmaturity. They are small for gestational age, have long nails and peeling yellow- or green-stained skin. Meconium staining of the skin is proportional to the length of exposure to meconium concentration.

Early MAS is characterized by proximal airway obstruction by secretions that must be rapidly cleared by endotracheal suctioning. Later, as the meconium is aspirated into distal small airways, air trapping, chemical pneumonitis, and atelectasis develop. Newborns with MAS present with signs and symptoms of respiratory insufficiency: tachypnea, nasal flaring, intercostal and supraclavicular retractions, wheezing, hyperaeration, hypercarbia, hypoxia, respiratory acidosis and cyanosis.

Anatomy and Physiology

Fetal or perinatal hypoxia and hypercapnia lead to vagal stimulation, causing increased peristalsis and relaxation of the anal sphincter ensuing passage of meconium and gasping, which can be aspirated into the tracheobronchial tree. Meconium is a thick green to black mucilaginous material present beyond 34 weeks of gestation, produced by a mature gastrointestinal tract in a full-term fetus. It consists of intestinal and epithelial cells, bile pigments, fatty acids, vernix, lanugo, and amniotic fluid. This tenacious aspirate induces neonatal hypoxia via central and small airway obstruction, via a ball-valve effect. Surfactant dysfunction ensues as a result of meconium fatty acids causing diffuse atelectasis from the higher minimal tension, which results in chemical pneumonitis and alveolar apoptosis induced by caspases activated by digestive enzymes and bile salts. Sustained hypoxia can provoke pulmonary hypertension in severe meconium aspiration. See Figure 12.1.

Imaging Findings

The radiographic findings vary according to the severity of meconium aspiration, which may not correlate with the clinical disease. The lung volumes may be normal to increased, with flattened hemidiaphragms in those with air trapping and compensatory hyperinflation, resulting in alternating asymmetric lucencies (Fig. 12.2). Partial or complete airway obstruction results in patchy subsegmental atelectasis that occurs peripheral to the obstructed bronchi, in a pattern of perihilar "rope-like opacities" (Fig. 12.3). Increased alveolar tension and airway blockage causes wall rupture leading to interstitial emphysema, pneumothorax or pneumomediastinum, which occur in 10 to 15 percent of patients, requiring mechanical ventilation (Fig. 12.4). Pneumopericardium is rare. Chemical pneumonitis and surfactant dysfunction lead to multifocal bilateral, asymmetric, and sometimes rounded opacities, representing acinar consolidation (Fig. 12.5).

Imaging Strategy

In infants with clinical signs of respiratory distress and MSAF, a chest radiograph should be obtained as soon as possible to assess the pattern of disease and help exclude other possible causes of respiratory insufficiency such as pneumonia or transient tachypnea of the newborn. Follow-up with portable chest radiographs is sufficient in those patients requiring mechanical ventilation. Chest CT may be used for the evaluation of suspected complications in patients undergoing mechanical ventilation, such as pneumothorax or pneumomediastinum. Features of chronic lung disease can be seen in prolonged mechanical ventilation.

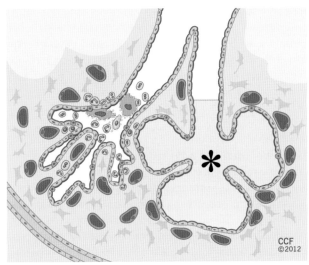

Figure 12.1. Illustration of pathophysiology in meconium aspiration. Meconium recruits acute phase reactants and airway and alveolar collapse as well as foci of air trapping (*)

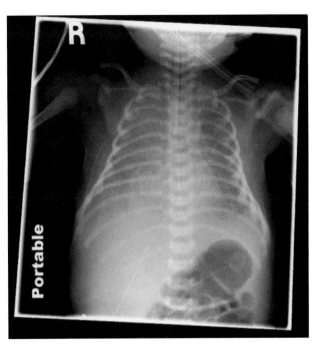

Figure 12.3. Frontal chest radiograph in a cyanotic newborn male with respiratory distress and meconium aspiration demonstrates alternating patchy lung opacities and asymmetric lucencies in both lungs, representing subsegmental atelectasis, acinar consolidation, and focal air trapping. The lungs are slightly hyperexpanded.

Related Physics

The density on a chest radiograph is largely created by blood-filled arteries and veins. A chest radiograph is considered normal if these vessels are sharply outlined, normal in size and architecture lying on a radiolucent background of air-filled lung. Spatial resolution in radiography is in part determined by the focal spot, which can be chosen by the operator. For infants, one should choose the smallest focal spot which in turn will render the highest resolution. Contrast sensitivity is determined by kVp control and noise control and can be augmented by decreasing the kVp to the lowest possible setting to allow for adequate penetration. This is easily done in the

newborn. Noise is a function of how many photons are liberated and how many are captured by the image receptor. Radiation dose can be lowered by using highly sensitive image receptors thereby not wasting any photons during

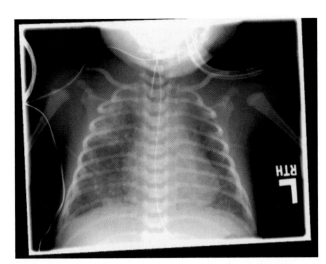

Figure 12.2. Frontal chest radiograph in a 1-day-old female born at 40 weeks gestation via vaginal delivery with meconium aspiration, perinatal cyanosis, and hypoxia shows perihilar rope-like opacities with slight lung hyperexpansion.

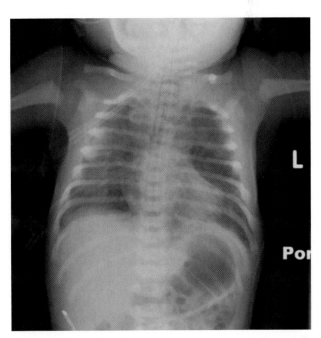

Figure 12.4. Frontal chest radiograph in a newborn male born at 40 weeks gestation with respiratory distress and meconium aspiration shows lucencies paralleling the mediastinal margins representing pneumomediastinum. There is a small right-sided pneumothorax.

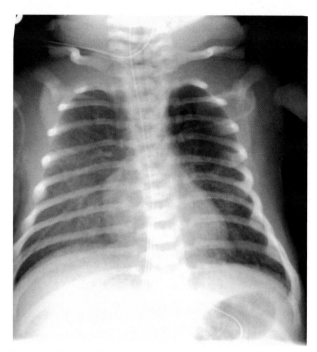

Figure 12.5. Frontal chest radiograph 9 days after meconium aspiration demonstrates residual subsegmental atelectasis.

the imaging process. Older imaging systems can only compensate for their decreased sensitivity by increasing mAs. Of all patients imaged, infants are the most sensitive to radiation insults.

Differential Diagnosis

- Neonatal pneumonia
- Severe transient tachypnea of the newborn
- Pulmonary hemorrhage
- Congenital lung masses

Common Variants

The severity of MAS varies according to the degree of meconium aspirate and respiratory distress, and the radiographic features correlate with the mechanical, chemical or hemodynamic sequela of the meconium reaching the different parts of the respiratory tract, which are not predictive of the clinical outcome.

Clinical Issues

Treatment is directed toward maintaining appropriate oxygenation, with mechanical ventilation commonly employed

for patients with severe disease and impending respiratory failure. New areas of air space disease should be identified promptly, with pulmonary toilet and chest physiotherapy usually being directed to the affected lung to help in resolving mucous plugs and clearing secretions that could result in atelectasis and superimposed pneumonia. Although meconium is sterile, which differentiates it from stool, it can predispose to pulmonary infection, so that antibiotics are administered routinely. Infants with severe meconium aspiration syndrome who require mechanical ventilation and have radiologic evidence of parenchymal lung disease are likely to benefit from early surfactant therapy. Because of the frequently associated pulmonary hypertension, close monitoring at the time of surfactant therapy is required to prevent the consequences of transient airway obstruction that may develop during the tracheal instillation of surfactant. Extracorporeal membrane oxygenation (ECMO) has been increasingly used to treat severe MAS as well as other associated causes of respiratory failure. Mortality rate for MAS is as high as 10 percent and up to 20 percent among those with severe parenchymal pulmonary disease or pulmonary hypertension.

Key Points

- Radiographic findings vary according to the severity of meconium aspiration, which may not correlate with the clinical disease.
- Radiographic features include perihilar rope-like opacities with lung hyperexpansion.
- Complications with mechanical ventilation are related to air block (pneumothorax, pneumomediastinum, or rarely pneumopericardium).

Further Reading

Cleveland RH. A radiologic update on medical diseases of the newborn chest. *Pediatr Radiol.* 1995;*25*(8):631–637.

Hedlund GL. Meconium aspiration syndrome. In: Kirks DR, Griscom NT, Ball WS Jr, et al., eds. *Practical Pediatric Imaging.* Third edition. Philadelphia, PA: Lippincott-Raven; 1998:712–715.

Lobo L. The neonatal chest. *Eur J Radiol.* 2006;*60*(2):152–158.

Newman B. Imaging of medical disease of the newborn lung. *Radiol Clin North Am.* 1999;*37*(6):1049–1065.

Strife JL. Meconium aspiration syndrome. In: Donnelly LF, Jones BV, O'Hara SM, et al., eds. *Diagnostic Imaging: Pediatrics.* Salt Lake city, UT: Amirsys; 2005:2–38-2–41.

CHAPTER 13

Transient Tachypnea of the Newborn

Raul Galvez Trevino, MD

Definition

Transient tachypnea of the newborn (TTN) is a benign and transient condition caused by prolongation of the normal physiological clearance of fetal lung fluid. This condition is also known as "wet lung" or type II respiratory distress syndrome better known as surfactant deficiency disease (SDD).

Clinical Features

Transient tachypnea of the newborn is one of the most common causes of respiratory distress, affecting approximately 1 to 2 percent of all newborns, with an equal sex distribution. The condition is usually a benign disease of large premature infants, near-term or term infants with mild to moderate signs of respiratory distress. There is mild cyanosis, with tachypnea (>60 breaths per minute), grunting, nasal flaring and rib retraction developing during the first 6 hours of life, with gradual increase and a peak at 1 day of age. Mild hypercarbia, hypoxia, and respiratory acidosis can be present. The course is self-limited with respiratory rates returning to normal by 2 to 3 days of age, with rapid clinical and radiological resolution, usually within 24 to 48 hours.

Anatomy and Physiology

Normal lung fluid is cleared through the bronchi by compression of the thorax during vaginal delivery (30 percent), through lymphatics (30 percent) and capillaries (40 percent). At birth, the pulmonary epithelium switches from predominantly facilitated chloride secretion to predominantly active sodium resorption, induced by the large release of fetal adrenaline, which occurs late in labor and is lessened in those undergoing cesarean section. Transient tachypnea of the newborn is thought to occur because of delayed clearance and resorption of fetal lung fluid from the pulmonary lymphatic system. The increased fluid and intrathoracic volumes causes a reduction in lung compliance and increased airway resistance. This results in tachypnea and muscle retractions. Infants at risk are those delivered by cesarean section because of the lack of the normal vaginal thoracic squeeze, which forces lung fluid out, those with a precipitous delivery, or hypotonic sedated infants. Prematurity, gestational diabetes, and hydrops are other conditions associated with TTN. A mild degree of pulmonary immaturity is also a central factor in the cause of TTN, with negative amniotic fluid phospatodylglycerol levels usually present in infants with TTN (Fig. 13.1).

Imaging Findings

The initial radiograph shows mild hyperinflation of the lungs with flattening of the hemidiaphragms that is better seen on the lateral views, which is a hallmark of TTN. Prominent perihilar interstitial markings representing the engorged lymphatics and interstitial edema with progressive clearance are common features identified early during the course of the disease. Fluid in the fissures is more common than small basilar pleural effusions causing mild blunting of the costophrenic and costodiaphragmatic sulci. Sometimes mild to moderate transient cardiomegaly is also present (Fig. 13.2). More severe cases show alveolar edema with patchy rounded alveolar opacities with perihilar distribution.

During the clearance phase, the alveolar fluid may appear as reticulogranular opacities, mimicking SDD, but this is temporary and shows rapid improvement. The resolution phase is established when the follow-up radiographs show decreased interstitial edema and resolving pulmonary vascular congestion. As fluid resorption follows a peripheral-to-central and upper-to-lower pattern, aeration of the lungs usually improves at the apices with progressive clearance toward the lung bases.

The chest film is usually normal within 48 to 72 hours (Fig. 13.3).

Imaging Strategy

Often TTN is a diagnosis of exclusion and other causes of tachypnea such as neonatal pneumonia, sepsis, congenital heart disease, surfactant deficiency, cerebral hyperventilation, metabolic disorders and polycythemia should be excluded first. Usually TTN is self-limiting; serial follow-up with portable frontal chest radiographs demonstrating signs of improvement are usually enough to document the reassuring features that are commonly seen with conservative management.

Related Physics

Chest radiographs are taken at the lowest kVp to augment photoelectric absorption while minimizing Compton

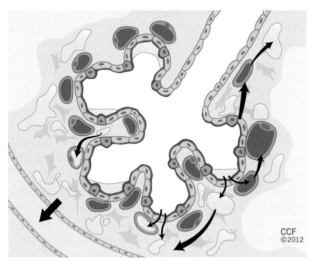

Figure 13.1. Illustration of pathophysiology of TTN. There is inefficient clearing of fluid from the airspaces and interstitium resulting in clinical and radiographic abnormality.

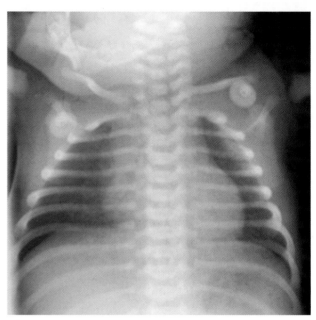

Figure 13.3. Follow-up radiograph obtained 48 hours later in the same child shows complete resolution and resorption of the pleural fluid and interstitial edema with a normal cardiomediastinal silhouette.

scattering. Newborn chest radiographs can take advantage of the lowest kVp as tissue thickness is small. Although Compton scattering is minimized, it is not entirely eliminated in newborn chest radiography. Compton scattering is the single largest contributor to dose and produces little useful information on the image while degrading low-contrast object detectability through photon scatter that hits the detector. Compton scattering will increase greatly as patient size and collimation increase. A grid will reduce the number of Compton photons reaching the detector by approximately 50 percent but the downside of this is that the detector senses fewer photons and in turn feeds back to the automatic exposure control telling it to increase the mAs, thus increasing patient dose by a factor of 3 to 5 (the Bucky factor). When a grid is not used, or one employs manual exposure techniques, one can reduce the dose to more acceptable levels. As a general rule, grids are not advised in children below 30 kilograms.

Differential Diagnosis

- Neonatal pneumonia (Group B streptococcal pneumonia)
- Surfactant deficiency disease (SDD)
- Congenital heart disease
- Meconium aspiration syndrome
- Congenital lymphangiectasia

Common Variants

Amniotic fluid aspiration is clinically and radiographically indistinguishable and should be suspected with moderate fetal distress or breech delivery, although this distinction is purely academic as both entities are treated conservatively.

Clinical Issues

Conventional treatment of TTN includes appropriate oxygen administration and continuous positive airway pressure in some cases. Most infants receive broad-spectrum antibiotic therapy until the diagnosis of sepsis or pneumonia is excluded. Antenatal glucocorticoids improve clearance of

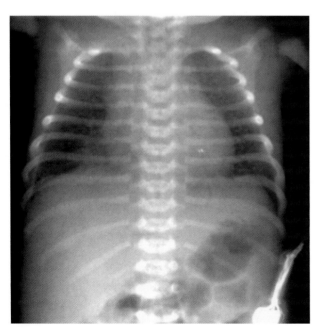

Figure 13.2. Frontal chest radiograph in a full-term baby girl born via cesarean section with tachypnea, grunting, and intercostal retractions shows mild interstitial edema, small bilateral pleural effusions and slight cardiomegaly, consistent with TTN.

retained fetal lung fluid through induction of the epithelial sodium channels, which facilitate ionic exchange and fluid resorption and may be used in treatment for preterm infants. Furosemide accelerates lung fluid resorption and pulmonary vasodilation, although no difference in decrease or duration of respiratory symptoms or length of hospital stay has been proven after its use.

Key Points

- Common condition in full-term infants undergoing cesarean section
- Mild interstitial pulmonary edema pattern
- Self-limiting with resolution in 48 to 72 hours adhering to the following pattern:
  - Peripheral-to-central lungs
  - Upper-to-lower lungs

Further Reading

Cleveland RH. A radiologic update on medical diseases of the newborn chest. *Pediatr Radiol.* 1995;25(8):631–637.

Hedlund GL. Wet lung disease. In: Kirks DR, Griscom NT, Ball WS Jr, et al., eds. *Practical Pediatric Imaging.* Third edition. Philadelphia, PA: Lippincott-Raven; 1998:711–712.

Lobo L. The neonatal chest. *Eur J Radiol.* 2006;60(2):152–158.

Newman B. Imaging of medical disease of the newborn lung. *Radiol Clin North Am.* 1999;37(6):1049–1065.

Strife JL. Transient tachypnea of the newborn. In: Donnelly LF, Jones BV, O'Hara SM, et al., eds. *Diagnostic Imaging: Pediatrics.* Salt Lake City, UT: Amirsys; 2005: 2–42–2–45.

Yurdakok M. Transient tachypnea of the newborn: what is new? *J Matern Fetal Neonatal Med.* 2010.

CHAPTER 14

Chronic Lung Disease of Prematurity

Rachelle Goldfisher, MD

Definition

All pulmonary disease that results from a neonatal respiratory disorder is called chronic lung disease. Bronchopulmonary dysplasia (BPD), which accounts for the vast majority of cases of chronic lung disease, is defined as the need for supplemental oxygen for at least 28 days after birth. This usually occurs in infants who are delivered at a gestational age of less than 30 weeks and who have a birth weight of less than 1.5 kilograms.

Clinical Features

Patients with chronic lung disease of prematurity usually have been treated for respiratory distress with positive pressure ventilation and oxygen; BPD develops in 20 percent. These patients typically continue to exhibit tachypnea, retraction, and rales. Recurrent wheezing, asthma-like symptoms and respiratory tract infections are common in survivors of BPD. Symptoms usually diminish over time with respiratory exacerbations becoming more infrequent as the patient becomes older. Although there has been improved survival of premature infants, the overall prevalence of BPD has not changed, rather a new pattern of lung injury is seen in patients born at an earlier gestational age.

Anatomy and Physiology

In the older, classic form of BPD, the structural integrity of the lung is maintained. However because of the aggressive mechanical ventilation and high concentrations of inspired oxygen, diffuse airway damage, smooth muscle hypertrophy, inflammation, and fibrosis occur. A newer form of BPD has developed as a result of the widespread use of antenatal corticosteroids and surfactant replacement. This newer form is a developmental disorder wherein the normal structure of the lung develops with fewer and larger alveoli.

Imaging Findings

Chest radiographs of infants with classic BPD demonstrated coarse reticular lung opacities, cystic lucencies, markedly disordered lung aeration with heterogeneous aeration, coarse strand-like areas of opacity, and intervening cystic lucencies ("bubbly" lungs). In the current era of surfactant replacement, BPD is increasingly a disorder of very low-birth-weight neonates with arrested alveolar and pulmonary vascular development, minimal alveolar septal fibrosis and inflammation, and more subtle radiographic abnormalities. Sequential chest radiographs often reveal a gradual and subtle progression from clear or minimally abnormal lungs into a hazy ground-glass opacity and ultimately into a relatively uniform pattern of coarse interstitial opacities without cystic lucencies. In those patients who eventually manifest "bubbly" lungs, the radiographic abnormality tends to be symmetric and the cystic lucencies smaller and more uniform than originally described with the classic form, however the appearance of the bubbly lungs of BPD is variable. The findings depend on the size of the bubbles and the degree of associated interstitial inflammation and fibrosis. Therefore, some patients may have small bubbles (Fig. 14.1) and others may have large bubbles especially at the lung bases (Fig. 14.2).

Imaging Strategy

Serial chest radiographs are usually sufficient for diagnosis and follow-up. Additional modalities are usually not

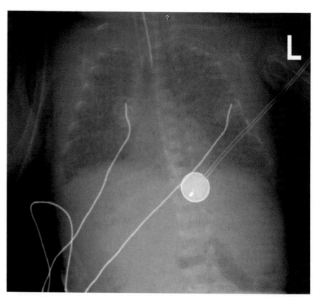

Figure 14.1. Single frontal radiograph of the chest demonstrates an endotracheal tube in the midtrachea. There are diffuse multiple small cystic lucencies throughout the lungs consistent with BPD.

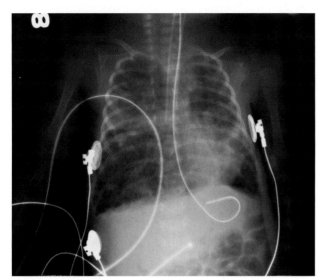

Figure 14.2. Single frontal radiograph of the chest demonstrates an endotracheal tube in the origin of the right mainstem bronchus. There is an enteric tube coursing within the esophagus and curled within the stomach. There are multiple bubbly lucencies with larger lucencies at the bases. There are also bilateral central streaky areas of segmental atelectasis and fibrosis, left greater than right.

required, however if the clinical course is atypical, chest CT can be obtained for further evaluation.

Physics

Babies in the newborn intensive care unit (NICU) can be subjected to many chest radiographs, depending on their length of stay and the severity of their illness. Premature infants are particularly vulnerable to the harmful effects of ionizing radiation as their length of stay is the longest and their cells are rapidly dividing. Precautionary parameters that must be considered are careful and tight collimation and kVp-mAs selection. First, one must ask if the imaging is necessary, and if so, which body part must be imaged. Gone are the "routine babygrams" of the past where the entire baby was X-rayed from head to toe-perhaps out of convenience, laziness, or ignorance about adverse effects from cumulative radiation exposure. Finally, we must move from the paradigm of "standing orders" and consider carefully the frequency of imaging in the NICU.

Differential Diagnosis

- Wilson-Mikity syndrome: the lungs are normally aerated the first few days of life and after a period of respiratory distress develop a coarse and nodular appearance without ventilator therapy.
- Respiratory distress syndrome: develops at birth in premature infants with surfactant deficiency and can

be reversed or improved with the administration of surfactant.
- Pulmonary interstitial emphysema: a manifestation of alveolar rupture usually caused by positive pressure ventilation where air then dissects into the interstitium and results in linear lucencies within the interstitium. These lucencies may be superimposed on chronic BPD.

Clinical Issues

In many infants, BPD results in substantial long-term morbidity, including increased airway reactivity, development of obstructive airway disease, poor growth, and an increased frequency of rehospitalization. Some lung function abnormalities may persist until adulthood. In very severe cases, death may result from progressive respiratory failure, cor pumonale, or superimposed infection.

No therapy to date has been shown to improve long-term outcome or decrease mortality. Currently, treatment is supportive and includes optimizing nutrition, prevention of injurious mechanical ventilation, judicious use of oxygen, and timely treatment of superimposed infections.

Key Points

- Affects premature infants less than 30 weeks requiring oxygen beyond 28 days of life.
- Prevalence of BPD has not changed, rather a new pattern of lung injury is seen in patients born at an earlier gestational age.
- Surfactant administration will not result in improvement.
- Appears as a hazy opacity progressing to coarse reticular pattern with small or large cysts (bubbly pattern).

Further Reading

Bancalari E. Changes in the pathogenesis and prevention of chronic lung disease of prematurity. *Am J Perinatol.* 2001;18:1–9.

Cleveland RH. A radiologic update on medical diseases of the newborn chest. *Pediatr Radiol.* 1995;25:631–637.

Jobe AJ. The new BPD: an arrest of lung development. *Pediatr Res.* 1999;46:641–643.

Newman B, Kuhn JP, Kramer SS, Carcillo JA. Congenital surfactant protein B deficiency: emphasis on imaging. *Pediatr Radiol.* 2001;31:327–331.

Northway WH Jr. Bronchopulmonary dysplasia: thirty-three years later. *Pediatr Pulmonol.* 2001;23(suppl):5–7.

Swischuk LE, John SD. Immature lung problems: can our nomenclature be more specific? *AJR Am J Roentgenol.* 1996;166:917–918.

CHAPTER 15

Pulmonary Infection

Beverly Wood, MD, PhD

Definition

Infection in the lung is considered pneumonia, caused by viral infection, bacteria, or fungus. Pneumonia is the result of inflammation of the air spaces (alveoli) of the lung with resultant fluid filling them and white cells that are the host's response to the infection.

Clinical Features

Symptoms and signs of lung infection vary according to the age of the patient. Infants may only show signs of respiratory distress, hypothermia, and temperature instability. Over 1 month of age, they may have fever and cough. Infected children usually have fever, cough, and difficulty breathing. Children usually have a preceding upper respiratory infection, followed by pneumonia with or without fever. Children with true tachypnea are likely to have pneumonia. Pain is present only when the pleura is involved, as that is the site of pain fibers, and there are no pain receptors in the lung.

The diagnosis of lung infection is usually made on the basis of radiography. Although crackles or rales on auscultation of the chest is characteristic of pneumonia, auscultation may be negative even when the radiography is positive; similarly there may be a positive physical exam with a normal chest radiograph in early pneumonia.

Anatomy and Physiology

The common causes of pneumonia are aspiration of infected droplets, hematogenous spread of infection, or infection of the lung occurring in a compromised host or compromised region of the lung. As pneumonia progresses, the fluid in the airspaces changes the attenuation of the X-ray beam so that progressive opacity (consolidation) is seen. Volume changes reflect bronchial obstruction with volume loss, or sometimes increase in volume of the affected lung. Pleural fluid is mobile early in its course and reflects gravity effect with patient positioning. However, the presence of fibrin in the fluid may render it immobile within several days so that it forms an organized collection around the lung.

Patients with immunocompromise: Pneumonias are typically caused by unusual organisms, and those that are slow to clear, or those that form necrotic areas are a hallmark of underlying immunocompromise. The sequence of events is altered from that described above. These pneumonias can occur because of an abnormality of the tracheobronchial tree or systemic immune compromise. Infecting organisms in these pneumonias are Aspergillus, Cytomegalovirus, TB, varicella-zoster, or Herpes virus infection. Another circumstance leading to pneumonia is cardiopulmonary bypass or absence of the usual airway screening mechanisms such as with a tracheostomy or absent (nonfunctional) cilia. Preexisting lung disease predisposes the lung to infection, including bronchopulmonary dysplasia, diminished chest wall function such as in severe scoliosis, neuromuscular disease with compromised cough and recurrent aspiration, gastroesophageal reflux, and inhalation of smoke.

Classification of pneumonia: Pneumonias can be classified by organism, location in the lung, or tissue response in the lung (interstitial, obstructive from small airway inflammation, or alveolar).

Causes of pneumonia: Viral pneumonia is often epidemic and is the most frequent pneumonia of children < 2 years of age. About 45 percent of childhood pneumonia is viral. Respiratory syncytial virus is a causative organism in this age group and is seasonal in occurrence. Bacterial pneumonia occurs in approximately 60 percent of children and is characterized by fever that is still present 72 hours after diagnosis (Fig. 15.1). Causative organisms are most frequently Streptococcus pneumoniae and Mycoplasma pneumoniae. Mycoplasma pneumonia occurs in children in crowded urban communities. Community-acquired pneumonia is usually MRSA (methicillin-resistant Staphylococcus aureus).

Mycobacterium tuberculosis most often presents with asymptomatic mediastinal lymphadenopathy with a positive PPD test; lobar airspace disease with lymphadenopathy is classic for TB but uncommon. Histoplasma capsulatum lives in soil and may cause pneumonia with adenopathy after inhaling spores; Coccidiodomycosis in soil in the West can be a cause of pneumonia; Cryptococcus from exposure to birds and occurring in children with HIV disease is another unusual infection. Pneumocystis carinii occurs in HIV+ children and Pseudomonas aeruginosa is an infection common to children with cystic fibrosis.

Complications of Pneumonia

Complications of pneumonia include necrotic pneumonia with abscess formation, pleural empyema, pneumatocele formation, respiratory compromise, and sepsis.

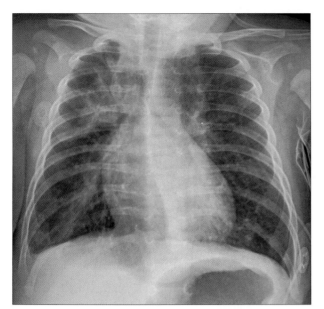

Figure 15.1. Frontal chest radiograph in a 3-month-old infant who presented with tachypnea and a cough in daycare during RSV season shows diffuse obstructive pattern of viral (RSV) pneumonia with multiple regions of atelectasis. The interstitium of the lung is thickened by inflammatory effect.

Imaging Findings

Pneumonia is thought to occur within 24 hours of infection. In the initial stages, a poorly defined increase in thickness of the interstitium reflects the early vascular congestion and edema. The alveoli rapidly fill with neutrophils, followed by erythrocytes, desquamated epithelial lining cells and fibrinous exudates. As the alveoli fill with fluid, the opacity of the usually air-filled lung increases and if the pneumonia is accompanied by a large amount of exudate, the bronchi may also fill with fluid, obscuring the initial air-bronchograms (Fig. 15.2).

The stage of resolution is seen as resorption of fluid and return of the lung to its normal architecture. Radiographically, the aeration of affected regions of the lung improves.

When the pneumonia is necrotizing (Fig. 15.3), there may be destruction of lung parenchyma with formation of one or several cysts, known as pneumatoceles. There may be interstitial scarring secondary to a fibrin response to destruction of the architectural components of the lungs. Scarring is usually interstitial, but with thicker interstitial bands than normally present.

Imaging Strategy

If pneumonia is suspected, a chest radiograph in frontal and lateral projections is recommended. This will indicate the presence of pneumonia and whether a parapneumonic pleural effusion is present. It can also demonstrate unusual features that point toward an unusual organism or immune compromise. If pleural effusion is suspected, chest CT is helpful to localize the effusion and characterize it by mobility and hyperemia of the pleura. Ultrasound is also effective in identifying and localizing the effusion and establishing the presence of septations in the pleural fluid. A CT scan helps to identify underlying congenital and bronchial abnormalities, which often predispose to pneumonia. (Fig. 15.4).

(A)

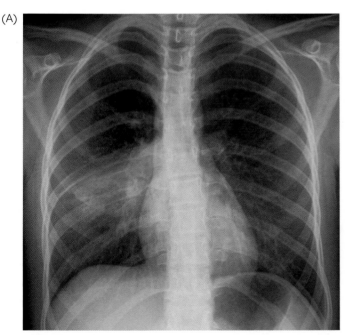

(B)

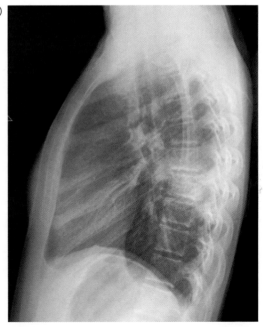

Figure 15.2. Frontal and lateral chest radiographs in a 12-year-old child who presented with cough, fever, and respiratory difficulty show consolidation of the right lower lobe secondary to bacterial infection. The pneumonia is in the exudative stage in which fluid fills the alveoli.

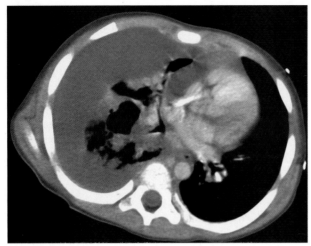

Figure 15.3. Contrast-enhanced axial CT image in a 30-month-old child who presented with tachypnea, cough, fever, and chest pain on the right after 6-week history of upper respiratory infection shows a right empyema and necrotizing pneumonia of Streptococcus pneumonia. On antimicrobial management and pleural drainage, the patient improved and the lung resumed normal architecture.

Related Physics

The chest radiograph can be taken in anteroposterior (AP) or posteroanterior (PA) projection. Portable chest imaging is almost always performed as AP for convenience as the patient is lying supine. For ambulatory imaging, it is more desirable to image upright against the chest board as PA, because there is less differential magnification, more highly calibrated automated exposure control (AEC) for chest techniques, a 72-inch subject-to-image distance (SID), and a grid that is tailored to the longer distance. The PA upright technique is performed at 72 inches versus 40 inches at the table to minimize differential magnification and scatter from the tube head. The AP image will selectively magnify the anterior structures including the sternum and anterior ribs. Conversely on the PA view the scapula will be magnified. The PA positioning deposits most of the dose at the posterior chest and not the breast. Supine AP imaging of sick children will be compromised by their inability to cooperate to maximize lung volumes, which will in turn lead to an artifactual increase in heart size. Automated exposure control is always used for PA upright imaging but is not an option for portable imaging.

Differential Diagnosis

- Atelectasis
- Asthma
- Chest mass

Clinical Issues

Much pneumonia is community-acquired and is related to current infecting organisms. As reported previously, underlying alterations in the airway and immunity are responsible for pneumonia. Some infecting organisms are extremely contagious, such as RSV, so that most infants in the early years develop the infection during community epidemics.

Patients placed on management protocols are likely to have a favorable outcome. Most cases of viral pneumonia resolve without treatment, while bacterial pneumonia responds to appropriate antimicrobial therapy. Immunocompromised children are likely to have more severe sequelae to infection and may also be slower to respond to treatment.

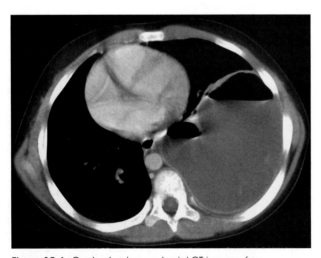

Figure 15.4. Contrast-enhanced axial CT image of an 11-year-old child with recurrent lung infection who presented with tachypnea and fever shows a large congenital lung cyst containing fluid. The bronchoscopy indicated an infection of the fluid with Streptococcus pneumoniae. Surgical removal of the cyst was effective in eradicating the recurrent infections.

Key Points

- Pneumonia in pediatric patients is often community acquired.
- Organisms causing infection may be virus, bacteria, or fungus.
- Underlying anatomic abnormality, ciliary dysfunction, or systemic immune deficiency may predispose the child to pneumonia.
- Three stages of pneumonia are early inflammation, filling of the alveoli with fluid and neutrophils, and clearing with residual interstitial thickening.

Further Reading

Tan TQ, Mason EO Jr, Wald ER, Barson WJ, Schutze GE, Bradley JS, et al. Clinical characteristics of children with complicated pneumonia caused by Streptococcus pneumoniae. *Pediatrics.* 2002;*110*(1):1–6.

The Red Book: Report of the Committee on Infectious Diseases. *American Academy of Pediatrics.* 2011.

CHAPTER 16

Mediastinal Masses

Daniel N. Vinocur and Edward Y. Lee, MD, MSc

Definition

Overall, the mediastinum is the most common location for primary thoracic masses in children. These may be caused by benign and malignant neoplasms, congenital anomalies and inflammatory conditions. Proper anatomic localization is key to providing a meaningful differential diagnosis.

Clinical Features

The clinical presentation varies according to the age of the patient, the size and location of the lesion, and whether chest wall or mediastinal invasion, mass effect or other complications are present. Mediastinal masses may be found incidentally on chest radiographs obtained for unrelated indications. However, up to two-thirds of patients are reportedly symptomatic. Children may present with irritability, anemia, weight loss or fever. However, dysphagia or cough and stridor may be present in cases of esophageal compression or airway involvement, respectively. Cephalic and cervical venous distention may be observed when superior vena cava flow is compromised. Chest pain, hoarseness, diaphragmatic paralysis, and the presence of Horner syndrome are usually indicative of malignant and often invasive mediastinal masses. Posterior mediastinal masses, specifically, neuroblastoma tend to be asymptomatic until local extension to neighboring structures or metastatic disease arises. Intraspinal extension may cause nerve root or cord compression leading to pain, paralysis, bowel and/or bladder dysfunction. Unusual paraneoplastic syndromes may uncommonly develop, such as opsoclonus myoclonus syndrome.

Anatomy and Physiology

The mediastinum is anatomically bordered by the lung parietal pleura, extending superiorly to the thoracic inlet and inferiorly to the diaphragm. It contains the heart, great vessels, airways, esophagus and numerous nerves, venous and lymphatic structures. A simplified, radiographically driven definition of the mediastinal compartments is provided by the modified Felson's classification. The anterior mediastinum extends from the posterior sternum to a line passing along the posterior margins of the heart and great vessels. The posterior mediastinum is bordered anteriorly by a line passing 1 centimeter posterior to the ventral margins of the vertebral bodies and posteriorly by the paravertebral gutters. The middle mediastinum is between the anterior and posterior mediastinal compartments (Fig. 16.1).

Imaging Findings

The various mediastinal masses are summarized according to mediastinal compartments in the Differential Diagnosis section. In this chapter, the five most common mediastinal masses will be specifically discussed and include: (1) prominent but normal thymus and lymphoma in the anterior mediastinal compartment; (2) foregut duplication cysts and lymphadenopathy in the middle mediastinal compartment; and (3) neuroblastoma in the posterior mediastinum.

Anterior Mediastinal Mass

The first step in assessing a presumed anterior mediastinal mass in a child is to exclude a normal thymus (i.e., pseudotumor). Unfortunately, thymic size and morphology are variable in infants and younger children (< 5 years old). However, several characteristic imaging findings have been described that can help identify a normal thymus including: (1) a notch or cleft at the inferior edge of the thymus (notch sign); (2) scalloping of the thymic margins by the ribs (wave sign); and (3) a flattened inferior border of its right lobe near the horizontal fissure (sail sign). A normal thymus should not cause mass effect over the main vessels or the adjacent airway. On cross-sectional imaging studies such as CT or MRI, the normal thymus should be homogenous. Heterogeneity, marked lobularity, or the presence of calcifications should raise concern. Lymphoma may appear as numerous discrete lymph nodes or as a conglomerate mass (Fig. 16.2). Calcifications are uncommon in untreated lymphoma and suggest an alternative diagnosis, such as germ cell tumor. The presence of an anterior mediastinal mass consisting of calcification, fat, and soft tissue is virtually diagnostic for germ cell tumor-teratoma.

Middle Mediastinal Mass

Foregut duplication cysts (bronchogenic cyst, esophageal duplication cyst, and neurenteric cyst) typically appear

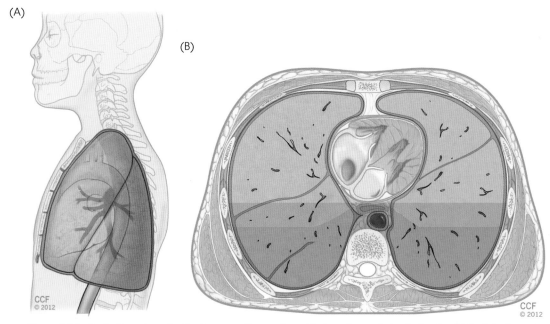

Figure 16.1. Illustration of mediastinal spaces. Figures A and B show the anterior (yellow), middle (blue), and posterior (red) mediastinal spaces and the structures housed by each.

as well-defined cystic masses on cross-sectional imaging studies such as CT or MRI (Fig. 16.3). Occasionally, given their proteinaceous contents, developmental cysts may simulate a solid mass on CT (higher than water attenuation, or > 15 Hounsfield Units (HU) and MRI (intermediate T1 and T2 signal intensities). In these cases, administration of intravenous contrast will reveal their nonenhancing nature. Vertebral segmentation anomalies are associated with neuroenteric cysts and may suggest the correct diagnosis. The imaging characteristics of mediastinal lymphadenopathy are usually nonspecific. However, certain features may suggest a specific diagnosis. Low-attenuation lymph nodes may be seen with necrotic neoplasm and certain infectious processes such

as tuberculosis and fungal disease. Calcified lymphadenopathy may be seen with sarcoidosis, tuberculosis, fungal infection, and osteosarcoma. Hyperenhancing lymph nodes may be found in Castelman disease and metastatic disease.

Posterior Mediastinal Mass

When large enough, thoracic neuroblastomas appear on radiographs as a posterior mediastinal opacity. Calcification is present in up to 25 percent of thoracic neuroblastomas. Posterior rib erosion or osteolysis may also be seen. On close inspection, the neural foramina may appear enlarged on the lateral view when intraspinal tumor extension is

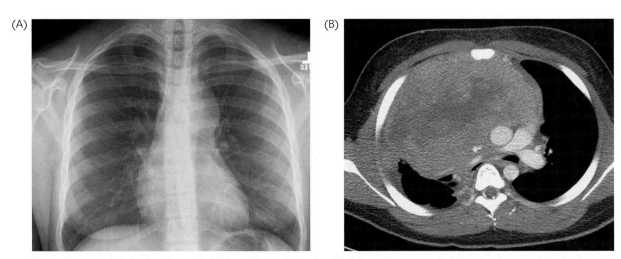

Figure 16.2. Frontal chest radiograph (A) in a 15-year-old male with fatigue shows a well-defined anterior mediastinal mass. Axial contrast-enhanced CT (B) demonstrates a large heterogeneous anterior mediastinal mass with extreme mass effect on the superior vena cava consistent with lymphoma.

(A)

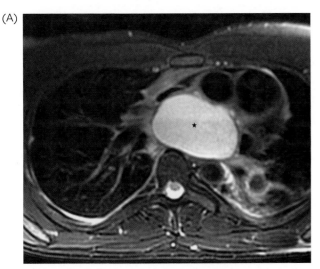

(B)

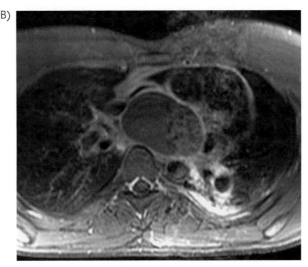

Figure 16.3. Axial FSE T2 image with fat saturation (A) and axial contrast-enhanced T1-weighted image with fat saturation (B) of a 20-year-old male with dysphagia resulting from a bronchogenic cyst demonstrate a well-circumscribed middle mediastinum hyperintense mass with no significant enhancement.

present. An MRI is helpful for characterizing the mass and confirming its intraspinal involvement. Thoracic neuroblastomas typically demonstrate a dumbbell configuration with a waist at the intervertebral foramen (Fig. 16.4).

Imaging Strategy

Most pediatric mediastinal masses can be initially identified on chest radiographs depending on their location and size. Further characterization is performed with cross-sectional imaging studies such as CT or MRI, allowing confirmation

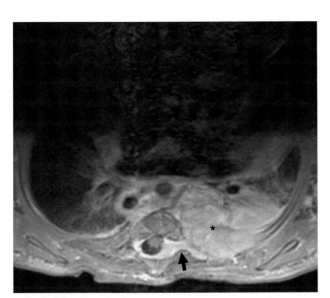

Figure 16.4. Axial contrast-enhanced T1 imaging with fat saturation in a 3-month-old male with irritability demonstrates a large posterior mediastinal mass invading the chest wall with prominent intraspinal extension through the neural foramen, with a characteristic "dumbbell" configuration consistent with neuroblastoma.

of the mass, evaluating the extent of disease, and the presence of complications such as airway or vascular compression. In general, anterior and middle mediastinal masses are evaluated with contrast-enhanced CT. Posterior mediastinal masses, which may demonstrate intraspinal extension, are typically imaged with MRI. Nuclear medicine studies have limited but well-defined roles for evaluating mediastinal masses in children and are typically performed for staging or follow-up evaluation for assessing residual or recurrent disease. Currently used nuclear medicine studies include I-131 MIBG (metaiodobenzylguanidine) for neuroblastoma staging, Tc-99m MDP (methylene diphosphonate) scintigraphy in the work-up of skeletal metastasis, and F-18 FDG PET (fluoro-deoxy-glucose) in staging and restaging of lymphoma, other neoplasms and inflammatory conditions.

Related Physics

The selection of appropriate parameters for pediatric CT balances the need for adequate soft-tissue differentiation with the ability to distinguish the edges of objects while minimizing patient dose. With mediastinal masses there is less need for high spatial resolution and more for high contrast-noise ratio that allows one to distinguish between fat, calcification, and soft tissue. The field of view (FOV) should be chosen to maximize the number of pixels that include the lesion. When viewing the image, a narrow window width (~2 to 300 HU) with center at approximately 50 HU will maximize differentiation between two tissues of similar density. The clinical indication for the study will dictate the choice of reconstruction kernel; high-resolution kernels are used for lung and bone and smooth kernels are used for mediastinum.

Differential Diagnosis

Anterior mediastinal mass:

- Prominent normal thymus (pseudotumor)
- Lymphoma (most common)
- Germ cell tumor (teratoma, choriocarcinoma, seminoma—latter is the most common primary malignant mediastinal germ cell tumor and is typically seen in adolescents and young male adults)
- Thymic cyst (thymoma rare to nonexistent in children)
- Cardiovascular (structural or anomalous vessel)

Middle mediastinal mass:

- Foregut duplication cyst (bronchogenic, esophageal, neuroenteric)
- Lymphadenopathy (fungal infection, tuberculosis, lymphoma, metastatic disease)
- Cardiovascular (structural or anomalous vessel)

Posterior mediastinal mass:

- Neurogenic tumors (neuroblastoma*, ganglioneuroblastoma, ganglioneuroma)
- Nerve sheath tumors (plexiform or peripheral neurofibroma, schwannomas)
- Spinal processes (diskitis, hematoma, lateral meningocele, extrameduallry hematopoiesis)
- Mesenchymal tumor

*Given its prevalence, the initial diagnosis in young children is neuroblastoma until proven otherwise. Approximately 15 percent of neuroblastomas occur in the posterior mediastinum, typically in patients younger than 2 years of age.

Key Points

- Normal thymus is homogenous, sharply marginated, has slightly convex borders, molds its contour to the ribs, without displacement of the adjacent airway or the vessels.
- True anterior mediastinal mass in a child is usually lymphoma or germ cell tumor.
- Posterior mediastinal mass in an infant is usually neuroblastoma.
- Mediastinal masses in children can be initially evaluated with chest radiographs for their location and then further characterized with CT or MRI.

Further Reading

Franco A, Mody NS, Meza MP. Imaging evaluation of pediatric mediastinal masses. *Radiologic Clinics of North America.* 2005;43(2):325–353.

Lee EY. Evaluation of non-vascular mediastinal masses in infants and children: an evidence-based practical approach. *Pediatr Radiol.* 2009;39(Suppl 2):S184–S190.

Lee EY. Imaging evaluation of mediastinal masses in infants and children. In: Medina LS, Applegate KE, Blackmore CC, eds. *Evidence-Based Imaging in Pediatrics.* New York, NY: Springer; 2010:381–400.

Slovis TK. *Caffey's Pediatric Diagnostic Imaging.* Eleventh edition. Philadelpia, PA: Mosby Elsevier; 2008: Chapter 79.

Cardiac

CHAPTER 17

Left to Right Shunts

Ramesh S. Iyer, MD and Randolph K. Otto, MD

Definition

In normal cardiac physiology, the pulmonary and systemic circulations function in series and supply each other in a 1:1 volumetric relationship. The term "shunt" refers to abnormal communication between these two circulations. Left-right shunts send a fraction of oxygenated pulmonary venous return directly back to the lungs (right-sided circulation) rather than supplying systemic (or left-sided) circulation. Systemic cardiac output is decreased by the shunted volume, thereby decreasing delivery of oxygenated blood to the rest of the body. The four primary types of left-right shunts are ventricular septal defect (VSD), atrial septal defect (ASD), atrioventricular septal defect (AVSD), and patent ductus arteriosus (PDA). See Figure 17.1.

Clinical Features

Clinical presentation of left-right shunts depends on the type of shunt as well as its size.

VSD: VSD is the most common type of pediatric congenital heart defect, accounting for approximately 20 percent of such malformations. Patients with VSD typically present in infancy or early childhood. As pulmonary vascular resistance declines in the neonatal period, there is a corresponding increase in flow diverted from the higher-pressure systemic left ventricle into the lower-pressure pulmonic right ventricle. A large VSD may result in congestive failure with dyspnea, tachypnea, and failure to thrive. A smaller VSD may have a delayed presentation and first be detected as a murmur at chest auscultation. Infectious endarteritis is a potential complication of VSD; antibiotic prophylaxis for dental procedures is recommended.

ASD: ASD is the most common shunt lesion detected in adulthood, with variable age of presentation, shunt direction and magnitude. The majority of ASDs produce asymptomatic murmurs throughout childhood. In adults, the most common symptomatic manifestation is dyspnea on exertion. Less common presentations include atrial arrhythmia and ischemic stroke from paradoxical embolization of venous thrombus. With ostium secundum defects, there is a male:female ratio of 1:2.

AVSD: The clinical presentation of AVSD, or endocardial cushion defect (ECD), is highly variable and dependent upon structural involvement. Large left-right shunts may present as infantile congestive heart failure, tachypnea, tachycardia, or failure to thrive. The child is at increased risk for pneumonia and other pulmonary infections. A loud murmur is auscultated with larger defects, usually with a VSD component. Of children with trisomy 21, 15 to 20 percent present with an AVSD of varying severity.

PDA: Small left-right shunts through a patent ductus arteriosus are usually asymptomatic throughout childhood. A large PDA, similar to a large VSD or AVSD, will cause symptoms of congestive heart failure in the infant. A continuous, machine-like murmur may be auscultated. There is a low but real risk of infectious endarteritis with PDAs of any size, necessitating antibiotic prophylaxis for dental work.

Anatomy and Physiology

VSD: The ventricular septum forms from complex fusion of multiple embryologic components. The membranous portion of the septum is situated in the left ventricular outflow tract, just below the aortic valve, and adjacent to the septal leaflet of the tricuspid valve. This is largely the site where fusion of these elements occurs. Membranous or perimembranous VSDs are thus the most common subtype, comprising 80 percent of such defects. Muscular septal defects are the next most common subtype, the result of excessive muscular resorption in the fetus.

Intraventricular blood may either exit the heart through the ipsilateral outflow tract, or cross the VSD and flow through the contralateral artery. The hemodynamic effects of the VSD are dependent upon the comparative resistances to flow between these two pathways. With small defects, there may be no or little left-right shunting because of the high resistance imposed by the defect itself (restrictive). With moderate and large VSDs, there is efficient circulatory transmission from the left ventricle to the pulmonary vascular bed. Flow across the VSD is primarily during systole.

ASD: Formation of the atrial septum is similarly a complex process. Growth, partial resorption and fusion of two tissue membranes, the septum primum and septum secundum, result in the normal fully formed atrial septum. Resorption of the fetal sinus venosus also contributes to formation of the right atrium. The three main subtypes of ASD, in descending order of frequency are ostium secundum, ostium primum, and sinus venosus defects. The circular or oval secundum defect is typically bordered by the edge of the fossa ovalis. The primum defect is located in the anteroinferior portion of the septum and is commonly part of an AVSD resulting from a disturbance in the embryology of the endocardial cushion, while the sinus venosus defect is situated at the superior portion of the interatrial septum near the superior vena cava.

The direction and degree of left-right shunting across an ASD depends in large part upon the differential compliance of the ventricles. In most patients, the thin-walled right ventricle distends more easily than the muscular left ventricle, facilitating rightward shunting. Flow across an ASD occurs primarily during diastole.

AVSD: AVSDs include a spectrum of disorders in the development of the endocardial cushion, with ensuing defects in the atrial and ventricular septa, and one or both atrioventricular valves. In a complete AVSD, there is communication of all four cardiac chambers through an ASD, VSD and a common atrioventricular valve. Bidirectional circulatory shunting may occur simultaneously, though left-right shunting typically predominates early on because of the lower afterload faced by the compliant right ventricle.

PDA: The ductus arteriosus plays a critical role in fetal life, allowing right ventricular output to bypass the nonfunctional fetal lungs and return to the placenta via the aorta. The ductus closes in most newborns within 72 hours of life, likely triggered by rise in systemic oxygen levels. In PDA, this arterial communication persists between the aorta and the main pulmonary artery.

As with other left-right shunts, the systemic circulatory resistance exceeds that of the pulmonary vasculature, allowing increased blood flow to the lungs. Unlike other shunts this flow occurs throughout the cardiac cycle.

In untreated left-right shunts, chronically increased pulmonary blood flow leads to both volume and pressure overload. The resultant vascular disease leads to pulmonary hypertension that can exceed systemic pressures. When this occurs there may be shunt reversal, or the Eisenmenger Syndrome, where right-left shunting can cause cyanosis.

Imaging Findings

The chest radiograph may be normal with small left-right shunts. Moderate to large shunts may cause cardiomegaly and "shunt vascularity," generally requiring a pulmonary to systemic flow ratio (Qp:Qs) greater than 2.5:1. Shunt vascularity refers to increased number and caliber of pulmonary vessels resulting from increased arterial flow (Figs. 17.2

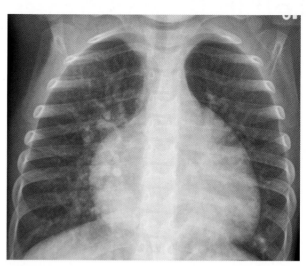

Figure 17.2. Frontal chest radiograph in a 3-year-old boy with atrial septal defect (ASD) shows moderate cardiomegaly including right atrial enlargement and prominent shunt vascularity. Note increase in number and sharp enlargement of pulmonary vessels bilaterally. The carina is not splayed and on the lateral view (not shown) the left atrium is normal.

and 17.3). The vessels in this condition are sharply defined, as opposed to the blurry vessels identified in pulmonary edema caused by venous hypertension.

On the frontal projection, an enlarged left atrium will splay the normal carinal angle greater than 90 degrees and in severe or long-standing cases may form an additional right heart border producing a "double-density" appearance. On the lateral projection, the large left atrium may project over the thoracic spine and will posteriorly displace both the left main bronchus and the esophagus. The latter feature may be demonstrated on an esophagram in select cases. All but ASD shows enlarged left atrium on chest radiography. ASD may feature right-sided cardiac chamber enlargement.

Aortic arch size may be used to distinguish between PDA and VSD. Although PDA is associated with a prominent aortic arch and an enlarged left atrium, VSD exhibits either a normal or small aortic arch along with left atrial enlargement.

Imaging Strategy

Echocardiography is the preferred modality for diagnosis of left-right shunts and can characterize type, location, cardiac, and hemodynamic function. Echocardiography can be performed during fetal or neonatal life. Cross-sectional imaging for further characterization of the defect may be performed with either MRI or CT angiography (Figs. 17.4 and 17.5). Because it provides exquisite functional and anatomic detail without ionizing radiation, MRI is often favored. Exams are gated to the cardiac cycle in order to limit motion degradation and evaluate cardiac function. "Black blood" sequences (spin-echo sequences or double-inversion recovery) and "bright blood" sequences

(A)

(B)

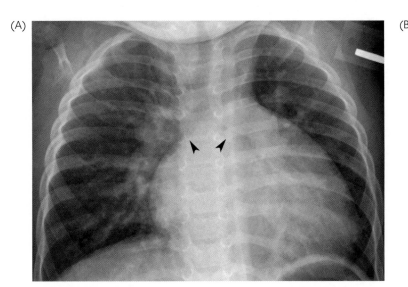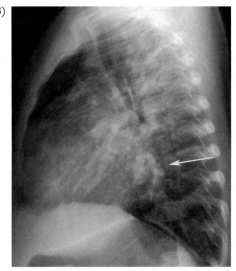

Figure 17.3. Frontal chest radiograph (A) in a 19-month-old girl with ventricular septal defect (VSD) shows moderate cardiomegaly and shunt vascularity. There is widening of the carinal angle (arrowheads). Lateral projection (B) shows projection of the left atrium (arrow) over the anterior margin of the thoracic spine, confirming left atrial enlargement.

(steady state free precession or GRE) are both utilized to demonstrate anatomic relationships and show dynamic findings (e.g., flow across a septal defect). Advantages of CT include greater availability, rapid acquisition time, and high resolution, with the downside of requiring ionizing radiation. With the advent and advancements in fetal and cross-sectional imaging, the role of radiography in left-right shunt diagnosis has waned. However, in some circumstances, the radiologist may be the first to suggest the possibility of left-right in a child presenting with respiratory distress or failure to thrive.

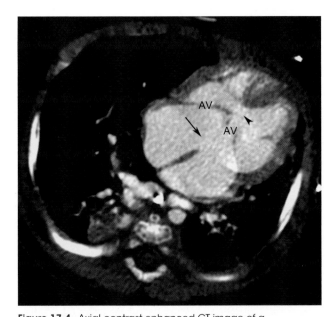

Figure 17.4. Axial contrast-enhanced CT image of a 3-month-old boy with trisomy 21 and an atrioventricular septal defect (AVSD) shows both atrial septal defect (arrow) and ventricular septal defect (arrowhead). Note the atrioventricular valves (label ""AV").

Related Physics

In performing cardiac catheterization for repair of left-right shunts, one should consider the following imaging variables: source-to-image-receptor distance (SID), source-to-object distance (SOD), object-to-image-receptor distance (OID), focal-spot size, geometric magnification and tube position relative to the table. The source is optimally placed as far from the patient as possible to limit the rate of skin entrance exposure. Likewise the optimal position for the image receptor is as close to the patient as possible—ideally in contact with the patient. This will permit capture of as many photons as possible allowing one to minimize the radiation emitted at source. General fluoroscopic units have two focal spots whereas many higher-end angiographic units have three. The user can control the focal-spot size based on the size of the anatomy of interest and patient. Small objects require smaller focal spots with the downside being that the anatomy may require higher tube output that could exceed the output limit of that filament. When smaller focal spots cannot be used, geometric magnification may be employed. This is accomplished by moving the patient closer to the source (or decreasing the SID while increasing the OID); when the object is halfway between the source and receptor, 2:1 magnification is achieved, which is the practical limit of geometric magnification, limited by focal-spot blurring. Geometric magnification can increase skin exposure by a factor as high as 4. Dose can be lessened by adding copper filtration (compensation filters) to harden the beam, thereby increasing penetration and lessening skin dose. When the X-ray source is below the patient the majority of back scatter is directed safely at the floor or laterally at lead table skirts. This will spare the operator and room staff from unnecessarily high scatter rates.

(A)
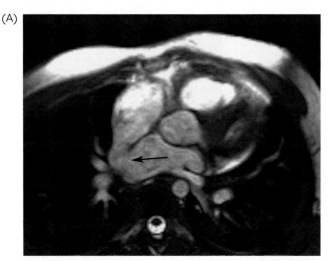

(B)
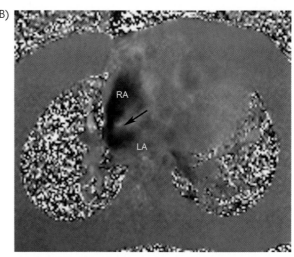

Figure 17.5. Steady state free precession ("bright blood") sequence from a cardiac MRI (A) in an 11-year-old boy with ASD, sinus venosus subtype "demonstrates the defect along the superior aspect of the atrial septum (arrow). Velocity-encoded in-plane phase contrast sequence (B) shows left-to-right flow (arrow) crossing the defect. Right Atrium (RA). Left Atrium (LA).

Differential Diagnosis

The specific anomaly will usually be identified and characterized on either echocardiography or cardiac MRI. If findings suggestive of left-right shunting are seen on a chest radiograph, the primary diagnostic considerations include VSD, ASD, AVSD, and PDA. Partial anomalous pulmonary venous return (PAPVR) is a left-right shunt that may be identical to an ASD on a chest radiograph, including a normal left atrium. The most common left-right shunt in trisomy 21 patients is AVSD.

Common Variants

VSD: Membranous or perimembranous VSDs are by far the most common subtype, comprising approximately 80 percent of all VSDs.

ASD: Ostium secundum defects account for the vast majority of ASDs (approximately 75 to 80 percent).

Patent foramen ovale (PFO) is another type of interatrial communication, technically not an ASD because it is present in all newborns. The foramen ovale is comprised of portions of both septum primum and septum secundum and acts as a one-way valve allowing right-left shunting during fetal life. In approximately 20 to 25 percent of individuals this foramen remains patent. The majority of people with PFOs remain asymptomatic throughout life. The most common presenting symptom is paradoxical embolization.

Clinical Issues

VSD: Small defects may close spontaneously in childhood. Moderate to large defects with significant left-right shunting require surgical closure.

ASD: Small defects may close spontaneously in childhood. Moderate to large defects with significant left-right shunting require repair. Ostium secundum defects are frequently amenable to treatment by placing an occlusion device via percutaneous transcatheter approach. The less common ASD subtypes cannot be closed by transcatheter occlusion and require surgical repair.

AVSD: Medical management is primarily directed at treating congestive heart failure, including diuretics and angiotensin-converting enzyme (ACE) inhibitors. However, virtually all symptomatic AVSDs require corrective surgery.

PDA: As with other conditions, significant left-right shunting causing congestive heart failure requires treatment. In newborns, indomethacin may be administered to promote ductus closure. For older children, surgical clipping or endovascular occlusion may be performed.

Key Points

- Symptomatic left-right shunts cause pressure and volume overload to right-sided cardiac chambers and the pulmonary vascular bed.
- Chest radiographic hallmarks of left-right shunts include cardiomegaly and shunt vascularity.
- Only ASD has a left atrium of normal size; the atrium is enlarged in all other left-right shunts.
- The aortic arch is large in PDA and normal or small in VSD.
- Diagnosis is most often made with echocardiography.
- Cardiac MRI and CT are useful for lesion characterization and functional information.

Further Reading

Donnelly LF, Jones BV, O'hara SM, et al. *Diagnostic Imaging: Pediatrics*. First edition. Salt Lake City, UT: Amirsys; 2005.

Higgins CB. Radiology of congenital heart disease. In: Webb WR, Higgins, CB, eds. *Thoracic Imaging: Pulmonary and Cardiovascular Radiology*. Second edition. Philadelphia, PA: Lippincott, Williams and Wilkins; 2004:679–706.

Samryn MM. A review of the complementary information available with cardiac magnetic resonance imaging and multi-slice computed tomography (CT) during the study of congenital heart disease. *Int J Cardiovasc Imaging*. 2004;*20*(6):569–578.

Sommer RJ, Hijazi ZM, Rhodes JF Jr. Pathophysiology of congenital heart disease in the adult. Part 1: shunt lesions. *Circulation*. 2008;*117*:1090–1099.

Wang ZJ, Reddy GP, Gotway MB, Yeh BM, Higgins CB. Cardiovascular shunts: MR imaging evaluation. *Radiographics*. 2003;*23*:S181–S194.

Yoo S-J, MacDonald C, Babyn P. *Chest Radiographic Interpretation in Pediatric Cardiac Patients*. First edition. New York, NY: Thieme; 2010.

CHAPTER 18

Tetralogy of Fallot

Mark R. Ferguson, MD

Definition

First recognized for its clinical significance in 1888 by French physician Etienne-Louis Arthur Fallot, the four established morphological features of tetralogy of Fallot (TOF) include a ventricular septal defect (VSD), infundibular pulmonary stenosis, an overriding aorta, and right ventricular hypertrophy.

Clinical Features

This condition arises with equal frequency between males and females and accounts for 10 to 11 percent of cases of congenital heart disease. The clinical manifestations are those of cyanosis often occurring in the first 6 months of life. Dyspnea, tachypnea, and ultimately clubbing of the fingers and toes may be seen. Infants may demonstrate a preference to lie with their knees to the chest that is equivalent to squatting seen in older children, which increases peripheral vascular resistance resulting in increased pulmonary blood flow. Polycythemia is common in affected children. A systolic thrill along the upper- or mid-left sternal border may be present. An ejection-type systolic murmur can also be heard in this location secondary to the pulmonary stenosis.

Anatomy and Physiology

The findings seen in TOF are all thought to be the sequelae of anterior malalignment of the conal septum resulting in a VSD, right ventricular outflow tract (RVOT) obstruction, and an overriding aorta (Fig. 18.1). Right ventricular hypertrophy develops secondary to the RVOT obstruction. This classic anatomic arrangement results in diminished blood flow to the lungs and increased flow to the body. Furthermore, there is a right-to-left shunt with poorly oxygenated blood coursing from the right ventricle through the VSD to the aorta. A right-sided aortic arch with mirror-image branching is associated with congenital heart disease 95 to 97 percent of the time; of these patients, 90 percent have TOF. Twenty-five to thirty percent of patients with TOF have a right-sided arch.

Imaging Findings

The classic radiographic appearance of TOF is a "boot-shaped" heart, secondary to right ventricular hypertrophy, and normal to diminished pulmonary blood flow with possibly a right-sided aortic arch (Fig. 18.2). However, affected patients may also have a normal chest radiograph. The four basic components of TOF can be demonstrated with CT, however MRI can show these components (Figs. 18.3 and 18.4) as well as provide functional information such as calculating the relative amount of blood exiting the right ventricle via the pulmonary artery versus crossing through the VSD and out the aorta.

> **IMAGING PITFALLS:** It is important to evaluate the right and left branch pulmonary artery anatomy, as stenosis of these vessels is often associated with TOF. In addition, coronary artery anomalies can occur; specifically a left coronary artery extending anteriorly across the RVOT, which can be at risk for injury during surgical repair.

Imaging Strategy

Typically a child with cyanosis or a heart murmur will have a chest radiograph. The child will then usually undergo echocardiography. Patients diagnosed with TOF by echocardiography will often go directly to surgery without further cross-sectional imaging. If further imaging is desired, MRI is the modality of choice. Utilizing various short axis, long axis, and oblique projections through the heart, the morphology and function of the chambers can be determined. Steady-state free precession cine sequences are often employed for this evaluation. Additionally, phase contrast imaging is critical to calculate blood flow and velocities through the vessels to determine the presence of regurgitation, stenoses, and relative flow. To map collateral vessels in patients with pulmonary atresia, MRA and CTA can be used (discussed below).

Related Physics

Patients with TOF may undergo angiography for staged transcatheter repair. In performing angiography using an image intensifier (II) receptor for diagnostic or therapeutic purposes, one should consider the following imaging variables: minification gain, brightness gain, field of view, electronic magnification, and electronic zoom. Minification

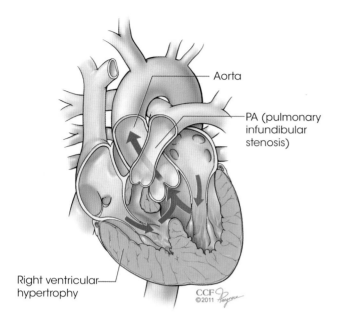

Figure 18.1. Illustration of tetralogy of Fallot components: 1. VSD 2. Infundibular pulmonary stenosis, 3. Overriding aorta, 4. Right ventricular hypertrophy.

gain is used by the system to create a brighter image for the receptor camera without using excessive radiation. This is accomplished in the II by focusing electrons from the input phosphor onto a much smaller output phosphor thereby concentrating electrons per unit area on the output phosphor. A second source of gain is called brightness gain, which is accomplished by accelerating the same electrons as they move from the input to output phosphor. The kinetic energy gained by these electrons is given back at the

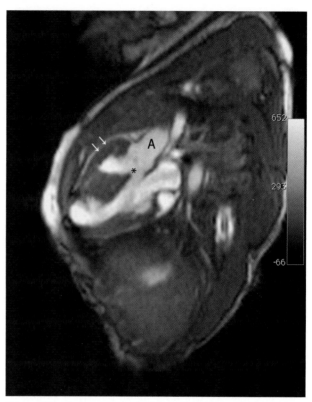

Figure 18.3. Three-chamber view of the heart showing a VSD and an overriding aorta. Also shown is right ventricular hypertrophy.

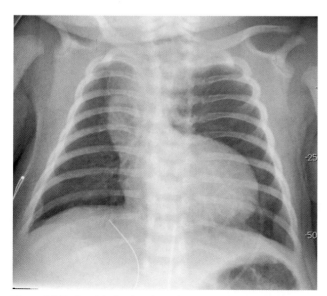

Figure 18.2. Frontal chest radiograph of a patient with tetralogy of Fallot demonstrating a "boot-shaped" heart with upturning of the cardiac apex, a right-sided aortic arch, and normal to diminished pulmonary vasculature.

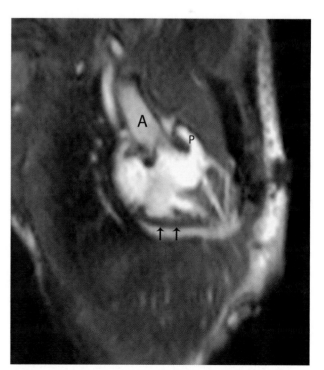

Figure 18.4. Right ventricle long-axis MR in a child with TOF shows the relative imbalance in size between the aorta and the small RVOT and pulmonary artery. Also shown is right ventricular hypertrophy.

output phosphor as elevated numbers of visible light photons picked up by the receptor camera. Most units have two or three magnification modes. Each stepwise decrease in field of view will result in magnification of pathology at the expense of increased radiation exposure rate up to a factor of 4. Likewise this will also result in the potential for higher spatial resolution. Electronic magnification on acquisition should not be confused with postacquisition image zoom; the former allows for increased spatial resolution whereas the latter merely magnifies existing pixels without added spatial resolution.

Differential Diagnosis

The differential diagnosis for a cyanotic patient with a chest radiograph demonstrating normal to diminished pulmonary blood flow includes:

- Double-outlet right ventricle with pulmonic stenosis (PS) and VSD
- Transposition of the great arteries with PS and VSD
- Single ventricle with PS
- Tricuspid atresia (with smaller VSD)

Common Variants

The previously described classic tetralogy of Fallot can result in significant right-to-left shunting with cyanosis (blue tetralogy). If there is less severe RVOT obstruction, shunting can be predominantly left-to-right (pink tetralogy). Furthermore, there can be complete obstruction of the RVOT, a scenario referred to as pulmonary atresia. With this condition, there can be variation ranging from simple atresia of the pulmonary valve with an intact main pulmonary artery to the absence of any normal pulmonary arteries. Blood flow to the lungs may therefore be dependent upon aorto-pulmonary collateral vessels (Fig. 18.5).

Another noteworthy variation is TOF with absent pulmonary valve syndrome. There is either complete absence of the pulmonary valve or a rudimentary rim of tissue with stenosis of the pulmonary annulus and infundibulum. The characteristic associated finding is aneurysmal dilatation of the central pulmonary arteries which can compress the adjacent bronchi and result in significant air trapping.

Clinical Issues

Surgical repair of classical TOF essentially revolves around closure of the VSD and relieving the RVOT obstruction. With advances in technique, the VSD repair can often be accomplished through a right atrial approach, and the RVOT obstruction can be reduced through a simple pulmonary valvotomy with limited or no transannular

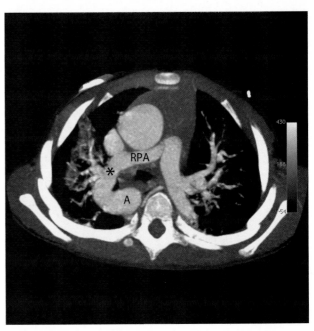

Figure 18.5. This CT angiogram of a child with TOF shows a large collateral vessel (*) extending from a right-sided descending aorta (A) to the right pulmonary artery (RPA) providing pulmonary arterial flow in a patient with TOF with pulmonary atresia.

incision. Previous approaches utilizing a larger right ventricular incision and a transannular pulmonary valvotomy left patients with a dyskinetic section of right ventricle and free pulmonary insufficiency that often necessitates a subsequent pulmonary valve replacement. As many of these patients are now being seen in follow-up, evaluation of pulmonary regurgitation and right ventricular end-diastoloic volume (RVEDV) are critical factors to interrogate. An RVEDV corrected for body surface area of 150 to 170 ml/m^2 is often considered the size at which further enlargement would be irreversible and therefore pulmonary valve repair/replacement is necessary.

Key Points

- Tetralogy of Fallot is the most common cyanotic heart lesion.
- The most common form of congential heart disease to have an associated right aortic arch is TOF.
- Four classic components of TOF: ventricular septal defect, infundibular pulmonary stenosis, overriding aorta, and right ventricular hypertrophy.

Further Reading

Bailliard F, Anderson RH. Tetralogy of Fallot. *Orphanet J Rare Dis.* 2009;4:2.

Ferguson EC, Krishnamurthy R, Oldham SA. Classic imaging signs of congenital cardiovascular abnormalities. *Radiographics.* 2007;*27*(5):1323–1334.

Frank L, Dillman JR, Parish V, Mueller GC, Kazerooni EA, Bell A, Attili AK. Cardiovascular MR imaging of conotruncal anomalies. *Radiographics.* 2010;*30*(4):1069–1094.

Gaca AM, Jaggers JJ, Dudley LT, Bisset GS III. Repair of congenital heart disease: a primer, Part 2. *Radiology.* 2008;*248*(1):44–60.

Kellenberger C. Tetralogy of Fallot and related conditions. In: Yoo SJ, MacDonald C, Babyn P, eds. *Chest Radiographic Interpretation in Pediatric Cardiac Patients.* New York, NY: Thieme Medical Publishers, Inc.; 2010:193–199.

Oosterhof T, Mulder BJM, Vliegen HW, de Roos A. Cardiovascular magnetic resonance in the follow-up of patients with corrected tetralogy of Fallot: a review. *Am Heart J.* 2006;*151*(2):265–272.

CHAPTER 19

Total Anomalous Pulmonary Venous Return

Adebunmi O. Adeyiga, MD and Laureen M. Sena, MD

Definition

Total anomalous pulmonary venous return (TAPVR) is a form of congenital heart disease in which the pulmonary veins do not drain into the left atrium and instead deliver pulmonary venous return to the right atrium, either directly or via a systemic venous connection. This condition accounts for approximately 1 to 3 percent of all congenital heart disease.

Clinical Features

The clinical features of TAPVR are dependent on the specific type and location of the anomalous venous connection, which may be obstructed to varying degrees. Patients with more severe obstruction usually present in the neonatal period with cyanosis, respiratory distress, and pulmonary arterial hypertension. Those patients with less pronounced obstruction, or no obstruction, can present later in life with mild cyanosis and right-sided volume overload or heart failure.

Anatomy and Physiology

The level of anomalous connection of the pulmonary venous confluence determines the classification of TAPVR (Fig. 19.1). Supracardiac connections (type I) are the most common and consist of a common pulmonary venous confluence draining to the left innominate vein via a vertical vein, or alternatively to the superior vena cava or azygous vein. Intracardiac connections (type II) consist of a direct connection to the right atrium or to the coronary sinus. Infracardiac connections (type III) consist of a connection to the inferior vena cava (either above or below the diaphragm), or to the portal venous system.

Total anomalous pulmonary venous return may be classified as a bidirectional shunt lesion. The anomalous pulmonary venous connection serves as an extracardiac left-to-right shunt. In all types of TAPVR, there is also intracardiac right-to-left shunting of blood via a patent foramen ovale or atrial septal defect, without which TAPVR would be incompatible with life. Types I and II are usually unobstructed and result in cyanosis with eventual congestive heart failure. In TAPVR type III, there may be obstruction of the pulmonary venous connection, usually as it passes through the hiatus of the diaphragm, or when

the ductus venosus closes if there is anomalous connection to the portal veins. In these cases, patients present early in life with marked cyanosis and pulmonary edema on chest radiographs.

Imaging Findings

A diagnosis of TAPVR can be confirmed by nonvisualization of the normal connection of the confluence of the pulmonary veins to the left atrium on echocardiography. Echocardiography can often delineate the specific anatomy of the anomalous pulmonary venous connection to a systemic vein. If there are more complex connections, CT or MR angiography can be complementary, especially mixed forms with pulmonary venous drainage to systemic veins above and below the diaphragm and when there is pulmonary venous obstruction.

When present, the classic radiographic appearance of TAPVR type I (unobstructed) is referred to as the "snowman" appearance (Fig. 19.2A). The head of the snowman is attributed to widening of the superior mediastinum because of the prominent vertical vein on the left and the dilated superior vena cava on the right. The enlarged cardiac silhouette (right heart enlargement) represents the body of the snowman. This appearance was more often visualized in the past because of later diagnosis after the newborn period. Currently, with advances in fetal ultrasound, the diagnosis is established earlier and this classic appearance is not often seen on newborn chest radiographs. Type II TAPVR (unobstructed) appears as right heart enlargement with increased pulmonary vascularity on chest radiography, similar in appearance to other left-to-right shunts such as a large atrial septal defect. Finally, the chest radiographic appearance of type III TAPVR usually has a normal- to small-sized heart with interstitial pulmonary edema and possible small pleural effusions (Fig. 19.2B) because of the common association of pulmonary venous obstruction with the infradiaphragmatic form of TAPVR.

Imaging Strategy

The chest radiographic findings in the different types of TAPVR are helpful, but are not specific enough to guide subsequent surgical repair. Both two-dimensional echocardiography and three-dimensional CT and MR

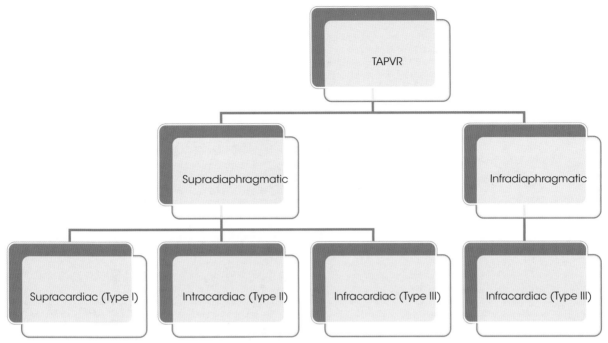

Figure 19.1. Flow diagram of the types of total anomalous pulmonary venous return.

angiography are therefore useful for definitive diagnosis and preoperative planning (Figs. 19.3, 19.4, and 19.5). Postoperatively, these patients are evaluated with echocardiography. Both CT and MR angiography are useful if there is suspected pulmonary vein stenosis, which is the most common complication following TAPVR repair.

Related Physics

Cardiac angiography was the mainstay in the past for diagnostic confirmation and is now reserved for selective therapeutic interventions. In using an image intensifier (II), potentially detrimental distortions must be understood. These include: lag, veiling glare, vignetting, and spatial distortions ("pin-cushion," "barreling" and "S"- distortion). Lag is

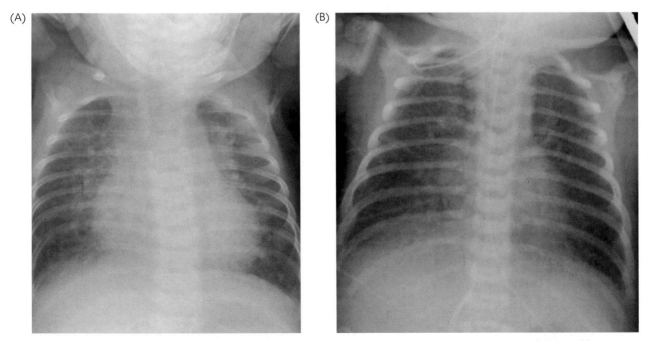

Figure 19.2. (A)Chest radiograph of a patient with tachypnea and poor feeding. Supracardiac (type I), with widening of the mediastinum and increased pulmonary blood flow.(B) Chest radiograph of a patient with tachypnea and poor feeding. Infracardiac (type III) with pulmonary venous obstruction, normal heart size, interstitial pulmonary edema, and small bilateral pleural effusions.

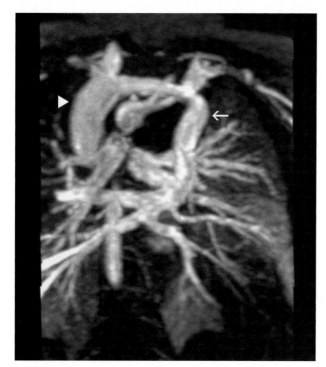

Figure 19.3. A 4-month-old male with failure to thrive and poor feeding. Oblique MIP image from MR angiography demonstrates a typical appearance of supracardiac (type 1) TAPVR. The pulmonary veins form a common confluence, which extends via a vertical vein (arrow) to the left innominate vein to a dilated SVC (arrowhead).

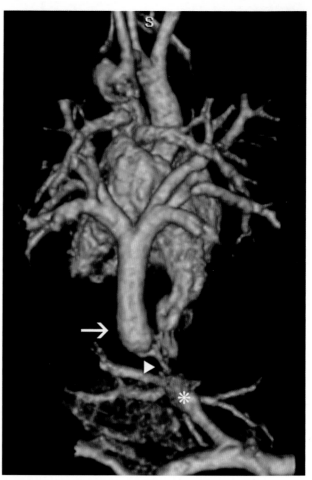

Figure 19.4. Newborn with tachypnea caused by infracardiac (type III) TAPVR. Posterior 3-D volume-rendered image from MR angiography demonstrating a common confluence of the pulmonary veins (arrow), which drains inferiorly to a constricted ductus venosus (arrowhead) to the left portal vein (asterisk). The closure of the ductus venosus results in pulmonary venous obstruction.

a phenomenon seen as blooming of the image when moving from chest to abdomen or vice versa. It is caused by the imaging system's inability to rapidly compensate for differing attenuation paths. Veiling glare is seen on the image as a wispy brightness overlaying the entire image and is caused by stray electrons from the input phosphor striking all portions of the output phosphor. Vignetting refers to diminished brightness of the image at the perimeter. This is caused by a lack of photons at the perimeter resulting in lower light output. Pin-cushioning and barreling are manifestations of imperfect focusing of input phosphor electrons onto the output phosphor creating curvilinear distortion of the margins: the margins are convex outward with barreling and concave outward with pin-cushioning. The issue of "S"-shaped distortion appears as wavy lines through the image caused by temporal instability of electrostatic focusing lenses within the II.

Differential Diagnosis
- Congestive heart failure:
    - Transposition of the great arteries
    - Truncus arteriosus
    - Hypoplastic left heart syndrome
    - Tricuspid atresia
- Chest X-ray of obstructed TAPVR:
    - Neonatal pneumonia
    - Meconium aspiration
    - Respiratory distress syndrome

Common Variants
Other forms of congenital heart disease may have associations with TAPVR, including atrioventricular septal defect, tetralogy of Fallot, or single ventricle. There is also a known association with heterotaxy (asplenia or polysplenia).

Clinical Issues
The key to survival for patients with TAPVR is early intervention, which consists of anastomosis of the pulmonary venous confluence with the left atrium. Pulmonary vein stenosis is the most common postsurgical complication, occurring in up to 20 percent of patients. Pulmonary vein stenosis, if untreated, may lead to pulmonary arterial hypertension.

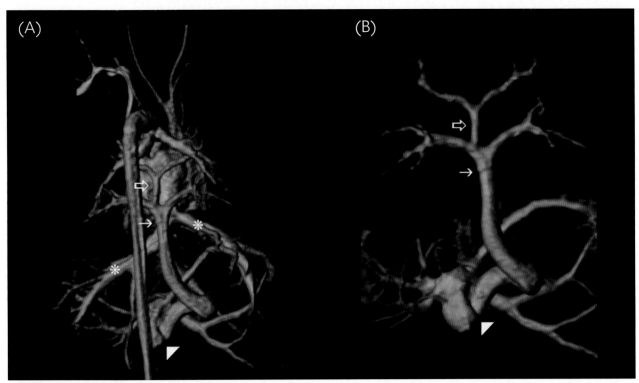

Figure19.5. (A and B) A 2-day-old male with heterotaxy and TAPVR. Posterior 3-D volume-rendered MRA images demonstrate infracardiac (type III) TAPVR to the portal vein. Small upper pulmonary veins form a confluence to a small vertical vein (open arrows), which then drains to a larger lower pulmonary vein confluence (arrows). Beneath the diaphragm, the tortuous pulmonary vein confluence drains to a dilated portal vein (arrowheads). Prior to birth, the pulmonary venous return to the heart passes from the portal vein via the ductus venosus to the inferior vena cava then on to the right atrium. After birth, the pulmonary venous return to the heart becomes obstructed when the ductus venosus closes and the blood must pass through the hepatic sinusoids to the hepatic veins (asterisks).

Key Points

- This disease features a congenital cyanotic cardiac lesion with bidirectional shunting.
- The entire pulmonary venous circulation is delivered to the right atrium via abnormal connection to the systemic venous system.
- Clinical presentation largely depends on the type of TAPVR and on the presence of obstruction.
- Early surgical correction is necessary for long-term survival.

Further Reading

Epelman M. Partial and total anomalous pulmonary venous connections. In: Yoo S, MacDonald C, Babyn P, eds. *Chest Radiographic Interpretation in Pediatric Cardiac Patients.* New York, NY: Thieme; 2010:206–214.

Fyler DC. Total anomalous pulmonary venous return. In: Fyler DC, ed. *Nadas' Pediatric Cardiology.* Philadelphia, PA: Hanley & Belfus; 1992:683–691.

Westra SJ. Total anomalous pulmonary venous return. In: Donnelly LF, Jones BV, O'Hara SM, et al., eds. *Diagnostic Imaging: Pediatrics.* Salt Lake City, UT: Amirsys; 2005:3-46-3-49.

CHAPTER 20

Transposition of the Great Arteries

Adebunmi O. Adeyiga, MD and Laureen M. Sena, MD

Definition

Transposition of the great arteries (TGA) is a form of congenital heart disease in which there is discordance of the ventriculoarterial relationship, but concordance of the atrioventricular relationship (Fig. 20.1). This form of ventriculoarterial discordance is also referred to as D-transposition of the great arteries, relating to normal D-loop configuration of the ventricles that occurred during embryological development.

Clinical Features

Approximately 5 percent of all congenital heart disease is TGA. There is a slight male predominance (60 percent). Without the presence of an underlying shunting lesion such as an atrial septal defect (ASD), ventricular septal defect (VSD), or patent ductus arteriosus (PDA), TGA is incompatible with life. The clinical presentation of patients with TGA is variable depending on the size and type of associated cardiac defects. Infants most commonly present with severe cyanosis shortly after birth and are tachypneic but do not appear to be in respiratory distress. If there is a coexisting shunt that allows for adequate admixture of the systemic and pulmonary circulations, infants may present with lesser degrees of cyanosis. Patients with an associated large VSD can develop pulmonary overcirculation and congestive symptoms as pulmonary pressures decrease after birth, especially in the absence of obstruction to the pulmonary outflow tract.

Anatomy and Physiology

In TGA, the aorta arises from the right ventricle and the main pulmonary artery arises from the left ventricle. There is a normal anatomic relationship between the atria and ventricles. As a result, deoxygenated blood from the systemic system enters the right atrium, passes through the tricuspid valve into the right ventricle, and then flows back into the systemic circulation via the aorta. Accordingly, oxygenated blood returns from the lungs via the pulmonary veins to the left atrium, passes through the mitral valve into the left ventricle, and then flows back into the pulmonary circulation via the main pulmonary artery. The systemic and pulmonary circulations are therefore parallel circuits that are not in communication, and physiologically, this results in cyanosis and variable pulmonary vascularity on chest radiography depending on the presence and degree of shunting. In order to sustain life, there must be admixture between the two circulations via an ASD, patent foramen ovale (PFO), PDA, or VSD.

Imaging Findings

Diagnosis of TGA is achieved with fetal echocardiography, during which there is an apparent parallel configuration of the great vessels, with the aorta arising from the anterior right ventricle and the pulmonary artery arising from the posterior left ventricle. The aortic valve is generally located anterior and to the right of the pulmonary valve. These findings may be confirmed with postnatal echocardiography.

Initially, neonates with TGA can demonstrate normal heart size and normal pulmonary vascularity. As pulmonary pressure decreases after birth, the heart enlarges and pulmonary overcirculation typically develops. The radiographic appearance of TGA is referred to classically as an "egg-on-a-string", in which the superior mediastinum appears narrow and the heart is oblong in configuration (Fig. 20.2). These findings result from thymic atrophy related to the stress of cyanosis, parallel relationship of the great arteries causing a narrow vascular pedicle and cardiomegaly (right atrial and left ventricular enlargement). Pulmonary vascularity can be normal to increased depending on the pulmonary vascular resistance, unless there is associated pulmonary stenosis, in which case pulmonary vascularity may be decreased.

Imaging Strategy

As the diagnosis of TGA is often made with echocardiography, CT and MR angiography are rarely needed for preoperative evaluation, but they are essential tools postoperatively (Fig. 20.3). Also, CT or MR angiography can be helpful for evaluation of postoperative complications following the arterial switch operation, such as narrowing of the anastomosis of the aorta or pulmonary artery, as well as branch pulmonary artery stenosis (Fig. 20.4). Because the operation also requires transfer of the

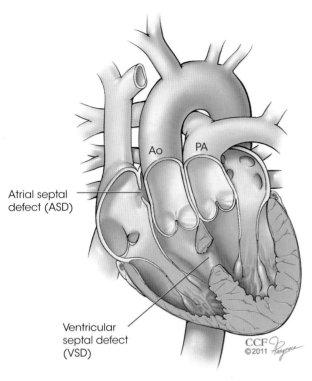

Figure 20.1. Illustration depicting the configuration of the heart in D-transposition of the great arteries with VSD. The main pulmonary artery arises from the left ventricle and the aorta arises from the right ventricle. The normal atrioventricular relationships are preserved. There is admixture across the VSD and the ASD. Deoxygenated blood (blue), oxygenated blood (red), mixed blood (purple).

coronary arteries, both CT and MR now play an important role in surveillance for possible coronary artery narrowing (Fig. 20.5).

Related Physics

Patients with complex congenital heart disease may undergo multiple imaging studies to define both the anatomic defects and the resultant physiologic disturbance and for surveillance postcorrection. Any imaging study must have excellent spatial resolution to characterize anatomy. Spatial resolution is measured in the "spatial" domain and recorded in units of distance (i.e., mm). Most often this is accomplished by imaging a test tool known as a line pair which is defined as a lead bar adjacent to an equal-sized bar of air. Line pairs have units of line pairs per distance (i.e., line pairs per mm). The test tool will have many sets of line pairs with varying sizes of bar patterns in an array from large to small. A consensus panel of experts will evaluate the images rendered from the bar patterns and determine the smallest pattern that can be visualized. Line pairs per millimeter and the number of lines and the size of the lines visualized are related by the Fourier transformation that moves one between "spatial" (mm) and "frequency" (line pairs per mm) domains.

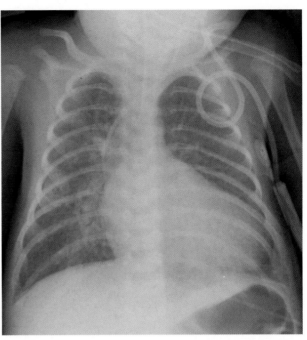

Figure 20.2. An 11-day-old female with unrepaired D-TGA with VSD. The heart is enlarged and there is evidence of pulmonary overcirculation. The superior mediastinum is relatively narrow because of the parallel relationship of the MPA and aorta arising from the heart and the very small thymus resulting from neonatal stress.

Differential Diagnosis

- Cyanosis with cardiomegaly and pulmonary overcirculation:
    - Truncus arteriosus
    - Tricuspid atresia
    - Other single-ventricle physiology

Common Variants

Transposition of the great arteries may be associated with other forms of congenital heart disease and approximately 50 percent are associated with a VSD. Other associations include pulmonary valvular stenosis, coarctation of the aorta, and interrupted aortic arch.

The ventriculoarterial discordance that defines transposition can occur with varying types of atrioventricular relationships. Although D-TGA is the most commonly encountered form of transposition, there is another classic but much less common form of transposition referred to as congenitally corrected TGA or L-TGA. The "L" refers to L-looping of the heart in utero, which results in an isolated form of ventricular inversion so that the right ventricle is positioned posteriorly and the left ventricle is positioned anteriorly. In L-TGA, the circulation through the heart is physiologic or "congenitally corrected" because there is both ventriculoarterial and atrioventricular discordance. Systemic venous return enters the right atrium, passes through the mitral valve into the morphologic left

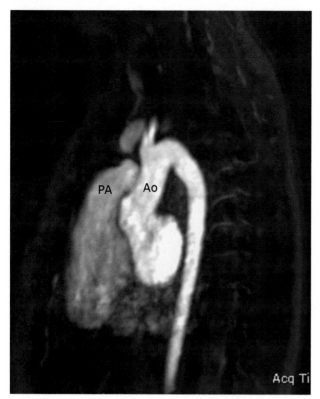

Figure 20.3. A 15-year-old male with D-TGA following the arterial switch operation. Sagittal oblique MIP image from MR angiography demonstrates a parallel configuration of the great arteries with the aorta (Ao) arising from the posterior LV and the main pulmonary artery (PA) arising from the anterior RV.

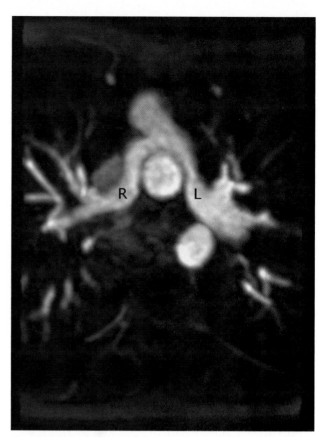

Figure 20.4. A 15-year-old male with D-TGA following the arterial switch operation. Axial oblique MIP image from MR angiography demonstrates the typical postoperative appearance of the pulmonary arteries, which are draped to either side of the ascending aorta resulting from the Lecompte maneuver as the MPA and aortic positions are switched during the operation. There is mild narrowing of the right pulmonary artery (R) as it courses between the SVC and aorta and moderate narrowing of the left pulmonary artery (L).

ventricle, and is then appropriately delivered to the pulmonary circulation via the main pulmonary artery. Pulmonary venous return enters the left atrium, passes through the tricuspid valve into the morphologic right ventricle, and is then appropriately delivered to the systemic circulation via

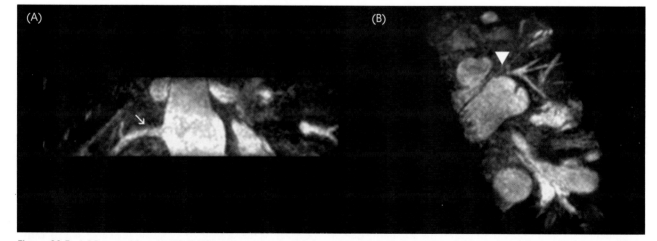

Figure 20.5. A 15-year-old male with D-TGA following the arterial switch operation. Oblique MIP reformatted images of the coronaries arteries from coronary MR angiography demonstrate (a) large caliber of the right coronary artery (arrow), and (b) near complete occlusion of the left main coronary artery origin (arrowhead). Distally the left main coronary artery trifurcates into the left anterior descending, first diagonal, and circumflex arteries, which are all small in caliber. On subsequent coronary CT angiography, numerous collateral arteries from the right coronary artery were noted to support the left coronary system.

the aorta. Although congenitally corrected TGA in isolation may be of little or no clinical consequence early in life, long-term outcome can be impacted by progressive right ventricular dysfunction and conduction abnormalities, which may require pacemaker insertion. Clinical presentation is also variable because of the presence of associated lesions including VSD, pulmonary stenosis, and Ebstein anomaly of the tricuspid valve.

Clinical Issues

Prior to definitive surgical intervention, neonates with severe cyanosis may require prostaglandin therapy in order to maintain patency of the ductus arteriosus for mixing of the systemic and pulmonary circulations. Balloon atrial septostomy is performed under fluoroscopic or echocardiographic guidance in emergent situations when there is inadequate admixture of the systemic and pulmonary circulations, especially when the interventricular septum is intact (i.e., there is no VSD) and the PDA closes.

Early surgical intervention with the Jatene arterial switch procedure is the preferred treatment option, which entails switching the great arteries so that they arise from the appropriate ventricle, as well as transfering the coronary arteries from the aorta to the neo-aorta (MPA) so that they are supported by the left ventricle. Prior to development of the arterial switch operation, which required full cardiac bypass and perfection of coronary artery anastomosis, patients typically underwent the atrial switch operation, using either the Mustard or Senning procedure. The Mustard procedure entails use of a baffle constructed from prosthetic material or pericardium that is placed intra-atrially to redirect the pulmonary and systemic venous blood flow to the appropriate ventricle. The intra-atrial baffle directs the systemic venous return to the left ventricle and pulmonary circulation, and the pulmonary venous return to the right ventricle and the systemic circulation. The Senning procedure redirects the venous blood flow in a similar manner, but uses the native atrial septum as the intra-atrial baffle.

Key Points

- Ventriculoarterial discordance with atrioventricular concordance in D-TGA results in parallel pulmonary and systemic circulations.
- Unless there is an associated shunting lesion for admixture of the systemic and pulmonary circulations, TGA is incompatible with life.
- There is a high association between TGA and VSD.
- Early surgical correction with arterial or atrial switch procedure is necessary for long-term survival.

Further Reading

Fyler DC. "Corrected" transposition of the great arteries. In: Fyler DC, ed. *Nadas' Pediatric Cardiology*. Philadelphia, PA: Hanley & Belfus; 1992:701–706.

Fyler DC. D-transposition of the great arteries. In: Fyler DC, ed. *Nadas' Pediatric Cardiology*. Philadelphia, PA: Hanley & Belfus; 1992:557–575.

Roman KS. Transpositions of the great arteries. In: Yoo S, MacDonald C, Babyn P, eds. *Chest Radiographic Interpretation in Pediatric Cardiac Patients*. New York, NY: Thieme; 2010:234–240.

Westra SJ. D-transposition of the great arteries. In: Donnelly LF, Jones BV, O'Hara SM et al., eds. *Diagnostic Imaging: Pediatrics*. Salt Lake City, UT: Amirsys; 2005:3-34–3-37.

CHAPTER 21

Truncus Arteriosus

Adebunmi O. Adeyiga, MD and Laureen M. Sena, MD

Definition

Truncus arteriosus is a rare congenital cardiac anomaly consisting of a single common great artery, which originates from the base of the heart and gives rise to the aorta, pulmonary arteries, and coronary arteries (Fig. 21.1). Truncus arteriosus is also described as a common arterial trunk or truncus arteriosus communis (TAC).

Clinical Features

The overall incidence of truncus arteriosus is approximately 5 to 15 per 100,000 live births, accounting for 1 to 2 percent of congenital cardiac defects. Patients with truncus arteriosus typically present within the first few weeks of life. Common presenting symptoms include tachypnea, costosternal retractions, and a heart murmur. Infants can develop progressive congestive heart failure with or without cyanosis. Truncus arteriosus is frequently associated with DiGeorge syndrome and deletion on the long arm of chromosome 22. These patients may present with immunodeficiency syndromes related to thymic hypoplasia/aplasia, or may present with convulsions or tetany resulting from altered calcium and parathyroid hormone levels in conjunction with parathyroid gland hypoplasia/aplasia.

Anatomy and Physiology

The primitive bulbus cordis normally separates into the aorta and main pulmonary artery between the third and fourth weeks of gestation. Failure at this stage of development results in a persistent truncus arteriosus. The truncus often overrides a high ventricular septal defect (VSD) and may also be associated with aortic arch anomalies, particularly a right-sided aortic arch or interrupted aortic arch. The associated semilunar valve or common truncal valve may have one to six cusps and may be regurgitant or stenotic because of thickened and dysplastic leaflets (Fig. 21.2).

Collett and Edwards developed a classification system for the different anatomic variants of truncus in 1949, which was based on the position of the pulmonary arteries. This classification system is no longer used by cardiac surgeons:

Type 1: Ascending aorta and short main pulmonary artery arise from base of truncus

Type 2: Branch pulmonary arteries arise directly from truncus posteriorly

Type 3: Branch pulmonary arteries arise directly from truncus laterally

Type 4: Branch pulmonary arteries arise from descending aorta ("pseudotruncus" or variant of tetralogy of Fallot with pulmonary atresia)

In 1965 Van Praagh and Van Praagh developed a modified classification system:

Type A1: Ascending aorta and short main pulmonary artery arise from base of truncus

Type A2: Branch pulmonary arteries arise separately from truncus

Type A3: Absence of one or both branch pulmonary arteries, with collateral supply to the affected lung via a ductus arteriosus or other collateral artery

Type A4: Truncus with interrupted aortic arch

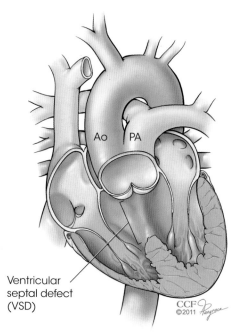

Figure 21.1. Illustration of truncus arteriosus, depicting a single common great artery, which gives rise to the aorta, pulmonary arteries and coronary arteries. Deoxygenated blood (blue), oxygenated blood (red), mixed blood (purple).

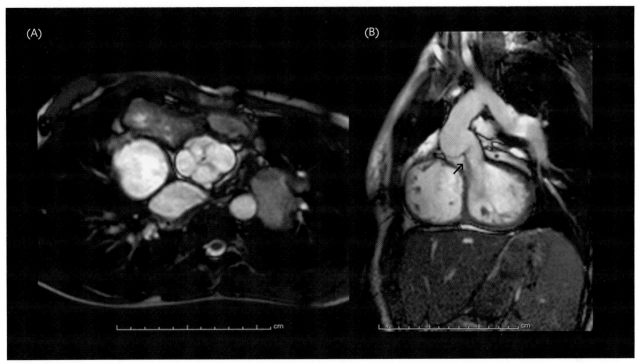

Figure 21.2. Axial (A) and coronal (B) oblique diastolic steady state free precession (SSFP) MR images through the truncal root in a patient with surgically repaired truncus arteriosus. The truncal root is dilated and the valve consists of four dysplastic leaflets. A central failure of coaptation results in significant regurgitation with a regurgitant flow jet (arrow).

Truncus arteriosus is considered a cyanotic lesion, with bidirectional intracardiac shunting of blood across the VSD, as well as extracardiac mixing of pulmonary and systemic circulations within the truncus. As pulmonary vascular resistance decreases after birth, pulmonary blood flow increases leading to pulmonary overcirculation and respiratory distress. Rarely, congenital stenosis of a coronary artery may lead to ischemic cardiomyopathy.

Imaging Findings

Prenatal diagnosis of truncus arteriosus may be made with visualization of a common great artery arising from the base of the heart on fetal echocardiography. Chest radiographs in infancy may demonstrate biventricular and left atrial enlargement with increased pulmonary vascularity (Fig. 21.3). The aortic arch is often right-sided and the superior mediastinum may be narrow as a result of thymic hypoplasia/aplasia. As an adjunct to echocardiography, CT and MR angiography are helpful for preoperative assessment of anatomy when the pulmonary arteries or the aortic arch are not completely evaluated, as well as for postoperative evaluation.

Imaging Strategy

Children suspected of having congenital heart disease should be assessed with echocardiography, which is the mainstay of diagnosis in these patients. Utilization of CT or MR angiography can assist with further delineation of the specific

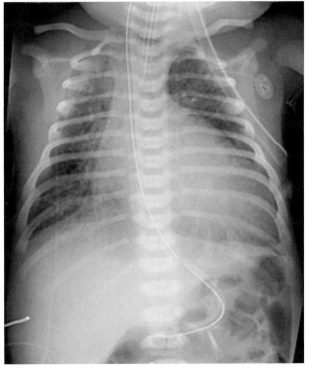

Figure 21.3. Frontal chest radiograph in an 11-day-old female with truncus arteriosus. The heart is markedly enlarged and there is prominent pulmonary blood flow. Also note the presence of a right-sided aortic arch.

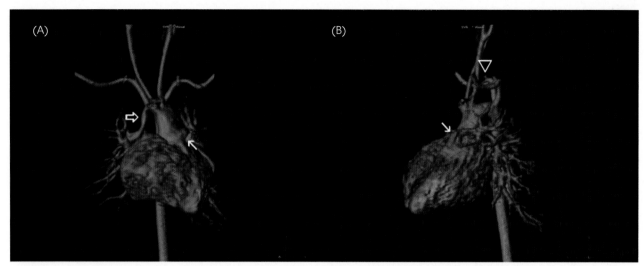

Figure 21.4. Anterior oblique (A) and lateral oblique (B) 3-D volume-rendered reformatted MR images in a 4-day-old male with a Type A3 truncus arteriosus. The right pulmonary artery arises from a right-sided duct-like collateral from the innominate artery (open arrow). The left pulmonary artery arises from the anterior aspect of the truncal root (arrow). Also noted is a left-sided aortic arch with an aberrant right subclavian artery (arrowhead).

anatomical relationships, including location of the pulmonary arteries, coronary anatomy, and the morphology of the aortic arch, especially when it is interrupted (Fig. 21.4).

Related Physics

Complex congenital heart disease is often first suspected from prenatal screening ultrasound (US) after which definitive fetal echocardiography is performed. Echocardiography gives information about structural anomalies as well as direction and velocity of flow. Historically, flow has been depicted on US in one of two ways, either in velocity (m/sec) or frequency (kHz), which represents the frequency of the Doppler shift. Either method is useful and the axes can be easily rescaled through a toggle switch on the unit. With persistent fetal connections, the Doppler shift represents a change in frequency of the transmitted to the received pulse and with flowing blood is proportional to the velocity of the moving red blood cells through the shunt. As Doppler is a vector, one obtains both magnitude and direction of flow through the shunt.

Differential Diagnosis

- Cardiomegaly and increased pulmonary blood flow with congestive heart failure on chest radiography:
  - Transposition of the great arteries
  - Large VSD with congestive failure
  - Common atrioventricular canal

Common Variants

There are many associated variants of aortic arch anatomy.

Clinical Issues

Truncus arteriosus is associated with a high mortality rate within the first year of life if untreated. Surgical repair of truncus arteriosus involves removing the pulmonary arteries from the truncus or duct supply and reestablishing pulmonary blood flow from the right ventricle (RV) with a right ventricle to pulmonary artery (PA) conduit (Fig. 21.5)). The truncal valve is maintained as the aortic valve and the VSD is closed. Often MRI is used

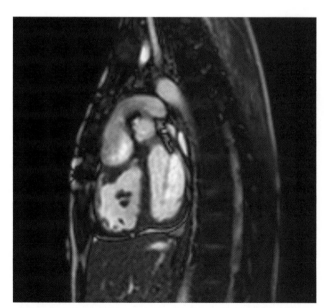

Figure 21.5. Sagittal oblique SSFP MR image in a patient with surgically repaired truncus arteriosus, demonstrating the proximal aspect of the RV-to-PA conduit.

postoperatively to evaluate the function of the truncal valve and RV-to-PA conduit. Patients may require multiple subsequent conduit revisions over time if the conduit becomes severely obstructed or regurgitant. Truncal valve dysfunction may also necessitate subsequent valve replacement.

Key Points

- Trucus arteriosus involves a rare congenital cyanotic cardiac lesion with admixture.
- Common arterial trunk overrides a VSD, supplying the coronary, pulmonary and systemic circulation.
- Decreasing pulmonary vascular resistance in the newborn can result in progressive pulmonary overcirculation and heart failure.
- There is a high mortality without surgical correction.

Further Reading

Anderson RH, Thiene G. Categorization and description of hearts with a common arterial trunk. *Eur J Cardiothorac Surg.* 1989;3(6):481–487.

Collett RW, Edwards, JE. Persistent truncus arteriosus: a classification according to anatomic types. *Surg Clin North Am.* 1949;29:1245–1270.

Fyler DC. Truncus arteriosus. In: Fyler DC, ed. *Nadas' Pediatric Cardiology.* Philadelphia, PA: Hanley & Belfus; 1992:675–681.

Kellenberger CJ. Truncus arteriosus. In: Yoo S, MacDonald C, Babyn P, eds. *Chest Radiographic Interpretation in Pediatric Cardiac Patients.* New York, NY: Thieme; 2010:185–188.

Marcelletti C, McGoon DC, Mair DD. The natural history of truncus arteriosus. *Circulation.* 1976;54(1):108–111.

Van Praagh R, Van Praagh S. The anatomy of common aorticopulmonary trunk (truncus arteriosus communis) and its embryologic implications. A study of 57 necropsy cases. *Am J Cardiol.* 1965;16(3):406–425.

Westra SJ. Truncus arteriosus. In: Donnelly LF, Jones BV, O'Hara SM, et al., eds. *Diagnostic Imaging: Pediatrics.* Salt Lake City, UT: Amirsys; 2005:3-42–3-45.

CHAPTER 22

Hypoplastic Left Heart Syndrome

Sjirk J. Westra, MD

Definition

Hypoplastic left heart syndrome (HLHS) is the most severe congenital cardiac anomaly, characterized by hypoplasia or complete atresia of the ascending aorta, aortic valve, left ventricle (LV), and mitral valve (Fig. 22.1).

Clinical Features

The incidence of HLHS is 1 to 3 per 10,000 life births, and males are two times more commonly affected than females. Hypoplastic left heart syndrome is a left-sided obstructive cardiac lesion leading to cyanosis and severe cardiac failure (cardiogenic shock after closure of the ductus arteriosus) within the first week of life. Without treatment, death occurs within days to weeks.

Anatomy and Physiology

The entire cardiac output enters a dilated pulmonary trunk, and perfusion of the systemic circulation can only occur by virtue of right-to-left shunting through a large ductus arteriosus (ductus dependency). Blood flow in the aortic arch (perfusing the head and neck vessels) and the hypoplastic ascending aorta (perfusing the coronaries) is in a retrograde direction. There is increased blood flow in the pulmonary arteries, leading to congestive heart failure. There is an obligatory left-to-right shunt through a patent foramen ovale, accounting for severe cyanosis.

Imaging Findings

The critical imaging finding of HLHS is hypoplasia of the left ventricle and ascending aorta, which exhibits retrograde blood flow (Fig. 22.1). Findings on radiography include cardiomegaly, pulmonary vascular (venous) congestion with interstitial fluid, hyperinflation and a narrow mediastinum, caused by stress-related thymic atrophy (Fig. 22.2). Echocardiography is usually diagnostic, with a prenatal diagnosis increasingly made. There is a diminutive (<5 mm) ascending aorta with retrograde flow, small thick-walled LV, small mitral valve (abnormally low Z-score is a prognostic indicator), dilatation of right-sided cardiac chambers and PA, and patent foramen ovale with left-to-right shunting. Performed after Norwood repair, CTA or MRA are helpful for assessment of residual stenosis in the neo-aorta, presence of coarctation and candidacy for Fontan procedure (Figs. 22.3 and 22.4). Cardiac catheterization with angiocardiography is reserved only for percutaneous interventions.

> IMAGING PITFALL: Echocardiography can severely underestimate the volume of the hypoplastic left ventricle, because of oversimplification caused by the application of the Simpson rule to a 2-D image. Cine MRI, because it is a truly three-dimensional technique, is much more reliable for ventricular volume calculation and hence, to predict which patients may undergo the preferred biventricular repair.

Imaging Strategy

The initial diagnosis of HLHS is made with echocardiography in the majority of cases. Postoperative MRI or CT is used to evaluate function of the univentricular heart and interventional angiography to address residua and sequelae of the Fontan repair (Fig. 22.5). Functional and morphological MRI is very valuable to investigate the altered hemodynamics of (partially) repaired complex cardiac anomalies and to detect complications (thrombosis, stenosis, kinking of vessels, etc.) (Fig. 22.6).

Related Physics

Anatomical MR imaging is done with a two-dimensional (2-D) balanced steady-state free precession (SSFP: cardiac-gated bright blood cine imaging) and double-inversion recovery fast (turbo) spin echo (FSE or TSE: black blood imaging) techniques in the standard cardiac vertical and horizontal long- and short-axis planes. Short axis cine images are used for subjective assessment of cardiac function (wall motion, myocardial thickening) and to measure systolic and diastolic ventricular volumes and hence, functional global cardiac parameters (cardiac output, ejection fraction). Extracardiac vascular structures are best imaged with a dynamic series of contrast-enhanced 3-D gradient-echo pulse sequences, reconstructed in multiple planes and with maximum-intensity projection (MIP) or volume rendering (VR). Phase contrast imaging is used to measure blood flow volumes across valves and within

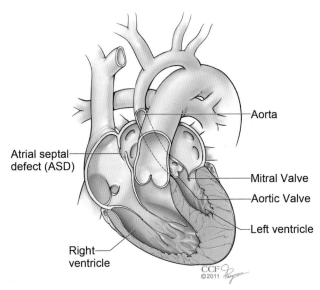

Figure 22.1. Illustration shows hypoplasia of left-sided cardiac chambers (including mitral valve), aortic valve and ascending aorta. Survival depends on patency of the ductus arteriosus.

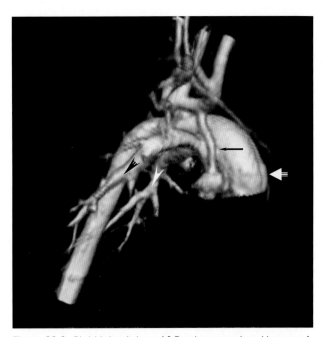

Figure 22.2. Right lateral view of 3-D volume-rendered image of CTA in newborn with HLHS shows large main pulmonary artery (large white arrow), the hypoplastic ascending aorta (small black arrow), and right and left branch pulmonary arteries (black and white arrowheads, respectively).

pulmonary artery branches and (Fontan) conduits, to estimate functional cardiac parameters such as regurgitant fractions, cardiac output and ejection fractions, systemic versus pulmonary perfusion and differential lung perfusion in postoperative patients.

Differential Diagnosis

- Left-sided obstructive cardiac anomalies:
  - Critical aortic valvular or supravalvular stenosis (Willams syndrome)
  - Severe infantile (preductal) coarctation
  - Interrupted aortic arch
- Severe heart failure in early infancy:
  - Cranial (vein of Galen) or hepatic arteriovenous malformations (characterized by a structurally normal heart and high cardiac output)
  - Neonatal cardiomyopathies
  - Coronary arteriovenous fistula, leading to early myocardial infarction

Common Variants and Complications

- HLHS with VSD
- Hypoplasia of aortic arch (preductal coarctation)
- Endocardial fibro-elastosis

Clinical Issues

Initial treatment of HLHS is with prostaglandin E1 to maintain patency of the ductus arteriosus. The feasibility of a complete (biventricular) surgical repair is critically dependent on the size and predicted function of the hypoplastic left ventricle. Palliative repair in patients who are not candidates for a complete repair is done initially through the Norwood surgery. This operation, typically done before 3 weeks of age, involves atrial septectomy, conversion of main pulmonary artery to neo-aorta as the main outflow

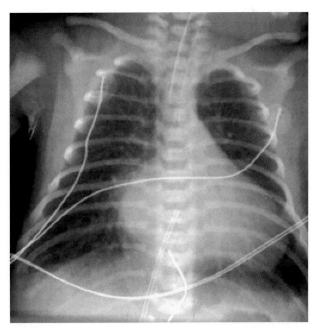

Figure 22.3. Frontal radiograph of newborn boy with hypoplastic left heart syndrome shows right-sided cardiomegaly, pulmonary vascular congestion and narrow mediastinum caused by stress-related thymic atrophy.

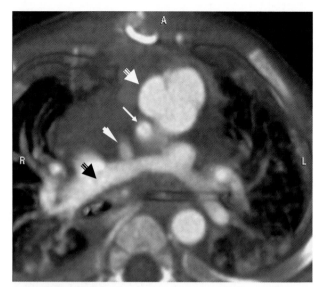

Figure 22.4. Axial contrast-enhanced CT image of 4-month-old boy following partial repair for HLHS shows large main pulmonary artery (large white arrow), hypoplastic ascending aorta (small white arrow), a patent modified Blalock-Taussig shunt (white arrowhead), and flow direction through a patent right-sided superior vena-cava-to-right pulmonary artery (Glenn) anastomosis (large black arrow).

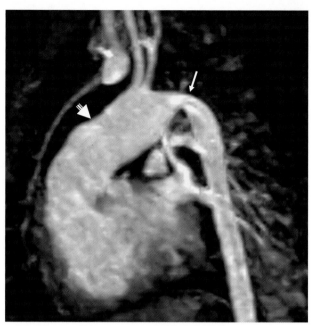

Figure 22.6. Sagittal oblique MRA of young child with hypoplastic left heart syndrome demonstrates dilated main pulmonary artery (large arrow), serving as the main cardiac outflow channel after Norwood repair. Note focal narrowing leading to obstruction in transverse aortic arch (small arrow). (Image courtesy of Laureen Sena MD)

channel of the (functionally) univentricular heart, and creation of a modified Blalock-Taussig shunt, to provide perfusion to the branch pulmonary arteries. Subsequent repair at the age of 4 to 6 months involves creation of cavopulmonary (Glenn) shunt(s)—the hemi-Fontan operation, with take-down of the Blalock-Taussig shunt. If possible, at the age of 1.5 to 2 years, a complete modified Fontan repair is performed. This operation involves the creation of an extra- or fenestrated intracardiac conduit to channel flow from inferior vena cava to the pulmonary arteries. Some centers favor primary cardiac transplantation over surgical palliation (Norwood, Fontan).

KeyPoints

- Hypoplasia of left-sided cardiac structures
- Cyanosis, cardiomegaly with increased vascularity
- Most common and severe cause of congestive heart failure presenting in early infancy
- Severe cardiogenic shock after ductus closure
- Complete biventricular repair (if possible) or three-staged surgical palliation (Norwood, Glenn, Fontan)
- CTA and MRI for all stages of repair for assessment of cardiac morphology
- Cine MRI and phase contrast MRA for functional evaluation

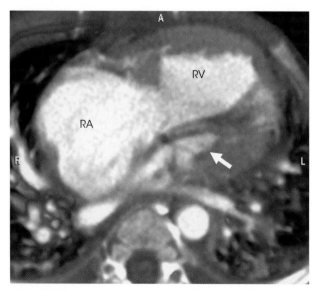

Figure 22.5. Axial contrast-enhanced CT image of 4-month-old boy following partial repair for HLHS shows relative hypoplasia of left ventricle (arrow) and severe dilatation of right atrium (RA) and ventricle (RV).

Further Reading

Bardo DM, Frankel DG, Applegate KE, Murphy DJ, Saneto RP. Hypoplastic left heart syndrome. *Radiographics.* 2001;*21*(3): 705–717.

Brown DW, Gauvreau K, Powell AJ, Lang P, Colan SD, Del Nido PJ, Odegard KC, Geva T. Cardiac magnetic resonance versus routine cardiac catheterization before bidirectional Glenn anastomosis in infants with functional single ventricle: a prospective randomized trial. *Circulation.* 2007;*116*:2718–2725.

Casolo G, Rega L, Gensini GF. Detection of right atrial and pulmonary artery thrombosis after the Fontan procedure by magnetic resonance imaging. *Heart.* 2004;*90*:825.

Dillman JR, Dorfman AL, Attili AK, Agarwal PP, Bell A, Mueller GC, Hernandez RJ. Cardiovascular magnetic resonance imaging of hypoplastic left heart syndrome in children. *Pediatr Radiol.* 2010;*40*(3):261–274.

Grosse-Wortmann L, Yun TJ, Al-Radi O, Kim S, Nii M, Lee Kj, Redington A, Yoo SJ, van Arsdell G. Borderline hypoplasia of the left ventricle in neonates: insights for decision making from functional assessment with magnetic resonance imaging. *J Thorac Cardiovasc Surg.* 2008;*136*:1429–1436.

Muthurangu V, Taylor AM, Hegde SR, Johnson R, Tulloh R, Simpson JM, Qureshi S, Rosenthal E, Baker E, Anderson D, Razavi R. Cardiac magnetic resonance imaging after stage I Norwood operation for hypoplastic left heart syndrome. *Circulation.* 2005;*112*:3256–3263.

Sundareswaran KS, Kanter KR, Kitajima HD, Krishnakutty R, Sabatier JF, Parks WJ, Sharma S, Yoganathan AP, Fogel M. Impaired power output and cardiac index with hypoplastic left heart syndrome: a magnetic resonance imaging study. *Ann Thorac Surg.* 2006;*82*(4):1267–1275.

CHAPTER 23

Anomalous Left Coronary Artery Origin

Lorna Browne, MD

Definition

The term "anomalous left coronary artery" refers to a congenital anomaly whereby the left coronary artery (LCA) arises from a location other than the left sinus of Valsalva. The two types of anomalous left coronary artery origin with the most serious clinical implications are LCA origin from the right sinus of Valsalva and LCA origin from the left pulmonary artery (ALCAPA).

Clinical Features

Severe ischemia results from narrowing of the proximal LCA in cases in which there is an interarterial LCA and coronary steal in patients with ALCAPA. LCA origin from the right sinus of Valsalva with an interarterial course is extremely rare (1 to 3 percent of population) and typically presents in adolescents or young adults with symptoms of myocardial ischemia (syncope or chest pain) associated with exertion. Anomalous origin of the LCA from the pulmonary artery is an extremely rare congenital cardiac abnormality. Collateral vessels from the normal RCA develop, however the connection between the LCA and low-resistance pulmonary circulation usually results in a vascular steal phenomenon into the pulmonary artery. Most cases of ALCAPA present at approximately 6 to 8 weeks of age with signs of ischemia and failure, including poor feeding and tachypnea, coinciding with the nadir of pulmonary vascular resistance and before significant collateralization has occurred. Approximately 15 percent of patients develop such extensive collateral circulations that presentation occurs much later, with rare cases of presentation during adulthood described. All other LCA anomalies are usually clinically silent.

Anatomy and Physiology

The right and left main coronary arteries (RCA and LCA) originate from the right and left aortic sinuses of Valsalva. These sinuses are located on the anterior and left sides of the aortic root, respectively, and face the pulmonary trunk (Fig. 23.1). The RCA arises slightly inferiorly to the LCA. The third aortic sinus, located rightward and posterior to the other sinuses, is known as the noncoronary sinus. The RCA courses in the anterior atrioventricular groove to the

inferior margin of the heart. The LCA divides into the left anterior descending coronary artery (LAD) and the left circumflex coronary artery (LCX). The LAD courses in the anterior interventricular groove to reach the apex of the heart, and the LCX courses at the margin of the heart before passing into the posterior atrioventricular groove.

The artery that supplies the posterior descending branch (PDB) over the inferior crux of the heart is considered to be the dominant coronary artery. In approximately 70 percent of individuals, the RCA gives rise to the PDB (RCA dominance); in 10 percent, the LCX artery gives rise to branches to the posterior right ventricle (LCX dominance); and in the remaining 20 percent, the PDB is supplied by branches from both RCA and LCX arteries (codominance). The right coronary artery supplies the right ventricular free wall and the inferior interventricular septum. The left coronary artery usually supplies the myocardium of the free wall of the left ventricle and anterior interventricular septum.

The left main coronary artery ostium usually arises perpendicularly from the center of the left sinus of Valsalva. Multiple anomalies of coronary artery origin have been described and all but two are clinically silent. The first with clinical importance includes anomalous LCA origin from the right sinus of Valsalva with either a course through the interventricular septum (transeptal), anterior to the right ventricular outflow tract (prepulmonic), behind the aorta (retroaortic), or between the aorta and pulmonary trunk (interarterial) to reach its normal myocardial territory in the interventricular groove. The second is anomalous origin of the LCA from the pulmonary trunk (ALCAPA).

Imaging Findings

Radiography: in ALCAPA, the chest radiograph (CXR) may show left atrial and left ventricular enlargement. Cardiac failure results in classic pulmonary edema. In the majority of types of anomalous LCA origins (including interarterial course of an anomalous LCA from the right coronary sinus) the CXR will be normal. In patients with an associated cono-truncal malformation, the CXR findings of repaired tetralogy of Fallot (elevated cardiac apex, right-sided aortic arch) or transposition of the great vessels (narrowed mediastinal silhouette) may be evident.

Echocardiography (ECHO): ECHO will often show the anomalous origin of the LCA from the right sinus, however proving the interarterial passage of an anomalous LCA is difficult as there is limited visualization of the LCA course. The passage of coronary flow into the pulmonary artery or the presence of diastolic flow in the pulmonary artery is suggestive of ALCAPA. Decreased myocardial systolic function, mitral regurgitation and left atrial and ventricular enlargement may suggest LCA anomalies.

Nuclear Medicine Perfusion Scan: nuclear medicine perfusion imaging is quite sensitive for ischemia and may demonstrate ischemia in the left coronary distribution in cases of ALCAPA or anomalous LCA from the right sinus. However, cardiomyopathies may also demonstrate a similar pattern of ischemia and normal near-maximal stress perfusion imaging has been reported in patients who have later died from interarterial course of the LCA.

MRI/CTA: noninvasive imaging with MRI or CTA is usually required for confirmation of coronary anomalies, and use of these modalities generally precedes conventional cardiac catheterization as a diagnostic test of choice (Fig. 23.1). Anomalously high and low take-offs of the coronary arteries are described when the ostia occur >10 millimeters above or below the sinotubular junction (Fig. 23.2). The LCA may originate from the wrong ostium and take a variety of anomalous courses (Fig. 23.3). A single coronary artery may arise from any aortic sinus and then has a variable course with multiple branches that follow the distributions of the RCA, LAD, and LCX. When the single coronary artery arises from the right sinus, the left main may travel interarterially between the aorta and pulmonary artery (Fig. 23.4).

The LCA usually arises from the leftward and posterior-facing sinus of the pulmonary trunk. In ALCAPA, collateral vessels from the normal RCA develop, however the connection between the LCA and the low-resistance pulmonary circulation usually results in a coronary steal phenomenon into the pulmonary artery. The left ventricle is usually enlarged and decreased left ventricular systolic function may be demonstrated on multiphasic imaging.

Imaging Strategy

Evaluation of the coronary arteries requires minimization of respiratory and cardiac motion and is therefore performed with breath-holding and ECG gating. Although higher heart rates are typical in children, beta blockade and vasodilating agents are not used routinely. Retrospective ECG gating provides high temporal resolution in children with faster heart rates and allows for the acquisition of different heart phases with at least one phase obtained during the period of relative cardiac quiescence. However, retrospective ECG-gated studies are performed at the expense of high-radiation doses (typically 5 to 10 mSV), which is of particular concern in pediatric patients. Weight-based kVp protocols and automatic dose modulation during acquisition should be employed to reduce radiation exposure. Prospective ECG gating can be performed routinely in older children with slightly slower and regular heart rates (approximately less than 75 bpm) and in younger children with faster heart rates using a "target mode." The use of prospective gating can significantly reduce radiation doses (typically 1 to 3 mSV). Dual-source CT scanners can adjust

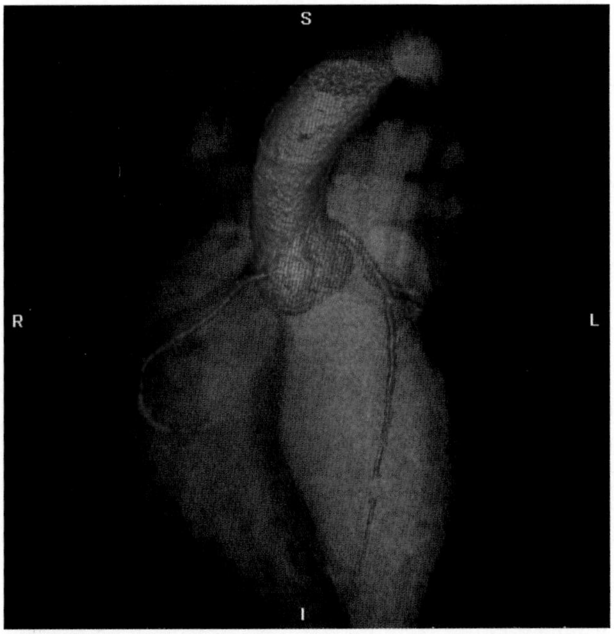

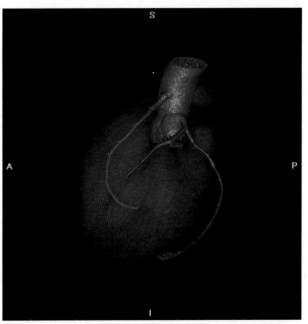

Figure 23.1. A 3-D volume-rendered image and axial MIP from a prospective ECG-gated CTA demonstrates normal origin of the LCA and RCA from the left and right coronary cusps.

Figure 23.2. A 3-D volume-rendered image from a prospective ECG-gated CTA in an asymptomatic patient demonstrates anomalously high origin of the RCA from the ascending aorta.

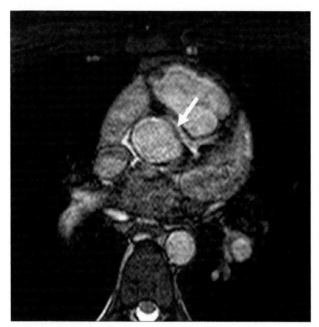

Figure 23.3. Axial oblique image from a respiratory navigator and ECG-triggered 3-D SSFP MR sequence in a child with chest pain demonstrates an anomalous origin of the LCA from the right coronary cusp and an interarterial (malignant) course between the aorta and pulmonary artery (arrow). The acute angle of origin may represent an intramural course of the proximal LCA.

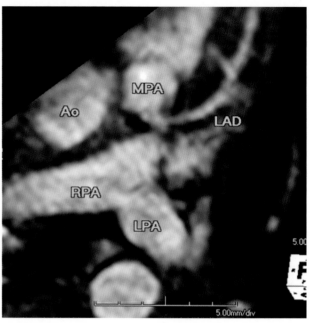

Figure 23.5. Axial oblique MIP image obtained from a respiratory navigator and ECG-triggered 3-D SSFP MR sequence in an infant with heart failure demonstrates anomalous origin of the left anterior descending artery (LAD) from the main pulmonary artery (MPA). Aorta (Ao), right pulmonary artery (RPA), left pulmonary artery (LPA).

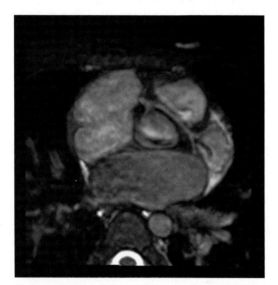

Figure 23.4. Axial oblique MIP image obtained from a respiratory navigator and ECG-triggered 3-D SSFP MR sequence in a teen with angina demonstrates a single coronary artery from the right coronary cusp that divides into RCA and LCA. The LCA passes interarterially before dividing into LAD and LCX arteries.

pitch based on heart rate. Faster rates result in a higher pitch, which also lowers the radiation dose.

Coronary artery anatomy evaluation on MRI is performed using a free breathing 3-D steady-state precession sequence (Fig. 23.5). Respiratory motion is minimized by using a respiratory navigator with image acquisition timed to occur during the period of maximum cardiac quiescence

(usually end-diastole for slower heart rates and end-systole for faster heart rates). This sequence allows relatively static evaluation of coronary artery anatomy with good spatial resolution (approximately 1-mm isotropic voxel sizes). Immediate perfusion imaging and 10-minute-delayed viability sequences can be also performed following the intravenous administration of gadolinium (0.1 to 0.2 mmol/kg) in cases positive for LCA anomalies, to assess for myocardial ischemia (decreased perfusion) and fibrosis (delayed myocardial enhancement).

Related Physics

Cardiac catheterization may be required for diagnostic or therapeutic intervention for anomalous coronary arteries. In ALCAPA the technique must be optimized in order to visualize the very small coronary arteries of an infant. Modes of operation include continuous fluoroscopy, high-dose-rate fluoroscopy, variable-frame-rate fluoroscopy, use of spot imaging, and operational mode variations. Continuous-mode fluoroscopy, as the name implies, will continuously expose the infant to radiation while imaging takes place. This mode is generally discouraged as it is unnecessary for adequate image quality. High-dose-rate fluoroscopy, by definition, includes systems that can exceed exposure rates in excess of 10 R/minute and are not used in pediatrics. Modern catheterization systems employ pulsed delivery of radiation in synchrony with image acquisition thereby lessening the total radiation burden to the patient. Pulse width and pulses per second delivered are user-controlled parameters, each of which can be employed to lower the radiation burden. The pulse width is the amount of time per second that the radiation is "on." Shorter widths deliver less radiation than longer pulses. Likewise, the number of pulses per second is proportional to the amount of radiation delivered whereby lower pulses per second lead to lower radiation at the expense of temporal resolution. Pulses per second can be tailored to the clinical indication. In conditions associated with high flow rates such as ALCAPA, higher pulses per second are necessary. Conversely, slower or venous rates can withstand lower pulse rates without sacrificing spatial or temporal resolution. The terms "variable-frame-rate" or "variable-pulse-rate" fluoroscopy, are synonymous. Operational mode variations exist between vendors. These include effective mA (real-time modulation of mAs based on attenuation), variable-beam filtration (real-time insertion or extraction of filters driven by noise), and various noise-reduction postprocessing techniques.

Differential Diagnosis

- Dilated cardiomyopathy (ALCAPA)
- Valvular (aortic stenosis or regurgitation)
  - Myocardial (severe right ventricular hypertrophy or hypertrophic cardioymyopathy)
  - Pericarditis, etc. in adolescence
  - ANOMALOUS LCA or RCA origin

Common Variants

Common variants include high/low take-off of the LCA above or below the left sinus of Valsalva and multiple ostia from the left sinus (individual ostia for both LAD and LCX).

Clinical Issues

Anomalous coronary artery takeoff and course may be discovered inadvertently during surgery for associated cono-truncal abnormalities such as tetralogy of Fallot or transposition of the great vessels or during cardiac valve repair in an older patient leading to surgical complications. Single coronary ostium may be predisposed to later development of atheroma.

Key Points

- Anomalous LCA from right sinus with an interarterial course is associated with a high incidence of sudden death in young adults after vigorous exercise.
- Anomalous LCA from pulmonary artery (ALCAPA) usually presents with heart failure at 6 to 8 weeks of age when the drop in pulmonary vascular resistance results in a steal phenomen from the LCA.
- In patients with a single coronary ostium, ostial atheroma can result in global ischemia.
- In patients with cono-truncal anomalies, accurate preoperative mapping of coronary pathways is important to avoid inadvertent injury during surgical repairs.

Further Reading

Baroldi G, Scomazzoni G. *Coronary Circulation in the Normal and Pathological Heart*. Washington, DC: Office of the Surgeon General; 1967.

Barth CW III, Roberts WC. Left main coronary artery originating from the right sinus of Valsalva and coursing between the aorta and pulmonary trunk. *J Am Coll Cardiol*. 1986;7:366–373.

Hirai N, Horiguchi J, Fujioka C, Kiguchi M, Yamamoto H, Matsuura N. Prospective versus retrospective ECG-gated 64-detector coronary CT angiography: assessment of image quality, stenosis, and radiation dose. *Radiology*. 2008;248:424–430.

Kim SY, Seo JB, Do KH, Heo JN, Lee JS, Song JW, et al. Coronary artery anomalies: classification and ECG-gated multi-detector row CT findings with angiographic correlation. *Radiographics*. 2006;26:317–333.

Sundaram B, Kreml R, Patel S. Imaging of coronary artery anomalies. *Radiol Clin N Am*. 2010;48:711–727.

CHAPTER 24

Myocarditis

Alan Vainrib, MD, Mark Goldman, MD, Michael Poon, MD, FACC, and Jeffrey Hellinger, MD, FACC

Definition

Myocarditis is a rare, sporadic nonischemic inflammatory disorder of the myocardium resulting in cardiac myocyte injury, which in turn may lead to myocyte necrosis, degeneration, or a combination thereof. Infrequently, the endocardium and/or pericardium may also be involved.

Clinical Features

The true incidence of pediatric myocarditis is unknown as most cases are subclinical. Based on autopsy data, the overall incidence of myocarditis may be as high as 10 in 100,000. Epidemics may occur in neonates infected with Coxsackie group B enterovirus (CBV). Presentation of myocarditis may be fulminant, acute, or chronic, with specific symptoms varying by age; the acute form is most common in pediatrics. Neonates and infants may present with a combination of fever, irritability, failure to thrive, feeding intolerance, respiratory distress, and sudden onset of congestive heart failure (CHF) with cyanosis or sudden cardiac death. Seventeen percent of infants dying of SIDS have underlying histopathologic evidence of myocardial infiltration; some may have polymerase chain reaction (PCR) evidence of enteroviridae or adenoviridae. In children and young adolescents to young adults, clinical presentation of myocarditis often includes constitutional and cardiac symptoms but onset tends to be more gradual. Constitutional symptoms include low-grade fever, chills, lethargy, myalgias, arthralgias, weakness, and poor appetite. Cardiac symptoms may include palpitations, chest pain, shortness of breath, dyspnea on exertion, easy fatigability, and orthopnea. There is often a history of upper respiratory tract infection or gastroenteritis within the month prior to the development of cardiac symptoms, although acute onset of CHF or ventricular arrhythmias may also occur. In older patients, symptoms can mimic myocardial ischemia or infarction. Physical exam findings include fever, tachycardia, arrhythmias, pallor, diminished pulses, CHF, murmur, and a pericardial friction rub (if there is concomitant pericarditis).

The electrocardiogram (ECG) is almost always abnormal, revealing sinus tachycardia, ventricular hypertrophy, ST segment changes, bundle branch blocks, and less commonly, atrioventricular (AV) block and prolonged QT interval. Cardiac enzymes, erythrocyte sedimentation rate, C-reactive protein, and white blood cell count may all be elevated. Viruses may be detected by culture or PCR from blood, nasopharyngeal mucosa, or stool specimens. Histopathology remains the gold standard for diagnosing myocarditis where myocardial tissue is obtained by endomyocardial biopsy (EMB) and interpreted using the Dallas Criteria, although sensitivity of EMB is invariably low (20 to 50 percent) because of sampling error. The Dallas Criteria defines *active myocarditis* as a myocardial inflammatory neutrophil or eosiniphil infiltrate with necrosis and/or degeneration of adjacent myocytes not showing features of ischemic changes found with coronary artery disease. *Borderline myocarditis* is defined as myocardial inflammatory infiltration with preserved and viable myocyte structure; no necrosis or degeneration is present.

Anatomy & Physiology

Myocarditis may be caused by infectious agents, autoimmune processes, and toxic exposures. Myocyte injury and cell loss may lead to: ventricular dilatation; mild, moderate, or severe globally depressed ventricular function with variable regional wall motion abnormalities; strain on the atrioventricular (AV) apparatus; AV valvular regurgitation; atrial dilatation; left- and right-sided CHF; arrhythmias; and sometimes death. Left ventricular dilatation with depressed contractility may lead to intracavitary thrombus formation with risk for systemic thromboembolism. Concomitant pericardial inflammation may cause pericardial thickening and/or pericardial effusion with or without cardiac tamponade. Viral infections are the most common etiology for developing myocarditis. Adenovirus (serotypes 2 and 5), CBV, and parvovirus b19 are among the most frequent viral organisms. Viral myocarditis is classified in acute, subacute, and chronic phases.

Imaging Findings

Chest radiography most often shows cardiomegaly, pulmonary edema, and pleural effusion. A large pericardial effusion may also be detected (Fig. 24.1). Echocardiography (ECHO) is performed with a transthoracic, two-dimensional technique. Findings include left ventricular (LV) enlargement, globally depressed LV function, and regional LV wall motion abnormalities. Less commonly, the right ventricle may also be enlarged with global dysfunction and regional wall motion abnormalities (Fig. 24.2). Other findings may include mitral regurgitation, tricuspid regurgitation, ventricular thrombus, pericardial effusion, and pleural effusions. Cardiac MRI (CMRI) is highly accurate in the diagnosis of myocarditis and has become an essential tool in the evaluation of suspected or known myocarditis (Fig. 24.3). The principal CMRI criteria for myocarditis are one or more regions of myocardial edema with corresponding abnormal wall motion, perfusion, and delayed hyperenhancement (DHE) in a nonischemic distribution, involving the intramyocardium (e.g., middle portion of the myocardium; Fig. 24.4). This is in distinction to myocardial ischemia, in which abnormal DHE is typically subendocardial. In addition, regions of abnormal myocardial perfusion and DHE do not follow a coronary arterial distribution. Delayed hyperenhancement is particularly useful in guiding a minimally invasive EMB. Cardiac CT angiography (CCTA) has a limited role given the required use of radiation and its restricted ability to assess myocyte physiology. Nevertheless, CCTA is valuable in evaluating coronary anomalies, congenital heart disease, and noncardiovascular thoracic anatomy, in addition to the myocardium. With a routine low-dose prospective ECG-gated CCTA protocol, regions of abnormal myocardial thickness, precontrast myocardial hypodensity (e.g., edema), and abnormal noncoronary patterns of myocardial enhancement (postcontrast) would suggest myocarditis. Abnormal enhancement may be accentuated if a low-dose rest-stress perfusion protocol is utilized (adolescents to young adults). If retrospective ECG gating is utilized, cardiac function can also be evaluated subjectively and ventricular end-systolic and end-diastolic volumes and ejection fraction can be quantified; abnormal global and regional myocardial wall motion and thickening could support the diagnosis of myocarditis. Finally, if a low-dose delayed phase is acquired, detection of noncoronary and nonischemic patterns of hyperenhancement would be highly suggestive for myocarditis. Cardiac radionucleotide imaging most commonly utilizes 2-deoxy-2-[^{18}F] fluoro-D-glucose (FDG) positron emission tomography (PET) combined with computed tomography (FDG PET-CT). In a cardiac PET-CT (CPET-CT) exam, increased hypermetabolic myocardial FDG activity localized to noncoronary distributions would be suggestive for myocarditis; abnormal activity may be global or regional. To provide a more comprehensive evaluation of cardiovascular structures and cardiac physiology, CPET-CT can be combined with coronary CTA. This however, is at the expense of increased radiation. Single photon emission CT (SPECT) Indium-111 is an alternative radionucleotide option for evaluation of myocarditis. Indium-111 is labeled to antimyosin (AM) antibodies. These antibodies bind to myosin released after myonecrosis occurs; increased activity will indicate regions of inflammation with myocyte injury. To plan and guide EMB, CCTA, PET-CT and cardiac SPECT (CSPECT) can all be used.

Imaging Strategy

Both chest radiography and ECHO are commonly obtained during the diagnostic evaluation of a pediatric patient with myocarditis. Chest radiography may be acquired with a single frontal projection or with frontal and lateral projections, depending on the age of the patient and clinical status. Although the chest X-ray and ECHO may not prove the diagnosis of myocarditis, they are essential for narrowing the differential diagnosis, suggesting potential etiologies, selecting additional imaging, and initiating clinical management. Cardiac MRI should be performed using a myocarditis protocol. Cardiac structure and function and myocyte physiology are all evaluated in one comprehensive examination, without radiation. A typical myocarditis protocol consists of: (1) ECG-gated T1-and T2-weighted dark blood sequences for cardiac structure and myocardial characteristics; (2) short- and long-axis cine sequences for qualitative assessment of myocardial wall motion and quantitative evaluation of ventricular end-systolic and end-diastolic volumes and ejection fraction; (3) real-time T1-weighted short axis perfusion sequence to assess global and regional myocardial blood flow; and (4) short- and long-axis delayed T1-weighted inversion recovery sequences to assess myocyte viability versus myocyte injury, necrosis, and/or scar. Radionucleotide imaging is recommended if MRI is contraindicated, nondiagnostic,

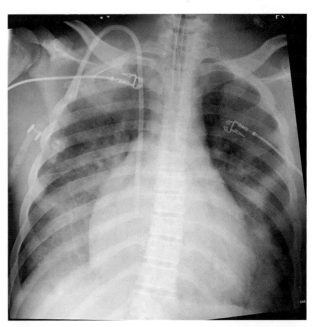

Figure 24.1. Frontal chest radiograph in an 8-year-old boy with end-stage renal disease and acute myocarditis who presented with acute CHF and uremia shows a small to moderate pericardial effusion and diffuse interstitial and alveolar pulmonary edema, greatest in the mid and lower lungs.

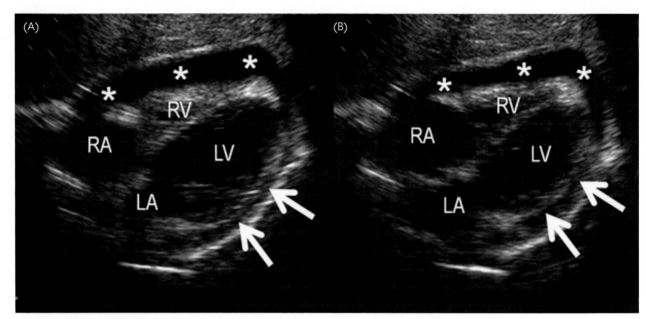

Figure 24.2. Diastolic (A) and systolic (B) static images from a four-chamber cine ECHO in a 17-year-old boy with early acute myocarditis who presented with a two-week history of constitutional symptoms, shortness of breath, and exercise intolerance show lack of myocardial thickening focally in the lateral wall of the left ventricle (arrows). Additional findings include a circumferential small pericardial effusion (asterisks) and secondary cardiac tamponade physiology. Right atrium (RA); left atrium (LA); right ventricle (RV); left ventricle (LV).

or not available. Although myocyte physiology is directly evaluated with both cardiac PET-CT and SPECT, FDG CPET-CT should be considered prior to CSPECT Indium111, given its advantages of greater spatial resolution, multiplanar projections, and assessment of noncardiovascular thoracic structures. Cardiac CT angiography is reserved for hemodynamically unstable or high anesthesia risk patients (precluding CMRI or CPET-CT) and when

the coronary arteries require evaluation. Surveillance ECHO and either CMRI or CPET-CT can be utilized to monitor clinical response to medical therapy and assess

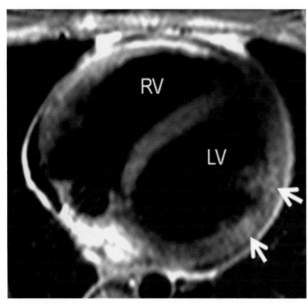

Figure 24.3. Transverse dark blood CMRI image in a child with myocarditis reveals two focal intramyocardial regions of mild hyperintensity (arrows) in the lateral wall of the left ventricle (LV). Right ventricle (RV).

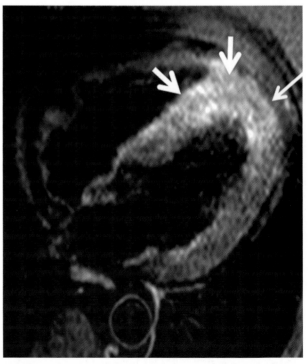

Figure 24.4. A ECG-gated T2-weighted transverse dark blood image in a 14-year-old girl with acute myocarditis who presented with low-grade fever, lethargy, myalgias, dyspnea on exertion, and easy fatigability 3 weeks following an episode of gastroenteritis reveals apical and apicoseptal hyperintensity consistent with myocardial edema (all arrows).

for complications, as per guidelines noted above for initial selection of diagnostic imaging modalities.

Related Physics

When performing cardiac catheterization for EMB it is important to be familiar with image-quality factors such as low-contrast object sensitivity, high-contrast object sensitivity (spatial resolution), temporal resolution, and image noise. Low-contrast object detection is necessary in differentiating the base of the heart from the diaphragm whereas detection of small contrast-enhanced coronary arteries against heart muscle would be an example of high-contrast spatial resolution. Temporal resolution allows visualization of structures in motion and is a necessary consideration for evaluation of decreased wall motion in myocarditis. The rapid heart rate in younger children poses a challenge in cardiac catheterization demanding higher temporal resolution. Image noise manifests as a mottled appearance of otherwise uniform structures and in general is a hindrance to low-contrast object detection. Image noise can be reduced by one of several techniques including increasing dose, image postprocessing, or real-time-frame-averaging.

Differential Diagnosis

Cardiomegaly and/or decreased ventricular function with CHF:

- Dilated cardiomyopathy
- Endocardial fibroelastosis
- Hypertrophic cardiomyopathy
- Myocardial sarcoma (primary)
- Left-sided obstructive lesions
- Anomalous left (ALCAPA) and right (ARCAPA) coronary arteries
- Carnitine deficiency
- Fabry disease
- Gaucher's disease
- Glycogen storage disease (e.g., Type II, Pompe disease)
- Hemochromatosis (autosomal recessive)
- Mitochondrial defects
- Muscular dystrophies
- Pericarditis (acute and chronic)
- Restrictive cardiomyopathies from diabetes, hemochromatosis (e.g., transfusion-related), Löffler's endocarditis, mediastinal radiation, myocardial metastasis, and postcardiac transplantation

Common Variants

In addition to CBV, adenovirus, and parvovirus, other viruses that may cause myocarditis include HIV, HCV, HHV6, and H1N1 influenza. Other infectious agents implicated in pediatric myocarditis include bacteria,

spirochetes, fungus, rickettsias, protozoa, and helminths. Bacterial myocarditis is relatively uncommon; however, myocarditis in pediatric patients may occur following acute rheumatic fever resulting from group A Streptococcus. The protozoan *Trypanosoma Cruzi* is the most common causative agent for myocarditis worldwide, endemic to Central and South America, causing Chagas' disease. Common autoimmune systemic diseases include collagen-vascular disorders, hypereosinophilia, giant cell myocarditis, and granulomatous disorders. Pediatric connective tissue disorders which may lead to myocarditis include systemic lupus erythematosus and mixed connective tissue disease. Eosinophilic myocarditis is a final common pathway of many systemic diseases such as vasculitis and hypersensitivity reactions. Toxic myocarditis may be caused by medical and nonmedical drugs and environmental exposures.

Key Points

- Myocarditis is a nonischemic inflammatory disorder of the myocardium, resulting in cardiac myocyte injury.
- Etiologies include viral infectious agents, autoimmune processes, and toxic exposures.
- Cardiac MRI shows hyperenhancement in a noncoronary and nonischemic distribution.
- Radionucleotide imaging and CCTA are utilized on a select basis.
- Endomyocardial biopsy may be required confirm the diagnosis.
- Immunosuppresive therapy may lead to substantial improvements in cardiac function and survival.

Survival of pediatric patients with myocarditis is good to excellent (69 to 97 percent). Most recover normal cardiac function without sequelae. Initial management includes supportive care, treatment of heart failure and arrhythmia, and administering immunosuppressive therapy. Advanced hemodynamic monitoring in an intensive care unit setting may include pulmonary artery catheterization, continuous ECG, invasive blood pressure monitoring, and sometimes extracorporeal membrane oxygenation (ECMO). Immunosuppressive therapy includes corticosteroids, cyclosporine, azathioprine, and/or intravenous immunoglobulin (IVIG); data for each is limited and there are currently no consensus guidelines using immunosuppressive therapy in the treatment of myocarditis. Corticosteroids have been shown to improve systolic function, ECG changes, and arrhythmias.

Further Reading

Aretz HT, Billingham ME, Edwards WD, Factor SM, Fallon JT, Fenoglio JJ, Olsen EG, Schoen FJ. Myocarditis: a histopathologic definition and classification. *Am J Cardiovasc Pathol.* 1987;*1*:3–14.

Durani Y, Egan M, Baffa J, Selbst SM, Nager AL. Pediatric myocarditis: presenting clinical characteristics. *Am J Emerg Med.* 2009;*27*: 942–947.

Kuhn B, Shapiro ED, Walls TA, Friedman AH. Predictors of outcome of myocarditis. *Pediatr Cardiol.* 2004;*25*:379–384.

McCrohon JA, Moon JC, Prasad SK, McKenna WJ, Lorenz CH, Coats AJ, Pennell DJ. Differentiation of heart failure related to dilated cardiomyopathy and coronary artery disease using gadolinium-enhanced cardiovascular magnetic resonance. *Circulation.* 2003;*108*:54–59.

Towbin J. Chapter 58. Myocarditis. In: Moss AL, Allen HD (Ed). Moss and Adams' heart disease in infants, children and adolescents: including the fetus and young adult. 7th edition. Philadelphia, PA. Wolters, Kluwer Health/ Lippincott Williams and Wilkins. pp 1207–1224.

Rasten-Almqvist P, Eksborg S, Rajs J. Myocarditis and sudden infant death syndrome. *APMIS.* 2002;*110*:469–480.

CHAPTER 25

L-Transposition of the Great Arteries

Sjirk J. Westra, MD

Definition

L-transposition of the great arteries (L-TGA) is a congenital cardiac anomaly characterized by inversion of the ventricles and great arteries. There is an abnormal connection between the atria and the ventricles (i.e., the right atrium is connected with the left ventricle and vice versa) and also between the ventricles and the great arteries (i.e., the left ventricle is connected with the pulmonary artery and the right ventricle with the aorta). This is called atrioventricular and ventriculoarterial discordance. Often, L-TGA is incorrectly referred to as "congenitally corrected transposition" because although the blood flow through the heart is directed physiologically, the right ventricle is ill-equipped to act as the systemic ventricle in the long term (Fig. 25.1).

Clinical Features

It is rare for patients with L-transposition to be completely asymptomatic. Associated abnormalities are common and determine the clinical presentation and prognosis. Ventricular septal defects (seen in 60 to 70 percent of L-TGA patients) may lead to congestive heart failure. Severe left ventricular outflow (subpulmonic) obstruction (in 30 to 50 percent) may cause cyanosis. Ebstein anomaly involving the left-sided tricuspid valve (in 30 percent) may present pulmonary edema and cardiac failure secondary to severe tricuspid regurgitation. Arrhythmias are also common, resulting from abnormalities of the conduction system. At older age, there is frequently a diminished exercise tolerance resulting from dysfunction of the systemic (morphologic right) ventricle.

Anatomy and Physiology

The right atrium connects via a right-sided mitral valve with a morphological left ventricle, which connects with the pulmonary artery without a subvalvular infundibulum. The left atrium connects via a left-sided tricuspid valve to a morphological right ventricle, which connects by way of a subaortic infundibulum with the aorta. The inverted ventricles and great arteries form an L-loop. The two great vessels lie side by side in (almost) the same coronal plane, without the normal spiraling course around each other. The coronary anatomy is typically the mirror image of normal (right-sided coronary gives rise to circumflex and anterior descending arteries). It is relatively common to find L-TGA in patients with dextrocardia and abdominal situs solitus.

Imaging Findings

The crucial imaging of findings of L-TGA to look for, through segmental analysis, is the double inversion and the L-loop of the great vessels, lying (almost) parallel to each other in the same coronal plane.

- Radiography: there is a straight upper-left border to the cardiac silhouette, caused by the left-sided position of the ascending aorta (Fig. 25.2).
- Echocardiography: identification of atria, ventricles, great arteries and their abnormal connections (segmental cardiac analysis); Note is made of the abnormal continuity between right-sided mitral and pulmonary valve annulus and the abnormal discontinuity between left-sided tricuspid valve and aortic valve annulus. The interventricular septum has an abnormally straight orientation rather than the normal curved course.
- CTA and MRI demonstrate the double discordance and the associated anomalies (Figs. 25.3 and 25.4). MRI is helpful for functional assessment of the systemic (morphological right) ventricle and to evaluate for regurgitation across the left-sided tricuspid valve, resulting from Ebstein anomaly (Figs. 25.5)

IMAGING PITFALLS: A common pitfall at cross-sectional imaging is failure to recognize the double inversion. The key is to notice the lack of normal spiraling of the great vessels around each other.

Imaging Strategy

Echocardiography is diagnostic in the majority of cases. Complementary tests are CT or MR, when there are associated abnormalities (VSD, subpulmonary stenosis, Ebstein). Functional evaluation of right ventricle (RV) function with dobutamine stress MRI is helpful in order to assess whether the RV can sustain the systemic circulation.

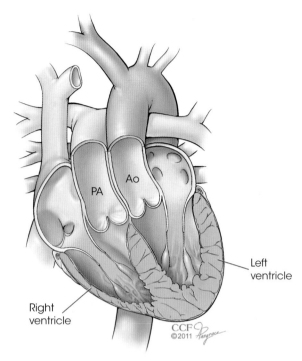

Figure 25.1. Diagram shows left-sided ascending aorta, connected to left-sided morphological (trabeculated) right ventricle. Right-sided pulmonary artery is connected to right-sided morphological left ventricle. A high VSD is commonly present.

Related Physics

The great vessel relationship can be easily evaluated with cardiac catheterization with attention to the following aspects of image processing: frame averaging, temporal recursive filtering, last image hold, edge enhancement and

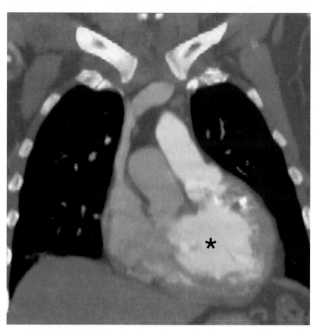

Figure 25.3. Coronal CTA of young child with L-TGA shows L-loop of ascending aorta, arising from a trabeculated left-sided morphological right ventricle (Star). Note also the abnormal side-by-side relationship of the great vessels.

smoothing, digital subtraction angiography (DSA), and roadmapping. Frame averaging is used as a method for reducing observed noise without the need to increase radiation with the downside being a slight decrease in temporal resolution. Temporal recursive filtering uses a method

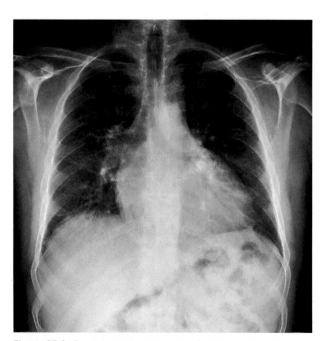

Figure 25.2. Frontal chest radiograph of adolescent male shows characteristic straightening of left upper-heart border, caused by L-looping of the embryological conotruncus.

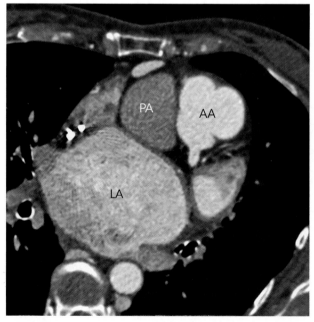

Figure 25.4. Axial cardiac CT image of 30-year-old male with L-TGA shows the pulmonary artery (PA) to lie to the right side of the L-looping ascending aorta (AA), with take-off of a coronary artery. Note also dilatation of the left atrium (LA), which resulted from massive regurgitation across the left-sided tricuspid valve from Ebstein anomaly (not shown).

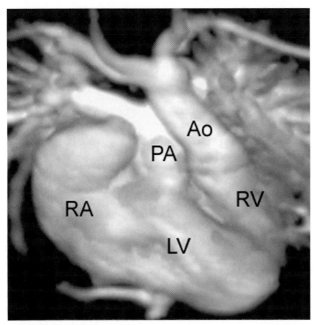

Figure 25.5. Oblique MRA shows abnormal side-to-side orientation of the main pulmonary artery (PA) and ascending aorta (Ao). Left ventricle (LV), Right ventricle (RV). (Image courtesy of Shi-Joon Yoo, MD.)

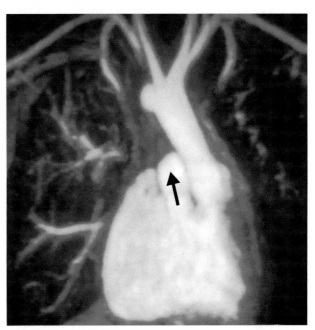

Figure 25.6. Young child with complex cyanotic congenital heart disease, with double-outlet right ventricle and L-transposition. Coronal MRA shows L-loop of ascending aorta, located to the left of the pulmonary outflow tract (arrow).

guided by the electrocardiogram whereby frames at like phases in the temporal sequence are added to currently acquired frames, effectively increasing signal and decreasing noise without increasing dose. There is a weighting factor that devalues older frames during the study. Last image hold freezes the last frame once fluoroscopy is stopped and saves it in memory for recall in viewing. This leads to shorter fluoroscopy times and obviates digital still images at a higher mAs, both contributing to decreased radiation dose to the patient. Edge enhancement and smoothing are techniques that can be employed real-time or during postprocessing to clarify edges while suppressing noise. Another technique most often used to image aortic root and coronary arteries is DSA. Here an image (mask) is taken before contrast medium is administered and shortly after the injection of the medium a digital run is acquired without change in imaging geometry. The mask is then subtracted offline from each frame in the run yielding a subtraction image containing only contrast-enhanced vessels. Roadmapping refers to the image obtained after a small bolus of contrast and is a technique used to plan the pathway for selective catheterization. This technique can theoretically decrease total fluoroscopy time during a longer or more complex procedure.

Differential Diagnosis

When the clinical presentation is that of congestive heart failure with increased pulmonary blood flow, the differential diagnosis includes isolated VSD, double-inlet ventricle, tricuspid atresia, and double-outlet right ventricle with subaortic VSD. When there is predominantly cyanosis with decreased pulmonary blood flow, the differential includes tetralogy of Fallot and related entities (Fig. 25.6).

When there is atrioventricular discordance with ventriculo-arterial concordance, the presentation is similar to D-TGA. "Crisscross heart" is a rare condition in which the inflow to the ventricles is maldirected.

Common Variants

L-transposition associated with ventricular hypoplasia, atrioventricular canal, straddling atrioventricular valves, aortic atresia, coarctation, or interruption.

Clinical Issues

The long-term prognosis of patients with L-TGA is critically dependent on the function of the systemic (morphologic right) ventricle and the development of tricuspid regurgitation. Surgical correction is aimed at correcting any associated abnormalities, such as the often-present VSD and subpulmonary stenosis. The balance between these two lesions (if both present) determines whether congestive heart failure or cyanosis is the most predominant presentation. Because the systemic (morphological right) ventricle is only perfused by a single coronary artery branch (the right coronary), investigators have shown limitations of myocardial perfusion because of a mismatch between oxygen supply and demand by the myocardium. Invariably, the function of the systemic ventricle deteriorates over time, which is aggravated by tricuspid regurgitation (either primarily, from an Ebstein-like deformity of the valve apparatus, or secondarily, from stretching of the valve annulus).

These problems have induced some to consider early repairs involving "reconnecting" the morphological left ventricle to the aorta, because this ventricle is better equipped to handle systemic blood pressures. This strategy involves a double switch procedure: a venous rerouting (analogous to the Mustard or Senning procedures that used to be performed for D-transposition), in combination with an arterial switch. In preparation for this, the left ventricle needs to be "prepared" to sustain systemic pressures, which can be accomplished by means of pulmonary artery banding. For this to be effective, this needs to be performed relatively early in life.

Functional cardiac MRI, in conjunction with high-dose dobutamine stress testing, is evolving to play a crucial role in the surgical decision process and is supplanting stress and/or dobutamine echocardiography for this purpose because MRI is more reliable and reproducible than echocardiography, and it is less dependent on availability of an adequate acoustic window.

Key Points

- L-TGA is rarely an asymptomatic lesion ("congenitally corrected transposition" is usually a misnomer).
- Clinical presentation is determined by associated abnormalities: VSD, subpulmonary stenosis, systemic aortic valve regurgitation, failure of the "systemic" RV.
- L-TGA is a relatively common finding in dextrocardia.

- Functional dobutamine stress MRI is helpful for assessing the systemic RV function.
- For symptomatic patients, an early double switch procedure may be considered. These patients require frequent follow up with cross-sectional imaging.

Further Reading

Chang DS, Barack BM, Lee MH, Lee HY. Congenitally corrected transposition of the great arteries: imaging with 16-MDCT. *AJR Am J Roentgenol.* 2007;*188*(5):W428–W430.

Lapierre C, Déry J, Guérin R, Viremouneix L, Dubois J, Garel L. Segmental approach to imaging of congenital heart disease. *Radiographics.* 2010;*30*(2):397–411.

Park JH, Han MC, Kim CW. MR imaging of congenitally corrected transposition of the great vessels in adults. *AJR Am J Roentgenol.* 1989;*153*(3):491–494.

Schmidt M, Theissen P, Deutsch HJ, Dederichs B, Franzen D, Erdmann E, Schicha H. Congenitally corrected transposition of the great arteries (L-TGA) with situs inversus totalis in adulthood: findings with magnetic resonance imaging. *Magn Reson Imaging.* 2000;*18*(4):417–422.

Tulevski II, van der Wall EE, Groenink M, Dodge-Khatami A, Hirsch A, Stoker J, Mulder BJ. Usefulness of magnetic resonance imaging dobutamine stress in asymptomatic and minimally symptomatic patients with decreased cardiac reserve from congenital heart disease (complete and corrected transposition of the great arteries and subpulmonic obstruction). *Am J Cardiol.* 2002;*89*(9):1077–1081.

Warnes CA: Transposition of the great arteries. *Circulation.* 2006;*114*(24):2699–2709.

CHAPTER 26

Aortic Coarctation

Melissa A. Daubert, MD and Jeffrey C. Hellinger, MD

Definition

Coarctation of the thoracic aorta is a focal, eccentric, obstructive narrowing involving the aortic isthmus, the portion of the distal aortic arch extending from the left subclavian artery (LSCA) origin to the ductus arteriosus. The narrowing results from an abnormal sling of fibromuscular ductal tissue encircling the aorta and is characterized by its location relative to the site of insertion of the ductus arteriosus: preductal, juxaductal, and postductal.

Clinical Features

The preductal type predominates in children less than 1 year of age, and the postductal type is more common in children greater than 1 year of age. Coarctation occurs in 1.8 to 9.8 percent of reported congenital heart disease, with most studies demonstrating an incidence of 5 to 6 percent. Males predominate with a male to female ratio of 1.2:1 to 2.3:1. Most cases of aortic coarctation occur sporadically, but both environmental factors and genetic causes may contribute. The clinical presentation and course depend upon the location of the coarctation, the rate of ductal closure, the severity of the coarctation, the presence of collateral circulation, and other concomitant cardiovascular abnormalities. Symptomatic neonates and infants often have associated congenital heart lesions; presentation may include lethargy, poor feeding tolerance, failure to thrive, congestive heart failure, renal insufficiency, and circulatory collapse (e.g., shock). Physical examination findings that may suggest hemodynamic compromise include respiratory distress, lethargy, cool extremities with poor capillary refill, and diminished pulses. Upper-extremity systolic hypertension relative to the lower extremity is a highly sensitive physical examination finding for coarctation and, if detected, can narrow the differential diagnosis.

Aortic coarctation diagnosed beyond infancy is usually isolated or accompanied by a bicuspid aortic valve (BAV; approximately 70 percent of patients). Presentation may include fatigue, exertional dyspnea, claudication, chest pain, headaches, dizziness, epistaxis, fevers, and/or asymptomatic hypertension. Important physical examination findings include a systolic ejection murmur at the left sternal border, diminished femoral pulses, and systolic blood pressure in the upper extremities greater than that of the lower extremities. It may also be possible to auscultate continuous bruits in the axillae and back (caused by collateral blood flow) and a systolic ejection click at the apex (reflective of a BAV).

Anatomy and Physiology

The ductal theory hypothesizes that as the LSCA migrates cephalad through the differential growth of the dorsal aorta, the ductal ostium from the sixth arch is pulled into the aorta, forming the circumferential sling; obstruction develops when there is postnatal constriction of the ductus arteriosus. Contributing to the ductal theory and lending explanation to the spectrum of thoracic aortic coarctation and their associated cardiovascular lesions is the hemodynamic theory. This theory hypothesizes that congenital lesions leading to decreased antegrade flow in the ascending aorta (e.g., left-sided obstructive lesions, left-to-right shunts) result in reversal of flow across the fetal isthmus, altering the "branch-point" angulation and accentuating LSCA cephalad migration.

The primary physiologic sequelae of coarctation is increased left ventricular afterload and decreased systemic perfusion with activation of the sympathetic and renin-angiotensin systems, resulting in increased blood pressure. In neonates and infants with coarctation (e.g., preductal type), systemic perfusion is dependent upon maintaining patency of the ductal arteriosus. Once the ductus closes, the inability to rapidly develop collateral blood flow and counter the rising afterload may lead to left heart dysfunction with chamber enlargement and congestive heart failure. Pulmonary hypertension with right heart dysfunction, renal insufficiency, and systemic shock may also develop. With isolated coarctation, when sufficient compensatory collateral flow develops to direct blood below the obstruction, clinical presentation is delayed until later in life (young child to adult, e.g., postductal type); collateral pathways include the subclavian, internal mammary, intercostal, cervical, scapular, and thoracodorsal arteries.

The associated congenital cardiovascular abnormalities may occur in 44 to 84 percent of patients with coarctation; the majority of these patients will present by 2 years of age. Such abnormalities include patent ductus arteriosus (PDA), BAV, tubular hypoplasia of the aortic arch, interrupted

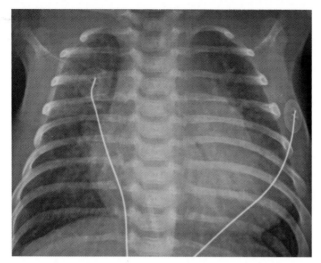

Figure 26.1. Frontal chest radiograph in a neonate with aortic coarctation shows cardiomegaly with moderate pulmonary venous congestion, suggestive for a left-sided obstructive lesion with congestive heart failure.

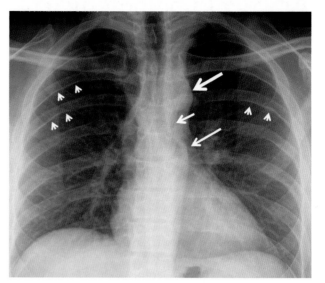

Figure 26.2. Frontal chest radiograph in an adolescent with coarctation shows "figure of 3" left upper mediastinal shadow (arrows) and both inferior rib scalloping and sclerosis (arrowheads), indicative of chronic coarctation with compensatory collateral flow.

aortic arch, atrial septal defects (ASDs), ventricular septal defects (VSDs), aortic valvular disease, mitral valvular disease, and transposition of the great arteries (TGA).

Imaging Findings

Diagnostic evaluation of coarctation focuses on structural morphology of the coarctation (location, length, degree of narrowing, and patency of the ductus arteriosus), physiology of the coarctation (pressure gradient, extent of collateral arteries), and the presence of associated congenital and acquired cardiovascular abnormalities (cardiomegaly, pulmonary venous congestion). Concomitant congenital cardiovascular anomalies must also be ruled out.

Chest radiography has moderate sensitivity (50 to 75 percent) for detection of coarctation depending on the age of the patient, the degree of narrowing, and the presence of associated cardiac defects. In the neonate and infant, the heart is typically enlarged and pulmonary venous congestion is present (Fig. 26.1). In the young child to young adult (e.g., isolated coarctation), findings include a prominent aortic arch and proximal descending aorta silhouette with a "figure of 3" contour, posterior rib scalloping and/ or sclerosis, and a heart size that is typically normal or mildly enlarged (Fig. 26.2). The waist of the "figure of 3" corresponds to the focal coarctation; the superior portion of the shadow reflects enlargement of the distal aortic arch and left subclavian artery proximal to the coarctation; the inferior portion of the shadow corresponds to poststenotic dilatation of the descending aorta distal to the coarctation. Rib scalloping and sclerosis occurs as a result of enlarged intercostal arteries and directly correlates with the severity and duration of coarctation.

Transthoracic echocardiography (TTE) is an ideal modality to assess for coarctation as it is noninvasive, requires

no radiation, and is readily performed. However, the acoustic window and diagnostic accuracy varies inversely with age and size of the patient. In neonates and infants, TTE has a sensitivity of 93 to 98 percent with positive predictive value as high as 97 percent and 100 percent, respectively. Grayscale imaging may reveal narrowing at the isthmus with posterior indentation. Color mapping can depict turbulent flow, and Doppler tracings show increased velocities across the coarctation; the pressure gradient is estimated using velocities in the modified Bernoulli equation (Fig. 26.3).

In older children to young adults, magnetic resonance imaging (MRI) with contrast-enhanced MR angiography (MRA; sensitivity 98 percent, specificity 99 percent) is superior to TTE for depicting the coarctation and the thoracic arterial system (e.g., caliber and course of the entire thoracic aorta, patency, caliber, and branching pattern of the aortic arch arteries and extent of collateral arteries; Fig. 26.4). Phase-contrast MRI is applied to measure the gradient across the coarctation and quantify collateral flow (Fig. 26.5). Computed tomography angiography (CTA) is a useful and sensitive alternative modality when MRI is contraindicated or unavailable, yielding 100 percent accuracy for detecting coarctation of the aorta. Collateral arteries are assessed with robust detail. The extent of systemic collaterals directly correlates with the pressure gradient across the aortic obstruction (Fig. 26.6). In general, noninvasive MRA and CTA have replaced catheter angiography in the diagnostic evaluation of aortic coarctation.

Imaging Strategy

The diagnostic algorithm for suspected coarctation is shown in Figure 26.7. Chest radiography is recommended as the

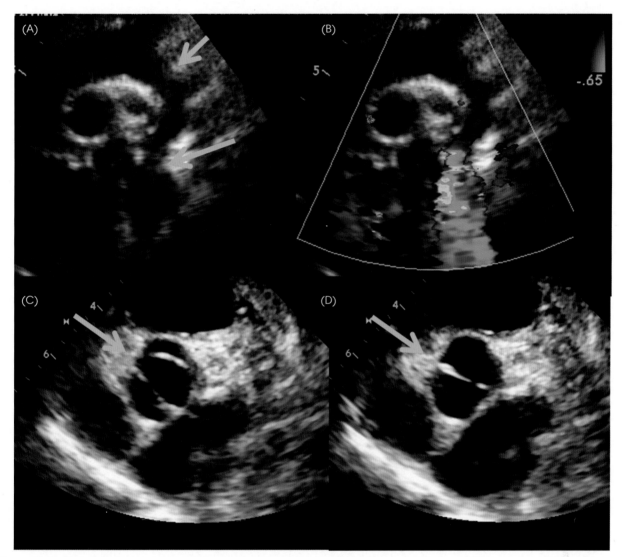

Figure 26.3. (A) Two-dimensional gray-scale suprasternal long-axis transthoracic echocardiogram (TTE) in a 3-year-old boy with asymptomatic upper-extremity systolic hypertension reveals mid aortic arch hypoplasia (short arrow) with narrowing at the isthmus (long arrow) and poststenotic dilatation, consistent with coarctation. (B) Color Doppler demonstrates accelerated velocity across the narrowing. The patient had a bicuspid aortic valve as shown in diastole (C) and systole (D).

first imaging modality. In neonates, infants, and young children, an echocardiogram (TTE) should be performed next. If TTE has a suboptimal acoustic window, MRI with MRA should subsequently be performed. For older children and adults, MRI with MRA is the initial study of choice. If MRI is not available or there are contraindications to MRI (or in the neonate or infant requiring MRI with MRA), then CTA with low-radiation-dose technique can be obtained. Following a positive MRI-MRA or CTA, echocardiography (if not previously obtained) is recommended prior to surgical or endovascular repair in order to assess cardiac morphology and function and exclude other cardiac anomalies. Conventional angiography is reserved for endovascular treatment with balloon angioplasty, stent placement, or both.

Related Physics

Several fluoroscopic applications can be employed for endovascular treatment of aortic coarctation. These include cine-fluorography, catheter-assisted intervention, biplane imaging, bolus chasing, and cross sectional cone-beam reconstructed fluoroscopic acquisitions. Cine-fluorography refers to continuous or pulsed real-time irradiation during the injection of intra-aortic iodinated contrast. It is used in suspected coarctation to produce an overview of the extent and location of the coarctation and associated pathology. One interventional procedure for coarctation includes balloon dilatation performed de novo in the fetus and for recoarctation following repair. Biplane may be useful for some cases in which there is unusual anatomy of the coronary arteries. Newer technologies

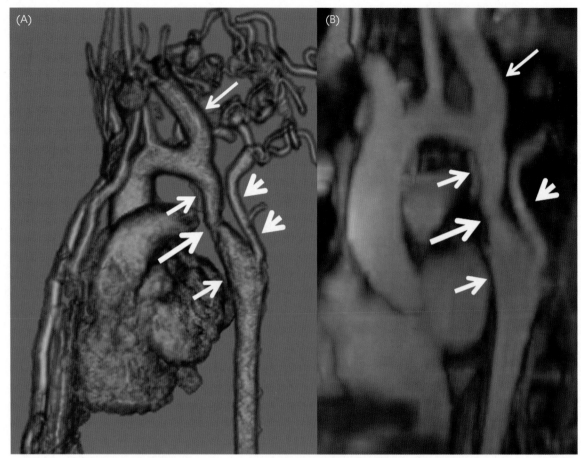

Figure 26.4. Volume rendering (A) and maximum-projection MR imaging (B) in a teen with coarctation show obstructive juxta-ductal narrowing (biggest arrow on left) with proximal and distal aortic dilatation (upper and lower arrows on left) and an enlarged left subclavian artery (top arrow on right). Note the well-developed supra-aortic collateral arterial network, which feeds into the descending aorta below the coarctation via a single dominant vertical mediastinal collateral artery (arrowheads).

have evolved to permit limited cross-sectional evaluation of the anatomy while in the catheterization suite using rotational acquisition of a cone beam (rather than a fan beam of CT), which is then reconstructed into axial images.

Differential Diagnosis

Aortic arch developmental anomalies:
- Tubular hypoplasia
- Interrupted aortic arch
- Shone's complex (supravalvular mitral membrane, parachute mitral valve, subaortic stenosis, and coarctation of the aorta)

Structural deficiency aortopathies:
- PHACE syndrome (posterior fossa brain malformations, cervicofacial hemangiomas, arterial anomalies, coarctation of the aorta, and eye abnormalities)
- Williams syndrome (supravalvular aortic stenosis)
- Noonan's syndrome

Autoimmune inflammatory aortopathies:
- Takayasu arteritis (adolescent to adult)
- Giant cell arteritis (adult)

Chromosomal abnormalities associated with coarctation of the aorta include:
- Turner (45 XO karyotype)
- Trisomy 13
- Trisomy 18

Acquired forms of aortic coarctation can be:
- Posttraumatic (e.g., undiagnosed injury resulting in luminal narrowing)
- Postsurgical (e.g., residual coarctation versus iatrogenic narrowing)
- After endovascular intervention (e.g., in-stent restenosis, stent kinking)

Common Variants

Aortic coarctation can present along a spectrum of disease. This can range from a critically ill newborn with severe

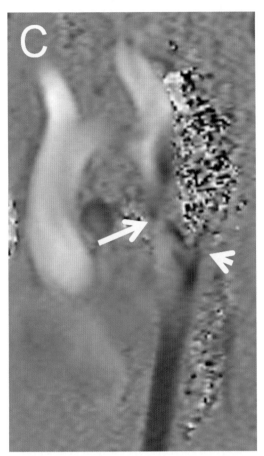

Figure 26.5. Phase-contrast imaging demonstrates turbulent signal across the narrowing (left arrow) and retrograde flow in the collateral artery (right arrowhead).

obstruction and heart failure to an asymptomatic adolescent with a systolic murmur, upper-extremity hypertension, and diminished lower-extremity pulses. In adults, the initial presentation may be with an aortic aneurysm proximal to a previously undiagnosed coarctation. It is important to determine if a recently diagnosed coarctation of the aorta is isolated or associated with other congenital heart lesions and/or part of a systemic syndrome or genetic disorder.

Clinical Issues

Early diagnosis (e.g., blood pressure screening) and intervention are paramount to minimizing morbidity and mortality. Untreated aortic coarctation in neonates and infants has an extremely poor prognosis (50 percent mortality rate) without urgent surgical intervention. Milder forms of coarctation of the aorta can take years or decades to become symptomatic. However, the long-term effects of systemic hypertension from aortic coarctation may lead to late cardiovascular complications (even after definitive treatment), reducing life expectancy as compared to the general population; in adults with untreated coarctation, nearly 90 percent of patients die by the age of 50 years. Chronically elevated blood pressure in the upper body results in left ventricular hypertrophy that can cause congestive heart failure in early to mid adulthood; elevated blood pressure is also associated with an increased incidence of premature coronary artery disease, ischemic heart disease, cerebral vascular accidents (e.g., ischemia, hemorrhage), aortic valvular disease (e.g., stenosis or insufficiency related to a BAV), aortic root dilatation, aortic aneurysms (e.g., proximal to a coarctation), acute aortic disease (e.g., dissection, rupture), and bacterial endocarditis.

In all patients, medical management focuses on controlling hypertension and optimizing cardiac function. In neonates and infants, if the ductus is patent with right to left flow (e.g., ductal-dependent systemic perfusion), prostaglandins

(A)

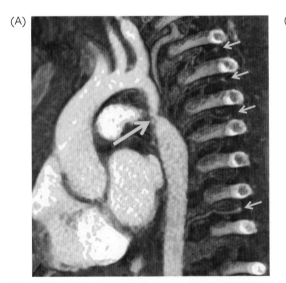

(B)

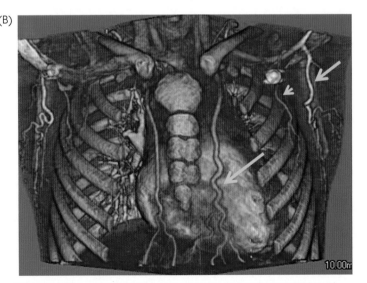

Figure 26.6. Volume-rendered contrast-enhanced CT image (A) in a child with coarctation demonstrates obstructive narrowing at the isthmus (long arrow). Enlarged intercostal arteries provide retrograde flow into the aorta below the coarctation (small arrows between ribs). The intercostal arteries receive flow from internal mammary (long arrow) (B) and other collaterals (other arrows).

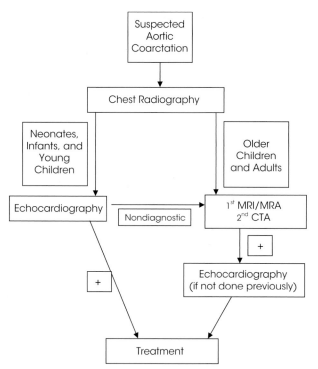

Figure 26.7. Diagnostic imaging algorithm for suspected aortic coarctation.

are initiated to maintain ductal patency. Definitive management requires surgical repair (e.g., resection with interposition graft). In select patients, endovascular therapy is an option with balloon angioplasty, stent placement, or both. Age at the time of coarctation repair is a predictive value for operative mortality (2 to 41 percent, highest in infants >1 year old), recoarctation (4 to 26 percent, highest in infants >1 year old), and residual hypertension (12.5 to 21 percent, lowest reported prevalence when operated between 1 and 5 years old). To optimize surgical outcome and minimize potential future cardiovascular risk, elective coarctation repair is recommended in early childhood (1 to 5 years of age) and should not be delayed past 10 years of age.

The prognosis in patients who have undergone surgical or endovascular repair of aortic coarctation is usually excellent. The presence of hypertension at the first postoperative evaluation and the development of postoperative paradoxical hypertension are additional risk factors for chronic hypertension and acquired cardiovascular disease.

These patients should be followed closely for recurrent coarctation, development of coronary artery disease, and progression of associated cardiac defects (e.g., calcific aortic stenosis and/or insufficiency of a bicuspid aortic valve).

Key Points

- Coarctation of the thoracic aorta is a focal, eccentric, obstructive narrowing of the isthmus.
- Types include preductal, juxaductal, or postductal, based upon the location relative to the ductus arteriosus.
- Preductal type predominates in children < 1 year of age; postductal predominates in children > 1 year.
- Associated congenital cardiovascular lesions are common (44 to 84 percent).
- Imaging strategy should include: TTE (> 90 percent sensitivity) in infants and young children; MRI-MRA (98 percent sensitivity) in older children and adults; Low-dose CTA (100 percent sensitivity) when MRI is contraindicated or unavailable.
- Early diagnosis of coarctation and associated cardiac abnormalities are essential to minimizing morbidity and mortality.
- Patients require lifetime surveillance for recurrent coarctation, hypertension, secondary cardiovascular complications, and progression of associated congenital heart defects.

Further Reading

Coarctation of the aorta. In: Gersony WM, Rosenbaum MS, eds. *Congenital Heart Disease in the Adult.* First edition. New York, NY: McGraw-Hill; 2002:93–108.

Ferguson EC, Krishnamurthy R, Oldham SA. Classic imaging signs of congenital cardiovascular abnormalities. *Radiographics.* 2007;27(5):1323–1334.

Hellinger JC, Cervantes LF, Medina LS. Congenital disease of the aortic arch: coarctation and arch anomalies. In: Medina S, Blackmore C, Applegate K, eds. *Evidence-Based Imaging in Pediatrics.* First edition. New York, NY: Springer; 2009:359–379.

Weber OM, Higgins CB. MR evaluation of cardiovascular physiology in congenital heart disease: flow and function. *J Cardiovasc Magn Reson.* 2006;8(4):607–617.

CHAPTER 27

Scimitar Syndrome

Lok Yun Sung, MD, Cheng Ting Lin, MD, Varghese Cherian, MD, MS, and Jeffrey C. Hellinger, MD, FACC

Definition

Anomalous pulmonary venous return is a rare congenital cardiac lesion (<1 percent of congenital heart disease) in which the pulmonary veins drain into systemic veins or the right atrium, resulting in a left-to-right cardiac shunt and admixture of deoxygenated and oxygenated blood. Normally, pulmonary veins drain into the left atrium, with a configuration of single bilateral superior and inferior pulmonary vein trunks. Partial anomalous pulmonary venous return (PAPVR) occurs when some, but not all of the pulmonary veins have aberrant drainage. Partial anomalous pulmonary venous return may be an isolated lesion or associated with other congenital cardiac as well as congenital pulmonary lesions.

Clinical Features

Clinical presentation of affected pediatric patients will vary depending upon the degree of shunting (e.g., number and size of anomalous veins), the level of anomalous connections, and the presence of associated lesions. With isolated PAPVR, neonates and infants are usually asymptomatic. As the pulmonary vascular resistance falls, a significant left-to-right shunt may lead to right heart volume overload, pulmonary hypertension, poor oxygenation, and right heart failure; rise in left atrial pressure may also lead to left heart failure with pulmonary venous congestion. Symptoms may include respiratory distress, tachypnea, feeding intolerance, and failure to thrive; initially acyanotic, the neonate may become cyanotic (e.g., decreased oxygen saturations). Diagnosis in young children to adults is primarily incidental (e.g., diagnosed on imaging studies). Significant left-to-right shunting over time can progress to right heart volume overload, enlarged right cardiac chambers, pulmonary hypertension, and decreased oxygenation; symptomatic patients may present with dyspnea, fatigue, variable acyanosis to cyanosis, arrhythmias (e.g., supraventricular from right atrial enlargement), hemoptysis (from pulmonary hypertension), and/or right heart failure. Additionally, patients may present with fevers and recurrent pneumonia related to associated underlying abnormal lung development and congenital lung lesions (e.g., bronchopulmonary sequestration).

Anatomy and Physiology

The embryologic lung buds initially drain via a venous plexus into developing systemic veins. The venous plexus eventually fuses with a developing common pulmonary vein (CPV, formed from a primitive left atrium outpouching); pulmonary and systemic venous primitive connections are obliterated. The CPV is resorbed into the wall of the left atrium resulting in variable pulmonary vein ostia and branching patterns. Partial anomalous pulmonary venous return results from a combination of abnormal development of the CPV (e.g., incomplete resorption) and its anastomoses with the primitive venous plexus, along with persistent connections to systemic veins.

In PAPVR, drainage may be into the superior vena cava (SVC), right atrium, coronary sinus, azygous vein, or the inferior vena cava (IVC). A hemodynamically significant shunt results in increased pulmonary blood flow (PBF) and cardiomegaly (e.g., right heart). Often, PAPVR occurs in isolation; the right lung is more commonly affected than the left. In right PAPVR, there may be an associated sinus venosus defect or potentially more complex pulmonary developmental anomalies in the spectrum of congenital pulmonary venolobar syndrome, including bronchopulmonary sequestration, scimitar syndrome, and horseshoe lung.

Concomitant bronchopulmonary sequestration is typically extralobar. By definition, there is systemic arterial supply from the descending thoracic or proximal abdominal aorta. In addition to the IVC or azygous vein, venous drainage in the setting of bronchopulmonary sequestration may also occur the hemiazygous vein.

Scimitar syndrome (e.g., hypogenetic lung syndrome) comprises 3 to 5 percent of all cases of PAPVR. Most commonly, the anomalous vein drains into the IVC at or below the level of the diaphragm (e.g., suprahepatic IVC). Less commonly, drainage may occur into the hepatic vein, portal vein, azygous vein, coronary sinus, or right atrium. The right lung is almost exclusively involved and is often hypoplastic or has partial agenesis, associated with dextroposition of the heart and ipsilateral decreased pulmonary blood flow. Additional anomalies associated with scimitar syndrome include bronchogenic cyst, bronchopulmonary sequestration, horseshoe lung, accessory diaphragm, and congenital diaphragmatic hernia. Frequently, there may be associated systemic arterial supply in the absence of an associated sequestration.

Imaging Findings

Chest radiography is used to assess the pulmonary vascularity and heart size and to exclude other potential pathology; radiographic findings will reflect the extent of anomalous drainage, degree of shunting, and associated lesions. Echocardiography with gray-scale and Doppler interogation, directly depicts the number, location and course of the pulmonary veins, determines the direction of blood flow, and excludes flow obstruction.

Magnetic Resonance Imaging and Angiography (MRI-MRA) and computed tomographic angiography (CTA) with advanced 2-D (e.g., multiplanar reformations, maximum-intensity projections) and 3-D (e.g., volume rendering) visualization techniques, directly assess the cardiac and venous morphology with superior detail, compared to echocardiography (Fig. 27.1). Distinct advantages of MRI include quantifying the shunt ratio and determining the direction of venous flow (using phase contrast imaging; Fig. 27.2). Additionally, CTA is useful for the visualization of the airway and lung parenchyma and assessment of associated pulmonary developmental anomalies (Fig. 27.3).

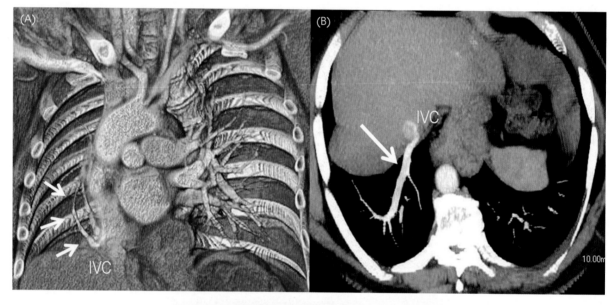

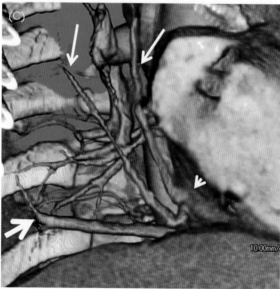

Figure 27.1. Anterior volume-rendered (VR) CTA display (A) from a 21-year-old male following pneumonia confirms two right middle lobe (RML) anomalous veins (arrows) draining into the supra-diaphragmatic inferior vena cava (IVC [on a and b]; arrowhead [on c]), corresponding to the scimitar veins seen on the chest radiograph. A third anomalous vein drains the posterior segment of the right lower lobe (RLL) into the IVC, as shown on the axial maximum-intensity projection display. Anterior (C) VR image demonstrates the relationships of the RML and RLL anomalous pulmonary veins. The two RML veins converge at a common ostium at the IVC, superior and anterior to the RLL vein. The RLL vein (fat arrow) drains into the left atrium.

In PAPVR, a significant shunt will manifest radiographically as increased pulmonary vascularity (e.g., increased caliber of arteries and veins with distinct margins) and cardiomegaly. Scimitar syndrome is distinguished by a curved vascular shadow (resembling a Turkish scimitar sword) medially in the right lower lung zone, with its apex extending from the midlung to the cardiophrenic angle—representing the anomalous draining common pulmonary vein. Additionally, there may be volume loss in the right lung, ipsilateral mediastinal shift, dextroposition of the heart, and diminished ipsilateral pulmonary vascularity (Fig. 27.4).

Imaging Strategy

In suspected PAPVR, chest radiography is recommended as the initial screening modality. Echocardiography should be performed next as it is noninvasive and is readily performed with high accuracy. If echocardiography cannot identify all veins or when more comprehensive imaging is required following the diagnosis of PAPVR, MRI-MRA or CTA is indicated. Of the two techniques, MRI-MRA is given first consideration as it utilizes no radiation or iodinated contrast material and can evaluate the shunt ratio and venous flow dynamics; CTA is indicated when MRI-MRA is contraindicated or not available or if detailed evaluation of the airway and lung parenchyma is also required. Cardiac catheterization is reserved for endovascular procedures or direct hemodynamic evaluation (e.g., flow, oxygen sampling, right heart and pulmonary pressures, shunt ratio quantification).

Related Physics

Cardiac catheterization for endovascular repair of Scimitar syndrome can involve large doses of radiation. For this reason one must be aware of federal and state regulations, some of which include advanced metrics such as dose area product (DAP) and Kerma area product (KAP), basic metrics such as entrance skin exposure, fluoroscopic time, peak and cumulative skin dose, and reporting of sentinel events. The DAP is the interventional reference point dose multiplied by the field size at the skin entry point. The interventional reference point is 15 centimeters above the patient support table. The KAP is similar to the DAP except it is the dose to air at the same interventional reference point and field size. Either can be used to quantify total radiation burden to the patient during a procedure and both are cumulative. Entrance skin exposure is the exposure rate at a given location on the skin multiplied by the total exposure time at that location. Skin dose is skin exposure multiplied by back scatter, which in most cases is a value between 1.3 to 1.5 centigray per Roentgen (cGy/R). Peak skin dose is measured at the skin location where the majority of irradiation has occurred. This is the location where skin damage would happen first if any were to occur. Cumulative skin exposure is equal to the average exposure rate during the case times the total beam on-time of the case. To determine cumulative, dose one simply multiplies the exposure rate and exposure time and back scatter factor for any patch of skin. In practice this is difficult in that the exposure rate at any given moment is difficult to estimate. In the case of Scimitar syndrome,

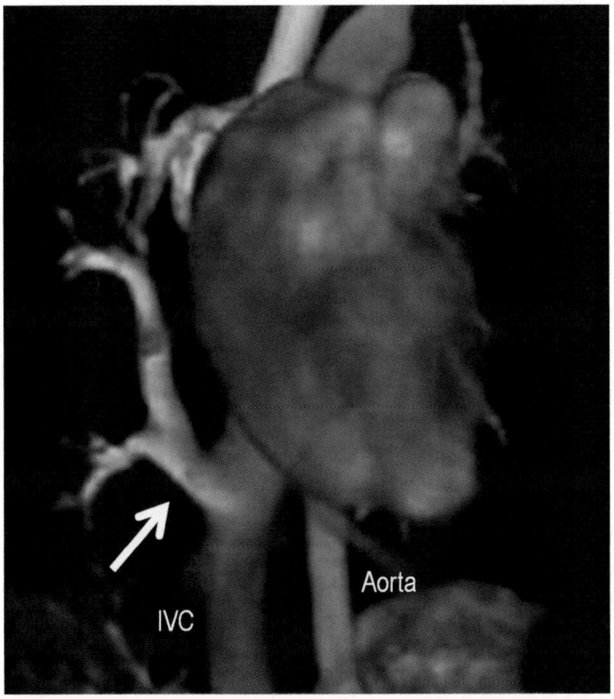

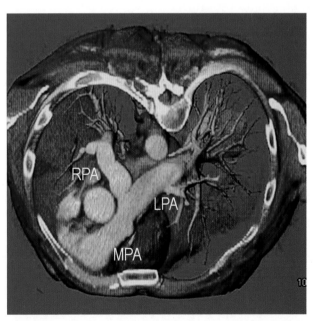

Figure 27.2. Coronal VR from MRI/MRA in a 14-year-old female with a hypoplastic right lung on chest radiography shows a common scimitar vein (arrow) draining the right lung, entering the IVC (IVC). Aorta (Aorta).

Figure 27.3. Axial cranial-caudal volume rendering generated from CTA in a teen with Scimitar syndrome shows moderate dilation of the pulmonary arteries with asymmetric pulmonary blood flow, related to the hypogenetic right lung. MPA: main pulmonary artery, RPA: right pulmonary artery, LPA: left pulmonary artery.

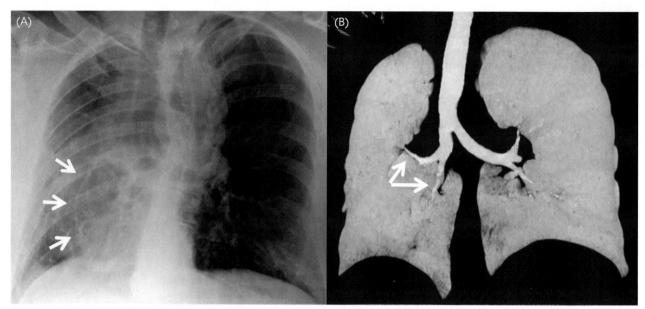

Figure 27.4. Frontal chest radiograph in a 21-year-old male following treatment for pneumonia reveals persistent cardiac dextroposition, rightward mediastinal shift, mild right lung hypoplasia, and two scimitar veins in the medial right lower lung field (arrows). A coronal minimum-intensity projection from the patient's chest CTA reveals right upper lobe agenesis with the right main bronchus dividing into right middle (smaller arrow) and lower lobar bronchi (larger arrow). Note the asymmetric smaller size of the right lung.

once the pertinent anatomy is defined, peak skin exposure is likely to occur on the posterior right chest in a line connecting the anatomy of interest to the skin surface. When peak skin dose exceeds 15 Gy, a sentinel event is reported to the Joint Commission.

Differential Diagnosis

Congenital venous disorders that may simulate PAPVR, with or without scimitar syndrome:

- Absence or interruption of the IVC with azygous continuation
- Anomalous unilateral single pulmonary vein
- "Meandering" aberrant pulmonary vein
- Pulmonary varix
- Pulmonary arteriovenous malformations (with either pulmonary or systemic arterial inflow; all have pulmonary venous outflow drainage)

Once PAPVR is identified, it should be determined whether the PAPVR occurs in isolation or occurs as one of the components of congenital pulmonary venolobar syndrome:

- Bronchopulmonary sequestration
- Isolated hypogenetic lung with normal venous drainage (pseudo-scimitar syndrome)
- Accessory diaphragm (diaphragm duplication with an aberrant pulmonary vein to the left atrium)
- Horseshoe lung

Common Variants

It is important on echocardiography, MRI-MRA, and CTA to follow the entire course of the pulmonary veins from their peripheral segments to their central drainage. Pulmonary veins that have anomalous peripheral drainage and/or take an aberrant course within the lungs prior to draining into the left atrium (e.g., normal central pulmonary venous connections) may simulate PAPVR (e.g., abnormal central pulmonary venous connections). Examples include an isolated single "meandering" pulmonary vein that drains directly into the left atrium and an anomalous unilateral single pulmonary vein (AUSPV) that receives all ipsilateral veins prior to draining into the left atrium. Pseudo-scimitar syndrome occurs when a right AUSPV is present along with ipsilateral right lung hypoplasia and cardiac dextroposition; radiographically the AUSPV may resemble the scimitar vein.

Clinical Issues

In the neonate and infant with significant PAPVR, medical management focuses on optimizing right and left heart function, improving tissue oxygenation, and controlling pulmonary hypertension. In older pediatric and adult patients with symptomatic PAPVR, medical therapy has similar objectives with the additional aims of treating and preventing arrhythmias and pulmonary infections. Surgical correction is necessary for all symptomatic, hemodynamically significant PAPVR. Surgical options include translocation of the anomalous vein(s) to the left atrium and when needed, creation of an intracardiac baffle. Initial postoperative imaging includes chest radiography and echocardiography. Indications for MRI-MRA and CTA in surveillance imaging are similar to preoperative criteria.

Key Points

- Anomalous pulmonary venous drainage in PAPVR may be into the SVC, right atrium, coronary sinus, azygous vein, or IVC.
- Scimitar syndrome is a combination of PAPVR, hypogenetic lung, and dextroposition of the heart; it almost exclusively involves the right lung.
- PAPVR results in left-to-right shunt physiology and admixture of deoxygenated and oxygenated blood.
- Initially, patients with PAPVR are acyanotic. Significant shunts will lead to increased PBF, right heart volume overload, pulmonary hypertension, and/or increased right heart chamber size; right heart failure may develop. Elevation of left atrial pressure may lead to congestive left heart failure; patients may become cyanotic.
- Chest radiography provides a direct window into the physiology of PAPVR.
- Confirmation of PAPVR is typically made by echocardiography. Selectively, MRI-MRA and CTA are used; both may incidentally detect PAPVR.

Further Reading

Haest RJ, van den Berg CJ, Goei R, Baur LH. Scimitar syndrome; an unusual congenital abnormality occasionally seen in adults. *Int J Cardiovasc Imaging.* 2006;*22*(3–4):565–568.

Ho ML, Bhalla S, Bierhals A, Gutierrez F. MDCT of partial anomalous pulmonary venous return (PAPVR) in adults. *J Thorac Imaging.* 2009;*24*(2):89–95.

Konen E, Raviv-Zilka L, Cohen RA, Epelman M, Boger-Megiddo I, Bar-Ziv J, Hegesh J, Ofer A, Konen O, Katz M, Gayer G, Rozenman J. Congenital pulmonary venolobar syndrome: spectrum of helical CT findings with emphasis on computerized reformatting. *Radiographics.* 2003;*23*(5):1175–1184.

Kramer U, Dörnberger V, Fenchel M, Stauder N, Claussen CD, Miller S Hegesh J, Ofer A, Konen O, Katz M, Gayer G, Rozenman J. Scimitar syndrome: morphological diagnosis and assessment of hemodynamic significance by magnetic resonance imaging. *Eur Radiol.* 2003;*13*(Suppl 4):L147–L150.

Najm HK, Williams WG, Coles JG, Rebeyka IM, Freedom RM. Scimitar syndrome: twenty years' experience and results of repair. *J Thorac Cardiovasc Surg.* 1996;*112*(5):1161–1168; discussion 1168–1169.

Wang CC, Wu ET, Chen SJ, Lu F, Huang SC, Wang JK, Chang CI, Wu MH. Scimitar syndrome: incidence, treatment, and prognosis. *Eur J Pediatr.* 2008;*167*(2):155–160.

Woodring JH, Howard TA, Kanga JF. Congenital pulmonary venolobar syndrome revisited. *Radiographics.* 1994;*14*(2):349–369.

Zylak CJ, Eyler WR, Spizarny DL, Stone CH. Developmental lung anomalies in the adult: radiologic-pathologic correlation. *Radiographics.* 2002;*22* Spec No:S25–S43.

Gastrointestinal

CHAPTER 28

Intestinal Malrotation and Midgut Volvulus

Grace Phillips, MD

Definition

The term "malrotation" refers to the abnormal or incomplete rotation and fixation of the bowel during embryogenesis whereby the duodenojejunal junction (DJJ) is in an abnormal location. Children with malrotation and malfixation of the bowel are at risk for midgut volvulus with resultant duodenal obstruction, superior mesenteric vascular compromise, intestinal ischemia, and necrosis.

Clinical Features

Eighty percent of patients with malrotation present within the first month of life. Midgut volvulus classically presents with bilious emesis and is often accompanied by abdominal pain and other symptoms of intestinal obstruction. Alternatively, affected children may present with failure to thrive, feeding intolerance, or intermittent reflux or vomiting. Volvulus resulting in bowel ischemia may cause hematochezia, melena, or malabsorption. Malrotation may be asymptomatic for many years and presentation in adulthood is well-documented.

Anatomy and Physiology

During normal embryogenesis, the midgut extends from the peritoneal cavity into the umbilicus. The bowel then undergoes 90 degrees counterclockwise rotation with respect to the superior mesenteric artery (SMA) and returns to the peritoneal cavity. If at this point there is an arrest in the sequence of normal bowel rotation and fixation, then the result is termed "nonrotation." The small bowel is positioned on the right and the colon is on the left. In the normal state the bowel would undergo an additional 180 degrees of rotation counterclockwise. The ligament of Treitz is a suspensory muscle group that arises from the right diaphragm crus and duodenum. It demarcates the transition between the duodenum and jejunum. The term "ligament of Treitz" is often used synonymously with the term "duodenojejunal junction". With complete rotation the DJJ, or ligament of Treitz, will be positioned posterior and to the left of the SMA, and the cecum will elongate and will be positioned in the right lower quadrant. The bowel will then become "fixed." The second to fourth portions of the duodenum, ascending and descending colon will

normally be "fixed" in the retroperitoneum. The transverse colon and sigmoid colon have omental and retroperitoneal attachments respectively with variable mesenteric attachments. The normal small bowel has a broad mesenteric attachment that extends from the ligament of Treitz to the cecum. If the last 180 degrees of rotation are incomplete, the result is a spectrum known as malrotation. Failures in the normal embryologic process of intestinal rotation typically result in either nonrotation or malrotation, in which the DJJ is to the right of the SMA and fails to ascend to the level of the pylorus. In malrotation, the cecum is also abnormal in position 80 percent of the time and may be within the right upper quadrant or left abdomen. The base of fixation of the mesenteric root in malrotation is subsequently narrow, which places the patient at risk for midgut volvulus (Fig. 28.1).

Imaging Findings

Radiographs:

- Usually normal in malrotation.
- With prolonged midgut volvulus there may be signs of bowel obstruction or of intestinal ischemia.

Fluoroscopy:

- Abnormal location of the DJJ below the pylorus or first portion of the duodenum and to the right of the left L1 pedicle
- Volvulus: either an abrupt cut-off of the contrast column where the duodenum passes under the superior mesenteric artery (SMA), or the bowel has a "cork-screw" appearance (Fig. 28.2)
- Proximal jejunal loops abnormally located within the right abdomen
- Jejunal loops in the right upper quadrant as an isolated finding is normal
- Cecum is unusually high or left of midline in 80 percent of people with malrotation

On ultrasound (US), CT, or MR:

- Indirect signs
- Superior mesenteric vein (SMV) anterior to or left of SMA (malrotation): sensitivity and specificity are low (Fig. 28.3)
- "Whirlpool" sign of mesenteric vessels (midgut volvulus; Fig. 28.4)

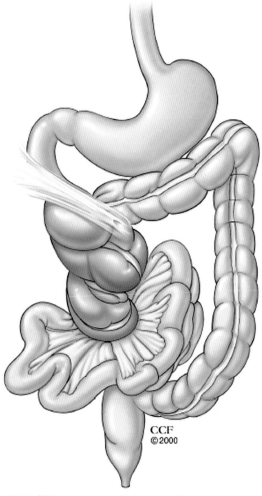

Figure 28.1. Midgut volvulus. Abnormal DJJ position (arrow) below the duodenum to the right of the spine leaves the small bowel free to twist. Obstruction may be complicated by pre-existing Ladd bands (arrowheads).

Imaging Strategy

Imaging of suspected midgut volvulus generally begins with conventional radiographs of the abdomen followed by upper GI (UGI) examination. Barium is typically used unless there is suspicion for bowel ischemia in which a nonionic water-soluble contrast agent would be preferable. If contrast is injected, the tube may be retracted into the proximal stomach during assessment of the course of the duodenum to be certain that it is not abnormally displacing the duodenum. Because the second to fourth portions of the duodenum are retroperitoneal, visualizing the second and fourth portions of the duodenum in the same posterior paraspinal plane on the lateral view is reassuring of a normally rotated and fixed duodenum. If the position of the DJJ is equivocal, an enema or small bowel follow-through (SBFT) may be performed to document the position of the cecum. However, this is of limited utility given that the cecum is fairly mobile in infants and is normally positioned in 20 percent of children with malrotation. In cases of duodenal atresia, a coexisting

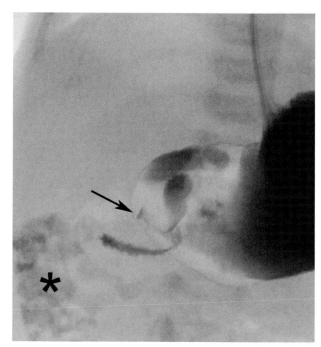

Figure 28.2. Oblique lateral image from UGI in a newborn with bilious vomiting shows a corkscrew configuration of the duodenum (arrow) as it spirals around the SMA and the jejunum is atypically positioned in the right abdomen (asterisk).

malrotation cannot be excluded by fluoroscopic examinations. A normally positioned DJJ may be displaced in patients with indwelling enteric tubes, abdominal masses, a grossly distended stomach, a grossly distended adjacent bowel, or a prior abdominal surgery.

Related Physics

It is important to choose the correct oral contrast when imaging a child for suspected high intestinal obstruction.

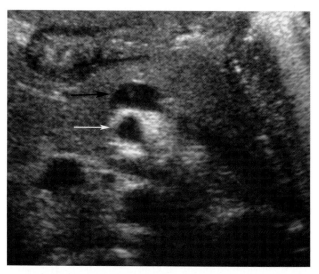

Figure 28.3. Transverse US image with Doppler in a newborn with bilious vomiting shows reversal of the SMA (white arrow) and SMV (black arrow) in a patient who later underwent UGI that showed malrotation without volvulus.

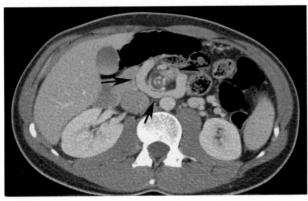

Figure 28.4. Axial oral and IV contrast-enhanced CT image in a teen with abdominal pain shows the classic "whirlpool" sign (arrows) of midgut volvulus from malrotation.

A commonly used choice is thin barium given by bottle, cup, or nasogastric tube. As many infants in distress will aspirate small amounts of contrast during the UGI, barium is the safest choice of contrast as its inert properties rarely cause significant pneumonitis if aspirated. The challenge comes with imaging a child with suspected esophageal or intestinal perforation as barium is not well-tolerated in the mediastinum or peritoneal cavity and leads to intense inflammation and subsequent adhesions. In this case a non-ionic water-soluble medium should be chosen. The numerical value of the agent refers to its iodine concentration and ionic agents are about two times the osmolarity as nonionic agents posing much greater risk in terms of fluid loss and chemical reactivity. Normal serum osmolality is approximately 300 mOsm/L so that the best choice for oral contrast when there is risk for both aspiration and extravasation is a nonionic agent with iodine concentration of approximately 180 mOsmL/ml. If one were to use ionic diatrizoate meglumine sodium with an iodine concentration of 370 mOsmL/ml at full strength, the osmolarity of 1,940 mOsm/L would create a six-fold osmolarity gradient with serum, leading to serious risk for dehydration and death. Similarly, aspiration of this agent would cause massive noncardiogenic pulmonary edema. In general it is best to avoid ionic contrast media for GI studies in children and to pay attention to the iodine concentration of nonionic agents and osmolarity that can lead to significant fluid shifts.

Differential Diagnosis

Congenital duodenal obstruction:
- Duodenal web, stenosis, or atresia
- Annular pancreas

Acquired duodenal obstruction:
- SMA syndrome
- Duodenal hematoma

Bilious emesis:
- Any obstruction distal to the ampulla of Vater

Common Variants

Ladd bands infrequently cause complete or high-grade duodenal obstruction. Volvulus in utero may result in bowel ischemia with possible resulting bowel perforation, stenosis or atresia. There may also be meconium peritonitis. Malrotation is found in association with heterotaxy, gastroschisis, omphalocele, and congenital diaphragmatic hernia. There is an increased incidence in children with Trisomy 21, as well as with the less common conditions of cloacal extrophy and prune belly syndrome.

Clinical Issues

Midgut volvulus is a true surgical emergency and therefore, rapid communication of positive radiographic results is essential. The finding of malrotation without volvulus should also be relayed directly to the referring physician so that appropriate therapy may be instituted.

Key Points

- Malrotation with midgut volvulus is a true surgical emergency.
- The radiologist plays a key role in the diagnosis of midgut volvulus, typically by UGI evaluation.
- Reversal of SMA-SMV relationship may be seen on US, CT, and/or MR but is not reliable.
- A normally positioned DJJ may be displaced in patients with indwelling enteric tubes, abdominal masses, a grossly distended stomach, a grossly distended adjacent bowel, or prior abdominal surgery.

Further Reading

Applegate KE, Anderson JM, Klatte EC. Intestinal malrotation in children: a problem-solving approach to the upper gastrointestinal series. *Radiographics.* 2006;26(5):1485–1500.

Fortuna RB. Midgut Volvulus. In: Donnelly LF, ed. *Diagnostic Imaging: Pediatrics.* First edition. Salt Lake City, UT: Amirsys; 2005:4:6–9.

Lampl B, Levin TL, Berdon WE, Cowles RA. Malrotation and midgut volvulus: a historical review and current controversies in diagnosis and management. *Pediatr Radiol.* 2009;39(4):359–366.

Shew SB. Surgical concerns in malrotation and midgut volvulus. *Pediatr Radiol.* 2009;39(Suppl 2):S167–S171.

Strouse P. Disorders of intestinal rotation and fixation ("malrotation"). *Pediatr Radiol.* 2004;34:837–851.

CHAPTER 29

Duodenal Atresia and Duodenal Stenosis

C. Anne Waugh Moore, MD

Definition

Duodenal atresia, duodenal web, and duodenal stenosis are all part of the same spectrum of developmental duodenal obstructions. In duodenal atresia, the intestinal lumen is completely obliterated whereas with duodenal stenosis, the duodenum is partially occluded or narrowed by a web or diaphragm. Intrinsic anomalies can coexist with extrinsic anomalies that also contribute to duodenal luminal narrowing, such as annular pancreas, Ladd bands, or preduodenal portal vein.

Clinical Features

The duodenum is the most common site of intestinal atresia. Duodenal atresia is more common than duodenal stenosis and can present prenatally with maternal polyhydramnios, a dilated fetal stomach and duodenum. Newborns present with vomiting, which is usually bilious (85 percent), without distention of the abdomen or small bowel loops. Vomiting can be nonbilious (15 percent) if the atresia is proximal to the Ampulla of Vater. Other presentations include feeding intolerance, dehydration, bile-strained aspirates from an oro-gastric tube and electrolyte imbalance. Approximately one-half of infants with duodenal atresia have other congenital anomalies such as Trisomy 21 (30 percent), annular pancreas (20 to 33 percent), the VACTERL association (Vertebral anomalies, gastrointestinal Atresias of the duodenum or anus, TracheoEsophageal fistulas, Renal anomalies, and radial ray Limb defects)., biliary anomalies, renal anomalies, imperforate anus, malrotation, preduodenal portal vein, congenital heart disease, and heterotaxy.

Anatomy and Physiology

The duodenal lumen obliterates by proliferation of epithelial cells during 5th and 6th weeks of embryologic development and recanalization is usually complete by the 10th fetal week. Duodenal atresia is thought to result from failure of the recanalization process. Most cases of duodenal atresia are distal to the Ampulla of Vater and involve the second or less often the third portion of the duodenum. Partial recanalization can result in duodenal stenosis or duodenal web. The most common extrinsic cause of high-grade partial duodenal obstruction is annular pancreas. There are three types of duodenal atresia. Type 1, the most common type, includes an intact intestinal wall and mesentery, septal, or membranous luminal obstruction and the proximal duodenal diameter is greater than distal duodenum. In type 2, the intestinal segments are separated by a fibrous cord. Type 3 includes two blind intestinal ends without intervening cord and wedge-shaped mesenteric defect (Fig. 29.1).

Imaging Findings

Prenatal ultrasound (US):
- "Double bubble"
- Polyhydramnios

Postnatal US:
- Distended fluid-filled duodenum with "gut signature" (Fig. 29.2)

Postnatal radiography:
- Double bubble (gas-distended stomach and proximal duodenum) and no distal bowel gas (atresia; Fig. 29.3)
- Double bubble with some distal bowel gas (stenosis, web or annular pancreas)

Imaging Strategy

Dilated fetal stomach and duodenum, as well as maternal polyhydramnios (40 percent), can be seen on prenatal US and is usually indicative of duodenal atresia or high-grade stenosis. This is easily confirmed with postnatal abdominal radiographs. An uncommon gastric or duodenal duplication cyst seen prenatally may be mistaken for a dilated duodenum. The fluid-filled stomach and duplication cyst together could simulate a fetal sonographic double bubble. In this case the postnatal plain films would fail to show a gas-dilated proximal duodenum, and postnatal US would demonstrate the characteristic "gut signature" of the duplication cyst. The classic radiographic appearance of duodenal atresia is the double bubble sign. This appearance results from air within the dilated stomach and duodenum proximal to the atresia. The marked dilation of the stomach and duodenum implies a longstanding in utero obstruction. With duodenal atresia, no distal small bowel gas is present except in the rare case of associated bifid common bile duct in which a bile duct drains on either side of the

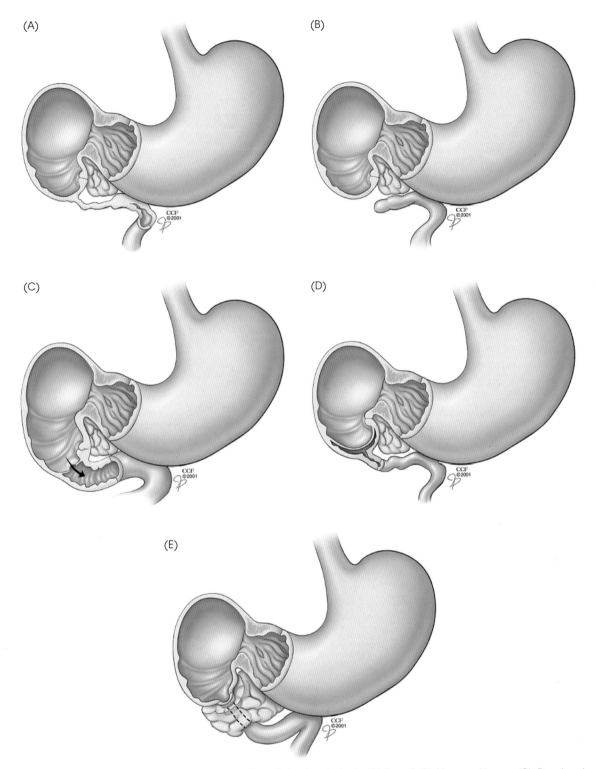

Figure 29.1. Spectrum of duodenal atresia and stenosis. Type 2 duodenal atresia (A). Type 3 (B). Narrowed lumen (C). Duodenal diaphragm (D). Annular pancreas (E).

atretic segment allowing some air to pass from the distended proximal duodenum into the distal duodenum and small bowel. Imaging beyond abdominal radiographs is usually unnecessary with duodenal atresia. The swallowed air provides excellent contrast for delineation of the point

of obstruction. The presence or absence of coexisting malrotation cannot be determined by performance of a fluoroscopic upper gastrointestinal exam. If performed, contrast, like the swallowed air, will not pass beyond the atresia. In duodenal stenosis, the stomach and proximal duodenum

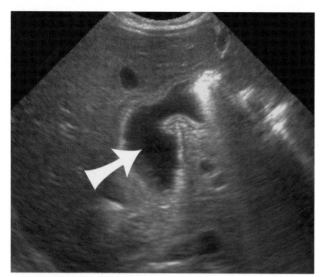

Figure 29.2. Transverse US image in newborn with multiple congenital anomalies and bilious vomiting shows dilation of the proximal duodenum (arrow) in duodenal stenosis.

are dilated and distal bowel gas is also present. In this situation, coexisting malrotation and midgut volvulus can be ruled out with an upper gastrointestinal exam prior to surgical repair of the stenosis (Fig. 29.4). A contrast enema may be requested to exclude other intestinal atresias preoperatively, especially if there is evidence of bowel obstruction beyond the duodenum.

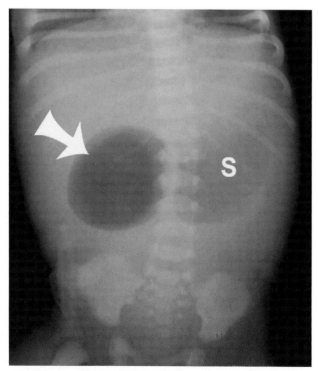

Figure 29.3. Supine frontal image of abdomen in a newborn with vomiting shows moderate dilation of the air-filled stomach (S) and proximal duodenum (arrow) with no distal bowel gas consistent with double bubble in duodenal atresia.

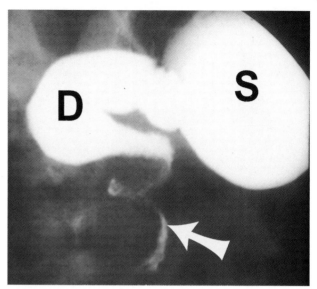

Figure 29.4. Upper GI image in an infant with bilious emesis shows dilation of the stomach (S) and proximal duodenum (D) with the "corkscrew" appearance of proximal jejunum (arrow) caused by malrotation with midgut volvulus.

Related Physics

Most newborns with duodenal atresia have been diagnosed prenatally by US and only a supine abdominal radiograph is performed for confirmation. In order to characterize the radiation output from the X-ray device as well as the radiation incident on the patient, several parameters have been developed. These include exposure, KERMA, and absorbed dose. Within each of these parameters there are classical as well as international units. The former is largely historical and has been rendered obsolete in modern scientific literature; international units are now universally accepted. The historical unit for exposure is the roentgen (R) and the international unit is Coulombs/kilogram (C/kg). Exposure is defined as the ability of the ionizing radiation to ionize air, which makes it easy to measure in the clinical setting. The acronym "KERMA" stands for kinetic energy released in matter, and it is the precursor to absorbed dose. The historical unit for KERMA is the Rad and the Gray (Gy) is the international unit. The relationship between Rad and Gy is given by [100 Rad = 1Gy = 1 J/kg], which is the amount of energy released in a kilogram of tissue. Absorbed dose has historical units of Rad and international units of Gy and is equal to the residual energy deposited in a small volume of tissue. Absorbed dose is one of the most important parameters when considering either acute or long-term effects of radiation.

Differential Diagnosis

- Annular pancreas
- Malrotation and midgut volvulus

■ Malrotation with obstructing Ladd bands coexisting with intrinsic duodenal obstruction

Common Variants

Annular pancreas and preduodenal portal vein coexist with some cases of intrinsic duodenal obstruction/stenosis. A double bubble may be seen on plain radiographs and a partial duodenal obstruction can be confirmed at upper gastrointestinal fluoroscopy. On abdominal ultrasound, the preduodenal portal vein and or circumferential annular pancreas can be directly visualized. Duodenal web is a complete or partial intrinsic obstruction by an intraluminal diaphragm. The web typically occurs in the second portions of the duodenum adjacent to the Ampulla of Vater and may extend into the third portion of the duodenum. Newborns present with bilious vomiting, feeding intolerance, and dehydration. In children and adults, duodenal web presents with recurrent or progressive vomiting, abdominal pain, and nausea. The appearance of duodenal web on plain radiographs and upper gastrointestinal exams varies depending on the degree of narrowing or obstruction. On plain radiographs, the appearance ranges from a normal to severely distended stomach and proximal duodenum, or a double bubble appearance. On upper gastrointestinal examination, an imperforate duodenal web can be completely obstructing and indistinguishable from duodenal atresia. Most duodenal webs can be seen on upper gastrointestinal exam as a curvilinear, thin filling defect extending across the duodenal lumen or may have a so-called wind-sock appearance resulting from the long-term effects of peristalsing bowel contents against an incompletely obstructing intraluminal web with subsequent stretching and extension of the web into the distal duodenal lumen (Fig. 29.5). The wind-sock appearance can be noted on ultrasonography as a fluid-filled and distended proximal duodenum.

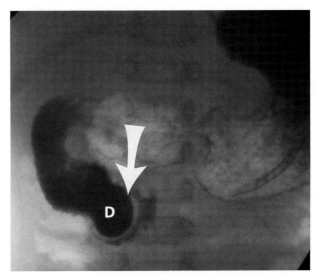

Figure 29.5. Upper GI image in an older child with persistent vomiting shows the contrast-filled dilated duodenum (D) to the level of a partially obstructing curvilinear filling defect (arrow) consistent with duodenal web.

between high-grade duodenal stenosis and malrotation with totally obstructed midgut volvulus can be difficult, if not impossible, and urgent exploratory surgery may be necessary. The proximal duodenum is typically more distended in duodenal atresia/stenosis than in isolated malrotation with acute midgut volvulus. The larger caliber of the proximal duodenum is likely because of the longstanding in utero obstruction of atresia/stenosis versus the acute obstruction in malrotation with volvulus. Occasionally (5 percent) of children with malrotation and midgut volvulus have coexisting duodenal obstruction and proximal duodenal dilatation. When the position of the duodenojejunal junction cannot be confirmed on upper gastrointestinal exam because of severe obstruction, surgical exploration is necessary to exclude malrotation with volvulus.

Clinical Issues

Patients with duodenal atresia first require medical management to correct fluid and electrolyte imbalance, a nasogastric tube to decompress the stomach, followed by early surgical repair. Duodenostomy is the most common surgical procedure. With surgical treatment, the survival rate is over 90 percent with mortality typically the result of other associated congenital anomalies. Partial or complete duodenal obstructions, in which malrotation is a diagnostic consideration and cannot be ruled out on imaging exams, are treated emergently. In the newborn with bilious emesis and a double bubble appearance on plain radiograph with no distal bowel gas, no further preoperative gastrointestinal imaging is recommended before surgical repair. If there is clinical concern for malrotation in an infant with distal bowel gas, a fluoroscopic upper GI study is the test of choice. However, differentiating

Key Points

■ Onset of symptoms, such as vomiting, is most often within hours of birth.

■ Thirty percent of patients with duodenal atresia have Trisomy 21, 20 to 33 percent have annular pancreas.

■ Duodenal atresia can also be part of the VACTERL association.

■ Classic radiographic feature of DA is double bubble sign.

■ Double bubble on the plain radiograph requires no further imaging; contrast is not advised in total obstruction.

■ If there is a double bubble and gas is seen beyond the duodenum, upper GI study is required to exclude malrotation and other causes of duodenal obstruction if surgical correction is to be delayed.

Further Reading

Bedard MP, Bloom DA. Embryology, anatomy, and physiology of the gastrointestinal and genitourinary tracts. In: Slovis TL, Adler BH, Bloom DA, et al., eds. *Caffey's Pediatric Diagnostic Imaging*. Philadelphia, PA: Mosby Elsevier; 2008:139–147.

Bloom DA, Slovis TL. Congenital anomalies of the gastrointestinal tract. In: Slovis TL, Adler BH, Bloom DA, et al., eds. *Caffey's Pediatric Diagnostic Imaging*. Philadelphia, PA: Mosby Elsevier; 2008:188–236.

Kraus SJ. Duodenal atresia or stenosis. In: Donnelly LF, Jones BV, O'Hara SM, et al., eds. *Diagnostic Imaging: Pediatrics*. Salt Lake City, UT: Amirsys; 2005:4-10–4-13.

Kraus SJ. Duodenal web. In: Donnelly LF, Jones BV, O'Hara SM, et al., eds. *Diagnostic Imaging: Pediatrics*. Salt Lake City, UT: Amirsys; 2005:4-14–4-17.

CHAPTER 30

Jejunal Atresia

Charles Maxfield, MD

Definition

Jejunal atresia is characterized by an abrupt complete occlusion of the lumen of the jejunum, resulting in complete bowel obstruction. It may be isolated or there may be multiple distal small bowel, or less often, colonic atresias.

Clinical Features

Jejunal atresia is often detected on prenatal ultrasound (US) on which it classically appears as a few progressively dilating loops of bowel associated with maternal polyhydramnios. Newborns with jejunal atresia present clinically with bilious vomiting and feeding intolerance. The abdomen may be scaphoid if the atresia is very proximal; more distal atresia may cause abdominal distension.

Anatomy and Physiology

Current theories regarding the etiology of jejunal and ileal atresia favor intrauterine intestinal ischemia as the cause of bowel injury resulting in intestinal stenosis or atresia. In some cases the ischemic event results in perforation of the bowel and spillage of the sterile succus or meconium into the peritoneal cavity resulting in meconium peritonitis or meconium pseudocyst formation. This is different from the developmental failure of recanalization that results in the spectrum of intrinsic duodenal anomalies including duodenal web, stenosis, and atresia. For this reason, jejunal and ileal atresias are not typically associated with other extraintestinal congenital anomalies with the exception of cardiac that can also contribute to the in utero ischemia. More often jejunal atresia is associated with more than one atresia, malrotation and midgut volvulus, gastroschisis, and cystic fibrosis with meconium ileus (Fig. 30.1).

Imaging Findings

- Several abnormally dilated loops of bowel rendering a "high" intestinal obstruction pattern or "triple bubble" (Fig. 30.2)
- Loop most proximal to the first atresia is the most grossly dilated (Fig. 30.3)
- No rectal gas on prone images

- Microcolon (unused colon) if more distal jejunal atresia early in gestation (Fig. 30.4)
- Some or normal amount of meconium in the colon if late or very proximal single atresia
- Microcolon with thick meconium in the terminal ileum if a complication of meconium ileus
- Intraperitoneal calcifications if in utero perforation results in meconium peritonitis or meconium pseudocyst

IMAGING PITFALLS: If proximal bowel loops are decompressed by vomiting or nasogastric tube suction, the classic appearance of a small number of gas-dilated loops may not be present.

Imaging Strategy

Even when the diagnosis of jejunal atresia is suggested by prenatal US, postnatal abdominal radiographs are usually obtained to confirm the suspicion as the radiographic findings are characteristic. Given the relatively high likelihood of having additional distal atresias, meconium ileus, or Hirschsprung's disease, a preoperative water-soluble contrast enema is typically performed. A UGI exam using barium is performed to exclude malrotation if surgery is to be delayed beyond the first day of life.

Related Physics

Many infants with high intestinal obstruction are previously diagnosed by prenatal US and the diagnosis is confirmed with newborn abdominal radiographs. In order to characterize the radiation risk to the patient, several parameters have been developed including equivalent dose, effective dose and peak skin dose. Equivalent dose is related to absorbed dose by a weighting factor that characterizes the potential harm from various types of radiation (the "radiation weighting factor"). This parameter has historical units of Rem and international units of Sievert (Sv). The radiation weighting factor has a higher value for particulate radiation such as alpha particles and neutrons and is equal to 1 for all photons (including X-rays and gamma rays), so that this parameter has limited use

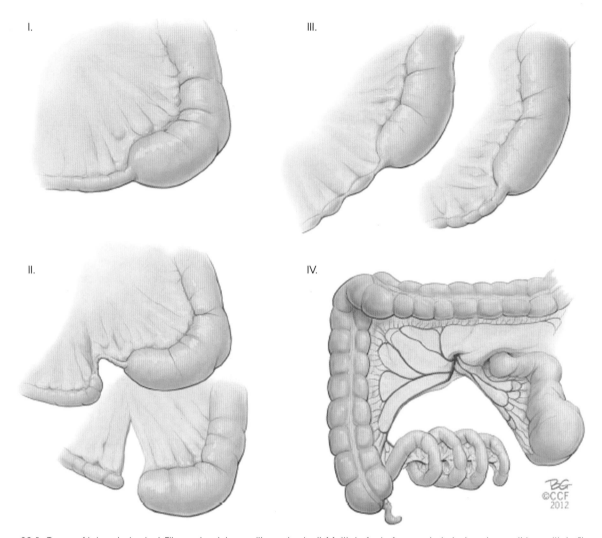

I.

III.

II.

IV.

Figure 30.1. Types of jejunal atresia. I. Fibrous track in a solitary atresia. II. Multiple foci of mesenteric ischemia result in multiple fibrous tracks. III. Combined fibrous tracks or stenosis with discontinuous loops from ischemia. IV. Multiple intestinal atresias including more distal ileal atresia will result in microcolon (unused colon) on enema.

in medical imaging and is more often used for industrial radiation accidents. Effective dose is related to absorbed dose by a weighting factor that characterizes the potential harm to an organ from various types of radiation ("tissue weighting factor"). This parameter also has historical units of Rem and international units of Sievert (Sv). The tissue weighting factor has larger values for organs that are more radiosensitive. The sum of all tissue weighting factors equals 1. Effective dose is used in diagnostic imaging to compare radiation risks between two competing imaging studies of the same organ or body part. This is the most important parameter in considering patient cancer risk. Peak skin dose has historical units of Rad and international units of Gray (Gy) and as the name implies is the maximum absorbed dose to a single point during an imaging exam. As a subset of the absorbed dose, this parameter is most useful in predicting acute skin injury during prolonged radiation such as during cardiac catheterization procedures.

Differential Diagnosis

- Partial duodenal obstruction: duodenal stenosis, duodenal web, or annular pancreas may have a "double bubble" pattern with some distal gas, which can mimic a third bubble very soon after birth. With time, gas will progress more distally.
- Malrotation with midgut volvulus can be excluded with UGI
- Duodenal atresia, stenosis, or web with malrotation have a "double bubble" pattern.

Common Variants

Small bowel atresia may present with a variable number of dilated loops, depending on how distal the atresia. The classic proximal jejunal atresia will produce a triple bubble appearance. Distal jejunal and ileal atresia will have more loops. A special variant of small bowel atresia is the

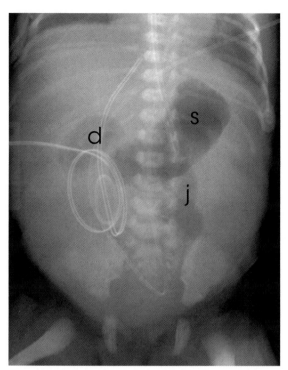

Figure 30.2. Supine abdominal radiograph in a newborn with vomiting demonstrates three distended loops of bowel in upper abdomen with no distal gas. The stomach (s) is normal, however the caliber of the duodenal bulb (d) and proximal jejunal loop (j) are larger than normal.

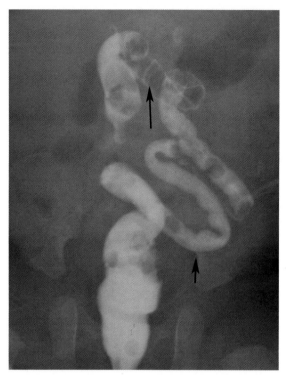

Figure 30.4. Frontal image from water-soluble enema in jejunal atresia shows "microcolon" (arrows) from an unused colon in fetal life. Continued instillation of contrast to fill the ascending colon and terminal ileum is needed to exclude meconium ileus or proximal colonic atresia.

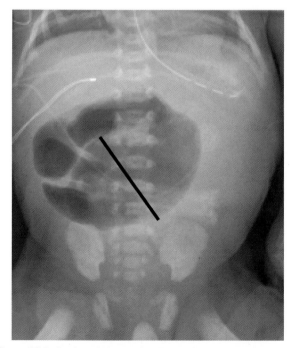

Figure 30.3. Supine abdominal radiograph in a newborn with vomiting shows few gas-distended loops of bowel; there is no distal bowel gas despite gross distention of one loop. The largest-caliber loop (black line) is typically immediately proximal to the atresia. The grossly large caliber indicates that the obstruction is chronic.

"apple peel" small bowel atresia that results from prenatal occlusion of the super mesenteric artery and infarction and absorption of the necrotic bowel. The distal ileum spirals around its only blood supply, a branch of the ileocolic artery that anastomoses with branches of the inferior mesenteric artery, producing an appearance resembling an apple peel.

Clinical Issues

Most infants undergo surgery within days of birth. In most cases, simple resection of the atretic segment with primary bowel anastomosis is performed. Some require resection with tapering enteroplasty, and complicated cases may require a temporary ostomy. The perioperative mortality rate for bowel repair is less than 1 percent. Most mortality is related to liver disease as a complication of total parenteral nutrition.

Key Points
- Ischemic etiology
- Three (triple bubble) or four dilated loops
- UGI to rule out malrotation
- Contrast enema to exclude coexisting Hirschsprungs, meconium ileus, additional small bowel atresias, or proximal colonic atresia

Further Reading

Berrocal T, Torres I, Gutiérrez J, Prieto C, del Hoyo ML, Lamas M. Congenital anomalies of the upper gastrointestinal tract. *Radiographics.* 1999;*19*:855–872.

Dalla Vecchia LK, Grosfeld JL, West K. Intestinal atresias and stenosis: a 25-year experience with 277 cases. *Arch Surg.* 1998;*133*(5):490–497.

Swischuk LE. *Imaging of the Newborn and Young Infant.* Fifth edition. Philadelphia, PA: Lippincott Williams and Wilkins; 2004.

CHAPTER 31

Distal Bowel Obstruction in the Newborn

Caroline Carrico, MD

Definition

Distal bowel obstruction in the newborn is a broad term used to describe any bowel obstruction from the distal jejunum to the anus. The most frequent causes are ileal atresia, meconium ileus (MI), Hirschsprung disease (HD), and functional immaturity of the colon. Anal atresia and anorectal malformations are less common. Isolated colonic atresia is rare.

Anatomy and Physiology

Jejunal and ileal atresias occur as a result of in utero bowel ischemia or from a perforation that is usually a secondary to high-grade long-standing obstruction. Small bowel atresias may therefore be found in newborns that also have meconium ileus, volvulus of the bowel, or less likely HD. Meconium ileus typically results from delayed passage of tenacious meconium through the ileocecal valve in patients with cystic fibrosis (CF). At birth, the colon is very small secondary to disuse and is given the term microcolon. Hirschsprung disease results from incomplete craniocaudal migration of the neural crest cells that form the ganglia of the enteric nervous system. The aganglionic bowel is not able to contract or relax normally. The lack of normal function results in bowel obstruction. Functional immaturity of the colon, small left colon or meconium plug syndrome are all names applied to the scenario of an newborn with normal histologic anatomy of the bowel without structural luminal narrowing and a temporary functional obstruction related to immaturity or environmental factors.

Clinical Features

Newborns with distal intestinal obstruction have similar clinical and radiographic presentations. The typical clinical presentation is that of a newborn with abdominal distension, emesis that is often bilious, and failure to pass meconium within the first 24 hours of life. Only 1 percent of normal term infants require 48 hours to pass meconium. Preterm infants that are otherwise normal may require as many as 9 days to pass meconium. Bilious emesis can occur with any obstruction distal to the ampulla of Vater. Because malrotation of the bowel with midgut volvulus can occur in utero and result in small bowel perforation, stenosis, or atresia, this critical diagnosis is considered in the assessment of newborns

with clinical symptoms and/or plain film findings suggestive of either proximal or distal bowel obstruction. Most newborns with MI have CF. The cause of MI in infants without CF is poorly understood. Hirschsprung disease occurs more often in infants with Trisomy 21 or with neurocristopathies. Delayed passage of meconium is often seen in preterm infants with normal anatomy and physiology in a condition known as functional immaturity of the colon. Peristalsis can also be impaired by maternal tocolytics. There is often a functional delay in bowel activity in infants of diabetic mothers.

Imaging Findings

Distal Jejunal or Ileal Atresia
Radiography:
  - Multiple loops of gas-filled bowel, too numerous to count
  - The single largest diameter loop is just proximal to the first atresia
  - +/- calcifications
  - Meconium peritonitis from in utero bowel perforation
  - Intraluminal enteroliths distal to first atresia (uncommon)
Contrast enema:
  - To look for coexisting colonic atresias prior to surgery and to rule out other causes of distal bowel obstruction
  - Microcolon if the obstruction is distal and occurred early in gestation (Fig. 31.1)
  - Normal colon with meconium in colon if the obstruction is very proximal or occured late in gestation
  - Small-caliber terminal ileum **without** meconium plugs in the terminal ileum
Upper GI:
  - May show malrotation of the bowel or may be normal

Meconium Ileus
Radiography:
  - Distal bowel obstruction
  - +/- bubbly lucencies in the right lower quadrant resulting from air mixed with meconium

- Calcifications:
- +/-intramural; +/- dysmorphic intraperitoneal calcifications (meconium peritonitis)
- +/- mass effect and peripheral calcifications from meconium pseudocyst

Contrast enema:
- Microcolon
- Meconium plugs in the terminal ileum (Fig. 31.2)
- Terminal ileum may be larger in caliber than the colon

Newborn ultrasound (US):
- Microcolon
- Dilated small bowel with poor peristalsis
- Hyperechoic layer of thick meconium adheres to the mucosa
- Lower and heterogeneous echotexture of more central luminal meconium
- Punctate foci of air within meconium
- Meconium peritonitis or meconium pseudocyst may result if there is bowel perforation from high-grade obstruction or focal small bowel volvulus (see Chapter 32)

Hirschsprung Disease
Radiography:
- Gas-filled loops of distended but normal-appearing bowel
- Loops of bowel are too numerous to count

Contrast enema:
- Nondistensible distal rectum and variable length of contiguous more proximal aganglionic colon
- Cone-shaped transition zone from small- or normal-caliber aganglionic colon to distensible distended meconium-filled normal bowel
- Rectosigmoid index is less than or equal to one: maximum diameter of the rectum divided by the maximum diameter of the sigmoid (Fig. 31.3)
- Irregular serrations or contractions of the aganglionic bowel (uncommon but specific finding)
- Enema may be normal

Total Colonic Hirschsprung Disease (TCHD):
- Normal-caliber colon, short (question-mark-shaped) colon or microcolon
- Microcolon with *intraluminal calcifications* in distal small bowel
- Colon is often featureless
- Colonic muscle spasms
- Easy reflux of contrast into small bowel
- May have spontaneous bowel perforation, pneumoperitoneum

Functional Immaturity of the Colon
Radiography:
- Gas-filled loops of bowel, too numerous to count
- +/- air-fluid levels

- Normal appearance of the colon
- Meconium to the level of the rectum

Contrast enema:
- Symptoms/signs resolve within hours of the water-soluble contrast enema

Small Left Colon Syndrome (a.k.a. Left-Sided Microcolon)
- Very small-caliber descending and sigmoid colon
- +/- intraluminal meconium
- Distensible rectum
- Sharp transition zone at the splenic flexure (abrupt, not cone-shaped) (Fig. 31.4)
- Dilated ascending and transverse colon, some small bowel distention

---

Differential Diagnosis
- Isolated colon atresia
- Anorectal malformation
- Multiple intestinal atresias
- Milk allergy colitis
- Hypoganglionosis
- Neuronal intestinal dysplasia type A or B
- Megacystis-microcolon-intestinal hypoperistalsis syndrome

Imaging Strategy
Plain radiographs of the abdomen show gaseous distension of multiple loops of intestine that are too numerous to count. Newborn colon typically does not have obvious haustral folds evident on radiographs, so unless there is gas in the rectum it is usually not possible to determine if the point of obstruction is in the small or large bowel. The imaging procedure of choice to differentiate between the various causes of distal bowel obstruction is a relatively low-osmolality water-soluble contrast enema. Water-soluble contrast has the added benefit of lubricating the meconium at the point of obstruction, so the contrast enema can be both diagnostic and therapeutic. The colon is not prepped prior to the contrast enema. A small rectal catheter is inserted and taped to the skin without inflating a balloon because of risk of rectal perforation; the stimulation from a balloon can override the transition zone in patients with HD. Contrast is dripped in by gravity rather than injected to lessen the risk of bowel perforation. Contrast enema is not performed in a newborn with pneumoperitoneum or active colitis. If the contrast enema is normal, an upper GI study is indicated to exclude malrotation with midgut volvulus. Also, UGI is indicated if the infant has jejunal or ileal atresia and corrective surgery is to be at all delayed. Jejunal and ileal atresia occur as the result of small bowel ischemia and as malrotation with midgut volvulus may be the underlying cause of the ischemia, volvulus can recur. Ultrasound of the abdomen

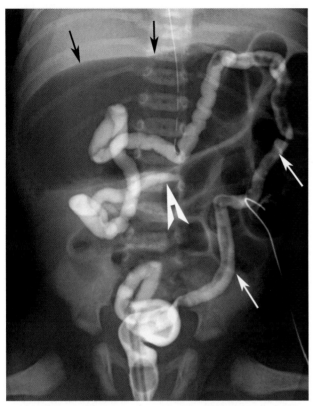

Figure 31.1. Frontal image from contrast enema in a child with small bowel atresia shows a very small colon (white arrows) with minimal meconium within the lumen. Contrast also partially fills the appendix and the extremely small-caliber distal ileum (arrowhead). The much larger-caliber gas-distended loops of small bowel proximal to the atresia are evident (black arrows). Image courtesy of James Crowe, MD

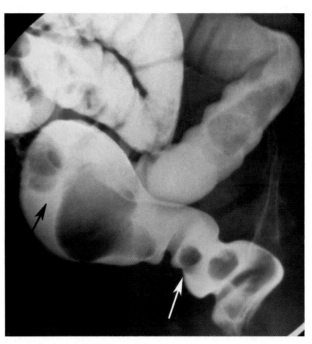

Figure 31.3. Lateral image from contrast enema shows the classic cone-shaped transition from nondistensible aganglionic rectum (white arrow) to the compliant normally innervated dilated sigmoid colon (black arrow) typical for HD. Normally the maximum diameter of the sigmoid colon is less than that of the rectum. Image courtesy of James Crowe, MD

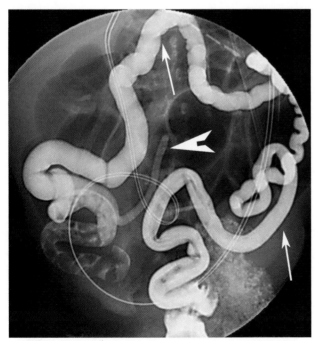

Figure 31.2. Frontal image from contrast enema in a newborn with meconium ileus shows a microcolon (white arrows) with minimal meconium filling defects in the rectosigmoid colon and distal ileum. The normal appendix (arrowhead) is filled with contrast. Image courtesy of James Crowe, MD

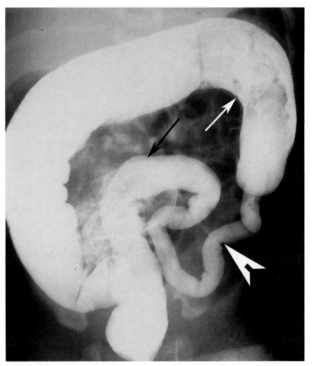

Figure 31.4. Frontal image from contrast enema in a newborn with small left colon syndrome shows abrupt transition from splenic flexure (arrowhead) to small sigmoid colon (white arrow) to normal rectosigmoid (black arrow). Image courtesy of James Crowe, MD

is used to further assess some infants with complicated meconium ileus and pseudocyst formation found on prenatal US or postnatal radiography.

Common Variants

- TCHD (3 to 12 percent): cone-shaped transition zone occurs at or proximal to the ileocecal valve; can resemble meconium ileus; often meconium in the terminal ileum is calcified.
- Ultrashort segment HD: limited failure of reflex relation of the internal anal sphincter and is rare.
- Complicated meconium ileus: MI can be complicated by bowel necrosis or small bowel perforation, which may result in coexisting small bowel atresia(s); spilled enteric contents can result in meconium peritonitis or meconium pseudocyst formation; typically requires surgical intervention.

Clinical Issues

Anorectal manometry can be used to assess for the presence of the rectosphincteric reflex in the newborn. Absence of this reflex is suggestive of HD, which can be further assessed by means of a suction rectal biopsy to identify enteric ganglia. Suction rectal biopsy may be falsely positive for aganglionosis that requires definitive diagnosis by full thickness biopsy. Hirschsprung disease can be seen in the setting of other pathology, either as an association or a contributing factor. Consider HD as a cause of appendix perforation in an infant. 'HD is associated with other neural crest anomalies that are known as neurocristopathies. A child with HD and shortness of breath may have central hypoventilation syndrome (Ondine's curse). HD is also associated with congenital neuroblastoma, a tumor of neural crest origin. There have been rare reports of skip segment HD, which may be related to transmesenteric migration of neural crest tissue. Nearly one-third of children with HD will develop enterocolitis. Contrast enema should be avoided during acute illness because of risk of bowel perforation. In TCH there is often a strong family history of aganglionosis. Consider HD in a newborn that fails to return to and maintain normal bowel function after a normal enema, a diagnosis of small left colon or meconium plug syndrome, or after usual treatment for presumed meconium ileus. Meconium ileus is seen almost exclusively in newborns with cystic fibrosis (CF), but only a minority of CF patients present with meconium ileus. Serial enemas, potentially with moderately hyperosmolar contrast agents can be performed once or twice a day if the infant is showing continued improvement and his/her fluid status is normal. Surgical decompression of the obstructed bowel is necessary if the enemas fail to relieve the obstruction or if the enema is complicated by bowel perforation. Untreated distal bowel obstruction can also result in bowel perforation.

IMAGING PITFALLS:

- The cone-shaped transition zone seen in HD does not correlate exactly with the surgical level of aganglionosis in all patients. In infants with long segment disease, the transition zone tends to underestimate the extent of disease.
- TCHD has a variable appearance on contrast enema. The colon may look normal, may be comma-shaped, short, or may be a microcolon. The standard diagnostic features of HD such as the abnormal rectosigmoid index and cone-shaped transition zone are usually absent in TCHD.
- Malrotation of the bowel with midgut volvulus can have an identical presentation. Abdominal radiographs are usually normal but can resemble proximal or distal bowel obstruction.

Key Points

- The clinical presentation includes abdominal distension, emesis that may be bilious, and failure to pass meconium
- Plain radiographs show numerous mild to moderately gas-distended loops of bowel or findings of high-grade distal bowel obstruction.
- Contrast enema shows microcolon with meconium ileus and some cases of distal jejunal or ileal atresia or TCHD.
- Cone-shaped transition zone in the colon and a rectosigmoid index of < 1 are classic findings of 'HD, except for TCHD, which may have a normal-appearing, short or microcolon.
- A baby with what appears to be small left colon, meconium plug syndrome, or meconium ileus who continues to act obstructed after normal treatment/time may have HD.
- If a contrast enema is performed to assess a distal bowel obstruction and the colon appears normal, UGI is indicated to exclude malrotation with midgut volvulus.

Further Reading

Bloom DA, Buonomo C, Fishman SJ, Furuta G, Nurko S. Allergic colitis: a mimic of Hirschsprung disease. *Pediatr Radiol*. 1999; 29 (1): 37–41.

Bloom DA, Slovis TL. Congenital anomalies of the gastrointestinal tract. In: Slovis TL, Coley BD. *Caffey's Pediatric Diagnostic Imaging*. 11th edition. Philadelphia, PA. 2007, pp 188–236.

Cowles RA, Berdon WE, Holt PD, Buonomo C, Stolar CJ. Neonatal intestinal obstruction simulating meconium ileus in infants with long-segment intestinal aganglionosis: radiographic findings that prompt the need for rectal biopsy. *Pediatr Radiol*. 2006;36(2):133–137. Epub 2005 Dec 3.

Jamieson DH, Dundas SE, Belushi SA, Cooper M, Blair GK. Does the transition zone reliably delineate aganglionic bowel in Hirschsprung's disease? *Pediatr Radiol.* 2004;*34*(10): 811–815.

Lang I, Daneman A, Cutz E, Hagen P, Shandling B. Abdominal calcification in cystic fibrosis with meconium ileus: radiologic-pathologic correlation. *Pediatr Radiol.* 1997;*27*(6): 523–527.

Reid JR, Buonomo C, Moreira C, Kozakevich H, Nurko SJ. The barium enema in constipation: comparison with rectal manometry and biopsy to exclude Hirschsprung's disease after the neonatal period. *Pediatr Radiol.* 2000;*30*(10): 681–684.

Roshkow JE, Haller JO, Berdon WE, Sane SM. Hirschsprung's disease, Ondine's curse, and neuroblastoma: manifestations of neurocristopathy. *Pediatr Radiol.* 1988;*19*(1):45–49.

Stranzinger E, DiPietro MA, Teitelbaum DH, Strouse PJ. Imaging of total colonic Hirschsprung disease. *Pediatr Radiol.* 2008;*38*(11):1162–1170. Epub 2008 Aug 5.

Swischuk LE. *Imaging of the Newborn, Infant, and Young Child.* Fifth edition. Philadelphia, PA: Lippincott, Williams and Wilkins; 2004:*400–408*;445–459.

Veyrac C, Baud C, Prodhomme O, Saguintaah M, Couture A. US assessment of neonatal bowel (necrotizing enterocolitis excluded). *Pediatr Radiol.* 2012;*42*(Suppl 1):S107–S114. Epub 2012 Mar 6.

CHAPTER 32

Meconium Peritonitis

Charles Maxfield, MD

Definition

Meconium peritonitis results from in utero perforation of bowel with spill of enteric contents into the peritoneal cavity typically causing multiple intraperitoneal calcifications. The perforation is often secondary to causes of bowel ischemia, infection, or high-grade obstruction, but in some cases, no etiology is evident. In those fetuses, the bowel defect heals; the GI tract remains patent and without obstruction and no further investigation or therapy is necessary.

Clinical Features

The peritoneal calcifications caused by meconium peritonitis may be discovered incidentally on prenatal ultrasound (US) or postnatal imaging performed for unrelated reasons. In others there may be coexisting prenatal or postnatal signs or symptoms of bowel obstruction. Rarely, the peritonitis results in adhesions that can cause bowel obstruction. Newborn males may present with a firm scrotal mass.

Anatomy and Physiology

Initially, the leakage of meconium (fetal stool) causes a sterile chemical peritonitis, which usually but not always results in radiographically and sonographically demonstrable calcifications. Calcifications distribute throughout the peritoneal cavity including through the patent processus vaginalis (more commonly on the right).

Imaging Findings

Abdominal radiographs usually demonstrate calcifications within the peritoneal cavity and in peritoneal recesses (Fig. 32.1). Occasionally the calcifications can extend into the scrotum via a patent processus vaginalis and present as a firm scrotal mass that is confirmed as dense calcification with posterior acoustic shadowing on US (Fig. 32.2). Less often, calcifications can extend into the thorax through normal anatomic communications. Calcifications may be amorphous, curvilinear, or irregular and all show posterior acoustic shadowing on US. Focally clustered calcifications, especially if curvilinear, may indicate the presence of a meconium pseudocyst, which represents a loculated perforation with rim calcification.

> **IMAGING PITFALLS:** Be certain that the calcifications are in the peritoneum, as opposed to intrahepatic, intravascular, intravesical, or within the bowel lumen.

Imaging Strategy

If the patient is asymptomatic, the calcifications may be an incidental finding and no further investigation is necessary. If there is bowel obstruction, UGI or contrast enema can be performed to diagnose the precipitating cause of the in utero perforation and resultant obstruction.

Related Physics

As meconium peritonitis is characterized by often subtle abdominal calcifications, radiography should be

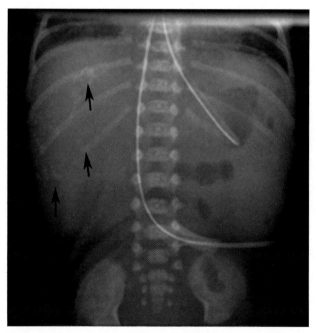

Figure 32.1. Supine abdominal radiograph in an asymptomatic newborn shows irregular calcifications clustered in the right upper quadrant of the abdomen (arrows) resulting from meconium peritonitis that required no further management. Ultrasound could be used to determine if these calcifications are intraluminal, intrahepatic, or intraperitoneal.

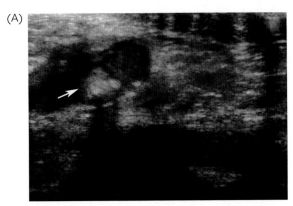 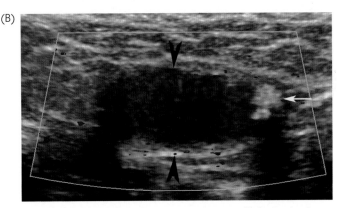

Figure 32.2. Transverse US (A) of the right scrotum in a newborn male with palpable extratesticular mass shows multiple shadowing foci (arrows) consistent with meconium peritonitis. Sagittal color Doppler (B) shows normal testis (arrowheads) and scrotal calcification adjacent to the lower pole (arrows).

optimized for photoelectric absorption for calcium. This may be accomplished through low-kVp imaging (~40) with similar technique to microcalcification detection in mammography. Mammographic technique can be emulated by using a small focal spot, low kVp, low grid ratio or no grid, and highly sensitive image receptors with superior spatial resolution. Of note, digital radiography (DR) and computed radiography (CR) cassettes have a limited intrinsic spatial resolution of 100 microns whereas many film-screen systems can detect as low as 10 microns, so it is possible that some calcifications below 100 microns detected on film-screen systems will be missed on DR/CR. In infants it is advisable to avoid the use of an antiscatter grid as a grid will needlessly raise the exposure and patient dose by a factor of 3 to 5 when compared to the same imaging study with the use of a grid. It is also advisable to use a kVp of 40 to 50 to maximize photoelectric interactions necessary for the detection of calcium. kVp is directly related to patient thickness, so that the lowest kVp can be used in the smallest patients or when tissue compression is employed. As patients start to approach adult size, the use of appropriate antiscatter grids and calibrated photo-timing systems should be considered. The use of CR or DR systems has several distinct advantages over film-based systems. The CR and DR systems permit the use of image-enhancement techniques such as noise reduction, edge enhancement, window and level capabilities.

Differential Diagnosis

Hepatic calcifications:

- Congenital cytomegalovirus (CMV)
- Parvovirus infections
- Hepatoblastoma: dedicated liver US and serum alphafetoprotein (AFP) levels can be used to assess for hepatoblastoma

Intraluminal bowel calcifications:

- Multiple intestinal atresias or total colonic Hirschsprung: associated with high-grade obstruction, and calcifications are more tubular
- Calcified meconium: occurs if meconium mixes with fetal urine. This can occur in boys with intermediate or high anorectal malformations or in girls with cloacal anomalies.

Clinical Issues

If the infant with meconium peritonitis is asymptomatic, no further investigation may be necessary. If the infant has clinical peritonitis or free air, then surgical exploration and repair is indicated. If the baby has a bowel obstruction, then a barium UGI or water-soluble contrast enema may be performed to characterize the small and large bowel before surgery.

Variants

A meconium pseudocyst results when meconium leaks from a fetal bowel perforation into a contained focal collection, rather than diffusely throughout the peritoneum. A meconium pseudocyst can present as a complicated cyst, detected incidentally on prenatal or postnatal ultrasound, or can occasionally present with pain or obstruction resulting from torsion.

Key Points

- Intraperitoneal meconium usually calcifies and causes a sterile chemical peritonitis.
- Results from in utero perforation, often from bowel obstruction and/or ischemia.
- Many infants are asymptomatic.
- Calcified meconium may migrate into the scrotum or, less likely, into the thorax.

Further Reading

Foster MA, Nyberg DA, Mahony BS, Mack LA, Marks WM, Raabe RD. Meconium peritonitis: prenatal sonographic findings and their clinical significance. *Radiology.* 1987;*165*(3):661–665.

Patole S, Whitehall J, Almonte R, Stalewski H, Lee-Tannock A, Murphy A. Meconium thorax: a case report and review of literature. *Am J Perinatol.* 1998;*15*(1):53–56.

Swischuk LE. *Imaging of the Newborn, Infant and Young Child.* Fifth edition. Lippincott, Williams and Wilkins; 2004.

CHAPTER 33

Necrotizing Enterocolitis

Beverly Wood, MD

Definition

Necrotizing enterocolitis (NEC) is an acquired disease that affects neonates believed to be related to bowel ischemia and activation of proinflammatory intracellular cascades that results in mucosal and deep intestinal wall necrosis. Neonates who are particularly vulnerable to NEC are those who have a history of asphyxia, hypotension, low APGAR scores, whole blood transfusions, formula feeding, sepsis, and other complications that can lower the blood flow to the intestine. Although infection is thought to play a key role in the development of NEC, it is unclear whether bacterial infection is an important initial factor or whether intestinal mucosal injury allows secondary bacterial invasion of the bowel wall.

Clinical Features

Symptoms and signs include abdominal distention, decreased bowel sounds, change in stool pattern, larger gastric residuals, and hematochezia. Progressive disease is characterized by bloody stools, lethargy, temperature instability, sepsis, and metabolic acidosis. In many infants the distended abdomen may be discolored (dusky purple-grey) and firm.

Anatomy and Physiology

Three intestinal factors are present in most infants who develop NEC: ischemic insult, bacterial colonization, and intraluminal substrate (enteral feedings). It is believed that an ischemic insult damages the intestinal lining, leading to increased intestinal wall permeability and bacterial wall invasion. Necrotizing enterocolitis rarely occurs before enteral feedings and is less frequent in breastfed neonates. *Escherichia coli* and *Klebsiella pneumoniae* are often present in the bowel flora of neonates affected with NEC. Once feedings are begun, ample substrate is present for proliferation of luminal bacteria to penetrate the damaged intestinal wall. Gas within the compromised bowel wall and its lymphatics is known as pneumatosis intestinalis. Necrosis begins in the mucosa and may progress to involve the full thickness of the intestinal wall, causing bowel perforation and subsequently peritonitis. Sepsis frequently occurs in neonates with NEC.

Imaging Findings

Radiography:
- Early radiographs of the abdomen may show focally dilated loops of bowel.
- Wall thickening causing separation of bowel and dysmorphic or elongated loops (Fig. 33.1).
- Fixed or persistent loop: aperistaltic and often ischemic, may precede perforation.
- Pneumatosis intestinalis appears as small sumucosal bubbly lucencies and smooth subserosal hyperlucent crescents or rings (Fig. 33.2).
- Portal venous gas: enters intestinal veins of compromised bowel with subsequent flow of gas into the superior mesenteric vein and portal venous system.
- Pneumoperitoneum: intraperitoneal free air is the result of intestinal ischemia and bowel perforation.

Ultrasound:
- Bowel wall thickening
- Decreased or absent bowel wall perfusion by color Doppler
- Bowel wall thinning (sloughed mucosa)
- Increased bowel wall echogenicity containing punctate echogenic foci of air (most specific if in the dependent part of the bowel wall)
- Focal fluid collections
- Portal venous gas
- Free intraperitoneal gas

Imaging Strategy

Serial abdominal radiographs are obtained usually with supine and cross-table or "shoot-through" lateral plain films. Imaging frequency of every 6, 8, or 12 hours depends on the severity of the disease clinically. Left-side-down decubitus views of the abdomen are most sensitive for free air and are often obtained if there is questionable free air on the cross-table lateral view. Ultrasound is useful to look for findings of bowel perforation or abscess, particularly if the neonate has a gasless abdomen, a persistent focal region with absence of bowel gas or if the neonate fails to improve with appropriate management. Feeding intolerance after recovery from medical or surgical treatment of NEC may result from stricture formation (Fig. 33.3). Small bowel follow-through to the level of the rectum can be used to assess for the presence or absence of obstruction from stricture or adhesions. Neonates with a surgical ostomy and mucous fistula after bowel resection from NEC typically undergo contrast enema with retrograde filling to the level of the mucous fistula to exclude stricture formation prior to ostomy takedown.

Related Physics

Doppler can be very useful in the evaluation of the premature infant with suspected NEC. It is important to recognize that arterial lines, most commonly umbilical arterial lines, can induce abnormal flow patterns in medium branch vessels such as the superior mesenteric artery (SMA) and renal arteries so that Doppler techniques are very important in the evaluation of aorta, renal arteries, as well as gut. Spectral Doppler will be optimized by meticulous technique that includes proper placement of the transducer, accurate placement of flow direction indicator, and correct choice of range gate size and location. When possible, the transducer should not be placed absolutely parallel to the vessel. Where angulation is not possible, some systems offer beam steering to create an angle between the transducer and the vessel. A less expensive alternative is to cant the transducer relative

to the vessel. Next, the flow direction indicator should be placed in the center of the vessel lumen aligned with the vessel axis. Third, a range gate is placed within the center of the lumen and size includes only desired volume to be sampled. With little or no angulation between the lie of the vessel and transducer, there will be little to no Doppler signal as there is no Doppler shift at this angle. Inaccurate

(A)

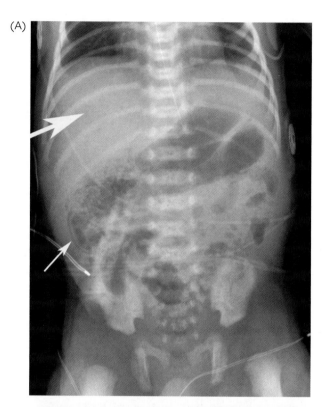

(B)

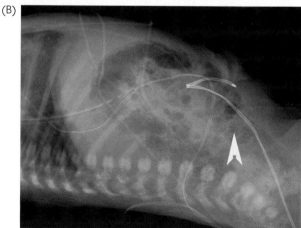

Figure 33.2. Supine frontal (A) and cross table lateral (B) abdominal radiographs in a 2-day-old baby born after premature rupture of membranes at a gestational age of 34 weeks show bubbly lucencies (arrowhead) and curvilinear lucent lines (thin arrow) consistent with pneumatosis intestinalis. The bubbly lucencies are indicative of submucosal air and the curvilinear lucencies are caused by air between the serosa and the bowel wall musculature. Branching lucencies over the liver on the frontal view are caused by portal venous gas (thick arrow).

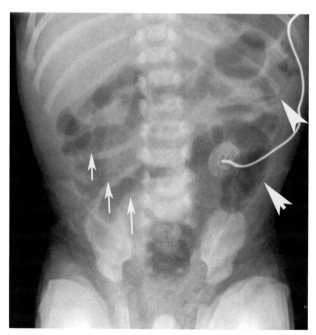

Figure 33.1. Frontal projection of the abdomen in a neonate with low Apgar scores at 1 and 5 minutes shows dilated, elongated, parallel loops of bowel (arrows) with separation of air within the bowel lumina indicating bowel wall edema. There is pneumatosis intestinalis seen in the walls of some of the loops of bowel in the left abdomen (arrowheads) raising the likelihood of NEC with compromise of the bowel wall.

angulation of the flow direction indicator will result in an inaccurate measurement of the angle to be used in the Doppler equation, in turn resulting in inaccurate flow estimation. Doppler angles between 30 and 60 are optimal as this is the shallowest section of the cosine curve (employed in the Doppler equation). The range gate is automatically paired with the flow indicator and is therefore best placed in the middle of the vessel lumen with the flow indicator. Changing the size of the gate will change the number of flow lamina sampled as flow is distributed parabolically throughout medium-sized vessels (such as newborn renal arteries, aorta, celiac, and SMA) with low flow at the walls related to friction and highest flow in the center. In large vessels such as the adult aorta, plug flow predominates, which effectively shows a "square" wavefront across the majority of the central portion of the vessel. Finally, with a larger gate, "spectral broadening" will occur as a broader range of velocities is sampled from the parabolic array of lamina.

Differential Diagnosis

Bubbly lucencies in the abdomen on abdominal radiography:

- NEC
- Ischemic bowel
- Normal gas mixed with stool (and otherwise normal bowel gas pattern)
- Meconium ileus (right-lower quadrant bubbles at terminal ileum)

Portal venous gas:

- NEC
- Bowel ischemia
- Air introduced iatrogenically via an umbilical venous line

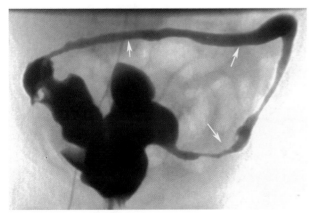

Figure 33.3. Frontal image from water-soluble contrast enema in a 2-month-old former preterm infant with a prior history of NEC and new feeding intolerance shows multiple long segment strictures in the colon (arrows) where the cecum and rectum are relatively spared. Subtotal colectomy was performed for post-NEC strictures.

Variants

Necrotizing enterocolitis totalis (NEC-T) is NEC that results in necrosis of 80 percent or more of the intestinal track. Preterm infants with lower gestational age, lower birth weight and intrauterine growth retardation are more likely to develop NEC-T. There may be a genetic predisposition. Feeding with primarily breast milk the week prior to the development of NEC has been retrospectively shown to significantly protect against NEC-T. Newborns who develop NEC-T usually have rapid and fatal progression of the disease once it is clinically evident. Bowel resection and bowel transplantation is a possible treatment.

Clinical Issues

Necrotizing enterocolitis is an important cause of morbidity and mortality in prematurely born neonates. Approximately 5 to 10 percent of preterm infants with very low birth weight develop NEC and the mortality for extremely low-birth-weight infants (<1000 g) with NEC is 15 to 25 percent. Length of hospital stay and mortality are higher in neonates with NEC than in neonates without NEC. Risk factors include prematurity, low birth weight, exposure to antenatal glucocorticoids, need for mechanical ventilator support, exposure to glucocorticoids and indomethacin during the first week of life, and low Apgar score at 1 and 5 minutes. A slowly progressive feeding regimen has been shown to reduce the incidence of NEC in neonates considered to be at risk. Clusters of NEC outbreaks occur and are usually not related to specific organisms. NEC can develop in term neonates where congenital heart disease is a predisposing factor. In this group risk factors include premature birth, hypoplastic left heart syndrome, truncus arteriosus, and episodes of poor systemic perfusion or shock.

Key Points

- NEC occurs in neonates with risk factors, most often premature birth.
- NEC is characterized by dilated, unchanging, dysmorphic bowel loops with pneumatosis intestinalis.
- Bowel necrosis may lead to perforation and intraperitoneal free air.
- Stricture formation in bowel affected by NEC may be the cause of feeding intolerance after recovery from the acute illness.

Further Reading

Coursey DA, Hollingsworth CL, Wriston C, Beam C, Rice H, Bissset G. Radiographic predictors of disease severity in neonates and infants with necrotizing enterocolitis. *AJR.* 2009;*193*:1408–1413.

Guthrie SO, Gordon PV, Thomas V, Thorp JA, Peabody J, Clark RH. Necrotizing enterocolitis among neonates in the United States. *J Perinatol.* 2003;*23*(4):278–285.

Sliva CT, Daneman A, Navarro OM, Moore AM, Moineddin R, Gerstle JT, Mittal A, Brindle M, Epelman M. Correlation of sonographic findings and outome in necrotizing enterocolitis. *Pediatr Radiol.*2007;*37*:274–282.

Thompson AM, Bizzarro MJ. Necrotizing enterocolitis in newborns: pathogenesis, prevention and management. *Drugs.* 2008;*68*(9):1227–1238.

Thompson A, Bizzarro M, Yu S, Diefenbach K, Simpson BJ, Moss RL. Risk factors for necrotizing enterocolitis totalis: a case-control study. *J Perinatol.* 2011;*31* (11):730–738.

CHAPTER 34

Esophageal Atresia & Tracheoesophageal Fistula

Amy N. Dahl, MD and Kristin Fickenscher, MD

Definition

Esophageal atresia (EA) is a congenital anomaly in which the upper esophagus is discontinuous with the lower esophagus. In 85 to 90 percent of cases, EA occurs in conjunction with a tracheoesophageal fistula (TEF), an abnormal communication between the trachea and the esophagus.

Clinical Features

The incidence of EA/TEF is approximately 1:3,500. Prenatally, EA may manifest as maternal polyhydramnios, however many cases remain undiagnosed in the prenatal period. Neonates with EA/TEF present in the immediate newborn period with coughing, gagging, vomiting, excessive drooling, cyanosis, and respiratory distress exacerbated by feeding. It is not possible to pass an enteric tube past the proximal esophagus into the stomach.

Anatomy and Physiology

Esophageal atresia with tracheoesophageal fistula is caused by failure of separation of the foregut into the trachea and esophagus before the sixth week of gestation. There are five types of EA/TEF. The most common type (>75 percent) is EA with a distal tracheoesophageal fistula that connects the trachea to the distal esophagus. In 10 to 15 percent of cases there is EA with no TEF. The third most common type is an isolated H-type or an N-type TEF that connects the trachea to the esophagus with no EA (5 percent). Up to 3 percent have EA with both proximal and distal TEF. The least common type is EA with a TEF to the proximal esophageal pouch (1 percent; Fig. 34.1).

Imaging Findings

Prenatal ultrasound (US):
- Polyhydramnios
- Distended proximal esophageal pouch
- Absence of a fluid-filled fetal stomach

Radiography:
- Air-distended proximal esophageal pouch
- Coiling of an enteric tube in the pouch (Fig. 34.2)
- Gasless newborn abdomen suggests EA with a proximal TEF, or isolated EA
- Signs of VACTERL association (Vertebral anomalies, gastrointestinal Atresias of the duodenum or anus, TracheoEsophageal fistulas, Renal anomalies, and radial ray Limb defects).

Imaging Strategy

Frontal and lateral chest radiography following attempted passage of a nasogastric tube is usually the first imaging exam. If needed, a small amount (1 to 2 cc) of relatively low-osmolality water-soluble contrast can be administered under careful fluoroscopic guidance into the proximal esophageal pouch to depict a proximal TEF or an H-type TEF (Fig. 34.3). It can also demonstrate the length of the proximal esophageal segment, which is important in surgical planning. TEF without atresia may be suspected in infants or children with recurrent respiratory distress or infections and esophagram can demonstrate the fistula. If contrast is present in the trachea without associated aspiration or identification of a fistula, then a pull-back tube esophagram (injecting iso-osmolar water-soluble contrast through a tube in the esophagus as the tube is withdrawn from the distal esophagus) may help demonstrate the fistula. At least 50 percent of the infants with EA have one or more additional anomalies in the VACTERL association. The workup typically consists of radiographic survey to look for skeletal anomalies, echocardiogram, and renal ultrasound. Occasionally, additional studies of the GI tract and spine US are required if anorectal malformations are present. Three-dimensional CT with virtual bronchoscopy may be useful for preoperative planning in some patients with complicated associated tracheal anomalies or tracheal stenosis.

Related Physics

Newborn fluoroscopy for EA must be undertaken with great care as the potential exists to deliver large doses of radiation in short periods of time. Most modern fluoroscopic equipment is capable of automatic selection and control of kVp and mA (X-ray tube current). Fluoroscopy can be employed to capture disordered peristalsis within the esophagus as well as abnormal wall motion of the trachea resulting from tracheomalacia. The patient is imaged supine in the lateral

(A) (B) (C)

(D) (E) (F)

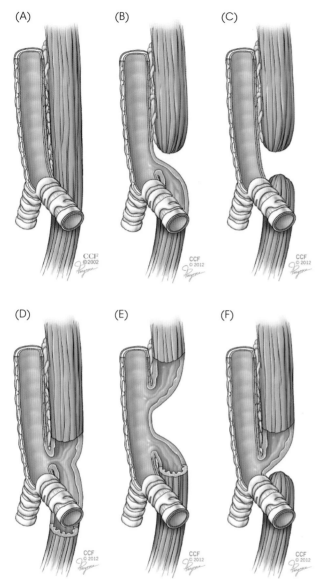

Figure 34.1. Spectrum of esophageal atresia and traceoesophageal fistula in order of frequency. Normal (A). Distal fistula (B). No fistula (C). H- or N-type fistula (D). Proximal and distal fistula (E). Proximal fistula (F).

projection and selection of frame rate must consider the balance between dose and image quality. Pulsed fluoroscopy is preferred to continuous fluoroscopy as it will further decrease dose; the pulse rate is adjusted to the lowest possible without compromising lesion detection.

Differential Diagnosis

- Traumatic enteric tube placement with pseudodiverticulum +/− pneumothorax or pneumomediastinum
- Esophageal web or rings
- Esophageal stricture
- Esophageal diverticulum
- Laryngotracheoesophageal cleft
- Congenital short esophagus with intrathoracic stomach

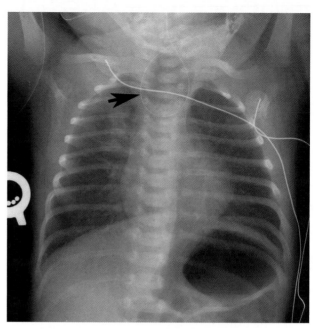

Figure 34.2. Frontal chest radiograph in a newborn with choking with feeds shows an enteric tube coiled in an air-distended proximal esophageal pouch (arrow). There is air in the stomach, which confirms a distal TEF. There are no associated vertebral anomalies.

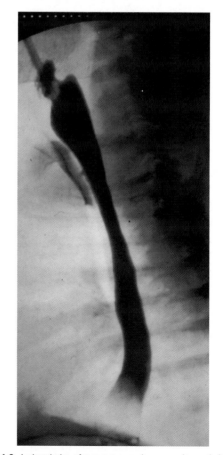

Figure 34.3. Lateral view from an esophagram in an infant with recurrent pneumonia where iso-osmolar contrast that is injected through an indwelling esophageal tube depicts an H-type TEF with contrast filling of the esophagus, fistula, and trachea.

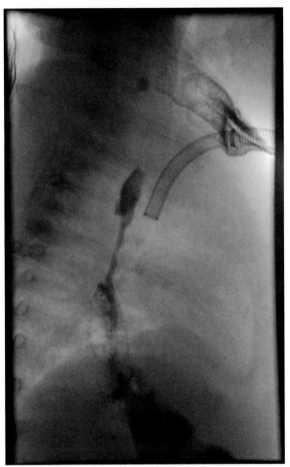

Figure 34.4. Lateral esophagram in a child postrepair for EA and TEF shows a long segment stricture which may be from postoperative scarring or from gastroesophageal reflux.

patients with EA/TEF have a right aortic arch, leading the surgeon to adopt a left rather than the preferred right lateral approach for open repair. Coexisting severe cardiac anomalies or very low birth weight increase mortality in infants with EA/TEF. The presence of a severe cardiac anomaly is the most significant factor. Respiratory and GI symptoms often persist following surgical repair. All patients have abnormal esophageal motility particularly in the distal segment, leading to reflux with poor clearance. Affected children may also develop esophageal stenosis resulting from anastomotic stricture, gastroesophageal reflux-induced strictures, postsurgical tracheal diverticulum, and recurrent TEF (Fig. 34.4). All patients have some degree of tracheomalacia. Image-guided esophageal dilation can be used to treat anastomotic esophageal strictures.

Key Points

- EA occurs in conjunction with TEF in 85 to 90 % of cases.
- Approximately 50 to 70 % of patients with EA/TEF have associated congenital anomalies of the VACTERL association.
- Most infants with an EA also have a distal TEF.
- Isolated EA without TEF is more likely to have a longer atretic segment, which makes primary repair more challenging.
- It is important to identify a right aortic arch, which will alter surgical approach.
- Failure to pass an enteric tube and a dilated proximal pouch are classic radiographic findings.

Common Variants

Fifty to 70 percent of patients with EA/TEF have associated congenital anomalies in the VACTERL association. Up to 10 percent of children with EA/TEF have associated syndromes or chromosomal anomalies, including Trisomies X, 13, 18, 21 and certain chromosomal duplications or deletions. Other associated syndromes include but are not limited to CHARGE syndrome, Feingold syndrome, DiGeorge syndrome, Pallister-Hall syndrome, anophthalmia-esophageal-genital syndrome, Fanconi anemia, and Opitz syndrome. Tracheoesophageal fistulas can also be induced by prolonged intubation or tracheostomy, erosive malignancy, infection or trauma.

Clinical Issues

Isolated EA without TEF is more likely to have shorter esophageal segments, making primary repair more challenging. Following gastrostomy tube placement, contrast instilled into the stomach will reflux into the distal esophageal segment and can help to define the length of the distal segment for esophageal repair planning. Five percent of

Further Reading

Al-Qahtani AR, Yazbeck S, Rosen NG, Youssef S, Mayer SK. Lengthening technique for long gap esophageal atresia and early anastamosis. *J Pediatr Surg.* 2003;38(5):737–739.

De Jong EM, Felix JF, de Klein A, Tibboel D. Etiology of esophageal atresia and tracheoesophageal fistula: "Mind the gap." *Curr Gastroenterol Rep.* 2010; 12:215–222.

Fitoz S, Atasoy C, Yagmurlu A, Akyar S, Erden A, Dindar H. Three-dimensional CT of congenital esophageal atresia and distal tracheoesophageal fistula in neonates: preliminary results. *AJR.* 2000;*175*(Nov):1403–1407.

Laffan EE, Daneman A, Ein SH, Kerrigan D, Manson DE. Tracheoesophageal fistula without esophageal atresia: are pull-back tube esophagrams needed? *Pediatr Radiol.* 2006; 36:1141–1147.

Okamoto T, Takamizawa S, Arai H, Bitoh Y, Nakao M, Yokoi A, Nishijima E. Esophageal atresia: prognostic classification revisited. *Surgery.* 2009;*145*(6):675–681.

Lederman HM, Demarchi GTS. Congenital esophageal malformations. In: Slovis TL. *Caffey's Pediatric Diagnostic Imaging.* Eleventh edition. Philadelphia, PA: Mosby Elsevier; 2008.

Wai-man Lam W, Tam PKH, Chan FL, Chan KL, Cheng W. Esophageal atresia and tracheal stenosis: use of three-dimensional CT and virtual bronchoscopy in neonates, infants, and children. *AJR.* 2000;*174*(Apr):1009–1012.

CHAPTER 35

Hypertrophic Pyloric Stenosis

Angelisa M. Paladin, MD

Definition

Hypertrophic pyloric stenosis (HPS) is an idiopathic acquired hypertrophy of the gastric outlet that presents in the newborn period. Abnormal thickening of the pylorus leads to gastric outlet obstruction.

Clinical Features

Hypertrophic pyloric stenosis is 2.5 to 5.5 times more common in boys than girls and has a higher incidence in first-born infants. Infants with HPS usually present 4 to 6 weeks after birth. Premature infants are rarely affected. Hypertrophic pyloric stenosis is rare in infants less than 1 week of age or greater than 3 months of age. Most have a normal feeding history with gradual onset of nonbilious vomiting that becomes projectile over time. Clinical exam of the right-upper quadrant may reveal a palpable rounded mass, the size of an olive. Surgical pyloromyotomy is the primary treatment.

Anatomy and Physiology

The normal pyloric antrum is 1 millimeter thick and terminates at the pyloric sphincter, marking the opening of the stomach into the duodenum. In children with HPS, a pyloric channel of variable length composed of hypertrophied muscle separates the duodenal bulb from the antrum (Fig. 35.1). The lumen of the rigid canal is filled with redundant mucosa that may herniate into the gastric antrum. The combination of redundant mucosa and the thickened pyloric muscle obstructs passage of the gastric contents.

Imaging Findings

Radiography:
  - "Caterpillar" sign: exaggerated contractions of gastric incisura with gastric dilation (Fig. 35.2)
Ultrasound (US):
  - Pyloric wall thickness greater than 3 millimeters
  - Pyloric length greater than 15 -millimeters (Fig. 35.3)
  - Delayed or failed transit of gastric contents through the pylorus

Upper GI
  - "String" sign: elongated pyloric channel outlined by a string of contrast (Fig. 35.4)
  - "Double track" of contrast in the pyloric channel related to barium passing between the redundant mucosa
  - "Shouldering" or bulging of the pyloric muscle mass into the distal antrum
  - Umbrella-shaped duodenal bulb resulting from the grossly enlarged pyloric musculature exerting mass effect on the duodenal bulb (Fig. 35.5)

IMAGING PITFALLS: For the most accurate evaluation of pyloric muscle thickness, US of the pylorus must be performed perpendicular to the axis of the pylorus for cross-sectional views, and longitudinal views must be aligned with the middle longitudinal plane such that the "double mucosal echo" is observed. If not properly orientated, oblique axial or off-side longitudinal images may falsely suggest muscle thickening. Pylorospasm can mimic HPS on US and measurement variability is an important clue. Pylorospasm is a dynamic process that resolves with time.

Imaging Strategy

Ultrasound should be the initial exam for 2- to 12-week-old children presenting with progressive and projectile nonbilious vomiting. The sensitivity and specificity are close to 100 percent for the US detection of HPS. A linear high-frequency transducer is used to obtain axial and longitudinal images through the center of the pyloric channel. Measurements of pyloric wall thickness and pyloric channel length are obtained after oral administration of water; placing a towel or blanket under the baby's left side will position the baby slightly right-side-down and will allow the recently ingested water now in the gastric antrum to act as an acoustic window for evaluation of size and patency of the pylorus. This also facilitates dynamic real-time evaluation of gastric emptying through the pylorus. If the pylorus is normal in appearance, other causes of vomiting, such as malrotation of the bowel, can be assessed. A transverse image to assess the superior mesenteric artery/vein (SMA/ SMV) relationship and to evaluate the position of the third

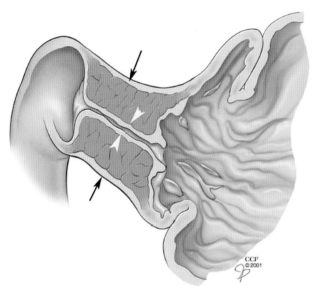

Figure 35.1. Hypertrophic pyloric stenosis. Elongated and thickened pyloric channel with marked luminal narrowing.

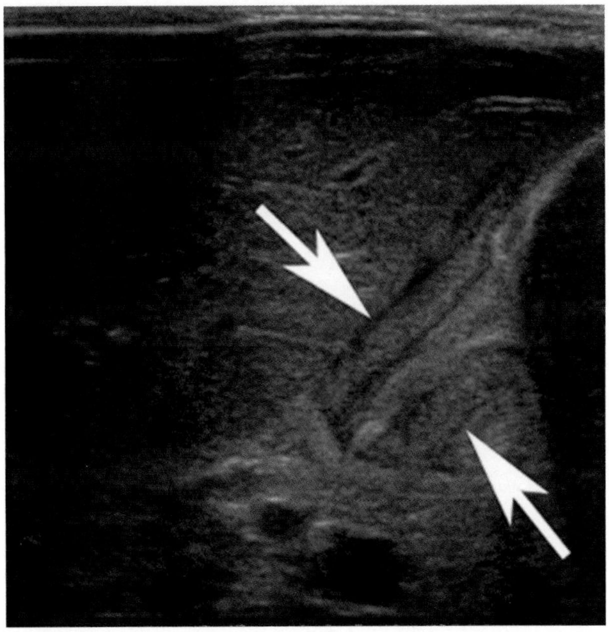

portion of the duodenum relative to the SMA and aorta may be obtained to evaluate for possible malrotation.

Related Physics
Ultrasound is the tool of choice for the diagnosis of HPS as it exquisitely demonstrates the anatomy of the gastric outlet and this along with strict measurement criteria will provide an accurate diagnosis in most cases. One characteristic feature that has been described is based on a

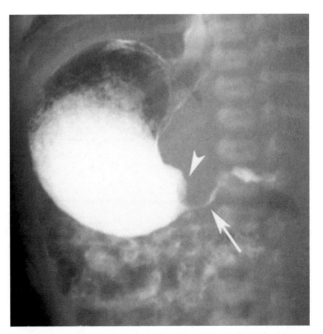

Figure 35.3. Transverse US of the right-upper quadrant in a 7-week-old term boy with projectile vomiting shows a longitudinal view of the elongated pyloric channel, with redundant mucosa and markedly thickened walls (arrows).

particular US artifact generated on the short-axis view of the pylorus. This "critical angle artifact" appears as twin anechoic wedge-shaped regions along the sides of the targettoid appearance of the pylorus in cross-section. This occurs because of sound reflected at shallow angles created by the smooth convex margin of the pylorus. This effect is most apparent with linear array transducers as the

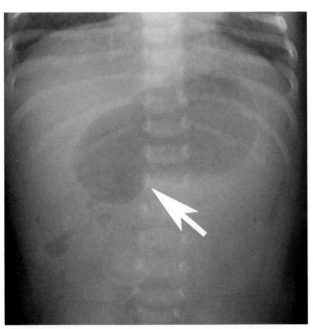

Figure 35.2. Supine frontal radiograph of the abdomen in a 6-week-old boy with projectile vomiting demonstrates gastric distension and signs of increased peristalsis (arrow), coined the "caterpillar" sign.

Figure 35.4. Lateral image from a UGI study in a 6-week-old male with projectile vomiting demonstrates shouldering of the antrum (arrowhead) and the "string" sign (arrow).

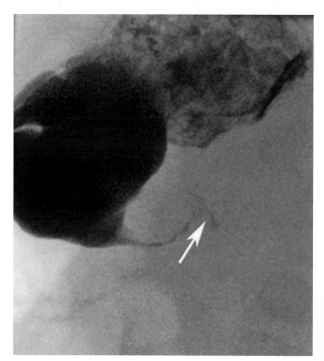

Figure 35.5. Lateral image from a UGI study in a 5-week-old girl with projectile vomiting demonstrates elongation of the pylorus (string sign) and an umbrella-shaped duodenal bulb (arrow).

insonating beam is nearly parallel to the lateral margin of the pylorus.

Differential Diagnosis

Nonbilious vomiting:

- Pylorospasm
- Gastroenteritis
- Gastroesophageal reflux
- Hiatal hernia
- Malrotation (usually bilious)
- Preampullary duodenal stenosis or web
- Gastric antral web

Common Variants

Hypertrophic pyloric stenosis can be isolated or can occur with other congenital defects, including esophageal atresia and tracheoesophageal fistula, renal abnormalities, Turner's syndrome, and trisomy 18. Premature infants present 4 to 6 weeks after birth—not their due date—and therefore the muscle thickness may be borderline normal because they are comparably smaller.

Clinical Issues

The clinical presentation varies with duration of symptoms. Initially, the infant has periodic forceful nonbilious vomiting, which may then become projectile, with an increase in frequency over time. Inadequate ingestion of oral intake may be followed by dehydration and electrolyte disturbances including hypochloremic alkalosis and sodium and potassium deficits. With a delay in diagnosis there may be extensive weight loss and complications related to dehydration.

Key Points

- Evolving acquired pathologic process with unknown etiology
- Common cause of gastric outlet obstruction in the newborn
- More common in males and first-born infants
- Presents with nonbilious vomiting that may become projectile
- US criteria are muscularis thickness > 3 millimeters and length > 15 millimeters, +/– mucosal hypertrophy
- Little to no passage of fluid though the enlarged pyloric channel over several minutes

Further Reading

Hernanz-Schulman M. Infantile hypertrophic pyloric stenosis. *Radiology.* 2003;*227*: 319–331.

Hernanz-Schulman M. Pyloric stenosis: role of imaging. *Pediatric Radiology.* 2009;*39*: 134–139.

Rohrschneider WK, Mittnacht H, Darge K, Troger J. Pyloric muscle in asymptomatic infants: sonographic evaluation and discrimination from idiopathic hypertrophic pyloric stenosis. *Pediatr Radiol.* 1998;*28*:429–434.

Spevak MR, Ahmadjian JM, Kleinman PK, Henriquez G, Hirsh MP, Cohen IT. Sonography of hypertrophic pyloric stenosis: frequency and cause of nonuniform echogenicity of the thickened pyloric muscle. *AJR.* 1992;*158*:129–132.

CHAPTER 36

Appendicitis

Angelisa M. Paladin, MD

Definition

Acute appendicitis is the most common surgical emergency in childhood and is the result of obstruction of the appendiceal lumen with secondary inflammation.

Clinical Features

One to 4 percent of children presenting to the emergency room with acute abdominal pain will have acute appendicitis. Perforation reportedly occurs in 16 to 39 percent with a median of 20 percent. Acute appendicitis can be a diagnostic challenge because the symptoms are similar to a variety of other conditions that cause acute abdominal pain and include nausea, vomiting, low-grade fever, crampy periumbilical or right-lower quadrant (RLQ) pain, and point RLQ or rebound tenderness. The classic history of pain beginning in the periumbilical region and migrating to the RLQ occurs in only 50 percent of patients. Laboratory findings show elevated white blood cell count (WBC)with increase in polymorphonuclear leukocytes.

Anatomy and Physiology

Appendicitis occurs when the appendix becomes inflamed and obstructed leading to infection and bacterial overgrowth. In grade-school-age children the luminal obstruction is often caused by lymphoid hyperplasia, foreign bodies, fecaliths, or parasites. Lymphoid hyperplasia could be related to viral infection, including upper respiratory infection and gastroenteritis. Fecaliths develop from inspissated feces, with progressive layering of fecal debris and calcium over time.

Imaging Findings

Primary findings on graded-compression ultrasound (US):
- Noncompressible, enlarged, fluid-filled, blind-ending tubular structure that originates from the cecum
- Maximal appendiceal diameter, from outside wall to outside wall, greater than 6 millimeters

Secondary findings:
- "Target" sign on axial plane (seen in early appendicitis): fluid-filled lumen surrounded by echogenic mucosa and submucosa and hypoechoic muscularis (Fig. 36.1)
- Periappendiceal fluid
- Hyperemia
- Periappendiceal echogenicity representing mesenteric fat inflammation
- Appendicolith: intraluminal echogenic focus with acoustic shadowing (Fig 36.2)
- Mesenteric lymphadenopathy
- Superior mesenteric vein (SMV) or portal vein thrombus

Primary findings on CT:
- Enlarged appendix > 7-millimeter transverse diameter
- Appendiceal wall thickening
- Wall enhancement greater than normal (uninflammed) bowel (Fig. 36.3).

Secondary findings:
- Periappendiceal fat stranding (Fig. 36.4)
- Focal cecal wall thickening
- Free fluid in RLQ or pelvis
- Appendicolith
- Periappendiceal abscess
- Mesenteric lymphadenopathy
- SMV or portal vein thrombus with or without hepatic emboli

IMAGING PITFALLS: The most common cause of a false-negative US diagnosis is lack of visualization of the appendix. This can be related to atypical location of the cecum, appendiceal perforation, or inadequate compression. Another potential source of error is the misinterpretation of the terminal ileum as the appendix. However, identification of the appendix as a blind-ending tubular structure will thwart this pitfall except in the uncommon cases of Meckel's diverticulitis. There is an overlapping range in maximal appendiceal diameter between an inflamed and uninflamed appendix. Therefore, secondary signs are very important. Young children may have clinical symptoms before changes are detectable by CT; US after a period of observation may be helpful.

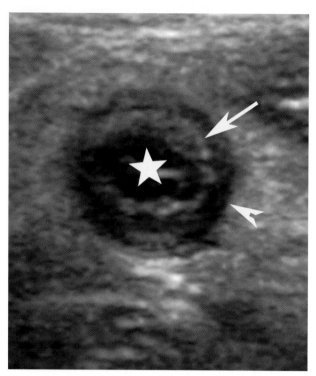

Figure 36.1. Transverse US image of the appendix tip in a 6-year-old boy with RLQ pain demonstrates a fluid-filled lumen (star) surrounded by echogenic mucosa and submucosa (arrow) and hypoechoic muscularis (arrowhead), the target sign.

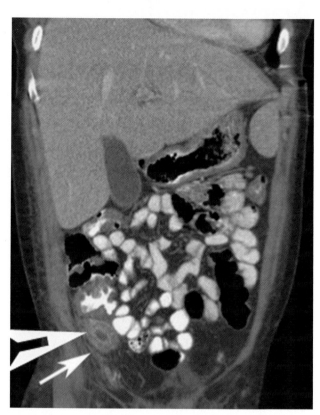

Figure 36.3. Coronal intravenous and oral contrast-enhanced CT image of the abdomen in an 8-year-old girl with RLQ tenderness shows an enlarged appendix with thick, hyperemic walls (arrowhead) and adjacent inflammatory fat stranding (arrow). The wall of the cecum is also thickened.

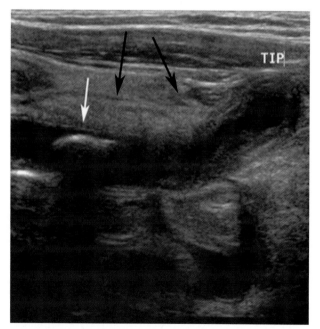

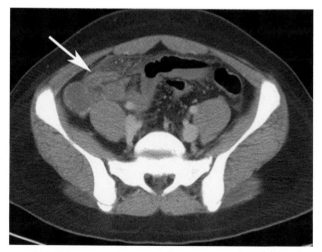

Figure 36.2. Sagittal US image of the pelvis in an 8-year-old girl with RLQ pain demonstrates an enlarged appendix measuring 1.4 millimeters in greatest transverse diameter. There is an echogenic appendicolith (arrow) near the tip and surrounding echogenic inflammatory changes in the periappendiceal fat (black arrows).

Figure 36.4. Axial intravenous and oral contrast-enhanced CT image of the abdomen in a 7-year-old boy with leukocytosis and generalized abdominal pain demonstrates an enlarged, hyperemic, thick-walled fluid-filled appendix with surrounding inflammatory changes (arrow).

On CT a fluid-filled loop of small bowel can be misinterpreted as appendicitis. Positive enteric contrast in the proximal appendix may abut and obscure an obstructing stone within the mid or distal appendix. Although the appendicolith may be obscured, surrounding inflammation should still be visible.

Imaging Strategy

Diagnostic imaging of appendicitis requires US and CT. Initial evaluation with US is recommended because of the lack of radiation and lower cost. Graded compression with a linear transducer is performed to localize the appendix. If the cecum is identified but the appendix is not found, coronal sonographic images may help visualize a retrocecal appendix. If the appendix is still not seen, then a curved transducer should be used to look deeper into the pelvis for complex free fluid or abscess formation secondary to a perforated appendix. If the appendix is not identified sonographically and clinical suspicion is low, CT can be delayed or averted in favor of clinical observation. If US is not diagnostic and clinical suspicion is high, an additional spiral, thin-section abdominal CT with IV and oral contrast can improve diagnostic accuracy and decrease the negative appendectomy rate. Coronal reformatted images may be used to cross-reference with axial images and increase the ease of detection of the appendix.

Related Physics

Ultrasound is the preferred first-line imaging tool for appendicitis except in those with larger body habitus. When CT is performed it is important to match beam width with patient size to avoid overirradiation. It is also prudent to maintain pitch at 1 to 1.3 in all patients. kVp and mAs are chosen from specialized pediatric protocol charts based on patient size or age. In general, lower kVp is used for smaller patients and higher kVp for the larger patients. In all cases the rotation time should be as short as possible (< 1 sec) in order to limit effects of patient motion. Image thickness should be between 1 to 3 millimeters and if multiplanar reformations are used, overlapping reconstruction interval of 50 percent of the slice thickness is advised. Scan length refers to the table travel distance for which axial images will be constructed and should be limited to the volume of interest (care should be taken to avoid testes in a male). When the order to rule out appendicitis is a common request, one can craft specialized techniques based on institutional preference and technology while incorporating the above factors.

Differential Diagnosis

Abdominal pain:
- Appendiceal or periappendiceal inflammation resulting from Crohn's disease or pelvic inflammatory disease
- Meckel's diverticulitis
- Ovarian or testicular torsion
- Gastroenteritis
- Epiploic appendagitis
- Intussusception
- Midgut volvulus

Enlarged tubular structure in the RLQ:
- Crohn's of the appendix
- Meckel's diverticulitis
- Tubovarian abscess
- Torsion of the fallopian tube
- Mucocele of the appendix

Common Variants

Tip appendicitis: obstruction of the appendiceal lumen can occur anywhere in the appendix. Only a portion of the appendix may be obstructed, resulting in localized inflammation distal to the point of obstruction. On US, the majority of the appendix will be normal in size. If the entire length of the appendix is not identified and the blind end confirmed, then this diagnosis may be missed.

Stump appendicitis: failure to invaginate the appendiceal stump into the cecum at the time of appendectomy creates the potential for recurrent inflammation. This possibility increases with a laparoscopic approach.

Clinical Issues

Early surgical intervention in patients with acute appendicitis is important to avoid perforation, which is associated with increased morbidity and mortality. Perforation rates are highest in preschool-age children (62 to 88 percent), likely related to delayed diagnosis or misdiagnosis. Laparoscopic appendectomy prior to perforation is the treatment for acute appendicitis. Nonsurgical treatment with antibiotic therapy is recommended if perforation has occurred and a phlegmon has developed, followed by delayed appendectomy. Percutaneous or surgical drainage is recommended if a well-defined periappendiceal abscess has developed. Patients with extensive and poorly defined collections usually require immediate surgical intervention.

Key Points
- Acute appendicitis is the most common surgical emergency in children.
- Only 50% have a classic history (pain beginning in periumbilical region migrating to RLQ).
- Maximal diameter of appendix from outside to outside wall is >6 millimeters (US) and >7 millimeters (CT).
- Entire length of the appendix must be visualized and be normal to exclude appendicitis.
- If appendix is not visualized with a linear transducer, a curved transducer is used to look deeper into the pelvis to assess for fluid collections or abscess from appendiceal perforation.

Further Reading

Birnbaum BA, Wilson SR. Appendicitis at the millennium. *Radiology.* 2000;*215*:337–348.

Kaiser S, Frenckner B, Jorulf HK. Suspected appendicitis in children: US and CT–a prospective randomized study. *Radiology.* 2002;*223*:633–638.

Levine CD, Aizenstein O, Wachsberg RH. Pitfalls in the CT diagnosis of appendicitis. *British Journal of Radiology.* 2004;*77*:792–799.

Sivit C, Siegal M, Applegate K, Newman K. When appendicitis is suspected in children. *Radiographics.* 2001;*21*:247–262.

Wan MJ, Krahn M, Ungar WJ, Caku E, Sung L, Medina LS, Doria AS. Acute appendicitis in young children: cost-effectiveness of US versus CT in diagnosis: A Markov decision analytic model. *Radiology.* 2009;*250*:378–386.

CHAPTER 37

Ileocolic Intussusception (Idiopathic)

Mohammed Bilal Shaikh, MD, Monica Epelman, MD, and Jeffrey C. Hellinger, MD, FACC

Definition

Intussusception is the invagination of a segment of bowel (intussusceptum) into the adjacent distal segment (intussuscipiens), causing bowel obstruction and compression of the associated mesenteric vasculature.

Clinical Features

Intussusception can be categorized as idiopathic or secondary to a pathologic lead point. Ninety percent are idiopathic, ileocolic, and occur in children less than 3 years of age. Less commonly intussusception is triggered by a pathologic lead point, usually in children less than 3 months or older than 3 years of age. Intussusception can have a variable clinical presentation, which overlaps with other acute abdominal pathologies. The characteristic presentation is a triad of vomiting, colicky intermittent abdominal pain (often severe), and red currant jelly stool. However, this triad is seen in fewer than 30 percent of cases. Other signs may include lethargy, diarrhea, bloody stools, and/or a palpable abdominal mass. Patients often have had a recent viral infection (e.g., upper respiratory, gastrointestinal).

Anatomy and Physiology

Intussusception may occur as a result of intestinal peristaltic dysmotility with or without focal bowel pathology. In the idiopathic subtype, the terminal ileum invaginates into the cecum and ascending colon (ileocolic). This is thought to be associated with hypertrophy of the normal lymphoid tissue in the Peyer patches which act as a nonpathologic lead point for the intussusception. In the pathologic subtype, common lead points include enteric duplication cysts, Meckel's diverticula, submucosal hematomas (e.g., Henoch-Schonlein Purpura, coagulation disorders, trauma), inspissated feces (e.g., cystic fibrosis), benign polyps (hamartomas), and malignant masses (e.g., lymphoma). As the abnormal bowel wall propagates into the "receiving" distal lumen, it pulls with it the proximal bowel and its mesentery, including mesenteric fat and vasculature (Fig. 37.1). The intussuscepted bowel is surrounded completely by the intussuscipiens and is often further compressed by the ileocecal valve. This is the basis for intestinal obstruction and vascular compression. With prolonged vascular compression, mesenteric venous drainage is impaired leading to venous congestion and bowel wall edema. Continued elevation of mesenteric venous pressure will impede mesenteric arterial flow, causing mucosal ischemia. If the vascular compromise persists, the end result is sloughing of intestinal mucosa and bleeding which, when mixed with mucus, yields the "red currant jelly" stool. Intermittent spontaneous reduction or partial reduction often occurs, which can account for the intermittent symptoms. If intussusception persists and is left untreated, it may lead to bowel infarction, perforation, sepsis, and death.

Imaging Findings

Radiography:
- Intraluminal mass or visualized intussusceptum
- Small bowel dilatation with absence of gas in the cecum and ascending colon
- Gas-filled small bowel loops in the expected location of the cecum
- Obscured lower-liver margin or right-upper abdominal mass (Fig. 37.2)
- Crescent sign: crescent of intraluminal air surrounding the rounded mass

Ultrasound (US), with a (sensitivity of 98 to 100%):
- Transverse US usually demonstrates a "target" or "doughnut" appearance with a hypoechoic outer rim of homogeneous thickness (intussuscipiens) and a central core consisting of the intussusceptum and adjacent mesentery (Fig. 37.3A)
- "Gut signature" represents hyperechoic mucosa adjacent to hypoechoic muscular layer and hyperechoic mesenteric fat
- Mass with a 3- to 5-centimeter diameter more likely ileocolic or colocolic
- Mass with < 2.5-centimeter diameter is likely caused by a small bowel-small bowel intussusception
- Mass often located just deep to the abdominal wall
- As bowel wall edema progresses, the number of detectable "layers" of the target may decrease
- "Pseudokidney" sign on sagittal projections caused by the relatively hypoechoic peripherally located

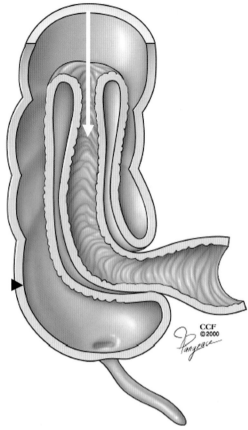

Figure 37.1. Intussusception. Intussusceptum (arrow) invaginates into the intussuscipiens (arrowhead).

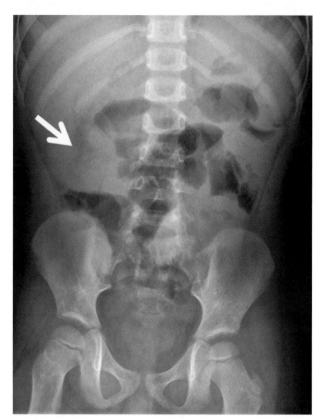

Figure 37.2. Supine frontal radiograph in a child with intermittent abdominal pain demonstrates a round, focal soft-tissue mass in the right mid-abdomen (arrow); cecum is not identified. Diagnostic US confirmed ileocolic intussusception.

bowel wall with a hyperechoic center resulting from intussuscepted mesenteric fat
- "Sandwich" sign: multiple alternating layers of bowel and mesentery may resemble a sandwich if the intussusception is imaged longitudinally (Fig. 37.3B)
- Free intraperitoneal fluid may be seen in greater than 50% of cases but is not definitely associated with perforation (anechoic fluid is likely reactive)

CT:
- Target appearance: outer layer of variable thickness (intussuscipiens), a hypoattenuating subjacent layer of mesenteric fat adjacent to the intussuscepted bowel (intussusceptum) (Fig. 37.4)
- Mesenteric lymph nodes may be drawn in with the mesenteric fat and vessels and seen within the intussusception on US or CT

Contrast enema:
- Intraluminal filling defect with a curvilinear leading edge with water-soluble contrast (Fig. 37.5) or air contrast used for reduction (Fig. 37.6)
- Successful reduction will reduce the mass and there will be free retrograde flow of contrast or air into the distal small bowel loops

Imaging Strategy

A high index of suspicion, based upon age, symptoms, and physical exam is essential for prompt imaging. Selection of diagnostic modalities depends upon the available technology and operator skill. Algorithms should strive for minimal patient radiation exposure, using the least invasive approach. Based on the presenting symptoms, radiography may be the initial modality obtained, particularly if the symptoms are very vague. Standard projections include a supine frontal and either an upright or left lateral decubitus projection to rule out free air. Prone positioning for abdominal radiographs moves air from the transverse colon into the cecum and ascending colon and can help with assessment of the cecum. When the patient's clinical presentation and/or radiographs suggest intussusception, US is performed. If the clinical pretest probability for intussusception is high, US could be performed as the first imaging modality. The entire abdomen and pelvis is examined. Once confirmed, and provided there are no contraindications, image-guided retrograde pressure reduction is performed using various techniques based upon operator skill. Image-guided reduction techniques include: pneumatic reduction with fluoroscopic guidance, water-soluble contrast enema with fluoroscopic guidance, or hydrostatic or pneumatic

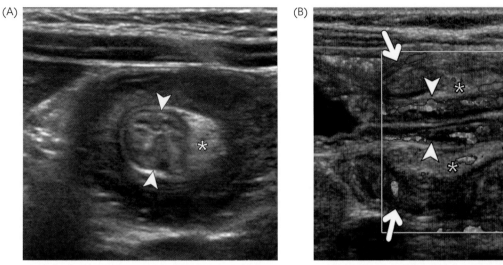

Figure 37.3. Transverse gray-scale US image of the right-upper quadrant (A) in a 6-month-old infant with colicky abdominal pain demonstrates the typical "target" or "doughnut" appearance of intussusception. Crescentic echogenic mesenteric fat (*) is noted adjacent to the intussusceptum (arrowheads) within the intussuscepiens. Sagittal color Doppler US image (B) shows blood flow to the intussuscepted bowel with some flow seen in the distended intussuscipiens. Note the alternating layers of intussuscepted bowel wall (arrowheads) and hyperechoic mesenteric fat (*) within the lumen of the distended bowel of the intussuscipiens (arrows). These alternating layers of bowel wall and mesenteric fat represent the "sandwich" sign.

reduction with US or fluoroscopic guidance. In clinically stable patients, some authors advocate the use of delayed, repeated reduction attempts if there is at least partial reduction with the first attempt. Following successful reduction, patients are clinically monitored prior to discharge as approximately 10 to 15 percent may recur. Suspected recurrence can be assessed with US. Image-guided reduction can be performed following a recurrence if there are no contraindications. The main complication from attempted enema reduction is bowel perforation. Most reported perforation rates are less than

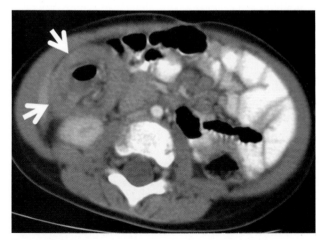

Figure 37.4. Axial oral and intravenous contrast-enhanced CT image in a child with abdominal pain shows a "target" sign of an intussusception in the ascending colon (arrows). Some gas is seen within the intussusceptum. There are enhancing mesenteric vessels in the mesenteric fat within the intussusception.

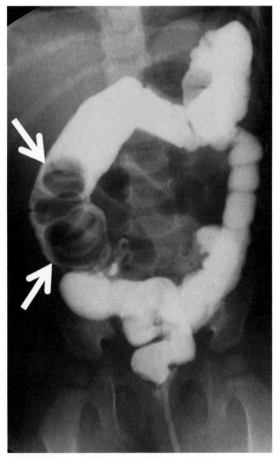

Figure 37.5. Frontal image from water-soluble contrast enema demonstrates a large filling defect in the cecum and ascending colon (arrows). Contrast fills the remainder of the colon and the appendix.

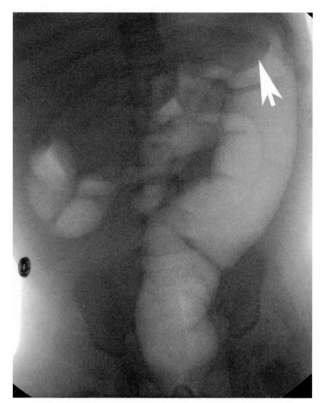

Figure 37.6. Frontal image from air enema reduction of intussusception shows the enema tip at the inferior margin of the image within the distal rectum. Air is insufflated, the pressure is monitored with a sphygmomanometer, and the progression of air within the bowel is visualized fluoroscopically. The insufflated air is abutting the leading edge of the intussusceptum (arrow) at the splenic flexure, creating an air crescent.

1 percent. An extremely rare but life-threatening consequence of perforation with air enema is tension pneumoperitoneum. This can be avoided by discontinuing the air enema as soon as the pneumoperitoneum is identified, by opening the tube to release the air from the bowel and, if needed, using a large-bore needle for percutaneous transabdominal emergency decompression.

Related Physics

Intussusception reduction can be performed in a variety of ways, using US or fluoroscopic guidance, and using air, water, or water-soluble contrast. Barium is generally avoided because of the risk for intestinal perforation during pressure reduction and the attendant risk of barium peritonitis. Modern fluoroscopic units use automatic brightness control to moderate the X-ray exposure rate and this mode is sensitive to the total attenuation along the imaging path. When air replaces solid or liquid bowel contents the exposure rate will decrease because the air has a lower attenuation than the material it is displacing. Water would be next in line whereby replacing solid bowel contents with water would increase the exposure rate over air but would still be less than for solid contents. The

highest exposure rates occur when intraluminal contrast agents such as water-soluble iodinated fluids or barium are used, higher for barium than for iodinated contrast. The dose rate effectively increases with the opacity of the intraluminal contents. For babies undergoing upper GI, water-soluble contrast can be diluted to achieve the lowest possible iodine level and osmolality, which in turn will minimize radiation exposure and also toxicity from aspiration or perforation. For all pediatric fluoroscopy, it is advisable to use magnification modes sparingly as X-ray output increases from a factor of 2 to 4 depending on modes chosen and specific equipment configurations. The choice between air and water-soluble iodinated contrast may be institution-specific with both media associated with similar success and perforation rates. A lower radiation dose is achievable with air than with positive contrast, primarily because of difference in physical density, however, it may be more difficult to detect an early perforation with air than with positive contrast.

Differential Diagnosis

- Colitis
- Bowel wall hematoma
- Intracolonic stool
- Midgut volvulus

Common Variants

Approximately 90 percent of cases are idiopathic and ileocolic, though approximately 10 percent have a recognizable etiology with a pathologic lead point (which itself warrants treatment or resection). In these cases, intussusception may be jejuno-jejunal, jejuno-ileal, ileo-ileal, and colocolic. When intussusception is encountered in these atypical regions, the radiologist must search for and attempt to exclude a pathologic lead point. Transient asymptomatic small bowel intussusceptions often occur. These tend to be smaller in diameter (less than 2.5 cm), involve a shorter segment of bowel of less than 3.5 centimeters, and show no pathologic lead point nor result in small bowel obstruction. Transient small bowel intussusceptions that occur and reduce spontaneously on real-time imaging are of no clinical significance. For patients with small bowel intussusception disease that results from the presence of a pathologic lead point and/or bowel complications, spontaneous reduction may not occur and small bowel obstruction or ischemia may result. Small bowel intussusception disease characteristically affects older children and the imaging appearance may mimic that of ileocolic intussusception potentially resulting in a delay in diagnosis and surgical treatment.

IMAGING PITFALLS
- If US confirms an intussusception, but no intussusception is found during reduction attempts then

there are three possible explanations: (1) the intussusception self-reduced; (2) the intussusception was isolated to the small bowel; or (3) the US result was a false-positive US (less likely). Immediately repeating the US may demonstrate a small bowel-small bowel intussusception that is not accessible by enema techniques.

■ Bowel wall thickening and mural stratification that occurs with colitis can mimic an intussusception when the bowel is image in cross-section, perpendicular to its long axis. Imaging in the long axis will allow for differentiation.

■ An edematous ileocecal valve may resemble an incompletely reduced intussusception by fluoroscopy.

■ Many lead points are not evident within the intussusception on US or CT.

Clinical Issues

The surgical team is the primary clinical managing service for patients with suspected intussusceptions and should be consulted prior to image-guided reduction attempts. Contraindications to image-guided reduction include: uncorrected hypotension, sepsis, peritoneal signs or bowel perforation/pneumoperitoneum. Surgical consultation is necessary prior to reduction attempts and the surgical team must be available for intervention should bowel perforation occur (<1 percent) or if the reduction attempt fails (10 to 20 percent).

Key Points

■ Characterized by invagination of proximal bowel (intussusceptum) into the distal bowel (intussuscipiens)

■ Ninety percent are idiopathic and ileocolic

■ Is one of the most common causes of an acute abdomen and bowel obstruction in the infant and young child

■ Can progress to bowel ischemia, infarction, and perforation if left untreated.

■ US is 98 to 100% accurate for the detection of intussusceptions.

■ Image-guided reduction is 80 to 90 percent successful.

Further Reading

Applegate KE. Intussusception in children: evidence-based diagnosis and treatment. *Pediatr Radiol.* 2009;39(Suppl 2):S140–S143.

Daneman A, Navarro O. Intussusception. Part 1: a review of diagnostic approaches. *Pediatr Radiol.* 2003;33(2):79–85. Epub 2002 Nov 19.

Daneman A, Navarro O. Intussusception. Part 2: An update on the evolution of management. *Pediatr Radiol.* 2004;34(2):97–108; quiz 187. Epub 2003 Nov 21.

Navarro O, Daneman A. Intussusception. Part 3: Diagnosis and management of those with an identifiable or predisposing cause and those that reduce spontaneously. *Pediatr Radiol.* 2004;34(4):305–312; quiz 369. Epub 2003 Oct 8.

Saverino BP, Lava C, Lowe LH, Rivard DC. Radiographic findings in the diagnosis of pediatric ileocolic intussusception: comparison to a control population. *Pediatr Emerg Care.* 2010;26(4):281–284.

CHAPTER 38

Liver Masses

Amy Mehollin-Ray, MD

Definition

Liver masses account for only 1 percent of pediatric malignancies and are subdivided by cell line of origin into epithelial types (hepatoblastoma, hepatocellular carcinoma [HCC]) and mesenchymal types (hemangioendothelioma, mesenchymal hamartoma, hepatic and biliary sarcomas). Of the malignant lesions, hepatoblastoma is the most common and is the third most common abdominal malignancy in children after neuroblastoma and Wilms tumor.

Clinical Features

A child with a liver mass typically presents with painless hepatomegaly or an abdominal mass, which may be detected by the parents or by the pediatrician. Alpha fetoprotein (AFP) levels are elevated in most tumors of epithelial origin. Hepatoblastoma has a peak incidence at 1 to 2 years of age, whereas HCC is rare under age 5 years, with a peak incidence in the teenage years. Liver tumors are about twice as common in males as females. Most children with hemangioendothelioma present by 6 months of age and many are diagnosed at birth with a male to female ratio of 1:2. The tumors of mesenchymal origin do not demonstrate elevated AFP levels, but hemangioendotheliomas may be associated with elevated endothelial growth factor (EGF) and may stain positive for glucose transporter protein1 (GLUT1) on histologic examination. Recently GLUT1 reactivity has been used to distinguish between hepatic infantile hemangioma (HIH; GLUT1-positive) and congenital hepatic vascular malformation with associated capillary proliferation (HVMCP; GLUT1-negative). The GLUT1-negative lesions are more likely to cause high-output congestive heart failure related to arteriovenous (AV) shunting within the hepatic mass or thrombocytopenia from platelet consumption (Kasabach-Merritt syndrome). Of the infants affected by GLUT1-positive lesions, 20 to 50 percent also have cutaneous hemangiomas.

Anatomy and Physiology

In general, isolated hepatic masses are more likely to affect the right hepatic lobe, related to its larger size. Hepatoblastoma is most often found to be a discrete mass, whereas HCC and hemangioendothelioma may either be discrete or multiple and diffuse. Hepatocellular carcinoma is more likely to occur in a cirrhotic liver, as in the adult, where the usual causes of cirrhosis in children include biliary atresia, cystic fibrosis, tyrosinemia, alpha-1 antitrypsin deficiency, and methotrexate therapy.

Imaging Findings

Hepatoblastoma:
- Ultrasound (US): well-defined solid mass with internal vascularity +/- calcifications
- CT: heterogeneous and enhances less than the normal liver (Fig. 38.1)
- MRI: variable signal related to areas of hemorrhage and calcification, with heterogeneous enhancement of the mass following intravenous gadolinium

HCC:
- May appear similar to hepatoblastoma, on a background of liver cirrhosis (Fig. 38.2)
- May be solitary or multifocal

Hemangioendothelioma (and related lesions):
- Varies according to the pathologic subtype
- GLUT1-positive lesions (HIH) are often multiple and diffuse (Fig. 38.3)
- GLUT1-negative lesions (HVMCP) are more likely to be solitary
- US: complex, predominantly solid mass with high-flow vascular structures on Doppler evaluation
- CT: peripheral enhancement with nodular puddling of contrast and centripetal filling on delayed images +/- central calcifications
- MRI: prominent flow voids

Imaging Strategy

The extent of disease in hepatoblastoma can be evaluated with CT or MR, although many centers favor CT as the chest can be imaged at the same time to rule out lung metastases. Hepatoblastoma is staged according to the PRETEXT system, which includes the number of involved liver segments, presence of vascular invasion and periportal lymph node metastases. These findings should be included in the imaging report to assist in surgical planning. Because

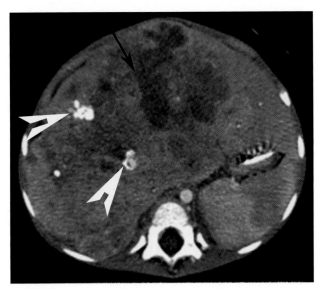

Figure 38.1. Axial contrast-enhanced CT image in a 2-year-old female with abdominal pain and elevated AFP shows a heterogeneous liver mass with areas of low attenuation, representing necrosis (arrow), and chunky calcifications (arrowheads) consistent with hepatoblastoma.

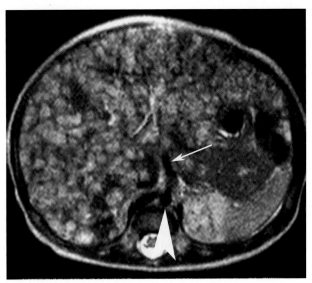

Figure 38.3. Axial single-shot T2 MR image in a 3-month-old male shows diffuse involvement of the liver with T2-hyperintense lesions. The hepatic arterial flow void (arrow) is almost equal in caliber to the abdominal aorta imaged below the celiac axis (arrowhead) in this patient with significant AV shunting consistent with hepatic infantile hemangioma.

of AV shunting in hemangioendothelioma there may be an abrupt decrease in the caliber of the abdominal aorta below the celiac axis origin. This finding may be easiest to demonstrate on coronal or sagittal reconstructions.

Related Physics

In abdominal tumor MR imaging it is often valuable to apply fat-suppression (FS) techniques in order to better define

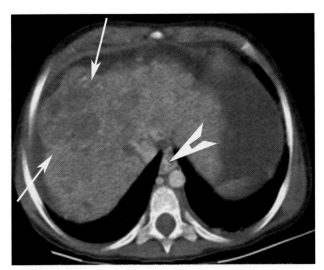

Figure 38.2. Axial contrast-enhanced CT image in a 7-year-old female with tyrosinemia and cirrhosis shows a heterogeneous mass within the right hepatic lobe (arrows). The underlying liver is shrunken and has a nodular surface. Esophageal varices (arrowhead) and ascites are seen secondary to portal hypertension. This patient also had multiple pulmonary metastases (not shown). Pathology revealed HCC.

tissue characteristics. This can be achieved by employing either chemical or "frequency-selective" FS, inversion recovery or the Dixon method in order of frequency of utilization and robustness of FS. Frequency-selective FS makes use of the fact that fat precesses at a slightly different frequency than water. In this method a radiofrequency pulse is applied at the frequency of lipid-based protons, followed by a phase-spoiling pulse that destroys the signal from these lipid-based protons thereby leaving only signal from water-based protons. Whereas chemical fat suppression relies on the difference in precessional frequencies of fat and water, inversion-recovery imaging relies on T1 recovery time differences; T1 of fat is shorter than water. In the inversion recovery method, a 180-degree inversion pulse is applied during the repetition time (TR) and when the fat signal decays and crosses the null point (ahead of water), the fast spin echo sequence is completed with a 90-degree followed by 180-degree pulse. Because the 90 and 180 pulses occur at the null point for fat, no fat signal is obtained. Dixon method uses the differences in chemical shift between fat and water. This method employs phase shifts (angles) of 0, 180 degrees, and -180 degrees to generate three image sets: true water, true fat, and the inverse fat images, the latter accounting for static field inhomogeneities. These three images are used to create decomposed images. The Dixon method is coupled with fast gradient echo techniques, generating images with acceptable signal-to-noise. Disadvantages of the respective methods include: imperfect signal reduction in fat from chemical FS, decreased signal to noise ratio (SNR) with inversion recovery, and time and expense of specialized deconstruction algorithms with Dixon.

Differential Diagnosis

- Hepatic adenoma: benign tumor of epithelial origin. Just as in adults, hepatic adenomas in pediatric patients are associated with steroid therapy, including oral contraceptives. Consequently, hepatic adenoma is typically seen in teenaged females, but can also occur in patients with Fanconi anemia, familial diabetes mellitus, and some forms of glycogen storage disease. Hepatic adenoma is not associated with an elevated AFP level. Patients may present with acute abdominal pain related to hemorrhage within the tumor. Imaging studies typically show intratumoral fat and hemorrhage, and fat-suppressed or in-and-out-of-phase MR imaging may be helpful.

- Mesenchymal hamartomas: occur in the same age group as hepatoblastoma but have a different appearance, typically a multicystic mass with septations that enhance like normal liver (Fig. 38.4). Mesenchymal hamartomas may also appear solid or mixed solid and cystic, but do not demonstrate hemorrhage or calcification. Being of mesenchymal origin, these tumors are associated with normal AFP levels. Because mesenchymal hamartomas may regress spontaneously, some centers simply observe these lesions. As there is a risk of transformation into undifferentiated embryonal sarcoma, an aggressive tumor with a poor prognosis, other centers recommend resection of mesenchymal hamartomas.

- Biliary rhabdomyosarcoma: the liver is an uncommon site for rhabdomyosarcoma but these tumors have a better prognosis than those arising in other sites. They appear as an intraductal enhancing mass causing biliary ductal dilatation that is depicted well with MR cholangiopancreatography (MRCP).

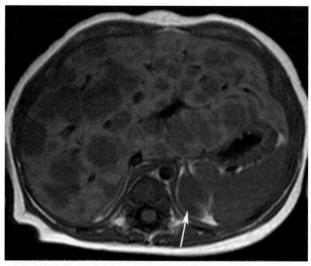

Figure 38.5. Axial T1 MR image of the liver in a 4-month-old female shows multiple hepatic lesions, which are hypointense to the normal liver parenchyma. There is a solid mass in the left suprarenal region (arrow), medial to the spleen. Findings are consistent with metastatic neuroblastoma.

- Metastatic disease: most often from neuroblastoma or leukemia/lymphoma. Multiple liver lesions in an infant should trigger a careful evaluation of the adrenal glands and retroperitoneum for a primary neuroblastoma (Fig. 38.5).

- Post-transplant lymphoproliferative disease: in the transplanted liver it appears as low-attenuation lesions within the enhancing liver parenchyma on CT.

- Fungal infection: immunocompromised patients, such as bone marrow transplant recipients, are prone to develop this. Low-attenuation lesions may involve the spleen and kidneys.

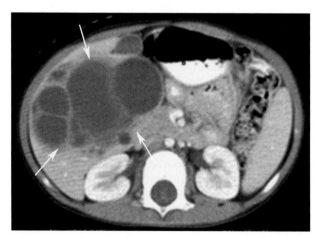

Figure 38.4. Axial contrast-enhanced CT image in a 4-year-old male shows a multicystic mass within the right hepatic lobe (arrows) with enhancing septations similar in attenuation to the surrounding liver consistent with mesenchymal hamartoma.

Common Variants

Hepatoblastoma is associated with several syndromes, including Beckwith-Wiedemann syndrome and other hemihypertrophy syndromes, familial adenomatous polyposis (FAP), neurofibromatosis type 1, and maternal exposures (including fetal alcohol syndrome and oral contraceptive use during pregnancy). Additionally, premature infants have a striking increased relative risk of hepatoblastoma. Fibrolamellar carcinoma is a variant of HCC that occurs in teenagers without cirrhosis and can mimic focal nodular hyperplasia (FNH), because both have a "central scar." The central lesion in FNH is actually a vascular anomaly, which will show high signal on T2-weighted MR images and will enhance briskly and early on dynamic contrast-enhanced MRI. The central scar in fibrolamellar carcinoma is truly a collagenous scar, with low attenuation on CT, low T1 and T2 signal on MRI, and poor contrast enhancement (Fig. 38.6). The central scar of fibrolamellar HCC may contain calcifications, which are not seen in FNH.

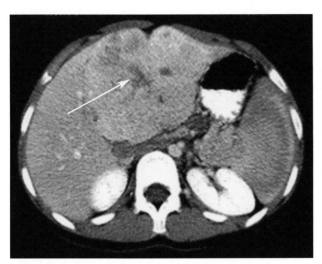

Figure 38.6. Axial contrast-enhanced CT image in a 14-year-old female with abdominal pain shows a heterogeneously enhancing mass in the left hepatic lobe with relative hypoenhancement of the central scar (arrow). Note that the underlying liver parenchyma is normal. Pathology revealed fibrolamellar HCC.

Clinical Issues

Hepatoblastoma and HCC are both treated with neoadjuvant chemotherapy prior to surgical resection. Inferior vena cava invasion was once considered a contraindication to resection of hepatoblastoma, but now the IVC may be resected en bloc and replaced with a prosthetic graft or venous autograft. Hepatic transplantation may be performed for large lesions. Chemoembolization is occasionally performed in patients who are poor candidates for surgery. Overall survival for hepatoblastoma is around 65 percent but is much poorer for HCC at around 25 percent. Many hemangioendotheliomas spontaneously involute and do not require any treatment. These cases are followed with US to document continued decrease in size and resolution. Symptomatic cases—those that cause congestive heart failure of consumptive coagulopathy—may be treated with high-dose steroids or interferon, or rarely with embolization or resection.

Key Points

- Most cases of hepatoblastoma and HCC have elevated AFP levels.
- Hemangioendotheliomas may show high-flow vascular structures resulting from AV shunting.
- In children under the age of 2 years, consider hepatoblastoma, hemangioendothelioma, metastatic neuroblastoma, and mesenchymal hamartoma.
- HCC typically occurs in children over 5 years of age with underlying cirrhosis.

Further Reading

Chung EM, Lattin GE, Cube R, Lewis RB, Marichal-Hernandez C, Shawhan R, Conran RM. From the archives of the AFIP. Pediatric liver masses: radiologic-pathologic correlation. Part 1. Benign tumors. *Radiographics.* 2010;*30*:801–826.

Emre S, McKenna GJ. Liver tumors in children. *Pediatric Transplantation.* 2004;*8*(6):632–638.

Finegold MJ, Egler RA, Goss JA, Guillerman RP, Karpen SJ, Krishnamurthy R, O'Mahony A. Liver tumors: pediatric population. *Liver Transplantation.* 2008;*14*:1545–1556.

Mo JQ, Dimashkieh HH, Bove KE. GLUT1 endothelial reactivity distinguishes hepatic infantile hemangioma from congenital hepatic vascular malformation with associated capillary proliferation. *Human Pathology.* 2004;*35*(2):200–209.

Silva AC, Evans JM, McCullough AE, Jatoi MA, Vargas HE, Hara AK. MR imaging of hypervascular liver masses: a review of current techniques. *Radiographics.* 2009;*29*:385–402.

Slovis TL, Bulas DI. Tumor and tumor-like conditions (masses) and miscellaneous lesions. In: Slovis TL, ed. *Caffey's pediatric diagnostic imaging.* 10th edition. St. Louis, MO. Mosby. 2003, pp 1494–1508.

Woodward PJ, Sohaey R, Kennedy A, Koeller KK. From the archives of the AFIP. A comprehensive review of fetal tumors with pathologic correlation. *Radiographics.* 2005;*25*:215–242.

CHAPTER 39

Biliary Atresia

Christopher Ian Cassady, MD

Definition

Bile duct obliteration in utero or in the early neonatal period will obstruct bile flow. This pathologic process is termed biliary atresia (BA) and is also known as *progressive obliterative cholangiopathy*.

Clinical Features

The etiology is unknown. Biliary atresia occurs in approximately 1 out of every 10,000 to 15,000 live births in the United States. The incidence is highest in Asia. Biliary atresia presents as persistent jaundice in the neonate past 14 days of life. Signs such as icterus, dark urine, and light/acholic stools are a result of conjugated hyperbilirubinemia. Surgery is the only cure for patients with biliary atresia. The type of biliary atresia indicates which surgical correction is required.

Anatomy and Physiology

The biliary system may be absent at any level from the intrahepatic radicles through to the common bile duct. The level at which there has been obliteration has important implications for surgical therapy. In a "correctable" atresia the surgeon can excise a distal obstruction that is isolated to the common bile duct and primarily anastomose the common hepatic duct to the small bowel. Most cases are ""not correctable as the obstruction includes the hepatic ducts. In these cases, the Kasai portoenterostomy is surgically created and allows direct drainage of bile from the surgically exposed intrahepatic ducts to the bowel. Once extensive liver damage has occurred, liver transplantation may be the only surgical option.

Imaging Findings

There are no prenatal imaging findings that anticipate biliary atresia except the absence of a gallbladder. In a neonate with conjugated hyperbilirubinemia, the differential diagnosis is broad. A variety of imaging modalities have useful findings that can help narrow the choices and point in some cases to biliary atresia.

Ultrasound (US):
- Gallbladder may be absent or small with a length of < 16 millimeters (16 to 18 mm is indeterminate (Fig. 39.1)
- The gallbladder wall may be irregular
- Triangular cord sign: the portal plate may be abnormally thick (> 4 mm) and echogenic. This is best evaluated as a measurement of the thickness of the anterior wall of the right portal vein proximal to its bifurcation (Fig. 39.2)
- The hepatic echotexture is normal early in the disease before fibrosis
- Bile ducts: extrahepatic ducts are not seen, intrahepatic ducts are not dilated (ductal dilation should prompt a search for other causes of biliary obstruction, such as bile plug, stone, or choledochal cyst)
- Splenomegaly may be the first sign of portal hypertension

Nuclear scintigraphy:
- Performed with Tc-99m labeled iminodiacetic acid (IDA) derivatives after premedication with phenobarbital (phenobarbital induces hepatic enzymes and increased radiotracer uptake and excretion into the bile)
- Good uptake of radiotracer but lack of tracer excretion from the liver into the bowel on 24-hour delayed imaging is supportive of the diagnosis of biliary atresia (Fig. 39.3)

MR cholangiography (MRC):
- Failure to demonstrate right, left, and common hepatic bile ducts
- Its use can be limited by cost, required sedation, and the limited relative spatial resolution of the images

Endoscopic retrograde cholangiopancreatography (ERCP):
- Has been used occasionally to evaluate ductal anatomy
- Special equipment is required for infants and cannulation of the papilla can be challenging because of small patient size

Percutaneous cholecystocholangiography:
- Most useful to demonstrate biliary anatomy and evaluate for BA
- Cholangiography performed in all cases prior to Kasai procedure in the operating room if this has not already been done percutaneously (Fig. 39.4)

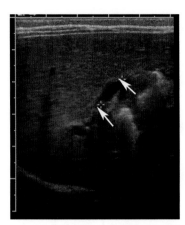

Figure 39.1. Transverse US image of the gallbladder obtained with a high-resolution linear transducer in a fasting newborn with jaundice demonstrates an abnormally short gallbladder length (arrows).

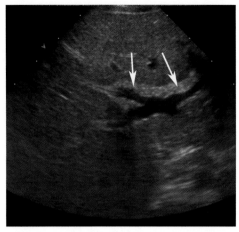

Figure 39.2. Transverse US image of the liver at the porta hepatis in a neonate with conjugated hyperbilirubinemia shows abnormally thick hyperechoic tissue paralleling and abutting the anterior wall of the proximal branches of the portal vein (arrows). This echogenic tissue represents the fibrotic and obliterated bile ducts coined the "triangular cord sign."

IMAGING PITFALLS

- In the setting of conjugated hyperbilirubinemia, gallbladder atresia should suggest biliary atresia, and prompt definitive diagnosis by biopsy and/or cholangiography to exclude the rare case of alternate pathology, such as Alagille syndrome, is indicated
- Patient should be fasting when the images are obtained to maximize gallbladder distension and visibility
- Presence of a normal-appearing gallbladder is less common but can exist in patients with BA
- Patients with altered liver function from neonatal hepatitis may have very poor uptake of the radiopharmaceutical by the liver (as a result the very small amount of radiopharmaceutical excreted into the bowel may not be detectable simulating biliary atresia)

Imaging Strategy

The preferred initial study is US because it is noninvasive, nonionizing, relatively inexpensive, and does not require sedation. Attention should be directed to the portal plate, ductal system, and gallbladder. Use of a high-frequency (13 MHz or higher) linear transducer is ideal. Although protocols vary, a reasonable approach after US would be to perform nuclear scintigraphy. Liver biopsy may also be indicated. In some cases US, nuclear medicine exams, and biopsy are all inconclusive. Percutaneous or intraoperative cholangiograms are used to confirm the diagnosis, particularly in patients who have a gallbladder. As technologies improve and costs change, MR imaging may play an earlier and important role.

Related Physics

The Diisopropyl Iminodiacetic Acid (DISIDA) or Hepatobiliary Iminodiacetic Acid (HIDA) scan is the definitive imaging study for the diagnosis of biliary atresia. The radiopharmaceutical used for the study is technetium 99m-labelled diisopropyl iminodiacetic acid, given intravenously. The administration is given as an amount of radioactivity in units of either Millicuries(mCi) or Bequerels (Bq). The new SI unit for activity is Bq, which equals one disintegration per second. A curie is equal to 3.7×10^{10} Bq. When computing the amount of activity at any time following administration one must use the decay equation as well as the decay constant for the isotope being used. The decay constant given by "λ" has units of 1/second and is unique for each isotope. The amount of radiation at time "t" after administration is given by:

$$N = N_0 \times e^{-\lambda t}.$$

Each radioisotope has an intrinsic parameter known as the physical half-life, which equals the time needed for one-half of the atoms to decay from radioactive to another state. For technetium 99m this is equal to 6 hours. When any radioactive isotope is injected into the human body, the decay rate becomes modified by biologic processes such as excretion; this modified half-life is known as the biological half-life. In a biologic system the reciprocal of the "effective" half-life (t_e) is equal to the reciprocal of the physical (t_p) plus the reciprocal of the biologic(t_b) half-life or:

$$t_e = 1/t_p + 1/t_b.$$

Differential Diagnosis

- Neonatal hepatitis (idiopathic or infectious) may be identical on scintigraphy to biliary atresia in some

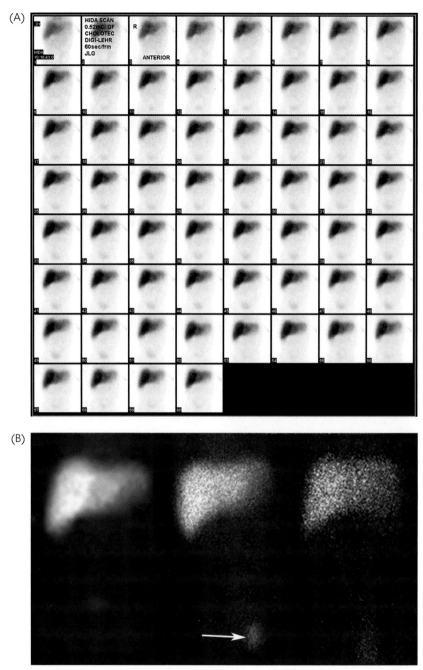

Figure 39.3. Nuclear scintigraphy with a TC-99m labeled iminodiacetic acid (A) in a neonate premedicated with phenobarbitol preparation shows very good hepatic uptake of the radiopharmaceutical, but no excretion into the bowel from the liver on the initial dynamic images. Delayed images obtained at 1 hour, 5 hours, and 24 hours (B) also lack any activity in the bowel. There is tracer activity in the bladder (arrow); urinary excretion of tracer is increased when liver function is impaired.

cases. In most cases of neonatal hepatitis, excretion of radiopharmaceutical into the bowel will be detectable.
■ Syndromes of intrahepatic bile duct paucity (e.g., Alagille syndrome) and other genetic causes of cholestasis (Byler disease; familial cholesterol degradation disorders) generally show no obvious findings on US.

■ Other causes of bile duct obstruction (choledochal cyst, bile plug syndrome) would be expected to demonstrate evidence of bile duct dilation on US.

Common Variants Practically, biliary atresia has been divided into two subtypes: correctable and noncorrectable. *Correctable (operable)* refers to patency of the bile ducts to the level of the common hepatic duct, in which there

higher failure rate if performed after the neonatal period. Eventually the majority of biliary atresia patients, including those who undergo early surgical intervention, later become candidates for liver transplantation.

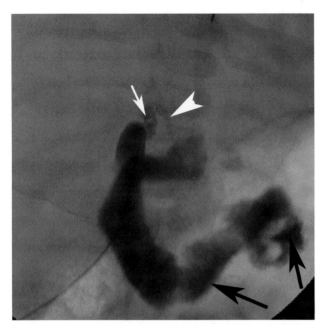

Figure 39.4. Frontal image from percutaneous cholangiography through a small gallbladder in a newborn with biliary atresia confirms patency from the cystic duct (white arrow) through the common bile duct (arrowhead) into the small bowel (black arrows), but fails to fill the intrahepatic ductal system, diagnostic of atresia above the insertion of the cystic duct. This noncorrectable BA requires a Kasai procedure.

is an adequate length of common hepatic duct to allow primary anastomosis with the small bowel. Unfortunately, this occurs in only 10 to 15 percent of cases. *Noncorrectable* form is defined by atresia of the ductal system proximal to the common hepatic duct. In some cases a small patent common bile duct may be present but not functional given the more proximal atresia. A portoenterostomy (Kasai procedure) or liver transplantation is needed for treatment. The most significant association with BA is congenital isomerism (heterotaxy), in particular polysplenia. In these cases, coexisting anomalies such as malrotation of the bowel or interruption of the inferior vena cava may complicate the operative treatment of biliary atresia.

Clinical IssuesThere is urgency to the work up and diagnosis of the patient with suspected BA. Because of the development of hepatic fibrosis, the Kasai procedure has a

Key Points

- US findings that are most suggestive of the diagnosis of biliary atresia include absent or small gallbladder with an irregular wall, nonvisualization of extrahepatic bile ducts, and the triangular cord sign.
- Nuclear scintigraphy studies may be falsely positive if the hepatic uptake of the radiopharmaceutical is poor resulting in excretion of an undetectable amount of radiopharmaceutical into biliary tract and bowel.
- Percutaneous or intraoperative cholangiography is the most direct diagnostic imaging exam and is performed prior to corrective surgery in infants with a gallbladder and presumed BA.
- Consider the possibility of BA in infants with congenital isomerism and hyperbilirubinemia.

Further Reading

Farrant P, Meire HB, Miele-Vergani G. Improved diagnosis of extrahepatic biliary atresia by high frequency ultrasound of the gallbladder. *British Journal of Radiology.* 2001;74:952–954.

Lee HJ, Lee SM, Park WH, Choi SO. Objective criteria of triangular cord sign in biliary atresia on US scans. *Radiology.* 2003;229:395–400.

Meyers RL, Book LS, O'Gorman MA, White KW, Jaffe RB, Feola PG, Hedlund GL. Percutaneous cholecysto-cholangiography in the diagnosis of obstructive jaundice in infants. *Journal of Pediatric Surgery.* 2004;39(1):16–18.

Poddar U, Bhattacharya A, Thapa BR, Mittal BR, Singh K. Ursodeoxycholic acid-augmented hepatobiliary scintigraphy in the evaluation of neonatal jaundice. *Journal of Nuclear Medicine.* 2004;45(9):1488–1492.

Takamizawa S, Zaima A, Muraji T. Can biliary atresia be diagnosed by ultrasonography alone? *Pediatric Surgery.* 2007; 42(12):2093–2096.

Tan Kendrick APA, Phua KB, Ooi BC, Tan CEL. Biliary atresia: making the diagnosis by the gallbladder ghost triad. *Pediatric Radiology.* 2003;33:311–315.

CHAPTER 40

Choledochal Cyst

Caroline Carrico, MD

Definition

Choledochal cysts are developmental malformations of the biliary tract that can involve the intrahepatic and or extrahepatic bile ducts and may be focal or diffuse, cystic or fusiform.

Clinical Features

Choledochal cysts are seen in girls more often than boys. The incidence in North and South America and Europe is approximately 1 in 100,000 to 150,000. The highest incidence is in Japan. The clinical features of choledochal cysts vary with age. Newborn hyperbilirubinemia that persists beyond 2 to 3 weeks of life and is accompanied by dark urine and light acholic stools is suggestive of cholestasis. Choledochal cysts are one of the surgically correctable causes of neonatal cholestasis. Large cysts may be palpable. Older children and adults may present with vomiting, fever, recurrent abdominal or right-upper quadrant pain, cholangitis, or pancreatitis. Conjugated hyperbilirubinemia is common, but is not always clinically apparent. Rupture of the choledochus is uncommon and affected patients usually present with vomiting and abdominal pain or distention. Classic peritoneal signs are often absent with bile peritonitis. Jaundice is also uncommon. Some patients form a contained bile pseudocyst after cyst rupture.

Anatomy and Physiology

Choledochal cysts and Caroli's disease are theorized to result from abnormal embryogenesis of the ductal plate and are included in the broad spectrum of ductal plate malformations (DPMs) that result in pediatric fibropolycystic liver disease. The ductal plate is a tubular column of bipotential hepatoblasts that encircles the portal venous branches. The ductal plate then duplicates forming two concentric layers. The space between the two cylinders becomes the lumen of the bile ducts. Through a complex series of remodeling, the intrahepatic bile ducts are formed. It is failure of normal remodeling that leads to a wide variety of DPM. Failure of normal remodeling of the small interlobular bile ducts results in abnormalities such as congenital hepatic fibrosis. When the malformation occurs at the level of the large extrahepatic and/or intrahepatic ducts, the result is formation of choledochal cysts and Caroli's disease, respectively. Additionally, an anomalous union of the pancreatic duct into the common bile duct 1 centimeter or more proximal to the ampulla of Vater has been found in many patients with a choledochal cyst. The pancreatic enzymes refluxing within the bile duct may contribute to ductal dilation seen with choledochal cysts. Stones and proteinaceous plugs can form in the common channel, which courses from the anomalous union to the ampulla of Vater. These obstructing agents can contribute to the proximal duct dilation. Pancreatic enzymes may weaken the cyst wall. High bile amylase levels have been reported in some cases of cyst rupture. This is compatible with a pancreatic and bile duct malunion.

The simplified Alonso-Lej classification system is illustrated in Figure 40.1 and has been modified by Todani as follows:

Type I: fusiform dilatation of predominantly the extrahepatic bile duct

    IA: cystic dilation of the choledochus, often with pancreatic duct and common bile duct malunion (pancreatobiliary malunion) and high-grade distal stricture

    IB: segmental dilation of a portion of the common bile duct (CBD).

    IC: fusiform or cylindrical dilation of the CBD usually with a pancreatobiliary malunion and low-grade distal duct stricture; the bile duct dilation may extend cephalad into the distal right and left hepatic ducts

Type II: diverticular dilation of the extrahepatic bile ducts

Type III: dilated distal CBD at the level of the duodenum wall (a.k.a. choledochocele), often associated with an obstructed ampulla of Vater

Type IV: multiple and/or intrahepatic involvement

Type IVA: cystic and or fusiform dilation of the CBD and intrahepatic ducts (left > right) with intraductal strictures common near the hepatic hilum and very distal near the ampulla (adults > children); pancreatobiliary malunion is common

Type IVB: multiple dilations of the extrahepatic bile ducts giving a beaded appearance

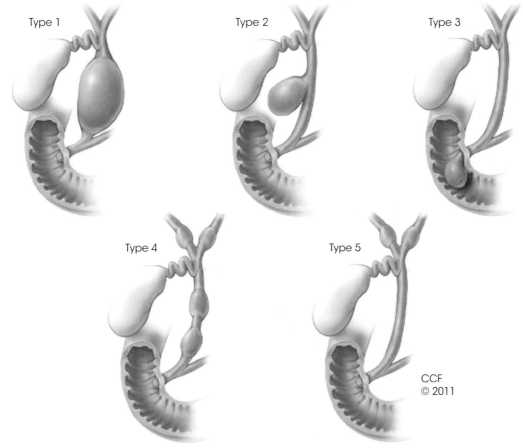

Type 1   Type 2   Type 3

Type 4   Type 5

CCF
© 2011

Figure 40.1. Classification system for choledochal cysts.

Type V: intrahepatic dilation, may be segmental, lobar (L >R) or diffuse and uncommonly has extrahepatic duct dilation

Imaging Findings

Postnatal ultrasound (US; *also seen on prenatal US):

- Cystic dilation of the intrahepatic and or extrahepatic bile ducts*
- Cyst extends to the porta hepatis* (Fig. 40.2A)
- Cyst is seen separate from the gallbladder* (Fig. 40.2B)
- Cyst communicates with the biliary system*
- On prenatal US the cyst usually gradually enlarges through gestation
- Fusiform dilation of the extrahepatic and or intrahepatic bile ducts (Figs. 40.3 and 40.4)
- Sludge and stones commonly found in the gallbladder, cyst or bile ducts and proximal intrahepatic bile ducts may be hyperechoic because of sludge
- No blood flow within the cysts on color Doppler for Todani types I to IV
- Central dot sign: blood flow is seen in the portal vein (the central dot) that is surrounded by the abnormally

formed and ectatic intrahepatic bile ducts in Caroli's disease and syndrome (Todani type V)
- Stones within the ducts (Caroli's >> choledochal cysts; adults > children)
- Free fluid in the abdomen or loculated bile pseudocyst can be seen after cyst rupture

Tc-99m imidodiacetic acid analog nuclear scintigraphy:

- Confirms that the cyst communicates with the biliary tree when it fills with excreted radiopharmaceutical (most cysts will fill)
- Bile leak into peritoneum if perforated

MRCP (MR cholangio-pancreatography), CT cholangiogram or ERCP (endoscopic retrograde cholangiopancreatography):

- Cystic or fusiform dilation of the intra- and or extrahepatic bile ducts (Fig. 40.5)
- Anomalous union of pancreatic and common bile ducts
- Common channel: the duct distal to the anomalous union of the common bile duct and the pancreatic duct (abnormal union is at least 1 cm above the ampulla of Vater)

(A)

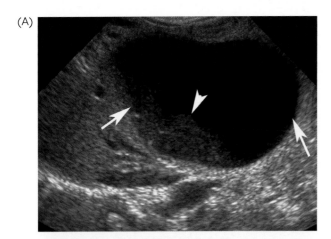

(B)

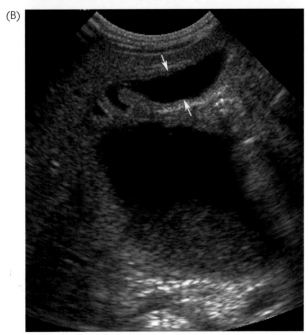

Figure 40.2. Sagittal US image (A) in an 8-day-old girl with hyperbilirubinemia and refusal to feed shows a large cyst (large arrows) with internal sludge (arrowhead) in the right-upper quadrant extending to the porta hepatis. Transverse US image (B) shows the cyst separate from the gallbladder (small arrows).

- Cyst or common channel stone: round filling defect within the duct
- If an MR contrast agent is used that is largely excreted by the liver into the biliary system, the "cysts" will typically fill with contrast because the cystic spaces in the choledochal cysts and Caroli's disease are the dilated bile ducts or are cystic spaces that communicate with the normal biliary system.

Imaging Strategy

Some choledochal cysts are detected on prenatal US. Postnatal US and MRCP are the primary diagnostic imaging studies performed to diagnose and follow up choledochal cysts and Caroli's disease. For primary workup and follow-up, MRCP is preferred over ERCP as it can define the extent of disease, look for pancreatobiliary malunion and coexisting stone disease without the risk of developing procedure-related hemorrhage, pancreatitis, or cholangitis as can occur after ERCP. Percutaneous or intraoperative cholangiography and ERCP can be used prior to surgery to define complex anatomy including anomalous pancreatic duct and bile duct union prior to surgical cyst excision. Also, ERCP can be used to extract obstructing stones in the extrahepatic ducts prior to definitive surgery. Some surgeons perform cholangioscopy for direct intraoperative assessment of the choledochal cyst. Imidodiacetic-acid-based nuclear scintigraphy (DISIDA) may be helpful to assess hepatobiliary function, anatomy, or to assess for biliary perforation.

Related Physics

Choledochal cyst may be confirmed with radionuclide DISIDA imaging. When using radioactive materials to image metabolic processes the materials can be produced in a variety of ways. Low-atomic-weight isotopes such as ^{15}O and ^{18}F can be produced using a linear accelerator or a cyclotron. Those of heavier weight can be produced by harvesting fission products from nuclear reactors. Some exotic species can be produced using neutron activation and commonly Tc-99 is produced using a molybdenum generator. In any of these processes quality control is important. One must have appropriate laboratory equipment to assure that contaminants are eliminated from the preparation. In large facilities, radionuclide production can be accomplished in-house; in smaller facilities these preparations are ordered on a daily basis from commercial suppliers.

Differential Diagnosis

- Obstructing choledocholithiasis
- Enteric duplication cyst of the duodenum
- Pancreatic pseudocyst
- Autosomal dominant polycystic liver disease (ADPLD) (rare) where cysts develop during adolescence and grow and do not communicate with bile ducts
- Spontaneous perforation of the bile duct
- Hepatic artery aneurysm

Common Variants

Caroli's disease is Todani type V. It is considered separately as it is usually isolated to the intrahepatic bile ducts and has an autosomal recessive mode of inheritance. The coexistence of Caroli's disease with congenital hepatic fibrosis is termed Caroli's syndrome. Autosomal recessive polycystic kidney disease (ARPKD) and congenital hepatic fibrosis have a genetic link on chromosome 6 and often coexist in the same patient. Caroli's disease is associated with ARPKD

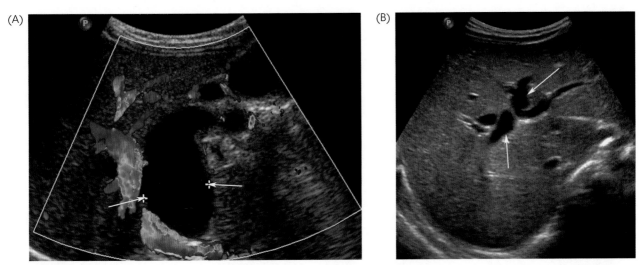

Figure 40.3. Transverse US image with color Doppler (A) in a 2-year-old girl with intractable emesis and elevated transaminases shows a grossly dilated common bile duct (2.3 cm) and forming a fusiform choledochal cyst (arrows) with sludge but without stones. Transverse US image of the liver above the level of the CBD (B) shows the dilatation extends to the central intrahepatic bile ducts (arrows).

more often than ADPKD or medullary sponge kidney. Patients with Caroli's disease usually present during childhood or as young adults. Signs and symptoms are likely secondary to bile stones and stasis and may include fever, crampy or recurrent abdominal pain, hepatomegaly, pruritus, acholic stools, and transient jaundice. The incidence of cholangiocarcinoma in Caroli's disease has been reported to be at least 100 times greater than that of the general population.

Clinical Issues

Because of stasis within the ectatic and sometimes obstructed biliary system, infection may result. Stone formation is most common in Todani type V (Caroli's disease). Long-term complications of untreated cysts can

also include the development of hepatic failure with cirrhosis and portal hypertension. Surgical excision of the cyst is the treatment of choice for choledochal cysts. The gallbladder is also removed, because of the increased risk of malignancy if left in situ. In some cases, the cyst involves the distal intrahepatic bile ducts and some degree of hepatic resection is required with formation of a Roux-en-Y hepaticojejunostomy. Liver transplantation may be needed for some patients with severe diffuse intrahepatic disease. The risk of developing cancer within a choledochal cyst or adjacent remaining bile ducts is considerably higher than in the general population. The rate of biliary malignancy in patients with choledochal cysts is as high as 18 percent in Japan. Additionally, authors from Japan report that patients with pancreatobiliary malunion have an incidence of gallbladder cancer that is

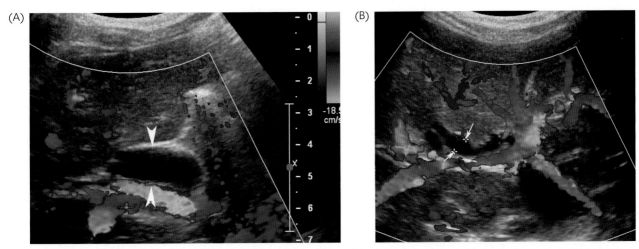

Figure 40.4. Transverse US image with color Doppler (A) in a 3-year-old girl with jaundice, abdominal pain, and vomiting shows a markedly dilated common bile duct (arrowheads). Transverse image above this level (B) shows intrahepatic bile duct dilation (arrows) in the left lobe of the liver.

(A)

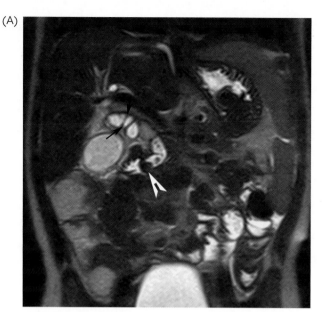

(B)

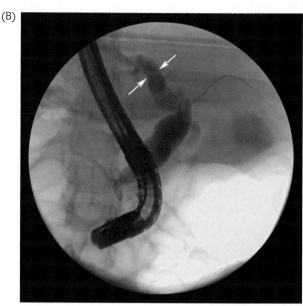

Figure 40.5. Coronal Haste thin-slice MRCP image (A) in a 3-year-old girl with jaundice, abdominal pain, and vomiting demonstrates a grossly dilated common bile duct (arrows) that contains multiple stones (arrowhead). Frontal ERCP image (B) shows duct dilation extending into the left lobe (arrows) consistent with choledochal cyst.

approximately 167 to 420 times that of the general population. Adenocarcinoma, squamous cell carcinoma, and adenoacanthoma have all been reported to occur within choledochal cysts. Malignancy is diagnosed at an average age of 27 years in men and a decade later in women. Metachronous malignancy of the bile ducts remote to the cyst excision has been reported as long as 19 years after cyst excision suggesting a need for long-term postoperative imaging surveillance.

Key Points

- Choledochal cysts are part of a group of disorders referred to as ductal plate malformations (DPMs).
- Choledochal cysts can be suspected on prenatal US.
- Postnatal US and MRCP are primary diagnostic studies.
- DISIDA can confirm choledochal cysts.
- Five types exist according to Todani classification.
- There is a high incidence of stones, stasis, and malignancy of the entire biliary tree.

Further Reading

Carrico CWT, Bisset GS III. Diseases of the pediatric gallbladder and biliary tract. In: Gore R, Levine MS, eds. *Textbook of Gastrointestinal Radiology*. Third edition. 2007. Philadelphia, PA. Saunders.

Chiang L, Chui CH, Low Y, Jacobsen AS. Perforation: a rare complication of choledochal cysts in children. *Pediatr Surg Int.* 2011;*27*(8):823–827.

Clifton MS, Goldstein RB, Slavotinek A, Norton ME, Lee H, Farrell J, Nobuhara KK. Prenatal diagnosis of familial type I choledochal cyst. *Pediatrics.* 2006;*117*(3):596–600.

Rozel C, Garel L, Rypens F, Viremouneix L, Lapierre C, Décarie JC, Dubois J. Imaging of biliary disorders in children. *Pediatr Radiol.* 2011;*41*(2):208–220.

Tanaka N, Ueno T, Takama Y, Fukuzawa M. Diagnosis and management of biliary cystic malformations in neonates. *J Pediatr Surg.* 2010 Nov;*45*(11):2119–2123.

Todani T, Watanabe Y, Toki A, Morotomi Y. Classification of congenital biliary cystic disease: special reference to type Ic and IVA cysts with primary ductal stricture. *J Hepatobiliary Pancreat Surg.* 2003;*10* (5):340–344.

Veigel MC, Prescott-Focht J, Rodriguez MG, Zinati R, Shao L, Moore CA, Lowe LH. Fibropolycystic liver disease in children. *Pediatr Radiol.* 2009;*39*(4):317–327.

CHAPTER 41

Neutropenic Colitis

Adam Zarchan, MD and Kristin Fickenscher, MD

Definition

Neutropenic colitis, also known as typhlitis, is a necrotizing colitis that occurs in immunosupressed patients, typically neutropenic cancer patients treated with chemotherapeutic agents, but may also be seen in patients after bone marrow transplant or with acquired immune deficiency syndrome.

Clinical Features

The reported incidence is variable but approximately 3 to 5 percent of cancer patients will suffer from typhlitis. The classic clinical triad includes abdominal pain, fever, and neutropenia. Other presentations include abdominal distention, nausea, vomiting, and watery or bloody diarrhea. The classic triad is not always present and not all patients are neutropenic. The presence of any one or more of these signs or symptoms in a pediatric oncology patient coupled with ascending colon wall thickness of greater than 3 millimeters is suggestive of typhlitis. Medical treatment is supportive and includes broad-spectrum antibiotics, antifungals, bowel rest, and total parenteral nutrition (TPN). Surgical intervention is reserved for complications such as bowel perforation or abscess formation. Mortality rates were previously as high as 10 to 20 percent, however with improved detection and management, recent pediatric mortality rates have been reported at 2.5 to 5 percent.

Anatomy and Physiology

The exact pathophysiology of typhlitis is unknown. Proposed mechanisms include injury to the mucosal lining related to cytotoxicity of chemotherapeutic agents, immunodeficiency with decreased resistance to normal intestinal bacteria, and impaired microvascular supply of the gut caused by inflammation and edema, which can lead to ulceration and necrosis of the mucosa.

Imaging Findings

- Abnormal bowel wall thickening ≥ 3 millimeters (wall thickness up to 30 mm has been reported; Fig. 41.1)
- Commonly localized to the cecum and ascending colon (Fig. 41.2)
- Involvement of the terminal ileum, remainder of the colon, rectum less common
- Pericolonic inflammatory fat stranding
- Free fluid
- Pneumatosis coli (Fig. 41.3)
- Abscess formation (Fig. 41.4)
- Free air if perforation has occurred
- Cecal distention
- Bowel obstruction

Imaging Strategy

In a patient with the appropriate history and clinical suspicion of typhlitis, ultrasound (US) or computed tomography (CT) may be performed to confirm the diagnosis. US evaluation of the bowel should be performed with a high-frequency linear transducer to assess the bowel wall thickness and with a curved array lower-frequency transducer used to evaluate for free fluid. CT is better for evaluating the complications of typhlitis including abscess formation and free air indicating perforation. CT should be performed with IV contrast when possible. Intraluminal oral contrast may help distend the bowel to reduce overestimation of bowel wall thickness measurements. Rectal contrast should be avoided if perforation is a clinical concern.

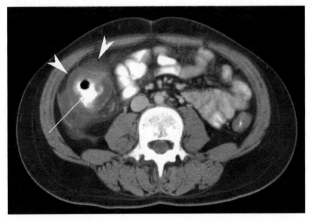

Figure 41.1. Axial oral and intravenous contrast-enhanced CT image of the abdomen in a 13-year-old female with acute lymphocytic leukemia (ALL), abdominal pain, and fever shows a dilated cecum (arrow) with bowel wall thickening (arrowheads) and pericolonic inflammation consistent with typhlitis.

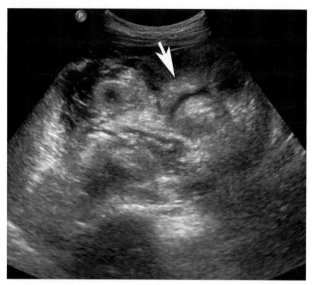

Figure 41.2. Transverse US image of the right-lower quadrant in a 3-year-old female with abdominal distention and sepsis while undergoing treatment for neuroblastoma demonstrates marked wall thickening of the cecum (arrow).

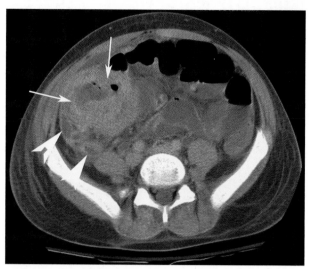

Figure 41.4. Axial intravenous contrast-enhanced CT image of the abdomen in a 15-year-old male with abdominal distention and acute myeloid leukemia (AML) and inability to tolerate oral contrast shows wall thickening of the distended, fluid-filled cecum (arrows) and there are two small right-sided pericecal abscesses (arrowheads).

Related Physics

The oncology patient with possible neutropenic colitis presents a challenge where optimal imaging may not be possible if the patient is too sick to drink oral contrast or has renal insufficiency and is unable to receive intravenous contrast. This may demand optimal CT imaging of soft tissues without the benefit of extrinsic contrast media. Bowel wall thickening, free fluid, and abdominal masses will be best seen using lower kVp that will optimize intrinsic soft-tissue contrast. The increase in noise will be offset by a modest increase in mAs and/or by increasing image thickness and largest collimation. In order to optimize low-contrast objects (which in the workup of the immunocompromised patient is needed to detect fungal infection or lymphoproliferative complications), images will be best viewed with narrow window at approximately 300 Hounsfield Units (HU) and level at approximately 40 HU.

Differential Diagnosis

- Graft versus host disease
- Pseudomembranous enterocolitis
- Infectious colitis
- Appendicitis
- Crohn's disease
- Ulcerative colitis

Clinical Issues

Any patient can develop appendicitis including the pediatric oncology patient. In a neutropenic patient with abdominal pain, the differentiation between typhlitis and appendicitis is important and imaging can be essential in making this distinction. Typhlitis can often be treated with medical management whereas acute appendicitis requires surgical intervention. Complications of typhlitis include bowel wall necrosis, gastrointestinal bleeding, sepsis, abscess formation and bowel perforation. Treatment of these complications typically requires more invasive therapy.

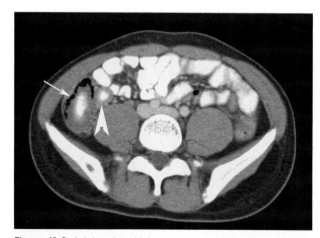

Figure 41.3. Axial oral and intravenous contrast-enhanced CT image of the abdomen in a 14-year-old male with abdominal pain while undergoing treatment for nasopharyngeal carcinoma shows pneumatosis of the thickened and distended cecum (arrow) and bowel wall thickening of the terminal ileum (arrowhead) consistent with typhlitis. The pericolonic fat stranding is minimal in this patient.

Key Points

- Necrotizing colitis in association with immunosuppression
- Bowel wall thickening ≥ 3 millimeters

- Typically involves the cecum and ascending colon, but can involve entire colon including the rectum or the terminal ileum
- Managed medically
- Exclude complications that would require more invasive treatment

Further Reading

Cloutier RL. Neutropenic enterocolitis. *Hematol Oncol Clin N Am.* 2010;*24*:577–584.

Gray TL, Ooi CY, Tran D, Traubici J, Gerstle JT, Sung L. Gastrointestinal complications in children with acute myeloid leukemia. *Leuk Lymphoma.* 2010;*51*(5):768–777.

McCarville MB, Adelman CS, Chenghong L, et al. Typhlitis in childhood cancer. *Cancer.* 2005;*104*:380–387.

Moran H, Yaniv I, Ashkenazi S, Schwarz M, Fisher S, Levy I. Risk factors for typhlitis in pediatric patients with cancer. *J Pediatr Hemantol Oncol.* 2009;*31*(9):630–634.

Schlatter M, Snyder K, Freyer D. Successful nonoperative management of typhlitis in pediatric oncology patients. *J Pediatr Surg.* 2002;*37*(8):1151–1155.

Thoeni RF, Cello JP. CT imaging of colitis. *Radiology.* 2006;*240*(3):623–638.

CHAPTER 42

Pseudomembranous Colitis

Jennifer L. Williams, MD

Definition
Pseudomembranous colitis (PC) is an infectious colitis caused by *Clostridium difficile* overgrowth. *C difficile* infection of the small bowel occurs with lesser frequency.

Clinical Features
Patients with pseudomembranous colitis present with fever, multiple episodes of diffuse watery diarrhea, and abdominal cramping. Nearly all patients with *C difficile* colitis have had recent antibiotic therapy. Other risk factors for the development of PC include chemotherapy, immunocompromised state, prior bowel surgery or prior hypotensive episode. Diagnosis is made with stool assay testing for C difficile toxin. Colonoscopy, if performed, reveals pseudomembranous plaques or nodules adherent to the mucosal walls.

First-line therapy is oral vancomycin and metronidazole. Electrolytes are monitored and replaced as needed. Most patients recover following initiation of therapy, but some may have recurrences. Untreated patients (and rarely treated patients) can develop complications including toxic megacolon or bowel ischemia. Patients who are refractory to medical management are treated with colonic resection.

Anatomy and Physiology
Antibiotic therapy results in alteration of the normal colonic flora. *C difficile*, in contrast to most normal colonic flora, is unaffected by common antibiotic regimens. As normal flora decline in numbers, *C difficile* will continue to thrive resulting in *C difficile* overgrowth. Exotoxins A and B are produced by *C difficile* and these bind to epithelial receptors resulting in alteration of the cell membrane and metabolism. There is subsequent sloughing of the colonic epithelium resulting in an inflammatory exudate of denuded necrotic cells known as pseudomembranous plaques. The exotoxins are directly responsible for the bowel injury.

Imaging Findings
Classic cases of pseudomembranous colitis involve the entire colon. Most often the rectosigmoid colon is involved but isolated involvement of the ascending colon or small bowel have been described. Skip area are uncommon. The degree of bowel wall thickening is usually more severe than that seen in other forms of colitis excluding Crohn's disease.

Radiography:
- Striking bowel wall thickening, with thumbprinting (Fig. 42.1)

CT:
- Bowel wall thickness averages between 10.7 and 14.7 millimeters (Fig. 42.2)
- Accordion sign: trapping of oral contrast between the haustral walls secondary to the marked bowel wall edema (Fig. 42.3)
- Target sign: hyperattenuation of the inner mucosal layer and outer serosa, separated by low-density edematous submucosa (Fig. 42.4)

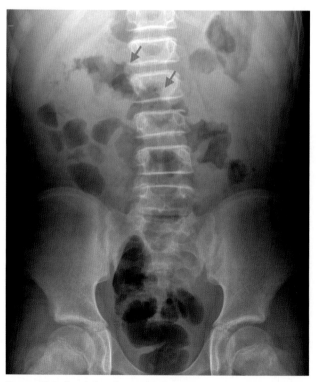

Figure 42.1. Frontal radiograph of the abdomen in a child with abdominal pain shows thumbprinting in the transverse colon indicative of bowel wall thickening (arrows).

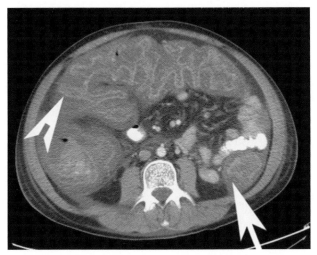

Figure 42.2. Oral and IV contrast-enhanced CT in a teen with abdominal pain and diarrhea show typical findings of pseudomembranous colitis including marked wall thickening (arrow) and mucosal enhancement (arrowhead) of the ascending, transverse, and descending colon with pericolonic edema and ascites.

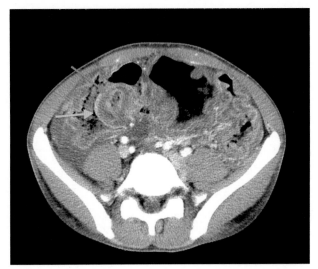

Figure 42.4. Oral and IV contrast-enhanced CT in a child with abdominal pain shows the target sign with hyperattenuation of both the inner mucosal layer (red arrow) and outer muscularis propria/serosa (yellow arrow). Common findings of *C difficile* colitis are also seen including bowel wall thickening and pericolonic edema/ascites.

- Relatively mild fat stranding surrounding the infected bowel
- Bowel lumen unusually large despite wall thickening
- Ascites common in PC (but rare in Crohn's)

Imaging Strategy

Evaluation should begin with a supine abdominal radiograph with an upright or left lateral decubitus view. CT with oral and IV contrast is frequently performed either to better evaluate plain-film findings or as the initial imaging modality. Positive or negative oral contrast agents can be used. Negative oral contrast agents allow better detection of mucosal enhancement. If an unlikely perforation is expected, positive contrast agents would better differentiate extravasated contrast material from ascites. Reformatted sagittal and coronal images of the abdomen and pelvis are recommended.

Related Physics

A useful and readily available technique for pediatric bowel imaging is CT enterography (CTE). Careful orchestration of CTE requires precise timing and judicious radiation delivery. Dilute oral contrast is given as a 0.2 percent solution over a set period of time to achieve adequate small bowel distension and opacification throughout its length. The slightly positive contrast contains an osmotic agent that acts to distend bowel such that the luminal Hounsfield Units (HU) are higher than water but lower than bowel wall enhancement. The speed of multirow scanners is such that no bowel paralytic is necessary (as in MRE). In addition, CTE may be superior to MRE for the younger child who would otherwise require sedation for MRI (oral contrast is a contraindication to sedation). In many patients, CTE may give more clinically reproducible results. Prone imaging will have advantages of less bowel motion and superior filling of the nondependent loops (such as transverse colon and rectosigmoid). Patient positioning can be tailored to the clinical indications. For children CTE must be optimized by employing appropriately sized field of view and by choosing girth-based tube kVp and mAs.

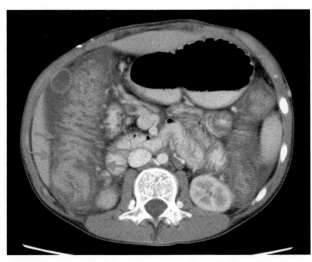

Figure 42.3. Oral and IV contrast-enhanced CT in a child with watery diarrhea shows marked bowel wall thickening with trapping of oral contrast between the haustra (accordion sign) throughout the transverse colon extending to the hepatic flexure (arrows). Note the ascites adjacent to the edematous bowel at the level of the hepatic flexure. Ascites are a common finding of pseudomembranous colitis but very rarely associated with Crohn's.

Differential Diagnosis

Inflammatory bowel disease:

- Crohn's disease (diagnostic clue is Crohn's disease usually lacks ascites and has skip areas)
- Ulcerative colitis (toxic megacolon occurs in patients with UC or PC)
- Infectious colitis: in particular cytomegalovirus, cryptosporidiosis, and salmonella
- Ischemic colitis

Common Variants

While pseudomembranous colitis usually involves the entire colon, segmentation of disease can be seen on occasion. In these cases there is typically involvement of the right colon and sparing of the left. There have been reports of *C difficile* enteritis in immunocompromised and postsurgical patients, however these are rare. It is theorized that colonic resection or bypass with ileostomy may result in colonization of small bowel, with increasing the likelihood of *C difficile* infection of the small bowel in that population.

Clinical Issues

With appropriate treatment, complications of PC are rare, however patients must be carefully evaluated for toxic megacolon and bowel perforation. Toxic megacolon occurs following damage to the muscularis propria and neural plexus by exotoxins. This results in loss of neuromuscular function and progressive dilation of the colon. Plain film demonstrates significant bowel dilatation. CT also shows bowel dilatation with thinning of the bowel wall and an ahaustral pattern in cases of toxic megacolon.

Key Points

- Pseudomembranous colitis most commonly occurs following antibiotic administration and is secondary to *Clostridium difficile* overgrowth.
- The distribution (pancolitis), degree of bowel wall thickening (more severe than most other forms of colitis), and associated findings (ascites and pancolonic edema) are very useful in distinguishing pseudomembranous colitis from other etiologies.

Further Reading

Applegate, K. Inflammatory and infectious diseases. In: Slovis TL, Adler BH, Bloom DA, et al., eds. *Caffey's Pediatric Diagnostic Imaging*. Philadelphia, PA: Mosby Elsevier; 2008:2188–2204.

Cotran RS, Kumar V, Collins T. *Pathologic Basis of Disease*. Sixth edition. Philadelphia, PA: W.B. Saunders Company; 1999.

Cronin CG, O'Connor M, Lohan DG, Keane M, Roche C, Bruzzi JF, Murphy JM. Imaging of the gastrointestinal complications of systemic chemotherapy. *Clinical Radiology*. 2009;54:724–733.

Horton KM, Frank CM, Fishman EK. CT evaluation of the colon: inflammatory disease. *Radiographics*. 2000;20(2):399–418.

Ruedi TF, Cello JP. CT imaging of colitis. *Radiology*. 2006;240(3):623–638.

Wee B, Poels JAD, McCafferty IJ, Taniere P, Olliff J. A description of CT features of Clostridium difficile infection of the small bowel in four patients and a review of the literature. *The British Journal of Radiology*. 2009;82:890–895.

CHAPTER 43

Inflammatory Bowel Disease

Eric J. Feldmann, MD, Monica Epelman, MD and Jeffrey C. Hellinger, MD

Definition

The two most common inflammatory bowel diseases (IBDs) in children, Crohn's disease (CD) and ulcerative colitis (UC), are chronic immune-mediated disorders that affect the gastrointestinal (GI) tract.

Clinical Features

The incidence of CD is 2.7 to 4.6 per 100,000 and of UC is 1.5 to 2.9 per 100,000. Differences reflect geographic variations with largest number of IBD cases occurring in the northern industrialized regions of Europe, the United Kingdom, and North America. Most recent studies demonstrate a slight female predominance for both CD and UC. Inflammatory bowel disease has a bimodal age distribution; the first peak is in the second and third decades with a smaller peak in the sixth and seventh decades.

Constitutional signs and symptoms include low-grade fever, sweats, fatigue, malaise, arthralgias, nausea, vomiting, anorexia, and weight loss, the latter occurring more commonly in CD related to small bowel malabsorption and food avoidance. Rarely, patients may present in septic shock in the setting of toxic colitis; this is encountered more frequently with UC in association with a dilated colon (toxic "megacolon"). Gastrointestinal symptoms include bloating, abdominal pain, diarrhea, bloody stools, rectal urgency (tenesmus), perianal discomfort, and fecal incontinence. Some patients with CD have oral aphthous ulcers and dysphagia. Crohn's disease ileitis results in non-bloody large-volume watery defecation related to malabsorption. If CD involves the colon the diarrhea is more likely to be bloody and mucopurulent. Ulcerative colitis results in bloody, small-volume, high-frequency defecation. Frequently GI complications from IBD occur with pathologic and clinical manifestation dependent on the subtype of IBD. With CD, common complications include fistulae (to segments of bowel, viscera, or skin), sinus tracts, phlegmon, and intra-abdominal abscesses. Ulcerative colitis may cause septic colitis +/- dilated colon "toxic megacolon," massive hemorrhage, and/or colonic cellular dysplasia with transformation to adenocarcinoma. Both CD and UC may be complicated by strictures and adhesions leading to bowel obstruction.

Extraintestinal manifestations (20 to 40%):
- Metabolic: growth failure and delayed puberty (CD>UC), osteopenia/osteoporosis
- Dermatologic: erythema nodosum, pyoderma gangrenosum
- Ocular: episcleritis, iritis, uveitis
- Pulmonary: chronic bronchitis, bronchiectasis
- Hepatobiliary: cholelithiasis (CD>UC), pericholangitis, primary sclerosing cholangitis (UC>CD), steatosis, chronic hepatitis
- Urologic: nephrourolithiasis (CD>UC)
- Hematologic: anemia, hyperhomocysteinemia
- Venous thromboembolism: extremity deep venous thrombosis, pulmonary embolism
- Rheumatologic: seronegative axial spondyloarthropathies (HLA-B27 antigen; ankylosing spondylitis, sacroiliitis), peripheral arthropathies

Anatomy and Physiology

The pathogenesis is a complex interaction of genetics, environmental triggers, infectious agents, and immunoregulatory dysfunction. Current evidence indicates that patients have genetic predispositions that cause a defective mucosal barrier, susceptibility to environmental antigens, native microflora and other infectious antigens, and an abnormal mucosal cellular immune response to these stimuli. This leads to impaired antiinflammatory regulation and an excessive, mucosal inflammatory response.

Crohn's Disease

Crohn's disease may involve any portion of the GI tract; the pattern of involvement is typically constant during a patient's lifetime. Most commonly, disease occurs in the ileum and cecum (40 to 50 percent) followed by disease restricted to the jejunum and/or ileum (30 percent) or colon (15 to 25 percent). Less commonly, CD may involve the oral cavity, esophagus, stomach, and duodenum. The rectum is often normal. For any diseased region, local bowel distribution is segmental with normal mucosa interspersed between pathologic regions (a.k.a. "skip areas"). The acute mucosal inflammation in CD leads to hyperemic mucosa with shallow ulcerations. Inflammation spreads to involve all layers of the bowel wall, resulting in transmural edematous thickening and loss of mural stratification. The initial inflammatory infiltrate progresses to a chronic, fibrosing inflammation, characteristically defined by the presence of noncaseating granulomas. The bowel wall thickening often becomes eccentric. Regional lymph nodes enlarge and may also have a granulomatous aggregate when granulomas are present in the affected bowel (40 to 50 percent). Longitudinal and transverse mural ulcers and fissures of variable depth connect. The pattern of ulcerations and fissures along with the intervening relatively preserved mucosa results in a characteristic "cobblestone" appearance grossly. Serosal involvement can lead to adjacent mesentery inflammation with edematous thickening and if chronic, fibrofatty proliferation of the adjacent fat may then develop (a.k.a. creeping fat). The transmural inflammation, fissures, and mesenteric involvement account for the high incidence of sinus tracts, fistulae, intra-abdominal abscesses, strictures, and adhesions in CD.

Ulcerative Colitis

Ulcerative colitis is primarily a mucosal disease. Disease may be limited to the rectum (proctitis), extend to the rectosigmoid or descending colon (left-sided colitis), or less commonly, extend into the transverse and ascending colon (pancolitis, 10 percent). Inflammation begins at and involves the rectum in >95 percent of cases. In the acute phase, inflammatory cells centered at the crypts of the mucosa form crypt abscesses. Inflammation leads to shallow mucosal ulcerations, which along with the inflammatory cellular infiltrate, extend into the lamina propria and submucosa. This leads to expansion of the lamina propia and submucosal fat proliferation, respectively. During the acute phase, inflammation may rarely extend into the muscularis propia with secondary hypertrophy. The combination of lamina propia inflammatory expansion, increased submucosal fat, and muscularis hypertrophy, results in bowel wall thickening which is typically symmetric. Subsequently, inflammatory mediators in the muscularis may lead to smooth muscle inhibition resulting in gross bowel distention. The term "toxic megacolon" refers to sepsis with bowel distention greater than 6 centimeters in diameter, typically in the transverse colon. The bowel wall usually appears thin in toxic megacolon. As the inflammation in UC progresses it spreads into adjacent regions with associated undermining of the mucosa and secondary ulceration resulting in retrograde extension into the more proximal colon without skip areas. In the chronic stage, submucosal fatty deposition contributes to apparent bowel wall stratification. As multiple mucosal ulcers connect, small islands of hyperemic and edematous mucosa positioned between channels of ulceration are spared. These islands of mucosa resemble polyps and are called "pseudopolyps." Chronic inflammation in UC typically leads to rigid wall thickening and foreshortening of the colon with atrophied mucosa and loss of the haustral folds. The affected colon resembles a lead pipe.

Imaging Findings

Radiography, US, fluoroscopy, CT, and MRI all may be utilized to evaluate patients with suspected IBD. Ultimately the diagnosis is made by endoscopic and/or histologic criteria.

Radiography:
- "Thumbprinting" (symmetric thickening of haustral folds/edema in bowel walls)
- Mesenteric thickening (mass effect)
- Ileus
- Toxic megacolon (UC>CD)
- Obstruction
- Pneumatosis (UC>CD) more likely asymptomatic pneumatosis "cystoides" intestinalis
- Pneumoperitoneum (perforation related to toxic megacolon)

Fluoroscopy:

Crohn's disease
- Segmental involvement (skip lesions)
- Aphthous ulcers
- Distorted folds
- Luminal narrowing/stenosis ("string sign"; Fig. 43.1)
- Strictures
- Pseudodiverticulae ("saccular outpouchings"; related to asymmetric, segmental distribution of disease)

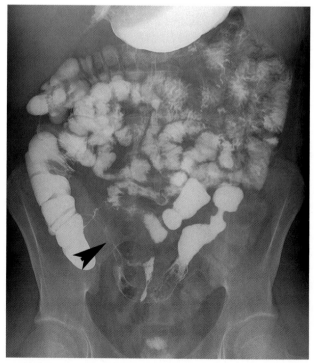

Figure 43.1. Frontal abdominal radiograph obtained during a small bowel follow-through in a 16-year-old with CD shows a markedly narrowed, but potentially distensible terminal ileum (arrowhead) consistent with the "string sign"; separation of the terminal ileum from the remainder of the bowel loops can be caused by wall thickening or represent fibrofatty proliferation.

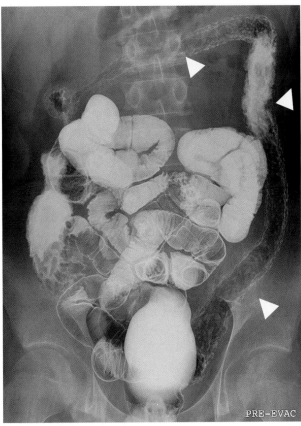

Figure 43.2. Barium enema in a 17-year-old with UC shows evidence of diffuse colitis with most pronounced changes involving the transverse and left colonic segments. Note the coarse, irregular, and granular appearance of the mucosa resulting from inflammation and ulceration (arrowheads).

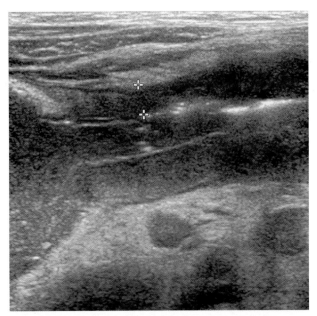

Figure 43.3. Transverse US of the right-lower quadrant with longitudinal imaging along the length of the terminal ileum (TI) in an 8-year-old boy with acute ileocecal CD demonstrates transmural wall thickening (between calipers). Note increased echogenicity of the surrounding fat reflective of inflammatory changes.

- Fistulae, anorectal ulcers, and sinus tracts (with abnormal regional transit or collections of barium)

Ulcerative colitis
- Wide presacral space
- Contiguous colonic involvement
- Mucosal granularity (Fig. 43.2)
- Spiculated bowel
- Collar button ulcers
- Double-tracking (from longitudinal ulcers)
- Pseudopolyps
- Postinflammatory filiform polyps in the healing phase
- "Lead pipe" colon (featureless bowel with colonic foreshortening)
- "Apple core" lesion/mass from secondary adenocarcinoma

US:
- Bowel wall thickening (Fig. 43.3)
- Dilatation
- Hyperemia (Doppler interrogation)
- Abscesses
- Phlegmon/fluid

CT and MRI:
- Mucosal and/or mural edematous thickening (with dynamic luminal narrowing, CD>UC)
- Hyperenhancement (Fig. 43.4)
- Engorged, tortuous vasa recta with wide spacing ("comb sign"; Fig. 43.5)
- Perienteric fat stranding (phlegmon)
- Bowel wall thickening without enhancement (chronic)
- Intestinal strictures (fixed narrowing; CD>UC)
- Mesenteric fat proliferation, "creeping fat" (CD; Fig. 43.6)
- Submucosal fat deposition, "halo" sign (UC)
- Mesenteric lymphadenopathy (CD)
- Bowel fistulae (CD>UC)
- Perirectal sinus, fistula, or abscess (CD)

Imaging Strategy

Diagnostic algorithms aim to evaluate intestinal and extraintestinal manifestations of disease in one comprehensive exam with the least invasive approach and radiation exposure. Abdominopelvic radiography is commonly the first modality obtained to assess patients with acute or recurrent GI symptoms. Depending on the presentation, US may then be considered as it is easy to perform and does not use radiation. Ultrasound can efficiently assess for bowel inflammation, dilatation, and secondary intra-abdominal abscesses, however performance will vary according to the sonographic window and operator skill.

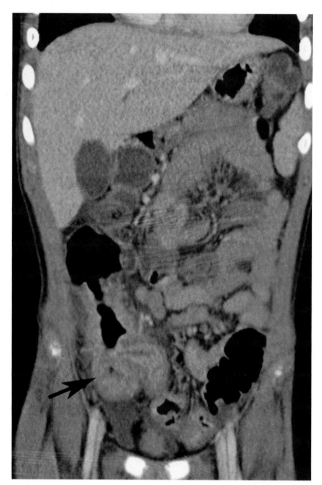

Figure 43.4. Coronal oral and intravenous contrast-enhanced CT reformation in an 8-year-old boy with CD shows wall thickening of the TI (arrow), mucosal hyperenhancement, and luminal narrowing.

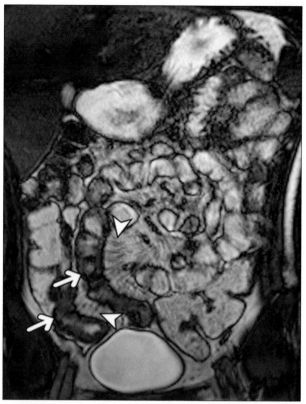

Figure 43.5. Oral and intravenous contrast-enhanced CT enterography coronal reformation in a 17-year-old with UC shows wall thickening and irregularity of the mucosa in the imaged descending and sigmoid colon (arrows). Note prominence of the adjacent pericolonic vasculature. The areas of low attenuation in the colonic wall (arrowheads) represent submucosal fat deposition.

Selection of additional modalities is based on whether the imaging goals are to evaluate morphology, function, or both. Fluoroscopy (UGI/SBFT) with postcontrast abdominal radiographs and fluoroscopic spot compression is used for functional and anatomic interrogation of bowel loops and assessment of contrast transit time. It can also be used to assess for fistulas or to look for strictures prior to capsule endoscopy. Capsule endoscopy, sigmoidoscopy, and conventional colonoscopy are recommended for direct visualization of bowel mucosa. Biopsy can be performed during traditional endoscopic procedures. Barium enema (BE) is relatively contraindicated in patients with moderate to severe colitis given the risk of bowel perforation. Often, CT is utilized for the initial diagnostic workup as well as for evaluation of emergent presentations or when MRI may be contraindicated or not available. In most pediatric acute abdomen evaluations, CT is performed with routine oral and intravenous contrast-enhanced technique. CT enterography is recommended for patients who can ingest a large amount of a negative bowel contrast agent or can have it administered via an enteric tube. For further localization and characterization of diseased bowel during acute flares or after treatment, in elective and nonemergent cases, MRI is recommended. When performed with enterography/colonography techniques, MRI is particularly useful to delineate the extent of inflammation and the presence of abscesses, fistulae, and strictures.

Related Physics

Eloquent MR enterography demands stringent quality assurance of measurable parameters for all equipment related to the magnet. Coil efficiency is measured by assessing its sensitivity to RF signals. An example of systematic error in coil sensitivity would be a fixed erroneous decrease in the coil sensitivity caused by the measuring instrument and not the coil. A random error would be one that occurs infrequently and without predictability such as those caused by fluctuations in the measuring tool sensitivity or interpretation by the operator. Because of random errors, one must perform repeat measurements to determine the truth of the value. With repeat measurements, accuracy refers to the difference between the true and measured value whereas precision describes the degree of difference

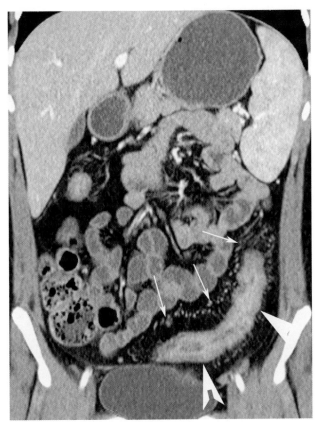

Figure 43.6. Coronal oral contrast-enhanced balanced steady-state free precession MR enterography image demonstrates focal wall thickening with associated fibrofatty proliferation, involving two ileal segments (arrowheads). Note the increased mesenteric vascularity with vascular dilatation, tortuosity, and wide spacing of the vasa recta, resulting in the "comb sign" (arrowheads).

between repeat measurements and has no relationship to truth. For coil sensitivity the plot of repeat measurements (x) against frequency of occurrence (y) forms a distribution curve. The Gaussian curve is the most common one encountered in imaging science and is characterized by the most probable value or mean value, mu, and standard deviation, sigma, the latter representing the width of the distribution in the x-axis. The median is that value that bissects the area of the distribution curve. The mode is the value in a series that occurs most often. In a Gaussian distribution the mean, median, and mode are one in the same. It is important to recognize that if test data should fall in a Gaussian distribution, certain predictions can be made regarding future measurements. The confidence interval is a statistical tool used to give a range between an upper and lower value where there is a certain percentage chance that the next measurement will lie within this range. When testing coil sensitivity, one would be concerned about measurements that repeatedly lie within either tail of the curve. Finally, propogation of error is a method by which individual errors from individual measurements can be combined to form an aggregate error.

Common Variants

- Backwash ileitis: rare involvement of the terminal ileum in ulcerative colitis from reflux of inflammatory contents through an incompetent, patulous ileocecal valve (more common with pancolitis and involvement of the cecum).
- Indeterminate colitis: in up to 20 percent of patients with colitis, histological specimens may show features of both CD and UC where it may not be possible to distinguish CD from UC.

Differential Diagnosis

Ileitis:

- Infectious: Campylobacter jejuni, Salmonella enteriditis, Yersinia entercolitica
- Secondary (from adjacent inflammatory process)
- Appendicitis
- NSAID-induced
- Eosinophilic

Colitis:

- Indeterminate (features of both CD and UC)
- Pseudomembranous
- Infectious: Campylobacter, Cytomegalovirus, Escherichia Coli, Salmonella, Shigella
- Neutropenic
- Radiation
- Ischemic
- Allergic (cow/soy milk hypersensitivity)
- Behcet's disease
- NSAID-induced
- Eosinophilic
- Stercoral proctitis/colitis (secondary to chronic fecal impaction)
- Acute self-limited (non-IBD colitis; no identifying etiology)
- Portal hypertension colopathy (venous congestion and not a true colitis)

Clinical Issues

Medical management for CD and UC is first-line therapy, targeting cellular inflammation with corticosteroids, salicyclates, and immunomodulators. Strictures and adhesions occur more commonly in CD. Perianal skin tags and anorectal ulcers, fissures, fistulae, and abscesses may occur in 30 to 50 percent of patients with CD. These are best evaluated with MRI. When assessing colitis, if the rectum is spared or there is perianal disease (e.g., skin tags, large hemorrhoids, abscesses or cutaneous fistulae), CD is much more likely than UC. Abscesses ≥ 4 centimeters in diameter may be considered for image-guided drainage (usually with US or CT). A simple fistula may respond to immunomodulators, but a complex fistula (e.g., with multiple connections) may require surgical management. Crohn's disease patients with strictures (chronic fibrosis) may be considered for surgical treatment or stricturoplasty. In pediatric patients, UC is more extensive with a higher rate of acute severe exacerbations. Approximately 30 to 40 percent of children will fail corticosteroids and require second-line medical therapy or colectomy. Surgery may be curative in 25 percent of patients refractory to medical treatment. With colitis, cellular dysplasia occurs as a response to inflammation. The risk for developing adenocarcinoma is directly related to the anatomic extent and duration of disease; this is highest for patients whose symptoms began during childhood, have pancolitis, or have frequent relapse. Estimated risk is 1 to 3 percent at 10 years, but may be as high as 30 percent by 30 to 35 years. Pancolitis patients may be considered at high risk after 7 years duration of disease. Pediatric patients who develop UC in the first decade of life should undergo yearly screening with invasive or noninvasive colonoscopy beginning in adolescence. Prophylactic colectomy may be considered in adults who developed UC as children. The anatomic extent of colitis also directly impacts the risk for toxic colitis ("megacolon"). Toxic colitis that is refractory to medical treatment may warrant subtotal colectomy with ileostomy.

Key Points

- CD is a segmental, transmural process, which may involve any portion of the GI tract.
- Transmural involvement in CD results in extraluminal complications, including fistulae, sinus tracts, phlegmons, and abscesses.
- UC is superficial and spreads in a continuous fashion, proximally from the rectum.
- UC may be treated and possibly cured surgically, whereas, only a fibrotic Crohn's with strictures may be considered for surgical treatment/stricturoplasty.
- Extraintestinal manifestations of IBD are common; prevalent associated disease includes primary sclerosing cholangitis, cholelithiasis, nephrolithiasis, IBD-related peripheral and axial arthropathies, and deep venous thrombosis.

Further Reading

Ausch C, Madoff RD, Gnant M, Rosen HR, Garcia-Aguilar J, Hölbling N, Herbst F, Buxhofer V, Holzer B, Rothenberger DA, Schiessel R. Aetiology and surgical management of toxic megacolon. *Colorectal Dis.* 2006;8(3):195–201.

Fidler J. MR Imaging of the small bowel. *Radiol Clin N Am.* 2007;48: 317–331.

Huprich JE, Rosen MP, Fidler JL, Gay SB, Grant TH, Greene FL, Lalani T, Miller FH, Rockey DC, Sudakoff GS, Gunderman R, Coley BD. ACR appropriateness criteria on Crohn's disease. *J Am Coll Radiol.* 2010;7(2):94–102.

Larsen S, Bendtzen K, Nielsen OH. Extraintestinal manifestations of inflammatory bowel disease: epidemiology, diagnosis, and management. *Annals of Medicine.* 2010;42:97–114.

Kucharzik T, Maaser C, Lügering A, Kagnoff M, Mayer L, Targan S, Domschke W. Recent understanding of IBD pathogenesis: implications for future therapies. *Inflamm Bowel Dis.* 2006;12 (11):1068–1083.

Tochetto S, Yaghmai V. CT enterography: concept, technique, and interpretation. *Radiol Clin North Am.* 2009;47(1):117–132.

Turner D. Severe acute ulcerative colitis: the pediatric perspective. *Dig Dis.* 2009;27(3):322–326.

CHAPTER 44

Gastrointestinal Duplication Cysts

Ramesh S. Iyer, MD

Definition

Gastrointestinal duplication cysts are congenital cystic or tubular anomalies of the gastrointestinal system. They typically share a smooth muscle wall and vascular supply with a portion of the native alimentary tract but usually do not communicate with the lumen of the native bowel and so are most often fluid-filled. They are lined by alimentary tract mucosa but the lining mucosa is not necessarily that of the adjacent native segment of the gastrointestinal tract.

Clinical Features

The majority of duplication cysts that become symptomatic do so in the first year of life. Presenting symptoms are dependent upon size and location of the duplication. Intrathoracic cysts may be large enough to cause cardiac or respiratory compromise, dysphagia, vomiting, or chest pain. Common abdominal manifestations include distension, vomiting, bleeding, pain, and a palpable abdominal mass. They are malleable and can extend into the lumen of the native bowel and act as a lead point for intussusception. Some cysts are small and lack ectopic gastric or pancreatic mucosa. These may be incidentally found at any decade of life.

Anatomy and Physiology

Multiple hypotheses have been proposed to explain the embryologic basis for gastrointestinal duplications. Unfortunately, no single theory can adequately account for all types of duplications. Proposed etiologies for duplication cysts include incomplete twinning, persistent diverticuli from fetal life, aberrant luminal recanalization, and sequelae of intrauterine vascular accidents. Enteric duplication cysts can be located anywhere from the tongue to the anus, but are most commonly located at the ileum and esophagus. They often contain ectopic gastric mucosa or pancreatic tissue. Ectopic gastric mucosa is most prevalent in esophageal duplication cysts and may result in peptic ulceration, hemorrhage, and anemia. Ectopic pancreatic tissue is most common in gastric duplication cysts and is associated with pancreatitis, caused either by inflammation of the pancreatic tissue within the cyst itself or by inflammation of the adjacent native pancreas. Pancreatitis and/or biliary obstruction can result from mass effect on the pancreas or bile ducts caused by duodenal duplication cysts.

Imaging Findings

The most common imaging modality used to evaluate enteric duplication cysts is ultrasound (US). The characteristic sonographic appearance is that of a double-layered wall ("double-wall" sign) or so-called "gut signature," consisting of an inner hyperechoic layer reflecting the mucosa-submucosa complex and an outer hypoechoic layer indicative of the muscularis propria (Fig. 44.1). These layers are usually relatively thick stripes that are confluent around greater than 50 percent of the cyst's circumference. The double-wall sign is often more conspicuous in the far field because of increased through transmission. Occasionally more than two layers in the cyst wall may be resolved sonographically. Wall layer morphology can be distorted or lost in the context of mucosal erosion or cyst perforation as can occur with ectopic gastric mucosa.

US:

- Double-wall sign or gut signature (described above)
- "Y-configuration" or split-muscle Y sign: formed at the junction of the hypoechoic outer wall of the cyst and the adjacent hypoechoic outer wall of the adjacent small bowel
- Fluid may be simple and anechoic
- Contents can be echogenic as a result of debris, proteins, or blood products within the fluid, with or without a fluid debris level
- Malleable with compression

CT:

- Fluid-filled cyst that is usually contiguous with the mesenteric side of the bowel wall (antimesenteric location has been described)
- Round or oval (Fig. 44.2) but may be tubular (especially colonic)
- May have submucosal mass effect on or protrude into the bowel lumen (Fig. 44.3)
- May change shape with compression or changes in patient position
- Contents are variable, rendering variable Hounsfield units

Fluoroscopy:

- Submucosal mass

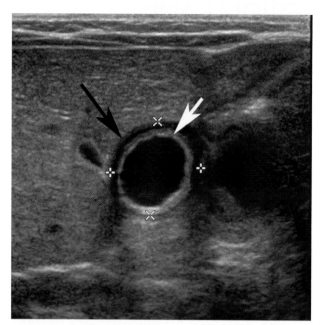

Figure 44.1. Transverse US image in a 12-year-old girl with renal anomaly demonstrates a round cyst in the region of the duodenum, abutting the liver adjacent to the gallbladder. A choledochal cyst could exist in this region, however, the cyst exhibits two concentric rings of inner hyperechogenicity (mucosa-submucosa complex) (white arrow) and outer hypoechogenicity (muscularis propria) (black arrow), representing the gut signature of a GI duplication cyst.

- May protrude into the lumen of the native bowel, potentially serving as a lead point for intussusception
- Esophageal and small bowel duplication cysts typically do not communicate with the native bowel lumen unless they have perforated
- Many tubular colonic duplications communicate with the native bowel lumen

Radiography
Esophageal duplication cysts present as mediastinal lesions of various sizes that are contiguous with the esophagus, right more so than left, inferior more often than superior.

MRI:
- Usually exhibit hypointensity on T1 and hyperintensity on T2, but the signal intensity is variable depending on the cyst contents
- Cyst wall is contiguous with the wall of the native GI tract

Imaging Strategy

Imaging strategy is highly dependent upon the reason for investigation and the level of the alimentary tract duplication. Many duplication cysts are found incidentally during prenatal screening sonograms or on a variety of postnatal imaging exams. Prenatally, duplication cysts lack the "gut signature" sonographically. Postnatal sonogram can confirm the diagnosis.

Esophageal duplication cysts are often detected on chest radiographs followed by cross-sectional imaging with either CT or MRI. If the mass extends posteriorly and there is an associated cervical or thoracic spine bony defect, then a rare neurenteric cyst should be considered. MRI would be most useful. Often an enteric or colonic duplication cyst is incidentally found on either CT or MR and further characterized with US, which is more specific than other cross-

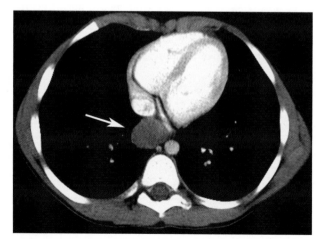

Figure 44.2. Axial contrast-enhanced CT image in a 9-year-old boy with a mediastinal mass on chest radiography demonstrates a mediastinal cyst (arrow) with water attenuation internally in the expected course of the esophagus. Differential considerations include bronchogenic cyst or less likely pericardial cyst.

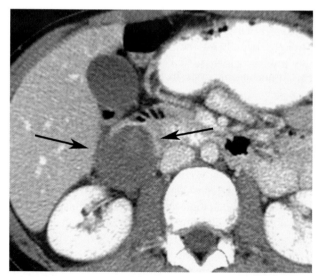

Figure 44.3. Axial oral and intravenous contrast-enhanced CT in an 8-year-old boy with intermittent abdominal pain reveals a cyst (arrows) arising from the descending duodenum with water-attenuation fluid internally. Differential considerations include choledochal cyst, mesenteric cyst, or less likely pancreatic pseudocyst. Ultrasound could be used to assess for gut signature in the wall of the cyst.

sectional modalities if the aforementioned characteristic double-wall or sonographic gut signature is demonstrated. In selected cases, barium administration through either a small bowel follow-through (enteric duplication) or an enema (colorectal duplication) may confirm the submucosal position of a suspected intramural lesion. Technetium 99-labeled pertechnetate scintigraphy may also be used to detect ectopic gastric mucosa in either intrathoracic or intra-abdominal duplication cysts.

Related Physics

Ultrasound has superior specificity in cystic masses by providing detailed information about the delimiting wall or border, which in the case of GI duplication cysts creates the gut signature. Imaging is optimized through the appropriate choice of transducer type, shape, and frequency. Transducer types are divided into linear and phased (sector) array. Linear transducers come in straight linear and curvilinear arrays, each with their own advantages. The phased array transducers have a square, round, or slightly rectangular surface with a smaller footprint (approximately 1 cm^2) to allow for easier access through smaller acoustic windows. Linear and curvilinear arrays offer excellent image coverage from the transducer surface down to maximum penetration depth. Phased array sacrifices near-field coverage in favor of wide coverage at depth. Either transducer type comes in a wide range of frequencies from 1 to 20 megahertz. Most transducers have a range of frequency options within one transducer head. The wider field of view in the near range coupled with the high frequency of a pediatric linear or curvilinear transducer permits excellent visualization of the gut anatomy in the near field and at depth in a child with suspected GI duplication cyst.

Differential Diagnosis

- Bronchogenic cyst (esophageal duplications and bronchogenic cysts are all part of spectrum of bronchopulmonary foregut malformations)
- Neurenteric cyst
- Pericardial cyst
- Cystic teratoma
- Lymphatic malformation (a.k.a. mesenteric cyst)
- Omphalomesenteric duct remnant cyst
- Ovarian cyst or teratoma
- Choledochal cyst
- Exophytic hepatic cyst
- Exophytic renal cyst

Clinical Issues

Some cysts may have local mass effect on the adjacent bowel and cause obstructive symptoms or act as a lead point for intussusceptions. Peptic ulceration or hemorrhage may occur in cysts that have ectopic gastric or pancreatic mucosa. The inflammation may affect adjacent structures. Most duplication cysts of the esophagus and small and large bowel are surgically resected to eliminate such potential complications. Malignant degeneration is rare but has been reported in the pediatric population. It can be difficult or impossible to distinguish esophageal duplication cysts from mediastinal bronchogenic cysts by imaging examination. Esophageal duplication cysts typically abut or are located within the wall of the esophagus and exhibit a mural smooth muscle layer without cartilage. Cartilage or respiratory epithelium within the wall of the cyst is typical of a bronchogenic cyst.

Key Points

- Gastrointestinal duplication cyst is a sporadic congenital abnormality of uncertain etiology.
- Duplication cysts an be found anywhere in the GI tract, but are most common in the ileum and esophagus.
- Most duplication cysts are round or oval fluid-filled cystic lesions with characteristic "gut signature" or "double-wall" sign on US.
- Some duplication cysts are tubular (mostly colonic) and communicate with the lumen of the native GI tract.
- Bronchogenic cysts and esophageal duplication cysts may be indistinguishable by imaging.

Further Reading

Berrocal T, Torres I, Gutierrez J, Prieto C, del Hoyo ML, Lamas M. Congenital anomalies of the upper gastrointestinal tract. *Radiographics*. 1999;19(4):855–872.

Hur J, Yoon CS, Kim MJ, Kim OH. Imaging features of gastrointestinal tract duplications in infants and children: from oesophagus to rectum. *Pediatr Radiol*. 2007;37(7):691–699.

Iyer CP, Mahour GH. Duplications of the alimentary tract in infants and children. *J Pediatr Surg*. 1995;30(9):1267–1270.

Kim YJ, Kim YK, Jeong YJ, Moon WS, Gwak HJ. Ileal duplication cyst: Y-configuration on in vivo sonography. *J Pediatr Surg*. 2009;44: 1462–1464.

Macpherson RI. Gastrointestinal tract duplications: clinical, pathologic, etiologic, and radiologic considerations. *Radiographics*. 1993;13(5):1063–1080.

CHAPTER 45

Henoch-Schönlein Purpura

Monther S. Qandeel and Laura Z. Fenton

Definition

Henoch-Schönlein purpura (HSP) is a pediatric nonthrombocytopenic vasculitis that typically affects the bowel, skin, joints, kidneys, and less often other organs.

Clinical Features

Most children affected are less than 12 years of age, the prevalence peaks in children age 5 years (range 2 to 20 years of age). The clinical diagnosis is based on the association of a palpable nonthrombocytopenic purpura (with characteristic predilection for the lower extremities and buttocks), arthritis (most commonly involving knees and ankles), and abdominal pain. Other GI symptoms include postprandial bowel angina, nausea, vomiting, upper and lower GI bleeding. Gastrointestinal manifestations may precede the characteristic rash in a minority of patients. In HSP, involvement of the kidneys (nephritis +/- nephrosis resulting in hematuria +/- proteinuria) occurs in approximately 50 percent, with varying severity. Scrotal swelling, erythema, and pain are present in 20 percent of HSP patients. The epididymis may be enlarged and indistinguishable on ultrasound (US) from acute infectious epididymitis. Many organs of the body are infrequently affected by this vasculitis. Cardiac involvement (rhythm abnormalities, myocardial infarction and myocardial dysfunction) is an infrequent, but potentially life-threatening, complication of HSP. Neurologic complications are rare. Mild symptoms such as headache, irritability, and behavioral alterations are often underestimated. Henoch-Schönlein purpura may cause stroke with propensity to involve the basal ganglia. Vasculitis of the gallbladder can result in acalculous cholecystitis or hydrops. Involvement of the vessels that support the biliary tree can result in bile duct stenosis and ultimately obstructive biliary cirrhosis.

Anatomy and Physiology

Although the disease has been described for over a century, the etiology has yet to be discovered. Histologically, there is small vessel necrotizing vasculitis with immunocomplexes and IgA deposition. In the intestine, submucosal and subserosal hemorrhage and edema can lead to intussusceptions that often spontaneously reduce. The small intestine is affected more often than the colon. Patchy mucosal erythema and petechiae may be visible at colonoscopy.

Imaging Findings

Fluoroscopy:

- Segmental bowel dilation, stenosis, or obstruction
- Hypomotility or ileus
- Bowel wall thickening with loss of mucosal fold pattern and separation of bowel loops ("picket-fence" pattern) or thumbprinting
- Skip areas with normal intervening bowel
- Intraluminal filling defects
- Small bowel-small bowel intussusception > ileocolic intussusception
- Stricture (late sequela) (Fig. 45.1)

CT:

- High-attenuation intramural hemorrhage
- Target sign
- Thickened bowel wall
- Dilated enhancing proximal mesenteric vessels in the region of abnormal bowel with small vessel vasculitis
- Free intraperitoneal air (if perforation)
- Intussusception

US:

- Bowel wall thickening can be circumferential (Fig. 45.2) or asymmetric
- Small bowel-small bowel intussusception (multilayered) more often than ileocolic (Fig. 45.3)
- Intraperitoneal fluid
- US features are not specific and are inconstant
- There may be increased renal cortical echogenicity and loss of corticomedullary differentiation

> **IMAGING PITFALLS**: GI symptoms may precede characteristic skin rash in a minority of patients, which may lead to a less directed workup.

Imaging Strategy

The clinical presentation of intussusception among children with HSP can be confusing because of overlap of symptoms

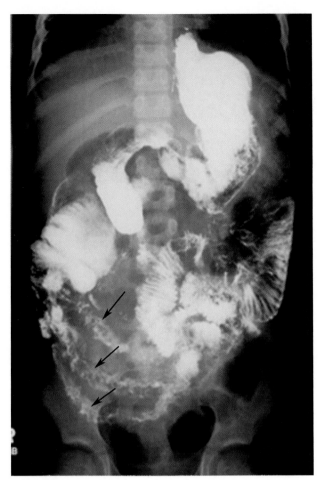

Figure 45.1. Small bowel follow-through image in a child with abdominal pain and rash shows long-segment distal small bowel wall thickening [[Note to Editor: arrows]] extending into the cecum with separation of these bowel loops in the right-lower quadrant. Findings are consistent with HSP.

from other abdominal manifestations of HSP. When abdominal symptoms are severe, small bowel-small bowel intussusception should be considered, which occurs in 5 to 15 percent of patients with HSP. The location and distribution of intussusception in children with HSP is as follows: ileoileal is 51.4 percent; ileocolic is 38.6 percent; jejunojejunal is

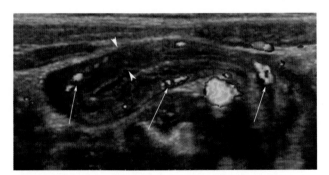

Figure 45.2. Transverse US image with color Doppler in a child with proven HSP shows small intestine wall thickening arrowheads and hyperemia arrows. Courtesy of Marthe Munden, MD, Texas Children's Hospital, Houston.

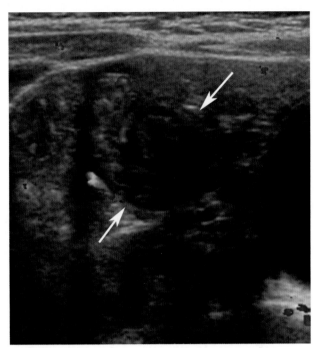

Figure 45.3. Transverse US image with Doppler in a child with abdominal pain shows small intestine-small intestine intussusception [[Note to Editor: arrows]]. Small bowel intussusceptions tend to be smaller in diameter (less than 3 cm) than ileocolic intussusceptions. Courtesy of Marthe Munden, MD, Texas Children's Hospital, Houston.

7 percent; and 3 percent are colocolonic. In contrast, nearly 90 percent of patients with idiopathic intussusception have ileocolic intussusception. The best modality to demonstrate intramural hematoma, ileus, peritoneal fluid, and intussusception in screening and follow-up is US. If US is nondiagnostic, then CT may be useful. When US or CT findings are diagnostic for a very distal ileoileal or any ileocolic intussusception, air enema (AE) should be considered as a potentially therapeutic procedure before laparotomy. As the majority of HSP-related intussusceptions are small bowel-small bowel, air enema (AE) or contrast enema (CE) cannot generate sufficient pressure across the ileocecal valve for reduction. Rare complications of HSP include spontaneous bowel perforation (most often ileal associated with steroid treatment), bowel obstruction, and small bowel stricture.

Related Physics

Ultrasound can be very helpful and diagnostic in certain intestinal diseases and will be optimized when bowel is fluid-filled as the presence of intraluminal gas will impede through transmission of sound. Equally so, US gel must be used as a coupling medium on the skin surface. In HSP there is marked bowel wall thickening, edema, and liquid intestinal contents, all of which lend themselves well to US imaging. The US energy moves through tissues through wave propagation. The types of waves include transverse, longitudinal, and shear waves though only the latter two are of interest to medical imaging. Longitudinal waves travel through the medium by compression alternating with rarefaction of the medium. In this way energy is moved in the direction of wave propagation. Ultrasound waves can be characterized by wavelength and frequency. The user chooses the frequency by choosing the transducer and the tissue defines the sound speed. In the human body, sound speeds vary from a low of 1,480 m/s in fat to 1,570 m/s in liver. Though we do not image bone, sound speed in bone is approximately 3,000 m/s. The wavelength then accommodates to satisfy the equation $c = f\lambda$. There will be loss of acoustic power when scatters are present within the tissue. In fluid-filled structures the attenuation tends to be very low and this is true for bowel, bladder, or cystic masses. Because attenuation is so severe in acoustics, a scale has been developed to characterize these massive power losses in an engineering shorthand called decibels. In the literature the acoustic power is described as acoustic pressure or more commonly acoustic intensity where [acoustic intensity ~ acoustic pressure^2] and is most often quoted in units of Watts/centimeter^2. Attenuation is proportional to the frequency of the transducer and echogenicity of the medium though which the sound travels given in units of decibels/megahertz/centimeter.

Differential Diagnosis

Intussusception:
- Meckel's diverticulum
- Lymphoma
- Polyp
- Duplication cyst

Hyperattenuating bowel wall thickening (hemorrhage):
- Traumatic intramural hematoma
- Bleeding diathesis
- Inflammatory or infectious colitis
- Hemolytic uremic syndrome

Common Variants

Reports and retrospective studies describe less favorable outcome in adults with HSP compared to children as a result of more frequent and severe renal and extrarenal involvement and complications. The same may be true for teenage children with HSP.

Clinical Issues

Usually HSP does not require more than supportive treatment, however cytotoxic/immunosuppressive therapy has been used to prevent complications.

Key Points

- Characterized by nonthrombocytopenic purpura that bowel, skin, and joints
- Renal involvement is present in 50%
- Many other organs can be, but rarely are affected (CNS manifestations may be under-reported).
- GI manifestations may precede characteristic rash.
- US is the best initial test for evaluation and follow-up of bowel wall thickening and intussusception.
- HSP-associated intussusception predominantly occurs in the small bowel (not ileocolic) and is not amenable to air enema reduction.

Further Reading

Chiaretti et al. Cerebral hemorrhage in Henoch-Schoenlein syndrome. *Child's Nervous System.* 2002;*18*(8):365–367.

Navarro et al. The impact of imaging in the management of intussusception owing to pathologic lead points in children: a review of 43 cases. *Pediatric Radiology.* 2000;*30*(9):594–603.

Schwab et al. Contrast enema in children with Henoch-Schonlein purpura. *Journal of Pediatric Surgery.* 2005;*40*(8): 1221–1223.

Siegel MJ, Coley BD. Esophagus and Gastrointestinal Tract. In: Siegel MJ, Coley BD, eds. *Pediatric Imaging.* Philadelphia, PA. Lippincott, Williams, and Wilkins. 2004, pp. 199–258.

Swischuk LE. Alimentary tract. In: Swischuk LE, ed. *Imaging of the newborn, infant, and young child.* Philadelphia, PA: Lippincott Williams & Wilkins; 2004:442–443.

Genitourinary

CHAPTER 46

Vesicoureteral Reflux

Michael Arch, MD

Definition

Vesicoureteral reflux (VUR) is abnormal retrograde flow of urine from the bladder into the ureter.

Clinical Factors

The prevalence of VUR is <1 percent in otherwise healthy children, substantially higher in children with history of febrile urinary tract infection (UTI) and prenatal hydronephrosis and is most often discovered during the workup of these problems. Newborn males have a higher incidence of primary VUR, but throughout childhood the condition is more common in females and decreases with age. Vesicoureteral reflux is more common in Caucasians than in African Americans. There is a significant increased risk in children and siblings of patients with VUR. Approximately 90 percent of children with reflux have sterile urine. Voiding dysfunction can occur with and complicate the treatment of reflux. Patients with UTI and VUR are at an elevated risk for pyelonephritis and subsequent problems related to renal injury, such as hypertension and renal insufficiency.

Anatomy and Physiology

Primary VUR is believed to result from abnormal angulation of the ureteral insertion at the ureterovesical junction (UVJ) and an inadequate length of intramural ureter. Pathologically, there is a deficiency or immaturity of the longitudinal muscle of the submucosal ureter. Reflux can also be secondary to any process that alters the normal mechanics at the UVJ such as the presence of a periureteral (Hutch) diverticulum. Vesicoureteral reflux can also occur secondary to bladder outlet obstruction and voiding dysfunction.

Imaging Findings

In 1985, the International Reflux Study Committee (IRSC) introduced a uniform system for the classification of VUR (Fig. 46.1). The grading system combines two earlier classifications and is based upon the extent of retrograde filling and dilation of the ureter, the renal pelvis, and the calyces on a voiding cystourethrography (VCUG). The IRSC also described a standardized VCUG technique to allow comparability of results. In a patient with VUR, the VCUG demonstrates contrast that is instilled into the urinary bladder refluxing into the ureter and in many cases to the pelvicalyceal system. Reflux may occur during bladder filling or during voiding. Approximately one-third of patients with VUR reflux only during the voiding phase of the study. Varying degrees of ureteric and renal pelvis dilation, calyceal blunting, and intrarenal reflux occur and should be vvassessed according to the grading system proposed by the IRSC (Figs. 46.2 to 46.5).

Other signs:

- Intraluminal lesions: ureteroceles, polyps
- Anterior or posterior urethral valves: urethral causes of bladder outlet obstruction
- Detrusor sphincter dyssynergy
- Periureteral diverticulum (Hutch)
- Ectopic ureteral insertion site
- DMSA (dimercaptosuccinic acid) scans demonstrate areas of infection or renal scarring, often occuring at the poles
- Hydronephrosis and hydroureter (low sensitivity and specificity

IMAGING PITFALLS: Potential false positives on VCUG include the bowel wall mimicking contrast in a ureter, residual contrast in the vagina after voiding, lines created by catheters or tubing, lines created by the costovertebral junctions and the bony ileopectineal line. Comparison with a scout view, oblique views or visualization during rotation should reliably differentiate these from VUR.

Imaging Strategy

Indications for renal-bladder ultrasound (US) include documented febrile UTI (sterile collection) in an infant or toddler, Society of Fetal Urology (SFU) grade III and IV prenatal hydronephrosis or a parent or sibling with a history of VUR. In an infant with first febrile UTI, only US is recommended to rule out anatomic abnormalies; VCUG is no longer indicated unless the US is positive according

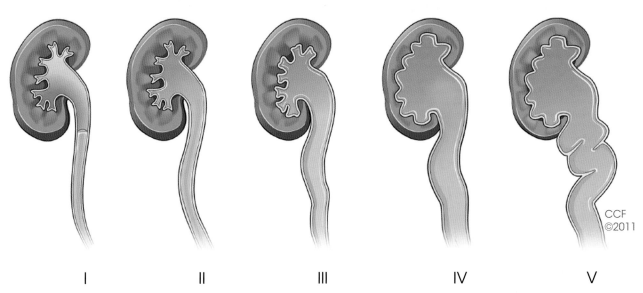

CCF
©2011

I   II   III   IV   V

Figure 46.1. International Reflux Study Commission grading system. **(I)** ureter only; **(II)** ureter and renal collecting system without calyceal blunting; **(III)** mild ureteric dilation and mild calyceal blunting; **(IV)** moderate ureteric and pelvic dilation and calyceal blunting with preservation of the papillary impressions; **(V)** severe ureteral and pelvic dilation with ureteral tortuosity and loss of the papillary impression in the calyces.

to the Subcommittee on Urinary Tract Infection, Steering Committee on Quality Improvement and Management latest practice guidelines. According to the 2010 American Urologic Association (AUA) guidelines, clinical observation is an option if no history of UTI in offspring and siblings of patients with VUR, or patients with low-grade (SFU grade I and II) prenatal hydronephrosis. Prenatal hydronephrosis is commonly expressed in terms of pelvic anteroposterior (AP) diameter. In the third trimester, 7 to 9 millimeters is mild, 10 to 14 millimeters is moderate,

and 15 or more millimeters is severe. Patients with mild prenatal hydronephrosis have a 12 percent incidence of pathology (including VUR) and require postnatal US at 1 to 4 weeks after birth, and if abnormal, VCUG. Newborns with moderate or severe prenatal hydronephrosis have

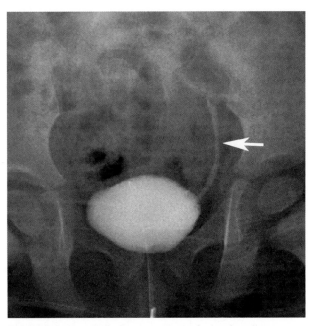

Figure 46.2. The VCUG shows contrast refluxing from the bladder into the distal left ureter (arrow) during early filling consistent with grade I VUR.

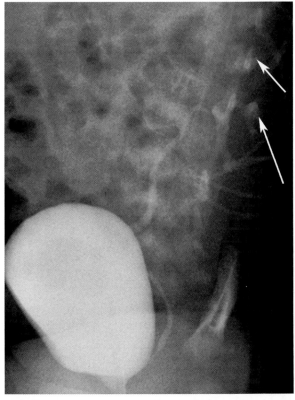

Figure 46.3. Oblique-view VCUG shows contrast in the left ureter and pelvicalyceal system and the fornices are sharp (arrows) consistent with grade II VUR.

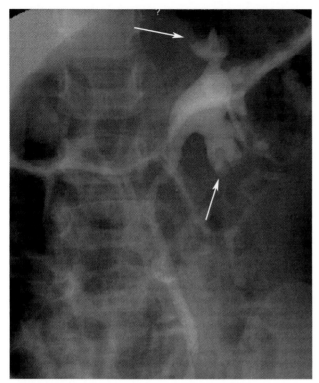

Figure 46.4. The VCUG shows contrast in the left ureter and pelvicalyceal system and there is mild calyceal blunting (arrows) with a normal-caliber minimally tortuous ureter consistent with grade III VUR.

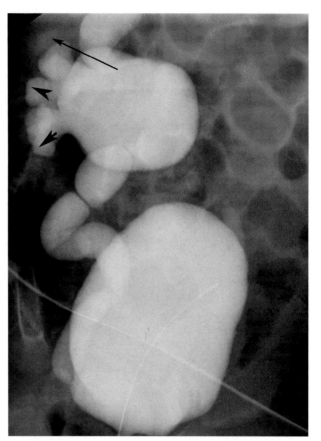

Figure 46.5. The VCUG shows contrast in the right ureter and pelvicalyceal system. The ureter is dilated and tortuous and the collecting system is severely dilated with loss of definite papillary impressions (arrowheads) consistent with grade V VUR. Intraparenchymal reflux is also present (arrow).

a high incidence of pathology (45 and 88 percent, respectively), and postnatal evaluation usually involves US, VCUG, and possibly nuclear medicine MAG-3 renogram. Radionuclide cystography (RNC) was traditionally recommended to screen siblings and to follow known VUR because of its historically lower radiation dose as compared to conventional continuous fluoroscopy. Newer fluoroscopy units have many dose-reducing features, including pulsed digital fluoroscopy, so radiation doses are now similar and performance of RNC has declined. In patients with known reflux, the AUA recommends annual US to monitor renal growth and assess for scarring. Follow-up VCUG or RNC is recommended between 12 and 24 months later, repeated until resolution of VUR or successful intervention. If there is a high clinical concern for scarring or if US is suggestive then DMSA scan is donerecommended.

Related Physics

Before the widespread implementation of lower-dose pulsed fluoroscopy units, RNC provided the lowest radiation dose to the child. To prepare the agent for a nuclear medicine study, first the radionuclide (Tc99m) is produced and then tagged to a molecule that will be metabolized (DTPA). Generally speaking, there are ranges of activity for each study that are based on patient weight or blood volume or in the case of a lung study, the tidal volume. The camera must be localized on the region of interest, which for RNC is the entire urinary tract from kidneys to urethra. As with all nuclear studies, the metabolic mode of uptake, organ distribution, and methods of physical and biological decay must be known and understood; for Tc99m, even though the physical half-life is six hours, the biologic half-life is much shorter as the radiopharmaceutical is rapidly excreted during the study. In general the shortest half-life dominates the effective half-life equation. Quality control procedures include screening for chemical contaminants, pyrogenic bioactive vectors (bacteria and viruses) and toxicity. Organ doses must be assessed by a qualified medical physicist and recorded in the patient record so that over a lifetime the potential cancer risk can be balanced against the benefits of future ionizing radiation studies. Unique in pediatrics, one must consider the radiation risk to surrounding family members during the time at which the child is radioactive. This risk can be ascertained by knowing the radioactive element being used, its dose rate at a fixed distance, and its mode of excretion and decay.

Differential Diagnosis

- Primary megaureter
- Ureterovesicle junction stenosis from ectopic ureter
- Dilated urinary tract in prune belly syndrome
- High urine output states

Common Variants

Vesicoureteral reflux may occur in kidneys with duplicated collecting systems and is usually through the lower pole ureter (that has orthotopic insertion at the bladder). Megacystis megaureter is an extreme form of VUR in which the majority of urine recirculates between the bladder and one or both ureters instead of emptying.

Clinical Issues

Often VUR will resolve spontaneously, particularly in young children with lower grades. The AUA recommends continuous antibiotic prophylaxis in children less than 1 year of age with history of febrile UTI and VUR, or grades III to V reflux with no history of UTI, and in children over 1 year of age with bowel/bladder dysfunction and VUR. Observation or antibiotic prophylaxis are both options for reflux grades I to II without history of UTI or children over 1 year of age with a single febrile UTI and reflux grade I to II. Patients who fail medical management or have renal scarring should be considered for surgical options, which include endoscopic UVJ injection therapies or open ureteric reimplantation. Contralateral VUR following UVJ injection therapy or open ureteric reimplantation can occur and is usually self-limited.

Key Points

- Normal US does not exclude VUR
- Five grades based on severity
- High spontaneous resolution, particularly in grades I–III
- Strong family history: screen siblings

Further Reading

Donnelly LF, Jones BV, O'Hara SM, et al., eds. Vesicoureteral reflux. In: *Diagnostic Imaging: Pediatrics*. Salt Lake City, UT: Amirsys; 2005:5–6–5–9.

Cendron, M. Antibiotic prophylaxis in the management of vesicoureteral reflux. *Adv Urol.* 2008;825475.

Lee RS, Cendron M, Kinnamon DD, Nguyen HT. Antenatal hydronephrosis as a predictor of postnatal outcome: a meta analysis. *Pediatrics.* 2006;*118*:586–593.

Skoog SJ, Peters CA, Arant BS Jr, Copp HL, Elder JS, Hudson RG, Khoury AE, Lorenzo AJ, Pohl HG, Shapiro E, Snodgrass WT, Diaz M. Pediatric Vesicoureteral Reflux Guidelines Panel summary report: clinical practice guidelines for screening siblings of children with vesicoureteral reflux and neonates/infants with prenatal hydronephrosis. *Jour Urol.* 2010;*184*:1145–1151.

Subcommittee on Urinary Tract Infection, Steering Committee on Quality Improvement and Management. Urinary tract infection: clinical practice guideline for the diagnosis and management of the initial UTI in febrile infants and children 2 to 24 months. *Pediatrics.* 2011;*128*;595.

Willi UV, Lebowitz RL. The so-called megaureter-megacystis syndrome. *AJR Am J Roentgenol.* 1979;*133*(3):409–416.

CHAPTER 47

Ureteropelvic Junction Obstruction

Lynn Ansley Fordham, MD

Definition

Ureteropelvic junction obstruction (UPJ) is congenital partial obstruction of the urinary tract at the transition between the renal pelvis and ureter.

Clinical Features

The most common cause of prenatal hydronephrosis is UPJ and it is seen in approximately 1 in 500 live births screened with prenatal ultrasound (US). It is more common in boys, more common on the left, and bilateral in 10 to 40 percent of cases. The degree of obstruction is variable. High-grade obstruction tends to present earlier in life with an abnormal prenatal US or palpable abdominal mass. Lower grades of obstruction may not present until later in life when the patient experiences back, flank, or abdominal pain, nausea and/or vomiting. Sometimes a mild UPJ is only symptomatic with ingestion of large amount of fluid with a diuretic agent such as beer or wine, which is termed "beer-drinkers hydronephrosis." Mild cases may be detected as incidental findings on studies performed for other indications.

Anatomy and Physiology

Either intrinsic narrowing or extrinsic compression can result in UPJ. The intrinsic stenosis is incompletely understood and thought to be related to errors in embryologic development. Other rare intrinsic etiologies include ureteral polyps and persistent fetal ureteral convolutions. Extrinsic obstruction, seen in approximately 10 percent of children with UPJ, is usually a result of crossing vessels, which can be renal arteries or veins (Fig. 47.1). The net result of either intrinsic or extrinsic etiologies is narrowing at the level of the UPJ with a variable degree of dilation of the renal pelvis.

Imaging Findings

- Enlarged renal pelvis out of proportion with calyces (Fig. 47.2A)
- Degree of dilation reflects a combination of the degree of the obstruction and the function of the kidney (poorly functioning kidney may have minimal hydronephrosis)

- Normal-sized or nonvisualized ureter
- Diminished or absent ureteral jet on color Doppler on affected side (Fig. 47.2B)
- Delayed wash out on diuretic MAG-3 renogram (Fig. 47.3)

> **IMAGING PITFALLS:** It is important to evaluate the contralateral kidney for any associated anomalies such as multicystic dysplastic kidney or evidence horseshoe kidney.

Imaging Strategy

The primary modality for anatomic evaluation of UPJ is US. Prenatal findings should be confirmed with postnatal imaging. Gray-scale and color Doppler imaging should both be utilized. The Society of Fetal Urology (SFU) grading system can be useful to communicate the degree of severity, which ranges from grade 0 (no renal pelvic dilation) to grade 4 (dilation of the renal pelvis and calices with parenchymal thinning). Measurements should be obtained of each kidney and of the transverse renal pelvis. Renal pelvis measurements greater than 15 millimeters are classified as severe hydronephrosis. Color Doppler is helpful in looking for aberrant vessels, which may be the etiology of the UPJ, and in identifying ureteral jets in the bladder. The timing of postnatal imaging depends on the degree of severity seen on the prenatal exam. Infants with severe hydronephrosis detected on prenatal US should have follow-up postnatal US at 48 hours of life to minimize false-negative exams from diminished renal excretion in the newborn. Children with mild to moderate hydronephrosis can be imaged at around 7 days of life. If the US is negative at 7 days of life, follow-up studies should be performed at approximately 6 weeks of age. The primary screening exam for UPJ is US in the older child and it can be performed at any time, preferably when the patient is symptomatic so that the maximal degree of dilation is identified. A voiding cystourethrogram (VCUG) is indicated in children with hydronephrosis to exclude vesicoureteral reflux (VUR) as a cause of collecting system dilation and to evaluate for obstruction at other levels, primarily posterior urethral valves in males. Diuretic renography is used to calculate differential renal function

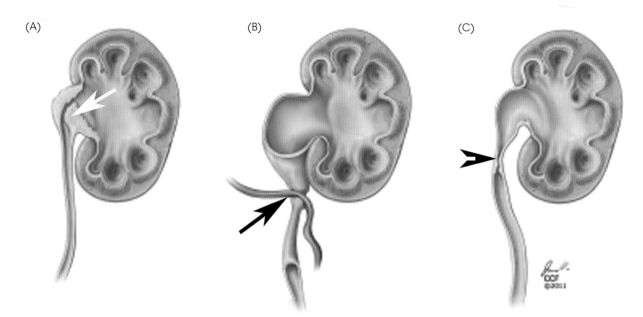

Figure 47.1. Theories of UPJ obstruction. Dilation of the renal pelvis and calices with (A) intrinsic tissue thickening at the junction of the ureteric bud and metanephric blastema (white arrow); (B) crossing vessel (black arrow); and (C) failure of complete canalization of the ureter (arrowhead).

and to evaluate the response to a diuretic. Technetium 99mTc MAG3 (Mercaptoacetyltriglycine) is administered intravenously and renal uptake and excretion are measured. This is followed by an intravenous diuretic agent such as furosemide with additional imaging obtained to measure washout of the radiotracer. A severely obstructed kidney will have both diminished differential activity and a delayed washout. The initial diuretic renogram is usually performed at approximately 6 weeks of life. Relative renal function is not a useful measure in patients with bilateral UPJ or an

otherwise compromised contralateral kidney. MRI can provide both anatomic and functional information. Routine anatomic imaging demonstrates the level of the obstruction. MR is more accurate than US in depiction of extrinsic compression caused by crossing vessels. MR urography (MRU) techniques provide 3-D reconstructed images showing the level of the obstruction and course of the ureters with their insertion into the urinary bladder. MRU is particularly useful in identifying ureteral strictures. Dedicated software is required to calculate differential function.

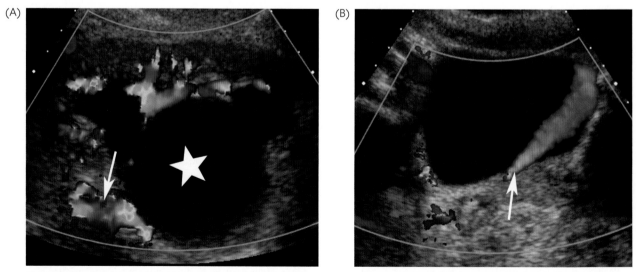

Figure 47.2. Sagittal US of the kidney with color Doppler (A) in a 17-year-old male with back pain after several caffeinated drinks demonstrates high-grade hydronephrosis with dilatation of the renal pelvis and calices (star) caused by a crossing vessel (arrow). Right parasagittal US of the bladder with color Doppler (B) shows a normal ureteral jet (arrow), however no jet could be found on the left suggesting a high-grade obstruction.

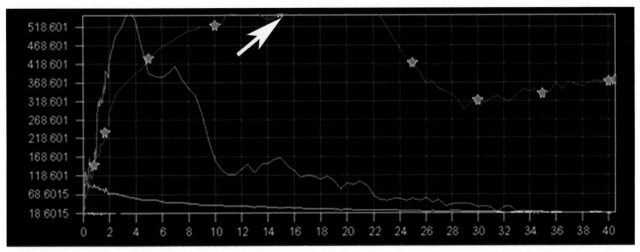

Figure 47.3. Diruretic MAG-3 renogram in UPJ obstruction demonstrates delayed washout at greater than 20 minutes (arrow) and split function of less than 40 percent.

Related Physics

Radiation from nuclear medicine studies such as MAG-3 can be detected using a variety of tools including gas-filled detectors, scintillation detectors, and others. Gas-filled detectors, though not capable of high-quality imaging, are useful for spills and unintended excretion of radioactivity into the environment. The most common gas-filled detector for this application is a Geiger counter, which simply answers the question of presence or absence of radiation. Among imaging devices, scintillation is the most common form of radiation detection. In gamma and SPECT cameras, sodium iodide crystal is used to create scintillation, whereas in PET imaging other crystals include barium fluoride, BGO, LSO and GSO (the actual chemical makeup and their profile are beyond the scope of this discussion). Other than medical imaging, scintillation well counters are used to confirm radioactivity of each prescribed dose prior to administration. Scintillators are also used in some types of contamination scenarios in a nuclear medicine department to determine which isotope has been spilled into the environment. This is done with the assistance of a pulse-height spectrometer.

Clinical Issues

The goal in UPJ management is preservation of renal function. The biggest challenge in UPJ management is deciding if an asymptomatic patient might benefit from surgical treatment and if so, when. Pyeloplasty is indicated for symptomatic patients, those with progression of hydronephrosis, and those with split renal function of less than 40 percent. Surgical options include open dismembered pyeloplasty, laparoscopic pyeloplasty, and robotic pyeloplasty. Identification of adjacent crossing vessels can be helpful in surgical planning. Postoperative patients are evaluated with serial US. If hydronephrosis does not improve, diuretic renography is performed to evaluate for residual or recurrent obstruction. Observation is an appropriate strategy in mild to moderate UPJ as many children will maintain a stable degree of dilation and some may improve over time. Serial US is performed at regular intervals with diuretic renography performed when there is any evidence of increased dilation. Decreasing split renal function or increase in delay in washout are indications for surgical intervention.

Differential Diagnosis

- Vesicoureteral reflux
- Massive urine output without obstruction
- Multicystic dysplastic kidney
- Extrarenal pelvis
- Distal obstruction of urinary tract: ureteral stricture, ureterovesical junction obstruction, bladder outlet obstruction, urethral structure and posterior urethral valves

Common Variants

Common associations include UPJ with pyelonephritis and UPJ with renal calculi.

Key Points

- The goal of UPJ management is to maintain renal function.
- All infants with prenatal hydronephrosis should have postnatal renal US.
- Timing of postnatal US is important to avoid false-negative exams.
- Diuretic renography using nuclear medicine or MR is important to provide a measure of differential renal function and severity of obstruction.
- Look for associated abnormalities in the contralateral kidney such as multicystic dysplastic kidney (MCDK).

Further Reading

Baek M, Park K, Choi H. Long-term outcomes of dismembered pyeloplasty for midline-crossing giant hydronephrosis caused by ureteropelvic junction obstruction in children. *Urology.* 2010.

Calder AD, Hiorns MP, Abhyankar A, Mushtaq I, Olsen OE. Contrast-enhanced magnetic resonance angiography for the detection of crossing renal vessels in children with symptomatic ureteropelvic junction obstruction: comparison with operative findings. *Pediatr Radiol.* 2007;37(4):356–361.

Darge K, Grattan-Smith JD, Riccabona M. Pediatric uroradiology: state of the art. *Pediatr Radiol.* 2011;41(1):82–91.

Karnak I, Woo LL, Shah SN, Sirajuddin A, Ross JH. Results of a practical protocol for management of prenatally detected hydronephrosis due to ureteropelvic junction obstruction. *Pediatr Surg Int.* 2009;25(1):61–67.

Little S, Jones RA, Grattan-Smith JD. Evaluation of UPJ obstruction before and after pyeloplasty using MR urography *Pediatr Radiol.* 2008;38(Suppl 1):106–124.

Mami C, Palmara A, Paolata A, et al. Outcome and management of isolated severe renal pelvis dilatation detected at postnatal screening. *Pediatr Nephrol.* 2010;25(10):2093–2097.

CHAPTER 48

Ureteropelvic Duplications

Caroline Carrico, MD

Definition

The term duplex kidney is applied to a kidney that has two separate renal pelvicalyceal systems in which each pelvis has its own ureter. The two ureters may join prior to inserting into the bladder, or each ureter may terminate separately. It is the separate termination of the ureters at the bladder that leads to potential problems.

Clinical Features

Duplex kidneys are more common in girls than in boys with an incidence of approximately 1 percent. It can be bilateral. The ureter that drains the upper pole moiety inserts ectopically: inferior and medial to the normal lower pole ureter at the bladder trigone. If the upper pole ureter joins with the lower pole ureter prior to bladder insertion, the combined distal ureter typically inserts at the normal location. The upper pole ureter is more likely to have a stenotic ureterovesical junction (UVJ) and obstruct. The dilated distal portion of the upper pole ureter may protrude into the lumen of the bladder as a ureterocele. Ectopic ureteral insertion and ureterocele formation can occur with single-system kidneys as well as with the upper pole of duplex kidneys. The division of the upper and lower poles of the kidney is not always equal. The upper pole ureter usually drains half or less of the total calyces. Duplex kidneys are not inherently pathologic, but their renal tissue, collecting systems and ureters are subject to the same pathology as normal single-system kidneys. Vesicoureteral reflux (VUR) often occurs within the (orthotopic) lower pole ureter. Simultaneous reflux into both ureters occurs when the two ureters join distally and share a common bladder insertion. If the upper pole (ectopic) ureter has a stenotic insertion then there may be compromise of renal function in the upper pole moiety. Multicystic dysplastic kidney may form in utero in an upper pole moiety that has a severely stenotic upper pole UVJ or atretic ureter. Prenatal hydroureteronephrosis may develop secondary to upper pole obstruction or lower pole reflux. Postnatal infection can occur within an obstructed or refluxing portion of the kidney. Duplex kidney may be detected during the workup of a urinary tract infection (UTI).

In girls, if the upper pole ureter inserts so inferior and medial to the normal bladder trigone that it inserts into the urethra, vagina, or onto the perineum there will be constant low-volume incontinence which is not usually noticed during the diaper-wearing years. The very slow but constant drip of urine is produced by what is usually a small upper pole moiety of a duplex kidney with a ureter that inserts into the urethra, vagina, or onto the perineum, usually periurethral. Uncommonly such ectopic insertion is associated with an ectopic and atrophic single-system kidney.

Anatomy and Physiology

There are two theories for multiplication of the renal collecting system. The two may coexist. In one there are multiple ureteric buds; in the other there is early fission of one or more ureteric buds. Duplication, triplication, or even quadruplication of the ureter can occur. The ureter starts to form as a bud from the Wolffian (mesonephric) duct called the metanephric diverticulum. The bud grows posteriorly and cephalad while the leading edge dilates. As it grows, it gathers mesoderm at its slightly dilated leading edge. This mesoderm is called the metanephric mesenchyme and ultimately becomes the renal parenchyma. The dilated end of the metanephric diverticulum becomes the renal collecting system. The more cephalad the origin of a metanephric diverticulum on the Wolffian duct, the more likely this higher bud will terminate ectopically, inside or outside of the bladder. In girls the upper pole ureter may insert into the urethra, vagina, or onto the perineum resulting in constant incontinence. In boys, the ectopic upper pole ureter inserts into the bladder or the urethra but always above the urethral sphincter. The lower pole ureter inserts into the bladder at the normal trigone.

Imaging Findings

Weigert-Meyer Rule (Fig. 48.1): The upper pole ureter inserts into the bladder more caudally and medially than the lower pole ureter. The lower pole ureter usually inserts closest to the normal trigone. The lower pole ureter may reflux; the upper pole UVJ may be obstructed (with or without ureterocele).

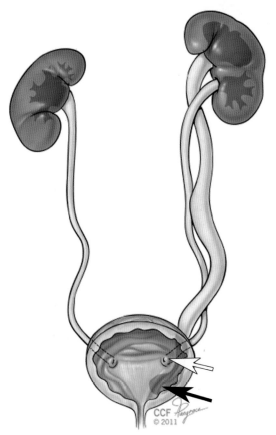

Figure 48.1. Duplication of the collecting systems and ureters. The upper pole ureter (black arrow) inserts ectopically below and medial to the lower pole ureter (white arrow) at the trigone.

US:

- Parenchymal bar separates the renal sinus fat on every longitudinal image if the upper pole moiety is large enough to be separated from the lower by sinus fat (Fig. 48.2).
- Upper pole pelvicalyceal system and ureter are dilated if the ureter is obstructed (Fig. 48.3) or if reflux is occurring into the ureter because it contains a common insertion with the lower pole ureter (Fig. 48.4); the latter may be intermittent.
- Lower pole pelvicalyceal system and ureter may appear normal or be distended from reflux (Fig. 48.5).
- Ureterocele: thin-walled intravesical dilated distal end of a ureter; it resembles a cyst that is contiguous with the wall of the bladder and distal ureter (Fig. 48.6); may be very small or quite large; can be so large as to fill much of the bladder lumen or may prolapse into the urethra or may decrease in size as the bladder volume increases and the urine within them is displaced into the more proximal extravesical ureter.

VCUG:

- Early filling images best reveal ureterocele (Fig. 48.7).

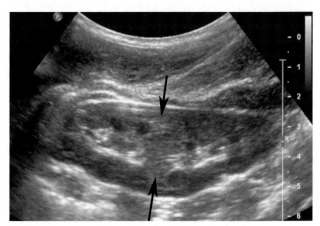

Figure 48.2. Sagittal US image of a duplex kidney shows a parenchymal bar (black arrows) that separates the hyperechoic renal sinus fat. There is no pelvicaliectasis.

- Ureterocele decreases in size and may be completely emptied as the intravesical pressure becomes greater with late filling.
- Urine in the distal intravesical portion of the ureter (ureterocele) is usually pushed back into the extravesical portion of the ureter as the bladder fills; may be completely decompressed with late filling or voiding; may evert into the extravesical ureter and resemble a bladder diverticulum on VCUG.
- Ureterocele can prolapse into the proximal urethra and interrupt voiding resembling a polyp on VCUG.
- Reflux into lower pole appears as "drooping lily" because an incomplete complement of renal calyces has been filled with contrast; location of the middle and lower pole calyces relative to the ureter resembles the flower (Fig. 48.8).

IMAGING PITFALLS

- An unobstructed upper pole moiety may be so small that it is not evident by US; kidney may look like a normal single-system kidney on US; contralateral duplex kidney with intravesical insertion of both ureters common.
- Extremely small (perhaps just one calyx), dysplastic and *unobstructed* upper pole moieties may lack normal concentrating ability and make a relatively large volume of poor-quality urine, which if draining into the urethra, vagina, or onto the perineum is very symptomatic; same physiology makes the tiny unobstructed upper pole difficult to detect on CT and MRU (delayed postcontrast images are often helpful).
- Dilated upper pole ureter may be so large in caliber as it passes through the bladder that it allows eversion of its ureterocele into its own distal ureter when the intravesical pressure becomes greater than the intraureteral pressure (during late filling or voiding) masquerading as a Hutch diverticulum on VCUG ("everting ureterocele").

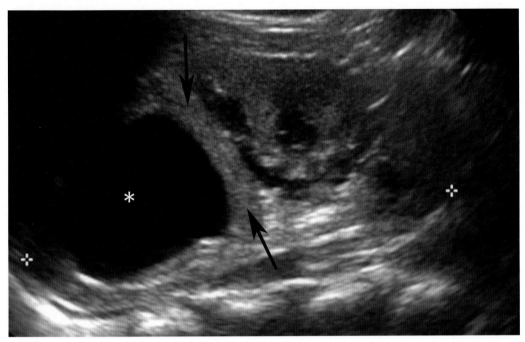

Figure 48.3. Sagittal US image of a duplex kidney with obstructed upper pole ureter shows gross dilation of the upper pole pelvicalyceal system (*). A parenchymal bar separates the upper and lower pole moieties (black arrows).

Imaging Strategy

Ultrasound and VCUG are both indicated, US for renal size, reflux-induced scarring, and signs of obstruction such as hydroureteronephrosis or ureterocele and VCUG to assess for ureterocele and VUR. VCUG is also used

to assess for development of VUR after cystoscopic incision of a ureterocele, after ureteric reimplantation or after a cystoscopic antireflux procedure. The more ectopic the insertion of the upper pole ureter, the more dysplastic the renal tissue that it drains. Renal scintigraphy can determine relative renal function to assist in presurgical planning. In a toilet-trained girl with constant low-volume urinary incontinence, infrasphincteric ectopic ureter is the likely diagnosis. The offending ureter is usually a very tiny upper pole moiety that is not obstructed. As the duplication is most often occult on US, contrast-enhanced MR urogram with

Figure 48.4. Frontal image from a VCUG shows filling of both the lower and the upper pole system (*) as both ureters join above the bladder with VUR into a single orthotopic ureter.

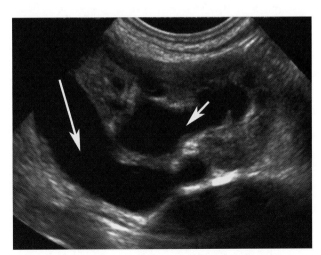

Figure 48.5. Sagittal US image of the kidney in a baby with prenatal hydronephrosis shows a duplex kidney with dilation of both the upper (long arrow) and lower pole (short arrow) pelvicalyceal systems.

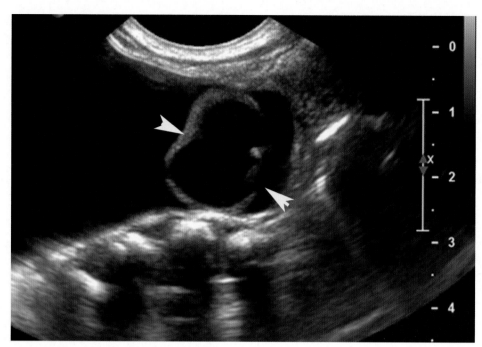

Figure 48.6. Sagittal US image of the bladder in a baby with prenatal hydronephrosis shows the upper pole ureter ends in a ureterocele (arrows).

delayed images may demonstrate function in the tiny upper pole and make the diagnosis. If the upper pole moiety is obstructed, the ureter may be seen to pass below the bladder on ultrasound. T2 MR urography images without contrast may easily show the course and insertion of a partially obstructed and extremely ectopic upper pole ureter.

Related Physics

Magnetic resonance imaging (MRI) has revolutionized imaging of pediatric obstructing renal disorders. The

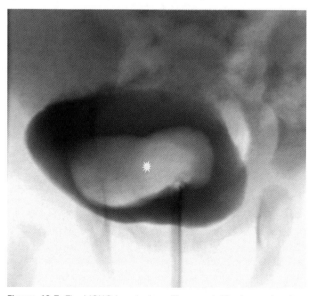

Figure 48.7. The VCUG in a baby with prenatal hydronephrosis shows the ureterocele as a bladder filling defect (*).

primary diagnosis of newborn renal disorders is often made on US and prior to MRI the imaging workup would include VCUG, intravenous pyelogram (IVP), and nuclear medicine MAG-3 studies. Multiple studies were necessary to provide both anatomic information (VCUG and IVP) and functional information (MAG-3); both could not be obtained with a single study. MRI can provide both contrast and temporal information through a technique referred to as MR urography allowing for single-source imaging without ionizing radiation. MRU includes anatomic conventional sequences (FSE T2 and inversion recovery) followed by multiphase dynamic contrast-enhanced sequences (FLASH) using the ultrafast application of radiofrequency pulses that allow for calculation of differential renal function.

Differential Diagnosis

- Crossed-fused ectopia (CREF): ectopic kidney's ureter inserts orthotopically on the contralateral side
- Adrenal hemorrhage: large hemorrhage may exert mass effect on the upper pole of the kidney, altering its shape resembling a dilated obstructed upper pole collecting system of a duplex kidney in which the normal kidney may be thought to represent only the lower pole moiety

Common Variants

The upper pole ureter may insert below the urethral sphincter in girls (infrasphincteric ectopic ureter). The

and the uppermost moiety is usually obstructed; the middle and lower units are prone to VUR. Quadruplication is rare with only 8 reported cases.

Clinical Issues

Upper pole ureterocele incision may result in return of normal function. However, ureterocele incision may convert an obstructed ureter into a refluxing ureter. Ureter excision and excision of associated upper pole tissue may be performed if the upper pole has insufficient function to warrant salvage. In the lower pole moiety VUR is common.

Key Points

- With duplex kidneys the lower pole ureter inserts orthotopically and is prone to reflux.
- The upper pole ureter may join the lower pole ureter at or proximal to the UVJ.
- The upper pole ureter may insert ectopically, inferior and medial to the normal trigone.
- Ureterocele forms from a stenotic insertion of the upper pole ureter at the bladder.
- Infrasphincteric upper pole ureter insertion is more common in girls and causes incontinence.
- Not all duplicated collecting systems are complicated by obstruction or reflux.

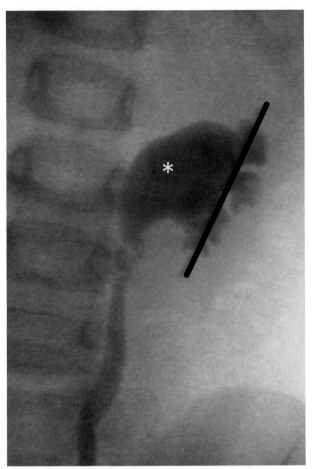

Figure 48.8. Frontal image from a VCUG shows VUR into the lower pole collecting system of a duplex kidney (*) contrast filling the pelvicalyceal system of the lower pole moiety resembles a drooping lily of a single system, however, a line drawn from the lowest to most superior calyx points toward the ipsilateral shoulder (line). If this were a typical single-system kidney with one ureter, the line drawn would usually point slightly to the contralateral side.

girls usually have normal toilet training and normal bladder voiding but are *always* mildly incontinent, with a slow drip of urine, day and night. Triplication of the ureter is uncommon but over 100 cases have been reported. Triplication is reported in girls more than boys, on the left more than the right. One of the ureters may end blindly

Further Reading

Berrocal T, Lopez-Pereira P, Arjonilla A, Gutierrez J. Anomalies of the distal ureter, bladder, and urethra in children: embryologic, radiologic, and pathologic features. *Radiographics.* 2002;*22*:1139–1164.

Carrico C, Lebowitz RL. Incontinence due to an infrasphincteric ectopic ureter: why the delay in diagnosis and what the radiologist can do about it. *Pediatr Radiol.* 1998;*28*:942–949.

Darge K, Grattan-Smith JD, Riccabona M. Pediatric uroradiology: state of the art. *Pediatr Radiol.* 2011;*41*:82–91.

Zerin JM, Baker DR, Casale JA. Single-system ureteroceles in infants and children: imaging features. *Pediatr Radiol.* 2000;*30*(3):139–146.

CHAPTER 49

Renal Ectopia and Fusion

Erjola Balliu, MD and Jeffrey Hellinger, MD, FACC

Definition

Renal ectopia is a congenital urologic abnormality whereby one or both kidneys are positioned outside of the retroperitoneal renal fossa and results from the disruption of normal embryogenesis and ascent of the kidney(s). Renal ectopia may occur with fusion to the contralateral kidney and fusion results in an abnormal number and configuration of renal moieties.

Clinical Features

Congenital renal ectopia and fusion are approximately twice as common in males as females. Horseshoe kidney is most common with an incidence as high as 1 in 400 to 600 births. The incidence of renal ectopia is 1 in 500 to 1,000 births. Crossed renal ectopia with fusion (CREF) occurs in 1 in 2,000 to 7,000 births. The majority of patients with renal ectopia with or without fusion are asymptomatic, however the ectopic kidney(s) may be palpable. Prenatal ultrasound (US) screening may lead to antepartum diagnosis, typically in the second or third trimester. Postnatally, diagnosis is typically made incidentally during imaging performed for other reasons. Uncommonly, patients may have asymptomatic renovascular hypertension detected during routine screening and physical examinations, which leads to diagnostic imaging. In symptomatic patients, presentation is often related to associated congenital anomalies, acquired urologic disorders, and secondary urologic complications. Associated anomalies include ectopic ureters, vesicoureteric reflux (VUR), cryptorchidism, hypospadias, Mayer-Rokitansky-Kuster-Hauser, and ureteropelvic junction obstruction (UPJ). Complications include UTI, renal calculi, ureteric obstruction, hydronephrosis, and mass effect on the pelvic structure including the bladder. Symptoms from complications include fever, abdominal pain, or hematuria.

Anatomy and Physiology

Early embryologic development of the right and left kidneys occurs in three phases: the pronephros, mesonephros, and metanephros. The first two urinary organs are rudimentary structures that normally involute. The metanephros develops into the kidney. Each paired metanephros is first seen by 5 weeks gestation and produces urine by 11 weeks gestation, contributing to the amniotic fluid.

Embryologically, the metanephros develops from a ureteral bud (metanephric diverticulum) and metanephric mesoderm cells (blastema). The ureteral bud (which grows from mesonephric duct at the junction with the cloaca) gives rise to the ipsilateral ureters, renal pelvis, and upper collecting system. As the ureteral bud grows, it extends into the metanephric blastema, triggering the formation of renal tubules, glomeruli, and nephrons. The developing metanephros is initially located in the pelvis with a ventral hilum. The metanephros undergoes relative cephalad migration to the expected retroperitoneal renal fossa as a result of asymmetric growth of the caudad portion of the embryo. As each kidney "ascends," it also rotates 90 degrees such that the renal hilum is directed anteromedially. Migration and rotation are completed by the 8th week of gestation.

Arterial blood supply to the kidneys varies as the developing kidneys ascend from the pelvis to the abdomen. Initially, renal arteries arise from the middle sacral and common iliac arteries. During renal migration, new local arteries arise from the aorta. Inferior branches typically involute, such that the kidney will most commonly have a single renal artery arising from the aorta at the level of its hilum. Renal veins undergo a similar pattern of embryogenesis in relation to the developing iliac and inferior cava venous system. Ectopic kidneys have variable arterial supply and venous drainage depending upon the location of the kidney. There are often numerous arteries and veins related to location and lack of branch involution.

Renal ectopia occurs when there is abnormal migration of a kidney, leading to an abnormal final location of the kidney. Renal ectopia occurs more frequently in the left kidney than the right. The ectopic kidney may be either ipsilateral (e.g., simple ectopia) or contralateral (e.g., crossed ectopia) to the normally positioned ureterovesicular junction (UVJ) and is typically located in the pelvis ("pelvic kidney") or low abdomen (Fig. 49.1A). Rarely, the ectopic kidney may be located superior to the normal renal fossa, in the upper abdomen or thorax. Associated renal malrotation is common, whereby the renal pelvis of the ectopic kidney is directed anteriorly. Crossed ectopia most commonly occurs with fusion to the contralateral kidney; less commonly it occurs without fusion and rarely will it manifest as a solitary crossed ectopic kidney or bilateral renal ectopia (Fig. 49.1B). Left-to-right crossed ectopia occurs with a greater frequency than right-to-left. In all types of

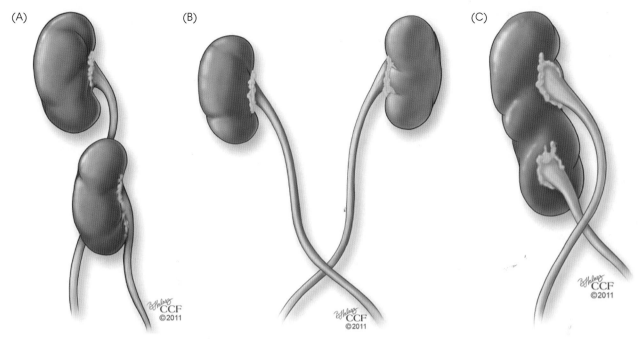

Figure 49.1. Spectrum of anomalies in renal ectopia and fusion. (A) Crossed ectopia without fusion. (B) Bilateral crossed ectopia without fusion. (C) Crossed fused renal ectopia.

renal ectopia, the ectopic kidney may have decreased function and may be hypoplastic. In such cases, the normally located kidney may have increased relative function along with compensatory enlargement.

Renal fusion anomalies arise from abnormal division of the metanephric mesoderm in the pelvis. It is theorized this may be related to malposition of the umbilical arteries. Common ectopic fusion anomalies include horseshoe kidney, cross-fused renal ectopia, and pancake kidney.

In a horseshoe kidney, early in embryogenesis there is abnormal ipsilateral migration and fusion of both kidneys. Fusion most commonly occurs at the lower poles, resulting in bilateral renal moieties connected by an isthmus of functional renal tissue or less likely fibrous tissue. Separate ureters drain ipsilaterally to the bladder. Renal malrotation is always present. Rarely, fusion may occur at the upper poles. The horseshoe kidney is typically located in the low abdomen, with a midline isthmus anterior to the distal abdominal aorta and inferior vena cava. Arterial blood supply and venous drainage are highly variable and branches may arise from the aorta, common or internal iliac arteries, phrenic artery, inferior mesenteric artery, and middle sacral arteries. Horseshoe kidneys have an increased incidence for Wilms tumor and are at increased risk for traumatic injury.

In CREF, the affected kidney and proximal ureter cross midline to the contralateral side (Fig. 49.1C). The ectopic kidney is usually positioned inferior to the normally positioned kidney. The UVJ remains at the original and normal side of the bladder. Fusion typically occurs between the upper pole of the crossed kidney and lower pole of the normally positioned kidney. Depending upon whether rotation has occurred, renal pelvi may either both face anteriorly or

in opposite directions. Less commonly the CREF may lie superior or transverse to the contralateral kidney or have extensive fusion to the contralateral kidney and lie in the pelvis or low abdomen, off midline.

The pancake kidney is the least common renal fusion anomaly. It has features of a horseshoe kidney and a CREF pelvic kidney, in that there is a single completely fused midline pelvic kidney with bilateral ureters that drain to the ipsilateral UVJ Arterial supply is typically from the aorta, iliac arteries, and/or middle sacral artery.

Imaging Findings

Simple ectopia:

- Empty renal fossa
- Pelvic, lower abdominal or thoracic location of the kidney (Fig. 49.2)
- Ipsilateral ureter insertion

Crossed-fused ectopia:

- Each ureter inserts at its native normal UVJ (Fig. 49.3)
- Upper pole of CREF is fused to the lower pole of the normal kidney (Fig. 49.4)

Horseshoe kidney:

- Upper or lower poles fused at the midline (Fig. 49.5)
- Each ureter inserts at the ipsilateral bladder trigone

Imaging Strategies

Ultrasound is the first-line modality to define anatomy postnatally and when new urologic signs are present in a newborn. If further evaluation is needed, dynamic MRU

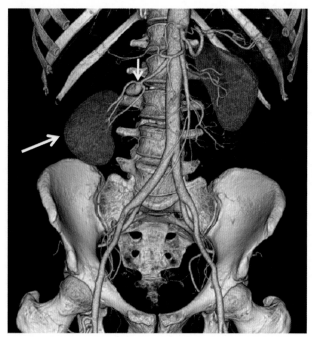

Figure 49.2. Volume-rendered coronal image from CTA in a 15-year-old asymptomatic female with renovascular hypertension demonstrates an ectopic, low-lying abdominal right kidney without fusion (large arrow) centered at L3–4. The left kidney lies in the expected renal fossa. The right renal artery is patent, however there is a small aneurysm (small arrow) centered at the hilar bifurcation of the right renal artery.

with arterial, venous, nephrographic, and urographic phases will best assess morphology and function and has largely replaced intravenous urography (IVU). Voiding cystourethrogram (VCUG) is usually performed for presumed solitary kidney, a history of febrile urinary tract infection/suspected pyelonephritis or hydroureteronephrosis. Radionucleotide imaging can also be performed to assess renal function and possible obstruction.

Related Physics

In order to accurately evaluate the renal parenchyma and vascularity in the newborn, the US transducer must support high-resolution B-mode, spectral and power Doppler. Despite the small size of the abdomen, the flank provides a sufficient acoustic window to support the larger face of the standard linear transducer that in turn is large enough to accommodate the complete length of the kidney. Parameters that must be individualized for accurate Doppler assessment include scale, baseline, pulse repetition frequency, wall filter, and transmit gain. Adjustment of scale sets the peak velocity; a scale that is too low will result in "aliasing" which is the misregistration of velocities below baseline (depicted as color in the high range above normal). Baseline is set to accommodate expected waveform; where there is bidirectional flow one would set baseline in the middle of the screen to show both above (positive) and below (negative) velocities and for higher positive velocities, the baseline should be positioned as low

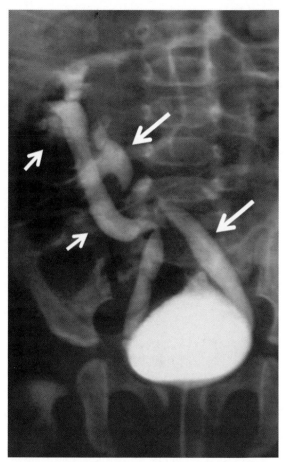

Figure 49.3. Frontal image from VCUG in a child with CREF demonstrates bilateral VUR into ureters draining the superiorly located right kidney (small arrows) and the inferiorly positioned crossed fused ectopic (native left) kidney (longer arrows). Note that the ureters maintain their native insertion into the urinary bladder.

as possible on the screen. Pulse repetition frequency (PRF) is automatically set on the color image once the B-mode image captures the region of interest in the field of view. Wall filter is adjusted to create a color image that optimizes color flow throughout the vessel without "bleeding" outside the vessel. Transmit gain must be balanced with receiver gain to minimize useless signal (noise) with useful signal (true flow).

Differential Diagnosis

- Unilateral renal agenesis with compensatory hypertrophy of the unilateral kidney
- Solitary duplex kidney (may mimic CREF except both ureters insert ipsilaterally; Fig. 49.4)

Common Variants

Once renal ectopia (with or without fusion) is identified one should look for associated congenital anomalies, secondary acquired disorders, and anatomic features that may suggest a syndrome. Renal ectopia can be seen with contralateral

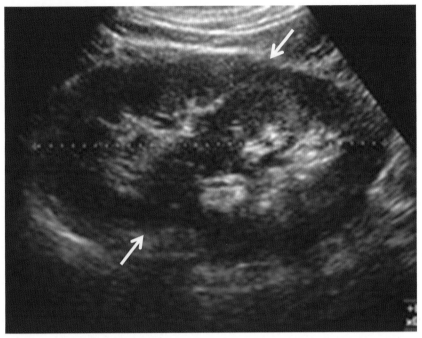

Figure 49.4. Sagittal US image in a child with CREF demonstrates symmetric fusion (arrows) of the kidneys simulating the appearance of a unilateral duplex kidney with contralateral renal agenesis.

renal dysplasia or agenesis, Müllerian agenesis, cardio-vascular, gastrointestinal, adrenal or skeletal anomalies, VACTERL or CHARGE syndromes. Horseshoe kidneys are associated with GU, cardiovascular, GI, and CNS anomalies, Trisomy 13, 18 and 21, and Turner syndrome. Renal ectopia also has a reported increased incidence of Wilms tumor in childhood. Congenital renal ectopia and fusion is associated with cardiovascular anomalies, imperforate anus, sacral agenesis and scoliosis.

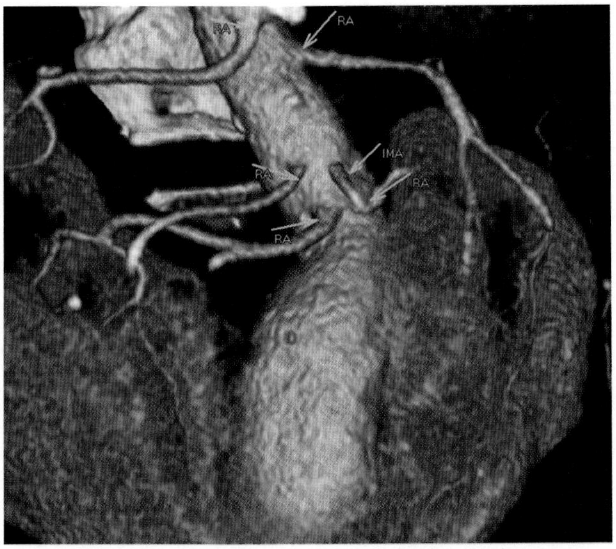

Clinical Issues

Prognosis is excellent in most cases without need for therapeutic intervention. The presence of associated anomalies and secondary urologic complications most often determines medical, interventional, or surgical management in childhood. As there are multiple renal arteries and veins supplying ectopic kidneys, CT angiography is useful in older patients with renal ectopia for investigation of hypertension or prior to repair of abdominal aortic aneurysm.

Figure 49.5. Coronal volume-rendered image from CT angiogram in an adolescent with systemic vasculopathy, demonstrates a horseshoe kidney with a midline parenchymal isthmus (arrow) connecting the bilateral lower poles. Note the three right and two left renal arteries (RA) and the inferior mesenteric artery (IMA).

Key Points

- Renal ectopia results from the disruption of normal renal embryogenesis and migration.
- Most patients are asymptomatic and diagnosed incidentally.
- Associated GU and non-GU anomalies and secondary complications impact clinical presentation and management.
- US is most commonly the first-line diagnostic imaging modality for symptomatic patients, followed by MRU and CTU.
- IVU, VCUG and nuclear medicine imaging are used on a select basis.
- Ectopic kidneys have multiple renal arteries and veins originating from regional visceral or aortoiliac branches.

Further Reading

Glodny B, Petersen J, Hofmann KJ, Schenk C, Herwig R, Trieb T, Koppelstaetter C, Steingruber I, Rehder P. Kidney fusion anomalies revisited: clinical and radiological analysis of 209 cases of crossed fused ectopia and horseshoe kidney. 2009;*103*(2):224–235. Epub 2008 Aug 14.

Guarino N, Tadini, B Camardi P, et al. The incidence of associated urological abnormalities in children with renal ectopia. *J Urol.* 2004;*172*:1757.

Koff SA, Mutabagani KH. Anomalies of the kidney. In: Gillenwater JY, Grayhack JT, Howards SS, Mitchell ME, eds. *Adult and Pediatric Urology.* Third edition. Philadelphia, PA: Lippincott Williams and Wilkins; 2002, 2129.

Moore KL. The urogenital system. In: *The Developing Human: Clinically Oriented Embryology.* Eighth edition. Philadelphia, PA: WB Saunders Company; 2008, pp. 244–260.

Van den Bosch CM, van Wijk JA, Beckers GM, et al. Urological and nephrological findings of renal ectopia. *J Urol.* 2010;*183*:1574.

CHAPTER 50

Posterior Urethral Valves

Loren Murphy, MD, J.C. Hellinger, MD, and Monica Epelman, MD

Definition

Posterior urethral valves (PUVs) are congenital obstructing posterior urethral membranes located at the distal aspect of the prostatic urethra and composed of connective tissue with some smooth muscle lined by stratified squamous epithelium. The precise etiology of valve formation is not known but it is theorized that the normal plicae colliculi may abnormally fuse anteriorly creating the obstructing valves; alternate theory is that they are a cloacal membrane remnant.

Clinical Features

The widespread use of prenatal ultrasound has enabled the prenatal diagnosis of PUVs, usually established during the second or third trimester. Outlet obstruction leads to decreased amniotic fluid production by the fetal kidneys and the resultant oligohydramnios decreases the space necessary for normal fetal development. Pulmonary hypoplasia and fetal structural deformities result in a constellation of findings known as Potter's syndrome. Physical findings may include flattened facies and epicanthal folds, hypertelorism, low-set ears, and micrognathia and limb deformities. Infants may present with respiratory distress with or without a pneumothorax at birth, weak urine stream, poor renal function and incomplete bladder emptying. The abdomen may be enlarged secondary to a distended urinary bladder or uriniferous ascites. Infants or older children may also present with urinary tract infection, voiding dysfunction, renal failure, urosepsis, failure to thrive, poor urinary stream or straining, shock, electrolyte imbalance (including life-threatening hyperkalemia) and hypertension.

Anatomy and Physiology

The exact pathogenesis of PUV is unknown, however, it is hypothesized that PUV may be caused by abnormal insertion of the Wolffian (mesonephric) duct into the fetal cloaca. The classification of PUV into type I, II, and III proposed by Young et al. in 1919 remains the most accepted classification, however some argue there is only one type of PUV. Type I valves account for 95 percent of the cases and originate distal to the veromontanum on the floor of the posterior urethra and fuse anterolaterally along the wall of the urethra while maintaining urethral patency posteroinferiorly in the prostatic urethra (Fig. 50.1). The thickness of the valves as well as the degree of obstruction is variable. The existence of Young Type II and III valves is debatable" and will not be discussed further. Valves occur in the prostatic urethra, proximal to the external urethral sphincter. In all types, renal and bladder function may be impaired by the longstanding and often high-grade obstruction caused by the valves in utero. However, some authors recently postulate that in addition to renal damage from outlet obstruction there may be a primary renal dysplasia contributing to later renal failure. In these patients there may be abnormal budding of the ureter from the Wolffian duct with resultant abnormal induction of mesenchyme akin to the mechanism in multicystic dysplastic kidney. Obstructive uropathy results from persistent high pressures; it is potentially reversible with early release of the obstruction or bladder decompression. Renal dysplasia is irreversible and ultimately will limit long-term renal function, with the risk for end-stage renal disease.

Imaging Findings

Prenatal/postnatal US or fetal MRI:

- Oligohydramnios
- Dilated, keyhole appearance of the posterior urethra (Fig. 50.2)
- Variable degrees of bladder dilation (Fig. 50.3)
- Bladder wall thickening and diverticula
- Pelvicaliectasis, ureterectasis
- Renal dysplasia: poor corticomedullary differentiation, increased echogenicity of the parenchyma with or without renal cysts (Fig. 50.4)
- Perinephric urinoma or uriniferous ascites from forniceal or bladder rupture, respectively, in the fetus may function as a protective mechanism for the developing kidneys by lowering the urinary tract pressures

Voiding cystourethrogram (VCUG):

- Abrupt caliber change between the posterior and anterior urethra, with a dilated posterior urethra and a relatively small bulbar and penile urethra; valves leaflets are usually but not necessarily seen (Fig. 50.5)

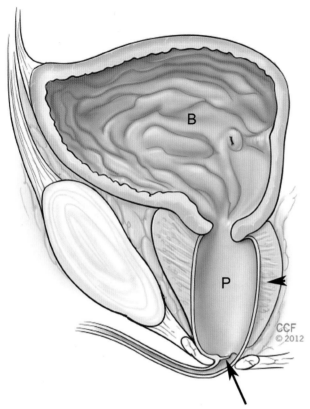

Figure 50.1. Anatomy of posterior urethral valves.
Verumontanum (arrowhead), valves (arrow), dilated posterior urethra (P), thickened bladder wall (B).

- Hypertrophic bladder neck (lucent ring)
- Thickened bladder wall with trabeculations
- Bladder diverticula
- Unilateral or bilateral vesicoureteric reflux

Imaging Strategy

A child suspected of having PUV should have a postnatal renal and bladder US. This will evaluate the degree of hydroureteronephrosis, the renal parenchyma for the presence of dysplastic changes and the thickness of the urinary bladder. Voiding cystourethrogram (VCUG) is performed to confirm the diagnosis. The images of the urethra must be obtained after removal of the catheter from the urethra and during a period of high urine flow in order to avoid a false-negative exam. Ultimately, cystourethroscopy is performed for direct endoluminal visualization of the valves and valve ablation. After valve ablation serial renal US and VCUG may be needed to assess renal growth and vesicoureteric reflux, respectively.

Related Physics

Fluoroscopy for PUV requires minimization of dose and study time in order to reduce radiation exposure to the testes. This mandates attention to imaging geometry. On

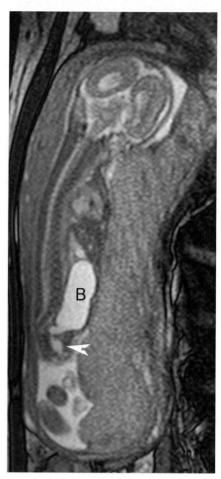

Figure 50.2. Sagittal T2 HASTE MR image in a fetus shows a significantly distended bladder (B) with a "keyhole" appearance of the dilated posterior urethra (arrowhead) with near-complete absence of amniotic fluid consistent with PUV.

a standard fluoroscopy machine, the X-ray tube lies below the imaging table at a fixed distance. The device is set up in "automatic brightness control mode" (ABC) which adjusts kVp and mAs to optimize dose at the image receptor. The image receptor is above the table and patient; if the image

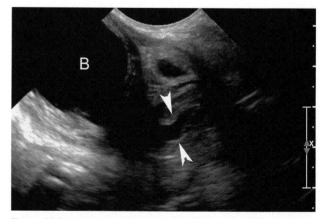

Figure 50.3. Postnatal sagittal US image of the bladder (B) angling the transducer toward the bladder neck in a newborn with PUV shows a dilated posterior urethra (arrowheads).

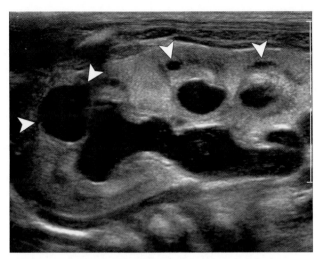

Figure 50.4. Postnatal sagittal prone US image in a newborn with PUV shows moderate to severe pelvicaliectasis and several parenchymal cysts (arrowheads) consistent with renal dysplasia.

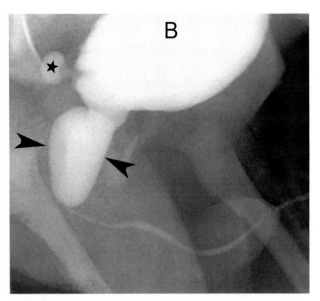

Figure 50.5. A VCUG image during early voiding after removal of the bladder catheter in a newborn with PUV shows a distended urinary bladder (B) with a small periureteral bladder diverticulum (star) without vesicoureteric reflux. There is marked dilation of the prostatic urethra (arrowheads) caused by the obstructing PUV. The urethra maintains patency posteriorly and there is significant narrowing of the anterior urethral caliber distal to the obstructing valves.

receptor is not in near contact with the patient the ABC will signal the generator to increase radiation output. In order to minimize radiation exposure it is imperative that the receptor be brought down to almost lie in contact with the patient. For the purpose of discussion the X-ray focal spot is defined as the "source" and in fixed-base fluoroscopy units resides 18 inches below the table. In C-arm units the distance could be less, which would significantly increase patient exposure. The patient is the "object" and the image receptor is the "image." For quality low-dose imaging, the source-to-object distance (SOD) should be maximized, and the source-to-image receptor distance (SID) should be minimized. The object-to-image receptor distance (OID) should also be minimized. Next, the radiation delivery must be switched from continuous exposure to pulsed radiation delivery, which is traditionally set in frames per second. In many cases frame rates as low as 3.25 to 7.5 frames per second can be used. Pulsed fluoroscopy can reduce exposures by a factor of at least 2 relative to continuous.

Differential Diagnosis

- Anterior urethral valves
- Anterior urethral diverticulum
- Post-traumatic or postoperative urethral stricture
- Prostatic hypoplasia with prune belly syndrome results in a large-caliber posterior urethra without obstruction (but may coexist with obstructing valves)
- Congenital megaurethra

Common Variants

Although a different entity, anterior urethral valves (AUVs) with or without anterior urethral diverticulum (AUD) are

part of the differential diagnosis of PUV. Both AUV and AUD are uncommon entities of unclear etiology. Some authors consider AUV and AUD to be two separate entities, although others believe these reflect a continuum of the same pathology. Causative theories include defective merging of the glandular and penile urethra, incomplete form of urethral duplication, faulty development of the corpus spongiosum, and congenital cystic dilation and rupture of the periurethral glands. Anterior urethral valves (AUV) consist of mucosal folds, which ascend and flatten against the urethral roof during voiding resulting in urethral obstruction. Unlike PUVs, AUVs involve the anterior urethra and are commonly found at the bulbar urethra, followed by the penoscrotal junction and the penile urethra. Clinical presentation is quite variable and may remain elusive. The VCUG shows dilation of the urethra proximal to the valves, while the urethra distal to the valves appears narrowed. The VCUG is also useful to exclude VUR which coexists in as many as 30 percent.

Clinical Issues

A PUV can be an isolated pathology or can be associated with additional urinary tract and extra-urinary pathologies. Thirty to fifty percent of patients with PUV will have secondary VUR; VUR results from increased bladder pressure (resulting from the outlet obstruction) and subsequent improper closing of the ureterovesical junction. Renal dysplasia is present in up to 60 percent of patients with prenatally diagnosed PUV; renal dysplasia will ultimately lead to chronic kidney disease (CKD). Approximately 10 to 15 percent of patients with CKD will develop end-stage renal disease. Associated extra-urinary anomalies include cryptorchidism, inguinal hernias, patent ductus arteriosus, mitral stenosis, imperforate anus, and scoliosis. Common therapeutic measures utilized in utero to relieve and/or prevent the deleterious effects of lower urinary tract obstruction (LUTO) include percutaneous vesicoamniotic shunting and in utero percutaneous cystoscopy. Percutaneous vesicoamniotic shunting, the most frequently used technique, entails the placement of a double pigtail catheter under US guidance, with one loop placed in the fetal bladder and the other loop in the amniotic cavity, facilitating drainage of fetal urine. These fetal interventions are believed to decrease perinatal mortality, however, long-term renal morbidity remains problematic. Postnatally, patients with PUV may have severe electrolyte abnormalities, requiring close serial monitoring. The serum creatinine concentration after birth reflects the maternal creatinine concentration; it often takes a few days to allow maternal influence to dissipate. In patients with severe obstruction, the bladder must be drained until definitive surgical intervention can take place. The surgical intervention of choice is cystoscopy with primary ablation of the valves. Intervention is limited by the size of the patient's urethral meatus in relation to the size of the cystoscope. After the procedure, the patient's renal and bladder function must be closely monitored. Renal damage resulting from PUV is responsible for the vast majority of end-stage renal disease in boys less than 4 years of age and renal transplantation necessary in boys less than 5 years of age.

Key Points

- Congenital condition exclusive to males
- Lower urinary tract obstruction
- Most cases are diagnosed in-utero with pre-natal US:
  - Oligohydramnios
  - Hydronephrosis
  - Bladder and posterior urethra dilation
- VCUG with urethral imaging is considered the diagnostic reference standard
- Following surgical intervention, continued monitoring for CKD is required

Further Reading

Ballek N, McKenna P. Lower urinary tract dysfunction in childhood. *Urol Clin N Am.* 2010;37:215–228.

Bernardes LS, Aksnes G, Saada J, et al. Keyhole sign: how specific is it for the diagnosis of posterior urethral valves? *Ultrasound in Obstetrics and Gynecology.* 2009;34:419–423.

Farhat W, McLorie G, Capolicchio G, Khoury A, Ba Gli D, Merguerian P. Outcomes of primary valve ablation versus urinary tract diversion in patients with posterior urethral valves. *Urology.* 2000;56(4):653–657.

Haeckel FM, Wehrmann M, Hacker Hw, Stuhldreier G, von Schweinitz D. Renal dysplasia in children with posterior urethral valves: a primary or secondary malformation? *Pediatr Surg Int.* 2002;18(2–3):119–122.

Krishnan A, de Souza A, Konijeti R, Baskin LS. The anatomy and embryology of posterior urethral valves. *J Urol.* 2006;175(4):1214–1220.

Wein AJ. Posterior Urethral Valves and Other Urethral Anomalies. In: *Campbell-Walsh Urology Ninth Edition Review.* Philadelphia, PA: Saunders/Elsevier; 2007.

CHAPTER 51

Urachal Abnormalities

Kamaldine Oudjhane, MD, MSc

Definition

Urachal abnormalities are caused by the persistence of part or all of the fetal allantois, a connection from the bladder dome to the umbilicus, as well as persistence of a portion of the ventral cloaca that contributes to formation of the urinary bladder.

Clinical Features

Subtypes of urachal remnants include: patent urachus, urachal cyst, umbilico-urachal sinus and vesico-urachal diverticulum (Fig. 51.1). They are more often encountered in males than in females, with a ratio of 2:1, however, in general urachal anomalies are uncommon. The clinical presentation varies with and reflects the location and patency of the residual urachal segment. In some neonates there may be retraction of the umbilicus during voiding; in others the abnormality resembles an umbilical hernia. Fluid may drain from the umbilical stump. Infection is the most frequent complication; development of malignancy is uncommon. A patent urachus (approximately 50 percent) is characterized by urine draining from the umbilicus, episodes of urinary tract infection (UTI), and recurrence of periumbilical inflammation. The patent urachus is associated with bladder outlet obstruction in up to 14 percent of affected infants where it acts as a pressure relief valve. Infection and inflammation often develop and may cause intermittent obstruction at one or the other of the patent urachus. This is termed an "alternating sinus." A urachal cyst (30 percent) is usually discovered incidentally or later in childhood and presents as a suprapubic mass with or without abdominal pain, fever, or dysuria. A urachal sinus (15 percent) can be suspected prenatally through identification of an edematous umbilical cord. After birth, wet umbilicus, nonhealing granulation tissue at the umbilical base or periumbilical tendern ess is typical. Patients with a urachal diverticulum (5 percent) are often asymptomatic. Relative stasis in the diverticulum will promote stone formation or infection and the diverticulum may be discovered during imaging assessment of UTI.

Anatomy and Embryology

The urachus derives from two embryonic structures: the ventral cloaca (precursor of the fetal bladder) and the allantois (the caudal end of the yolk sac). This vestigial remnant normally involutes before birth, leaving a fibrous cord termed the "median umbilical ligament" that extends in the midline from bladder to umbilicus between transverse fascia and the parietal peritoneum. If the fetal urachus merges with one of the obliterated umbilical arteries then any urachal remnant would deviate from midline to the side of the involved obliterated umbilical artery. Thus not all urachal remnants are midline.

Imaging Findings

- Urachal remnant: elliptical hypoechoic cystic structure in the midline very close to the anterior superior surface of the bladder between the bladder and umbilicus (Fig. 51.2)
- Urachal cyst: hypoechoic structure along the midline with well-defined wall
- Infected urachal cyst: may contain debris, thick hyperemic wall, +/− mural calcifications
- Urachal sinus: thickened tubular structure extending from the umbilicus toward the bladder, incompletely patent at the bladder
- Urachal diverticulum: best depicted on US or cystography with a full bladder, contiguous with the bladder dome, extending toward the umbilicus
- Pyourachus (US): hypoechoic necrotic material surrounded by severely thickened and hyperemic wall (Fig. 51.3A) best illustrated on color Doppler US (Fig. 51.3B)
- Pyourachus (CT): cone-shaped palpated suprapubic mass extending from umbilicus to bladder dome, with the largest end at bladder dome, increased wall thickness (Fig. 51.4) and subcutaneous inflammatory changes
- Voiding cystourethrography(VCUG): patent urachus identified with full bladder as an open channel from the bladder
- Urachal neoplasm (adenocarcinoma): mixed cystic and solid mass with mural nodularity, most have calcifications, lack of adjacent inflammation, but possible presence of perilesional spiculations that extend into the perivesical fat; bladder is often invaded and there may be pelvic lymphadenopathy; distant metastatic disease may be present at diagnosis to liver, lung, brain, ovaries, bones, and omentum

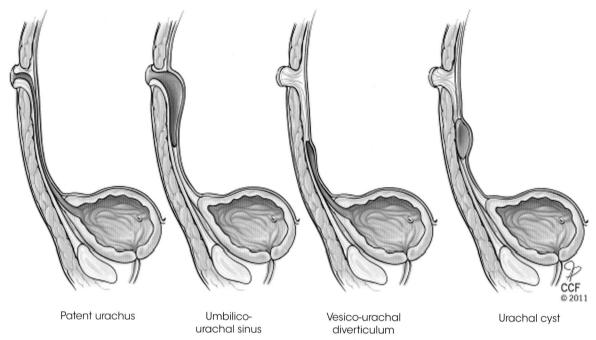

Patent urachus   Umbilico-   Vesico-urachal   Urachal cyst
                        urachal sinus   diverticulum

Figure 51.1. Spectrum of urachal anomalies.

Imaging Strategies

The best and often the only imaging exam needed for assessment of possible urachal abnormalities is US. VCUG may demonstrate patency of the urachus or help differentiate urachal cyst from urachal diverticulum if the US findings are not conclusive. Preoperative VCUG may underestimate the length of the urachal remnant as inflammatory changes may intermittently obstruct the lumen. Additionally, VCUG is extremely useful to rule out coexisting causes of bladder outlet obstruction such as posterior urethral valves, urethral stricture, or obstructed urogenital sinus malformation. Fistulography may help outline the depth of urachal sinus

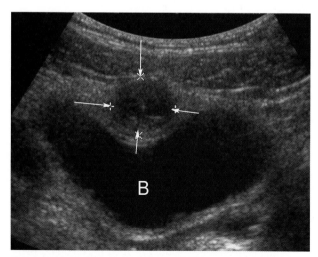

Figure 51.2. Transverse US of the bladder in an infant with vomiting shows a round structure with heterogeneous internal echotexture (arrows) with mass effect on the anterosuperior surface of the bladder (B) consistent with a urachal cyst.

but is rarely needed. CT may be indicated to further assess a complex mass seen on US and help differentiate infection from malignancy by looking for secondary signs or response to antibiotic therapy and/or percutaneous aspiration.

Related Physics

Ultrasound is uniquely suited to pediatric urologic imaging as the urinary bladder serves as a large anechoic acoustic window. The urachal remnant lies at the dome of the bladder and on US is seen as a hypoechoic mass adjacent to the backdrop of an anechoic fluid-filled bladder, thereby maximizing lesion contrast. The level of echogenicity of a lesion is relative to the number of "scatterers" within a unit volume of the lesion. When the scatterers are much smaller than the wavelength, this is known as Raleigh scattering and is ~ fourth power of the frequency. Speckles in the US image appear on a gradient from white to black and changes within an image where smaller speckles are seen nearer to the transducer or at shallower depths. This is because higher-frequency or shorter wavelengths are present at the shallower depths but are attenuated at greater depths leaving only the lower frequencies (longer wavelengths) that form larger speckle patterns. The strength of the echo is coded in the brightness of each speckle and in turn is dictated by the amount of constructive and destructive wave interference.

Differential Diagnosis

- Omphalitis (umbilical stump infection)
- Granulation tissue of the umbilical stump
- Omphalomesenteric duct patent tract, sinus or cyst

(A)

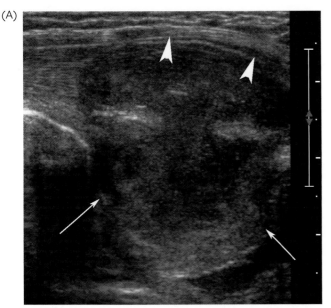

(B)

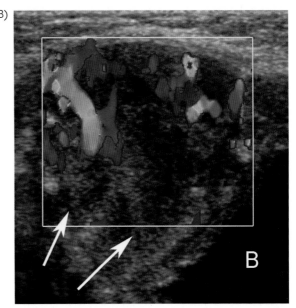

Figure 51.3. Sagittal US of the lower abdomen (A) in an 8-week-old female infant with 2-week history of vomiting and a palpable suprapubic mass shows a complex mass in the space of Retzius (arrows) displacing the rectus muscles (arrowheads) anteriorly. Transverse US with color Doppler (B) shows extensive hyperemia of a thick-walled structure (arrows) that is contiguous with the urinary bladder (B) with displacement of the bladder to the left consistent with infectious complication of urachal remnant.

- Umbilical cord hemangioma
- Bladder neoplasm
- Lipoma in the space of Retzius

Common Variants

Off-midline location of the remnant results from fusion of the urachus with one umbilical artery remnant.

Clinical Issues

The clinical presentation is variable. In the neonate, a patent urachus usually manifests as a variable amount of

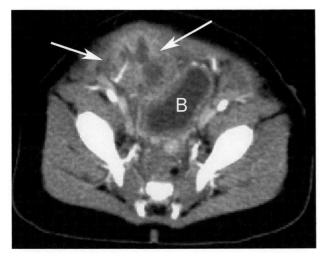

Figure 51.4. Axial contrast-enhanced CT image in a child with fever and abdominal pain depicts a mass (arrows) extending to the right of midline between the bladder (B) and the anterior abdominal wall musculature with a necrotic center surrounded by a thick enhancing wall consistent with pyourachus.

intermittent urine discharge through the umbilicus. The other types of urachal abnormalities are brought to medical attention through infection: fever, lower abdominal pain and tenderness, voiding symptoms, palpable suprapubic mass, and UTI. Hematuria is a rare presentation of urachal cyst and may be a sign of infection or malignancy. Perforation into the peritoneum with subsequent development of peritonitis, abscess or fistulization to bowel is rare.

Malignant neoplasms occur after the fourth decade, mostly in men (75 percent); however malignancy within an urachal remnant has been reported in persons as young as 15 years of age. Hematuria with pelvic pain and dysuria are the most common symptoms reported with malignant degeneration. Other less common symptoms include suprapubic pain with voiding, painful pelvic mass, dyspareunia, low back pain, and mucinuria. Complete surgical excision of the urachal remnant with a cuff of bladder is the treatment of choice; this prevents recurrence of infections and the risk of malignancy.

Key Points

- Urachal anomalies are secondary to failure of involution of the urachus; they include urachal sinus, cyst, diverticulum, and fistula.
- Preferred imaging modality is US.
- Pyourachus may simulate the US appearances of adenocarcinoma.
- CT may assist with the differential diagnosis.
- Antibiotic therapy usually clears the infection but often surgical resection of the entire urachus tract and a cuff of the bladder is needed for definitive therapy.

Further Reading

Cappele O, Sibert L, Descargues J, Delmas V, Grise P. A study of the anatomic features of the duct of urachus. *Surg Radiol Anat.* 2001; *23*:229–235.

Little DC, Shah SR, St. Peter SD, Calkins CM, Murphy JP, Gatti JM, Gittes GK, Sharp RJ, Andrews WS, Holcomb GW 3rd, Ostlie DJ, Snyder CL. Urachal anomalies in children: the vanishing relevance of the preoperative voiding cystourethrogram. *J Pediatr Surg.* 2005;*40*(12):1874–1876.

McCollum MO, MacNeily AE, Blair GK. Surgical implications of urachal remnants: presentation and management. *J Pediatr Surg.* 2003;*38*(5):798–803.

Yu JS, Kim KW, Lee HJ, Lee YJ, Yoon CS, Kim MJ. Urachal remnant diseases: spectrum of CT and US findings. *Radiographics.* 2001;*21*(2):451–461.

CHAPTER 52

Multicystic Dysplastic Kidney

Lynn Ansley Fordham, MD

Definition

Multicystic dysplastic kidney (MCDK) is a renal dysplasia resulting in a collection of cysts with connective tissue without any functioning renal tissue.

Clinical Features

Increasingly, MCDK is being diagnosed on prenatal ultrasound. The incidence is approximately 1 in 4,000 live births. It can be an isolated finding but is also associated with contralateral renal anomalies such as ureteropelvic junction obstruction, vesicoureteric reflux, renal agenesis, or anomalous renal position. Also, MCDK can be associated with posterior urethral valves or prune belly syndrome. The entire kidney is usually involved although segmental disease is also described. Bilateral MCDK is reported and is not currently compatible with life. The risk of malignant transformation into Wilms tumor is low and highly curable. Multicystic dysplastic kidney is expected to regress with the kidney becoming progressively smaller over time. Nephrectomy is indicated for hypertension.

Anatomy and Physiology

The etiology of MCDK is unknown. The most accepted theory is a failure of ureteral bud contact with the metanephric mesenchyme that leads to obstruction and secondary dysplastic changes (Fig. 52.1). Other proposed etiologies include genetic anomalies, teratogens, and intrauterine infection. The end result is a disorganization of the renal parenchyma with noncommunicating cysts surrounded by fibromuscular connective tissue.

Imaging Findings

- Multiple anechoic cysts of varying size (Fig. 52.2A)
- DMSA confirms lack of renal function on the affected side (Fig. 52.2B)
- Echogenic tissue between the cysts (Fig. 52.3)
- Can be associated with contralateral renal anomalies
- Postnatal compensatory hypertrophy of contralateral kidney
- Should regress over time (Fig. 52.4)

IMAGING PITFALLS: It is important not to miss contralateral UPJ obstruction or vesicoureteric reflux. Progressive regression should be documented on follow-up ultrasound exams.

Imaging Strategy

The primary tool for imaging children with MCDK is renal ultrasound (US). Follow-up US is recommended to confirm regression of the dysplastic kidney and to evaluate the contralateral kidney for compensatory hypertrophy, signs of obstruction or scarring caused by vesicoureteric reflux.

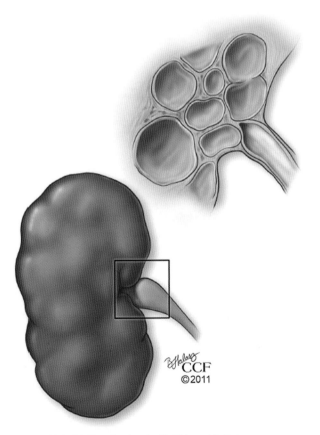

Figure 52.1. Multicystic dysplastic kidney. Multiple noncommunicating cysts replace the renal parenchyma. One theory describes failure of contact between the ureteric bud and metanephric mesenchyme as a cause (inset).

(A)

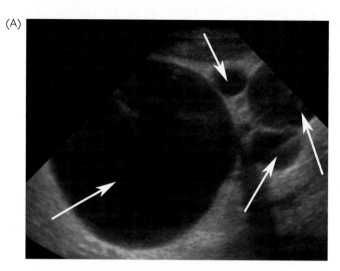

(B)

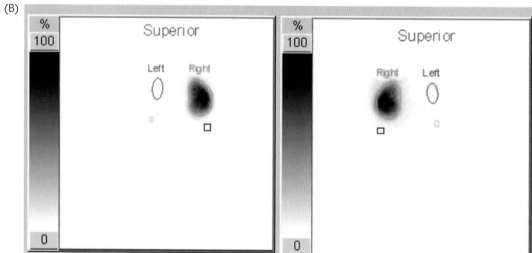

Figure 52.2. Sagittal US image (A) in a 1-day-old infant with prenatal diagnosis of hydronephrosis shows cysts of different sizes (arrows) which completely replace the normal renal parenchyma. There is no normal renal parenchyma. The DMSA (B) confirms lack of renal function on the left, with normal function on the right.

At the time of initial diagnosis VCUG should be performed to evaluate for vesicoureteric reflux. Nuclear medicine DMSA study should also be performed at the time of diagnosis to confirm lack of renal parenchyma and function in the affected kidney. Nuclear medicine MAG-3 diuretic renogram may be utilized to evaluate for renal obstruction in MCDK if there is an identifiable renal pelvis. MRI and MR urography may also be appropriate alternatives in the evaluation in centers that can perform these studies on children.

Related Physics

In order to accurately evaluate the renal parenchyma and vascularity in a fetus, the US transducer must support high-resolution B-mode, spectral and power Doppler. With B-mode imaging one may increase image signal by either increasing the transmit power or the receiver gain. Transmit power must be balanced with receiver gain to minimize useless signal (noise) while respecting that by

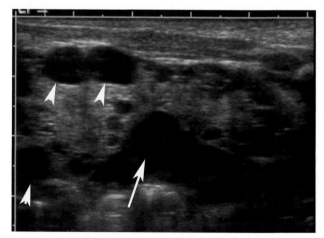

Figure 52.3. Sagittal US image in a newborn with imperforate anus and MCDK shows a dilated renal pelvis which could be mistaken for hydronephrosis (arrow). The renal cysts (arrowheads) vary in size and are separated by echogenic connective tissue.

(A)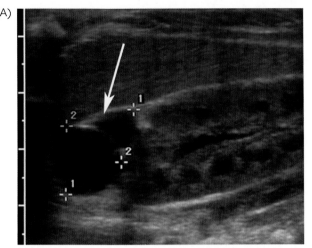

(B)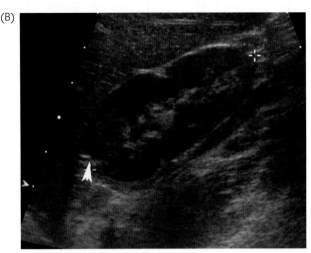

Figure 52.4. Sagittal US image (A) in a newborn with a multiloculated mass (arrow) in the upper pole of the right kidney shows cysts of different sizes without communication in this segmental MCDK. A normal adrenal gland was identified on other images (not shown). The DMSA showed no activity in the upper pole (not shown). Sagittal US image 2 years later (B) shows involution of the segmental MCDK that can be seen as a small triangular echogenic area above the normal remaining kidney (arrowhead).

increasing the transmit gain there will be an increase in power and heat deposition to the fetus. The indices for power and heat deposition are referenced as mechanical index (MI) and thermal index (TI). In general, both indices should be < 1 for obstetrical imaging. In practice one should begin the imaging session by choosing "obstetrical imaging protocol," which is a preset algorithm that includes a safe MI and TI. Using the algorithm, the transmit power button is rarely adjusted during B-mode fetal US to avoid increasing power deposition to the fetus. There is a greater risk of exceeding the MI and TI with fetal Doppler imaging as the unit produces much higher acoustic intensities and that by increasing "gain" one is actually increasing transmit as well as receive gain which translates as increased mechanical stress and heat deposition to the fetus. For this reason one should avoid Doppler interrogation of the heart/great vessels during first trimester.

Differential Diagnosis

- Severe ureteropelvic junction obstruction
- Cystic mesenchymal hamartoma or Wilms tumor
- Polycystic kidney disease (autosomal recessive or dominant)
- Glomerulocystic disease

Common Variants

Multicystic dysplastic kidney generally involves the entire kidney without an identifiable renal pelvis. Occasionally, there is an identifiable pelvis and calices in addition to the dysplastic cysts, which is termed the hydronephrotic form of MCDK. Also, MCDK may be confined to a segment of the kidney or can be bilateral.

Clinical Issues

If MCDK fails to regress over time in order to exclude the possibility of a "missed" cystic neoplasm, then it is resected.

Key Points

- Sporadic congenital condition
- Follow over time to confirm involution
- Carefully evaluate contralateral kidney and reminder of GU tract
- Follow contralateral kidney for appropriate growth
- Look for associated syndromes if bilateral

Further Reading

Hains DS, Bates CM, Ingraham S, Schwaderer AL. Management and etiology of the unilateral multicystic dysplastic kidney: a review. *Pediatr Nephrol.* 2009;*24*(2):233–241.

Ismaili K, Avni FE, Alexander M, Schulman C, Collier F, Hall M. Routine voiding cystourethrography is of no value in neonates with unilateral multicystic dysplastic kidney. *J Pediatr.* 2005;*146*(6):759–763.

Kiyak A, Yilmaz A, Turhan P, Sander S, Aydin G, Aydogan G. Unilateral multicystic dysplastic kidney: single-center experience. *Pediatr Nephrol.* 2009;*24*(1):99–104.

Mattioli G, Pini-Prato A, Costanzo S, Avanzini S, Rossi V, Basile A, Ghiggeri GM, Magnasco A, Leggio S, Rapuzzi G, Jasonni V. Nephrectomy for multicystic dysplastic kidney and renal hypodysplasia in children: where do we stand? *Pediatr Surg Int.* 2010;*26*(5):523–528.

Schreuder MF, Westland R, van Wijk JA. Unilateral multicystic dysplastic kidney: a meta-analysis of observational studies on the incidence, associated urinary tract malformations and the contralateral kidney. *Nephrol Dial Transplant.* 2009;*24*(6):1810–1818.

Autosomal Recessive Polycystic Kidney Disease

Linda Bloom MD, Kassa Darge MD, PhD

Definition

Autosomal recessive polycystic kidney disease (ARPKD) is a genetic hepatorenal disorder characterized by dilation of the renal collecting ducts and congenital hepatic fibrosis.

Clinical Features

The incidence of ARPKD is approximately 1 in 20,000 live births. In the most severe form, neonates present with fatal pulmonary hypoplasia caused by oligohydramnios, which results from impaired fetal renal function. Less severely affected patients may present with bilateral flank masses, severe systemic hypertension, or symptoms secondary to hepatic fibrosis with portal hypertension or Caroli's disease.

Anatomy and Physiology

In ARPKD the kidneys are symmetrically enlarged as a result of dilated distal tubules and collecting ducts. Ten to ninety percent of the ducts may be affected, accounting for the spectrum of disease severity. Some infants have disease limited to a small fraction of the tubules in the medullary pyramids; in others the entire medulla is involved. In most children there is diffuse medullary involvement with patchy cortical involvement. Macrocysts are likely to be present in the cortex or medulla in children with both cortical and medullary disease. Hepatic ductal plate malformation may result in ectatic or malformed bile ducts and fibrosis resulting from a progressive destructive cholangiopathy.

Imaging Findings

Fetal ultrasound (US):
- Grossly enlarged echogenic kidneys
- Macrocysts in the kidneys are rarely seen in utero
- Small or nonvisualized urinary bladder
- Oligohydramnios

Neonatal US:
- Kidneys may be more than four standard deviations above the mean in size for age
- Increased renal size for age but normal renal contours
- Multiple interfaces that increase the medullary echogenicity (Fig. 53.1)
- Diffusely echogenic kidneys
- Reversal of the normal corticomedullary differentiation
- When imaged perpendicular to the tubules with a linear transducer, the stacked dilated tubules resemble multiple small cysts

Childhood US:
- Some tubules dilate to form macrocysts in the medulla
- Kidneys have a lesser degree of enlargement relative to body size, especially after 3 years
- May show macrocysts in the medulla or cortex (Fig. 53.2)
- Hemorrhage or infection uncommon
- Nonshadowing echogenic foci are renal calcifications or acoustic interfaces at the cyst walls
- Congenital hepatic fibrosis: present in all but variable and clinically apparent over time
- large left lobe
- diffusely increased liver echogenicity
- coarsened parenchymal echotexture secondary to fibrosis
- splenomegaly
- "central dot" sign in Caroli's disease/syndrome (portal branch surrounded by dilated bile duct)
- bile duct dilation

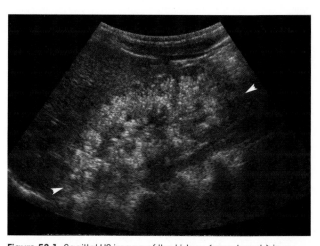

Figure 53.1. Sagittal US image of the kidney (arrowheads) in a child with ARPKD shows many minimally dilated tubules that cause multiple interfaces and increased echogenicity of the medulla.

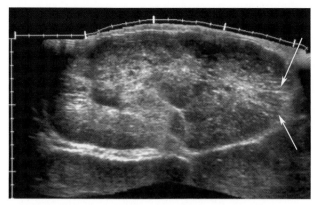

Figure 53.2. Sagittal panorama US image of the kidney in a neonate with ARPKD reveals massive enlargement of the kidney. Medullary echogenicity is greatly increased and there is reversal of the normal neonatal corticomedullary differentiation. There is some cortical involvement, particularly in the lower pole (arrows).

MRI:

- Enlarged kidneys
- Decreased T1, increased T2 signal intensity (SI)
- +/– cortical or medullary cysts
- Bile duct dilation (Fig. 53.3)

Imaging Strategy

Ultrasound is an essential tool in diagnosis and monitoring of ARPKD and the hepatic pathology. High-frequency linear transducers can be used to assess the architecture of the kidney and appreciate the dilated ectatic renal tubules and further characterize the extent of renal involvement (medullary +/– cortical) and liver disease. A lower-frequency curved transducer is often needed to visualize the entire kidney length in one image. Color Doppler US may reveal multiple renal twinkling artifacts resulting from cyst wall calcifications if present. For extrarenal disease, color

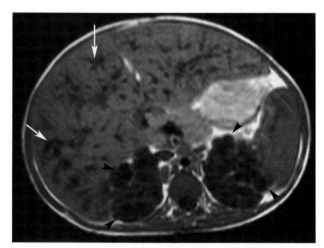

Figure 53.3. Axial T1 MR image of the upper abdomen in a child with ARPKD not only demonstrates the bilateral macrocystic changes of the kidneys (arrowheads), but also diffuse intrahepatic bile ductal dilation (arrows).

Doppler can assess for portal hypertension and varices. In the prenatal or postnatal period, MR may be used to help distinguish ARPKD from other renal cystic diseases with similar US findings. Also, MR is useful in assessing associated hepatobiliary disease. MR cholangiography (MRCP) can provide a global assessment of the extent of biliary disease and can evaluate for complications such as cholangitis and bile stone formation. Renal and hepatic US and MR without contrast are recommended as a baseline evaluation with follow-up imaging examinations performed every 1 to 2 years unless earlier assessment is required.

Related Physics

Two "beneficial" artifacts help to characterize cystic lesions on US. The first is reverberation artifact that is characterized by bright regularly spaced horizontal lines through the image deep to the cystic structure. This results from the sound pulse being trapped within the cyst and bouncing between near and far walls, with the amplitude diminishing with depth. The second is "through transmission enhancement," which is increase in echogenicity (amplitude) deep to the cystic structure. This occurs because the sound traveling through the cyst is unattenuated and the time-gain compensator being unaware of this enhances all signals based on depth. Therefore, the unattenuated signal through the cyst is more greatly amplified than normal tissue adjacent to the cyst, making the deeper tissue brighter. One artifact that may be encountered with cystic renal disease is shadowing related to the coexistence of a highly attenuating calculus. Shadowing results from acoustic impedence mismatch at the surface of the calculus resulting in near total reflection with no sound energy traveling through the calculus. When imaging structures with smooth rounded borders, "refraction" may occur related to a nonorthogonal direction of the imaging beam at the surface. This in turn will cause the US beam to be redirected away from its desired path such that echoes reflected will be misregistered in the image. The refraction phenomenon can underestimate the true length of the kidney and can be reduced with prone technique.

Differential Diagnosis

- Autosomal dominant polycystic kidney disease (ADPKD)
- Bardet Biedl syndrome
- Bilateral renal vein thrombosis

Common Variants

The severity of renal and hepatic involvement is inversely related. Generally, those with the renal predominant phenotype present earlier than those with the hepatic predominant phenotype.

Clinical Issues

Mortality rate is highest in neonates with severe disease diagnosed with a history of oligohydramnios because of pulmonary hypoplasia. Renal transplantation prior to age 18 years (mean 7.6 years) is usually required for those diagnosed in the perinatal period. The majority of patients with renal predominant disease with cortical and medullary involvement develop end-stage renal disease by adulthood. Those with predominant liver disease present with hepatosplenomegaly and have progressive hepatic dysfunction, increased risk of ascending cholangitis, and complications from portal hypertension such as splenomegaly, formation of varices, and gastrointestinal bleeding.

Key Points

- Inherited progressive disease
- Bilateral renal enlargement from tubular ectasia
- Varying degrees of hepatic duct malformations and congenital hepatic fibrosis
- US shows symmetrically enlarged, echogenic renal medulla with poor or reversed corticomedullary differentiation
- Some simple cysts may be present
- MRCP is performed to assess the liver and biliary system

Further Reading

Avni FE, Hall M. Renal cystic diseases in children: new concepts. *Pediatr Radiol.* 2010;*40*(6):939–946.

Bisceglia M, Galliani CA, Senger C, Stallone C, Sessa A. Renal cystic diseases: a review. *Adv Anat Pathol.* 2006;*13*(1):26–56.

De Bruyn R, Gordon I, McHugh K. Imaging of the kidneys, urinary tract and pelvis in children. In: Adam A, Dixon A, eds. *Grainger & Allison's Diagnostic Radiology.* Philadelphia, PA: Elsevier Churchill Livingstone; 2008:1553–1558.

Garel L. Renal cystic disease. *Ultrasound Clin.* 2010;*5*(1):15–59.

Park SJ. Retention of iodinated contrast material within renal cysts in a patient with autosomal dominant polycystic kidney disease. *British Journal of Radiology.* 2012;*85*:e53–e55.

Rizk D, Chapman AB. Cystic and inherited kidney diseases. *Am J Kidney Dis.* 2010;*42*(6):1305–1317.

Turkbey B, Ocak I, Daryanani K, et al. Autosomal recessive polycystic kidney disease and congenital hepatic fibrosis (ARPKD/CHF). *Pediatr Radiol.* 2009;*39*(2):100–111.

Wilson PD. Polycystic kidney disease. *N Engl J Med.* 2004;*350*(2): 151–164.

Autosomal Dominant Polycystic Kidney Disease

Linda Bloom, MD and Kassa Darge, MD, PhD

Definition

Autosomal dominant polycystic kidney disease (ADPKD) is an inherited multisystem disorder characterized by bilateral renal and extrarenal cyst formation.

Clinical Features

Incidence is 1 in 500 to 1,000 live births. Ten percent of cases are sporadic. All patients with ADPKD develop renal cysts, but presentation ranges from clinically silent disease to severe neonatal disease. Most patients become symptomatic as adults in the fourth or fifth decade of life, but some do present in infancy and childhood. Patients may present with flank or abdominal mass, hematuria, urinary tract infection, or hypertension. Progressive renal insufficiency may necessitate hemodialysis. Extrarenal manifestations are more common in adults and include cysts in the liver, pancreas, spleen, seminal vesicles and lung. Intracranial berry aneurysms are reported in 10 to 30 percent of patients with ADPKD. Coronary and aortic aneurysms also occur.

Anatomy and Physiology

The kidneys become progressively enlarged bilaterally as numerous micro- and macrocysts develop in the cortex and medulla. Cysts may originate from any segment of the nephron.

Imaging Findings

Prenatal or infant ultrasound (US):
- Macrocysts
- Diffusely echogenic enlarged kidneys without visible cysts

Child or adult US:
- Normal US does not exclude ADPKD as cysts may not appear until the fourth decade
- Micro- and macrocysts form in the cortex and medulla, usually by 36 years of age (Fig. 54.1A)
- Cysts distort renal contours
- Initially may be unilateral, especially in childhood, ultimately bilateral in nearly all
- Comet-tail artifacts, likely resulting from milk of calcium in small cysts, may be seen in childhood
- Macrocysts in other organs common in adults but uncommon in children
- Complex cysts from hemorrhage or infection

CT/MRI:
- Simple cysts usually do not enhance (cysts originate from nephrons, so some may enhance)
- Hemorrhagic cysts (90 percent of adults)
- Increased density on CT
- Variable signal intensity on MRI (Fig. 54.1B)
- May develop wall thickening or mural calcification
- Perinephric hematoma (rare rupture into perinephric space)
- Wall may thicken and enhance if infected
- Renal calculi

Imaging Strategy

The study of choice to evaluate renal and hepatic involvement is US; age-related diagnostic criteria assess the number of cysts and family history. Ultrasound offers a variety of tools including tissue harmonic imaging, power Doppler, and color flow. CT and MRI are useful in detecting extrarenal manifestations such as cerebral, coronary or aortic aneurysms and extrarenal cysts. Performing US on the parents may also be useful if the parents are not previously diagnosed. An MRI scan of the brain may be necessary if tuberous sclerosis (TS) is considered in the differential diagnosis, particularly in patients less than 5 years old without a positive family history. The TS gene (TSC2) is immediately adjacent to the ADPKD gene (PKD1) and the two entities may coexist. This is known as a "contiguous gene syndrome."

Related Physics

One US dilemma is trying to achieve high resolution at depth, and this is particularly problematic when imaging the large retroperitoneal kidneys in ADPKD. Tissue harmonic imaging has been developed to allow one to image at a fundamental frequency as well as the first harmonic (twice the fundamental frequency) through the simple push of a button. Harmonic origins can be understood by using the analogy of a gentle wave approaching a beach. When the wave is in deep water, the peak and trough travel at the same speed, maintaining a sinusoidal shape. As the wave

(A)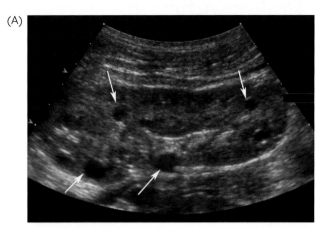

(B)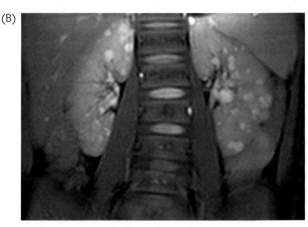

Figure 54.1. Sagittal US (A) of the kidney in a child with ADPKD shows a few scattered macrocysts (arrows) but the renal size, echogenicity, and the corticomedullary differentiation are normal for age. Coronal T2 MR image (B) shows cysts are more numerous and conspicuous than on the US.

approaches shallow water the trough is slowed down by bottom friction while the crest continues on, causing the wave front to steepen. In medical US, peak pressure travels at a slightly higher velocity than trough pressure. When the pulse is launched it has a true sinusoidal shape, but as it moves away from the transducer, the positive pressure peak overtakes the trough, causing the sinusoid to develop a steep downslope. Fourier transformation converts the waveform to its frequency components, assigning a higher frequency for the steep downslope than for the pure sinusoid. Because this phenomenon happens at depth, there is no attenuation along its path, allowing us to make use of the fact it originated at depth and has a higher frequency to produce higher-resolution images. To remove the fundamental frequency information, one can either apply a narrow-band pass filter or send in an equal and opposite fundamental pulse (pulse-inversion harmonic imaging) to cancel it out by destructive interference. One advantage is the availability of fundamental and harmonic imaging with the touch of a button and no need to change transducers. The other is the ability to achieve high resolution at greater depths. Disadvantages are that the higher-frequency harmonic echoes returning do suffer attenuation resulting in decreased signal strength that will decrease slightly the available depth of penetration over fundamental imaging.

Differential Diagnosis

- Glomerulocystic kidney disease
- Tuberous sclerosis
- Von Hippel-Lindau disease
- Autosomal recessive polycystic kidney disease (ARPKD)

Common Variants

- Type 1: mutation of the PKD1 gene located on the short arm of chromosome 16; 85 percent of patients;

ADPKD type 1 has an earlier onset, and more numerous and larger cysts than other forms
- Type 2: mutation of the PKD2 gene located on chromosome 4 [c1]
- Glomerulocystic form of the disease is seen most often in the prenatal population and in infants; kidneys may be small, normal, or large in size, are diffusely hyperechoic and may have a few subcapsular macrocysts

Clinical Issues

Autosomal dominant polycystic kidney disease is a progressive disease, with kidney size increasing throughout life because of increase in number and size of cysts. Complications include the development of hypertension (third or fourth decade of life), infection of or hemorrhage into cysts, renal calculi formation, and end-stage renal disease. Renal stones and infection are often sources of flank pain. Subarachnoid hemorrhage from cerebral aneurysm rupture may be fatal. Other vascular concerns include complications from coronary artery aneurysms or thoracic aorta dissection. When people with ADPKD develop renal cell carcinoma it is usually at a younger age than in the general population. It is more likely to be multicentric and to present bilaterally, but may be metachronous.

Key Points

- ADPKD is an inherited progressive multisystem disorder.
- Cysts may be present at birth, but may not develop until late 30s.
- The kidneys are enlarged with scattered micro- and macrocysts.
- Hepatic cysts are the most common extrarenal manifestation.

- Congenital cerebral aneurysms are associated with ADPKD.
- Renal cell carcinoma: younger patent age, multicentric, may be bilateral.
- Genetic focus immediately adjacent to TS gene so the two diseases may coexist.

Further Reading

Avni FE, Hall M. Renal cystic diseases in children: new concepts. *Pediatr Radiol.* 2010;*40*(6):939–946..

Bisceglia M, Galliani CA, Senger C, Stallone C, Sessa A. Renal cystic diseases: a review. *Adv Anat Pathol.* 2006;*13*(1):26–56.

De Bruyn R, Gordon I, McHugh K. Imaging of the kidneys, urinary tract and pelvis in children. In: Adam A, Dixon A, eds. *Grainger & Allison's Diagnostic Radiology.* Philadelphia, PA: Elsevier Churchill Livingstone; 2008:1553–1558.

Garel L. Renal cystic disease. *Ultrasound Clin.* 2010;*5*(1):15–59.

Park SJ. Retention of iodinated contrast material within renal cysts in a patient with autosomal dominant polycystic kidney disease. *British Journal of Radiology.* 2012;*85*:e53–e55.

Rizk D, Chapman AB. Cystic and inherited kidney diseases. *Am J Kidney Dis.* 2010;*42*(6):1305–1317.

Turkbey B, Ocak I, Daryanani K, et al. Autosomal recessive polycystic kidney disease and congenital hepatic fibrosis (ARPKD/CHF). *Pediatr Radiol.* 2009;*39*(2):100–111.

Wilson PD. Polycystic kidney disease. *N Engl J Med.* 2004;*350*(2):151–164.

CHAPTER 55

Wilms' Tumor

Marguerite T. Parisi, MD, MS

Definition

Wilms' tumor (nephroblastoma) is a malignant tumor of primitive metanephric blastema seen predominantly in children.

Clinical Features

With approximately 500 new cases diagnosed each year in the United States, Wilms' tumor accounts for approximately 6 percent of all childhood cancers and is the most common pediatric primary renal cancer. Wilms' tumor has a peak incidence at 3 years of age, is uncommon after age 6 years, is rarely seen in adults, and is slightly more common among African-Americans and girls. An asymptomatic mass is the most common clinical presentation of Wilms' tumor although coincidental trauma is present in up to 10 percent. Hematuria and pain (the latter from tumor necrosis) are other clinical manifestations. Hypertension resulting from renin production by the tumor may be present in up to 25 percent.

Although Wilms' tumor usually develops in healthy children, 10 percent of cases occur in individuals with known, predisposing syndromes including:

- WAGR syndrome: Wilms' tumor, aniridia, genitourinary malformation and mental retardation
- Denys-Drash syndrome: male pseudohermaphroditism and nephritis
- Beckwith-Wiedemann syndrome: macroglossia, exopthalmos, gigantism
- Perlman syndrome: fetal gigantism with multiple congenital anomalies
- Bloom syndrome: immunodeficiency and facial telangiectasia
- Soto syndrome: cerebral gigantism
- Trisomy 18
- Other predisposing factors include hemihypertrophy, cryptorchidism, hypospadius, sporadic aniridia, horseshoe kidney, and nephroblastomatosis
- Familial Wilms' tumor (FWT), in which cases run in families, siblings, or cousins, though rare (1% of cases), has also been reported

Anatomy and Physiology

Wilms' tumor is typically unilateral, although bilateral disease occurs in approximately 5 to 10 percent of cases.

While the exact etiology of Wilms' tumor is unknown, development is thought to involve changes in a number of genes including WT1, WT2, FWT1, and FWT2, located on chromosomes 11p13, 11p15, 17q, and 19q, respectively. In those with predisposing conditions or syndromes, Wilms' tumors tend to develop at an earlier age. Wilms' tumor is classified into either favorable (90 percent of cases) or unfavorable (anaplastic) histologic subtypes. Unfavorable histologic subtype occurs in 10 percent of patients but accounts for almost 50 percent of tumor deaths.

Imaging Findings

Radiography:
- Noncalcified retroperitoneal mass; mass effect

US:
- Large, well-defined hyperechoic renal mass, often heterogeneous as a result of hemorrhage, fat, necrosis, or rarely (<10%), calcifications
- The most reliable method for assessing the presence and extent of tumor invasion into renal vein or inferior vena cava (IVC), the presence of which will modify surgical approach

CT:
- Large, intrarenal mass that enhances but to a lesser degree than adjacent normal parenchyma. Heterogeneous attenuation may be secondary to hemorrhage, fat, or in <10%, calcifications (Fig. 55.1)
- Typically does not cross midline; tends to displace rather than encase vessels
- Can identify regional nodal disease, extracapsular extent, presence of invasion of the renal vein or IVC, and hematogenous spread to lungs or liver
- Crucial to determine if contralateral disease is present (5 to 10%)

MRI:
- Typically low or isointense to normal renal parenchyma on T1 and hyperintense on T2
- Enhances following IV gadolinium administration but to a lesser degree than normal renal parenchyma
- Permits assessment of caval patency and multifocal disease

(A)   (B)

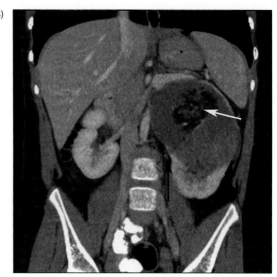

Figure 55.1. Axial (A) and coronal (B) contrast-enhanced CT images in a child with a large abdominal mass show a large Wilms' tumor, containing both fat (white arrow) and calcifications (arrowheads), showing the "claw" sign (black arrows) confirming its renal origin.

F-18 FDG PET:

- Often FDG-avid; but FDG is unlikely to play an important role in staging as:
  - FDG unable to distinguish favorable from unfavorable histologies
  - Not useful in the detection of small pulmonary nodules
- Adjunctive, primarily problem-solving role:
  - In therapeutic response monitoring to differentiate residual disease from postsurgical change
  - Useful in those with atypical recurrent disease

Imaging Strategy

At diagnosis:

- US: typically screening study; used to assess for renal vein and/or IVC invasion
- CT: to define the extent of the primary tumor and assess for metastatic disease
- MRI: may be used in assessment of primary tumor; need for additional CT chest scan
- Functional imaging:
  - Tc-99m MDP bone scans: not routinely performed as osseous metastatic disease is a late occurrence in Wilms' tumor
  - F-18 FDG-PET: not useful in staging evaluation

Therapeutic disease monitoring:

- Abdominal US classically used for assessment of nephrectomy bed in those with unilateral disease at diagnosis
- CT chest scan to assess for pulmonary metastatic disease
- FDG-PET as an adjunctive tool in certain circumstances as listed above

Screening studies in those with predisposing conditions:

- Abdominal US should be performed at time of diagnosis of any of the predisposing conditions or at 6 months of age (whichever is earlier) followed by serial US every 3 months until the patient reaches 7 years, after which the risk of developing Wilms' tumor significantly decreases
- Some have advocated an initial CT at 6 months of agein this patient group although the risks of associated radiation should be considered

IMAGING PITFALLS
- Even with the advanced state of current imaging, synchronous bilateral Wilms' tumor will go undiagnosed in up to 7% of cases. Correct diagnosis of bilateral disease is of paramount importance as management is changed from performance of a primary nephrectomy to biopsy followed by chemotherapy and renal parenchyma-sparing surgical procedures.
- Neuroblastoma can invade the kidney, mimicking Wilms' tumor. I-123 MIBG scans, which are positive in >90% of neuroblastomas but negative in those with Wilms' tumor, can be used to distinguish these entities (Fig. 55.2).

Related Physics

One common challenge in pediatric imaging is the differentiation between Wilms' tumor and neuroblastoma, two vastly different tumors with regard to behavior, management, and prognosis. Ultrasound generates specular acoustic reflection to show the interface between Wilms' tumor and renal parenchyma generating the "claw" sign, which confirms its intrinsic renal origin. The claw sign is produced by differential acoustic impedance between the native tissue and the mass. This in turn causes some of the sound to be

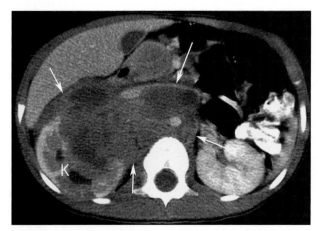

Figure 55.2. Axial contrast-enhanced CT image in a 5-year-old with abdominal pain demonstrates a large noncalcified mass (arrows), either arising from or invading the right kidney (K). The mass crosses midline and encases the vessels, favoring neuroblastoma over Wilms' tumor.

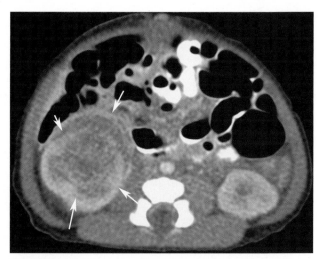

Figure 55.3. Axial contrast-enhanced CT image in a newborn with mesoblastic nephroma demonstrates a solid, noncalcified mass (arrows) arising in the right kidney. Patient age suggests the diagnosis, as imaging features of this pathologic entity are indistinguishable from those of Wilms' tumor.

reflected back to the transducer because of an acoustic impedence mismatch. Acoustic impedence is in turn the product of sound speed and tissue density. Further, sound speed is inversely related to tissue compressibility (e.g., stiffer tissues have higher sound speeds). With neuroblastoma there is a similar phenomenon with acoustic mismatch, but it is the shape of the specular reflector that differentiates neuroblastoma from Wilms' tumor; the interface is rounded for neuroblastoma, which is outside the kidney but it is sharp (producing the claw) for Wilm's which originates in the kidney. It is important to understand that this differentiation is only possible because of the high spatial resolution afforded by high-frequency transducers in the small patient.

Differential Diagnosis

- Multilocular cystic nephroma: fluid-filled cystic mass with multiple thin septations, can be difficult to distinguish from Wilms' tumor.
- Mesoblastic nephroma or congenital mesoblastic nephroma: commonly referred to as fetal renal hamartoma, has similar imaging characteristics to Wilms' tumor but occurs in the first few months of life (Fig. 55.3). Ninety percent are diagnosed by 1 year of age.
- Clear cell sarcoma of the kidney (CCSK): difficult to distinguish radiographically from Wilms' tumor, CCSK accounts for 4 percent of childhood renal malignancies, is characterized by aggressive behavior, with higher relapse rates and mortality than Wilms' tumor. Unlike Wilms' tumor, this neoplasm tends to metastasize to bone; consequently Tc-99m MDP bone scan is indicated in staging.
- Rhabdoid tumor of the kidney: most aggressive malignant renal tumor of childhood; accounts for 1 to 2 percent of pediatric renal neoplasms. Typically

diagnosed in the first year of life and like CCSK, this mass is radiologically indistinguishable from Wilms' tumor. Rhabdoid tumor metastasizes to brain, lung, and liver; thus cranial imaging is warranted.

- Renal cell carcinoma (RCC): solid intrarenal mass that is radiologically indistinguishable from Wilms' tumor. Ring-like calcifications can occur, atypical for Wilms' tumor. Less than 2 percent of cases of RCC occur in children; mean age of presentation is 9 years compared to 3 years for those with Wilms' tumor. Renal cell carcinoma is associated with von Hippel-Lindau syndrome. Compared with Wilms' tumor, RCC is more likely to be bilateral and to metastasize to bone.
- Renal lymphoma: renal involvement by lymphoma can result from direct retroperitoneal extension or by hematogeneous spread and on imaging is characterized by single or multiple homogeneous hypoattenuating masses, often with associated lymphadenopathy. Renal involvement is most commonly seen with non-Hodgkin's lymphoma, especially Burkitt's.
- Neuroblastoma: younger age at diagnosis; typically suprarenal, often calcified (85 to 95 percent on CT), encases rather than displaces or invades vessels; can invade the spinal canal; metastasizes most commonly to bone and bone marrow, unlike Wilms' which tends to spread hematogenously to the lungs.

Common Variants/Precursors

Nephroblastomatosis, a condition in which multiple nephrogenic rests (persistent embryologic renal parenchyma/metanephric blastema) are present, occurs most often in neonates and is considered a precursor lesion to Wilms'

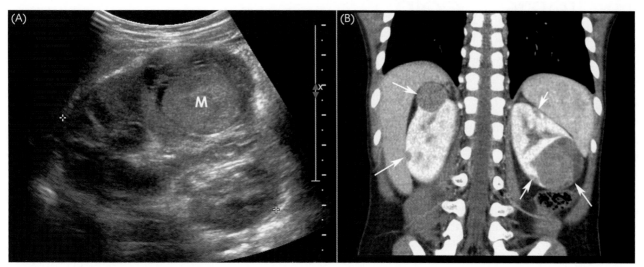

Figure 55.4. Sagittal US image (A) in a 3-year-old with abdominal mass shows a dominant mass in the lower pole (M). Multiple masses were suspected bilaterally. Axial contrast-enhanced CT image (B) demonstrates multifocal nephroblastomatosis with largest lesions in right-upper and left-lower poles (arrows) corresponding to US findings.

tumor. Not only do children with nephroblastomatosis have an increased incidence of Wilms' tumor but nephrogenic rests are found in approximately 40 percent of unilateral and 99 percent of bilateral Wilms' tumors. Nephroblastomatosis is unifocal (rare), multifocal (Fig. 55.4) or diffuse. On CT, macroscopic nephrogenic rests appear as low-attenuation peripheral nodules with poor enhancement relative to normal parenchyma; on MR, the nodules are of low signal intensity on both T1- and T2-weighted images. The diffuse form demonstrates a thick hypoechoic band on US which distorts the renal collecting system and is nonenhancing on CT or MRI.

Clinical Issues

Disease staging in Wilms' tumor is surgical as follows:

- Stage I: tumor limited to the kidney; completely resectable; renal capsule intact
- Stage II: tumor infiltrates beyond kidney; completely resectable (includes local spillage confined to the flank)
- Stage III: residual tumor confined to the abdomen without hematogeneous spread
- Stage IV: hematogeneous spread
- Stage V: bilateral disease

Unilateral Wilms' tumor is treated in North America by nephrectomy, followed by chemotherapy. Presurgical chemotherapy (as in Europe) may be used to improve outcome by promoting tumor shrinkage. In some cases, local radiation of the tumor bed is advocated; whole abdomen radiation is used when there is gross tumor spillage at surgery or in the presence of peritoneal implants. Bilateral disease is treated with preoperative chemotherapy and tumor resection with parenchyma-sparing surgery.

Key Points

- Large heterogeneous tumor arising from the kidney; "claw" sign may be present
- Calcifications rare (8 to 10%)
- Displaces rather than encases vessels but may invade the renal vein or IVC
- Bilateral in 8 to 10%
- Metastasizes to lung (20%); bone metastases rare
- Predisposing syndromes or conditions in up to 15%
- Disease staging is surgical

Further Reading

Aquisto TM, Yost R, Marshall KW. Best cases from the AFIP: anaplastic wilms tumor: radiologic and pathologic findings. *Radiographics.* 2004;24(6):1709–1713.

Cotton CA, Peterson S, Norkool PA, Takashima J, Grigoriev Y, Green DM, Breslow NE. Early and late mortality after diagnosis of Wilms' tumor. *J Clin Oncol.* 2009;27(8):4819.

Geller E, Kochan PS. Renal neoplasms of childhood. *Radiol Clin North Am.* 2011;49(4):689–709.

Lowe LH, Isuani BH, Heller RM, Stein SM, Johnson JE, Navarro OM, Hernanz-Schulman M. Pediatric renal masses: Wilms' tumor and beyond. *Radiographics.* 2000;20(6):1585–1603.

McHugh K. Renal and adrenal tumors in children. *Cancer Imaging.* 2007;7:41–51.

Moinul Hossain AK, Shulkin BL, Gelfand MJ, Bashir H, Daw NC, Sharp SE, Nadel HR, Dome JS. FDG positron emission tomography/computed tomography studies of Wilms' tumor. *Europe J Nuc Med Mol Imaging.* 2010;37(7):1300–1308.

CHAPTER 56

Hydrometrocolpos

Stuart Morrison, MB, Ch.B, FRCP

Definition

Various combinations of Latin terms are used to categorize developmental anomalies of the female reproductive system that result in obstruction at the level of the fallopian tubes, uterus, and vagina, and the associated retained products. These terms include: "hydro" (water or a simple fluid); "hem" (blood); "colpos" (vagina); "metra" (uterus); and "salpinx" (fallopian tube). An accumulation of blood in the uterus is called "hematometria," whereas distention of the vagina by retained blood products is termed "hematocolpos." The term "hydrocolpos" describes a fluid collection in the vagina; "hydrometrocolpos" includes the uterus.

Clinical Features

Hydrocolpos can present prenatally, in the neonatal period or at puberty and is included in the differential diagnosis of a midline pelvic unilocular cystic mass in a female fetus. Obstruction of the adjacent ureters by the distended obstructed vagina can lead to prenatal hydroureter and hydronephrosis. Rarely, severe cases of urinary obstruction result in oligohydramnios secondary to decreased fetal urine production. In the newborn, hydrocolpos presents as a bulging cystic mass at the introitus separating the labia. Less commonly a newborn female presents with a palpable midline cystic abdominopelvic mass. In newborn girls, hydrocolpos is second in frequency to renal enlargement (from multicystic dysplastic kidney or hydronephrosis) as a cause of abdominal mass. Peripubertal girls may present with cyclic abdominal pain and absence of external evidence of menstruation. This pain is secondary to repeated menstruation with retention of menstrual products within the obstructed uterine cavity and/or vagina.

Anatomy and Physiology

The paramesonephric (Müllerian) ducts appear at 6 weeks gestational age. They lie lateral to the mesonephric (Wolffian) ducts in both male and female embryos. Prior to 7 gestational weeks the embryonic genitalia are the same for both sexes. In females, the caudal end of the Müllerian ducts fuse together by about 9 gestational weeks to form the uterus and the most superior portion of the vagina. The bilateral fallopian tubes remain separate. The vagina is formed from elements of the Müllerian ducts and the urogenital (UG) sinus. The Sertoli cells in the testis secrete Müllerian-inhibiting substance that acts locally to prevent development of the Müllerian ducts in the male. The gonads develop completely separately and first appear on the genital ridge of the posterior coelom. In the female fetus and newborn, maternal estrogens stimulate the uterine and cervical glands to produce mucus that can accumulate in and distend the vagina if there is obstruction to outflow. In the pubertal girl the endometrium of the uterus responds to estrogen and progesterone in a cyclic pattern of proliferation and secretion. Withdrawal of the sex hormones produces shedding of the endometrium (menses) which may accumulate in and distend the uterus to a lesser extent than the vagina. Causes of vaginal obstruction include an imperforate hymen, transverse vaginal septum, and vaginal atresia. Imperforate hymen produces a low vaginal obstruction and can present with hydrocolpos in the fetus, newborn, or adolescent. A congenital transverse membrane or septum is the most common cause of vaginal obstruction and can occur at any level in the vagina but usually in the upper or middle thirds. A longitudinal vaginal septum is associated with failure of fusion of the Müllerian ducts, is not obstructive and usually not symptomatic (Fig. 56.1).

Imaging Findings

US and MRI:

- Dilated ovoid vagina is seen as a midline fluid-filled structure located between the urinary bladder and rectum
- Composition of the fluid is variable as is the US appearance: purely sonolucent, diffuse internal echoes, or fluid debris level
- Distended vagina can be extremely large in patients with hydrocolpos (Fig. 56.2)
- Simple or complex fluid can also occasionally be found distending the fallopian tubes (Fig. 56.3)
- Uterus and cervix may be more easily seen on MRI because of superior displacement of the uterus into the upper abdomen (Fig. 56.4)
- Fluid within the uterine cavity may be anechoic (hydrometria) or contain blood (hematometria)

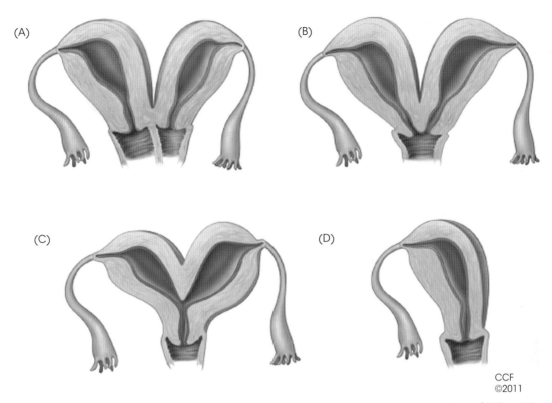

Figure 56.1. Spectrum of Müllerian anomalies. (A) Uterus didelphys with vagina duplex. (B) Uterus didelphys. (C) Uterus bicornate. (D) Uterus unicornate.

- Uterus has a much thicker wall than the thin-walled vagina and is less distensible so it remains smaller in size (Fig. 56.5)
- Ureteric or bowel obstruction may occur as a result of extrinsic compression

Imaging Strategy

Prenatal US first identifies the abdominopelvic cystic mass of hydrocolpos. Later in pregnancy, fetal MRI may offer additional information and increase diagnostic confidence if clinically indicated. Postnatal assessment with US is also

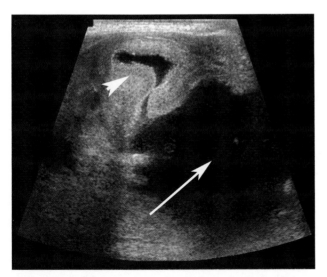

Figure 56.2. Sagittal pelvic US in a newborn with palpable lower abdominal mass demonstrates complex fluid and debris in the massively but irregularly dilated vagina, uterine cavity, and cervical canal (white arrow). The uterus (white arrowhead) is atypically but relatively hyperechoic, is displaced anteriorly and has a much thicker wall than the vagina.

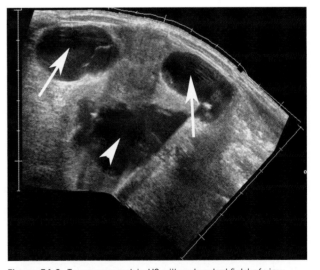

Figure 56.3. Transverse pelvic US with extended field of view in a newborn with palpable lower abdominal mass shows two anterior separate fluid collections that represent dilated fluid-filled fallopian tubes—hydrosalpinx (white arrows). The more posteriorly situated fluid collection is the enlarged fluid-filled thin-walled vagina—hydrocolpos (white arrowhead). The uterus is located between the hydrosalpinx (asterisk).

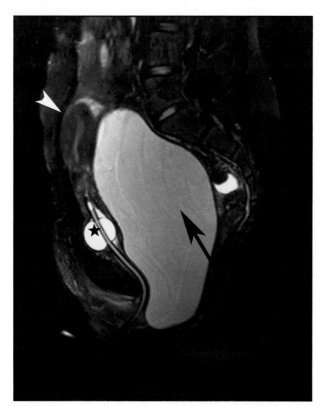

Figure 56.4. Sagittal T2 fat-suppressed pelvic MR image in a 13-year-old girl with abdominal pain and delayed menarche shows a massively distended fluid-filled vagina (black arrow) that occupies the majority of the pelvis and extends into the lower abdomen at the L5 level. The uterus (arrowhead) is displaced cephalad and is located anterior to the superior aspect of fluid-filled vagina. Foley catheter (star) is present in the decompressed bladder.

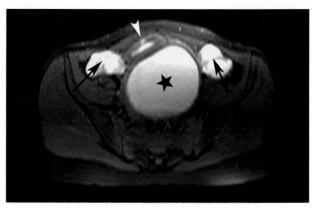

Figure 56.5. Transverse T2 fat-suppressed MR image in a 13-year-old girl with abdominal pain and delayed menarche shows the midline vagina (star) and bilateral fallopian tubes (black arrows) are dilated, fluid-filled and have thin walls. The uterus (arrowhead) is displaced anteriorly, immediately behind the anterior abdominal wall.

performed. Transperineal scanning of the newborn using a high-frequency linear transducer can be very helpful to identify more precisely the level of vaginal obstruction. Postnatal renal and bladder US is indicated because of the high association of congenital renal anomalies. Urinary tract obstruction can be a direct result of the mass effect of the distended obstructed vagina, or it can be coexistent as a result of common UG sinus obstruction. If US cannot provide complete renal, uterine, and vaginal anatomic information both for diagnosis and treatment planning, then MRI is needed.

Related Physics

The superior soft-tissue contrast and detail obtained from high-resolution MR imaging make it a very useful tool used to sort out genitourinary pathology in pediatrics. MRI can be thought of as two subsystems, the "transmit" side and the "receive" side. This section is focused on the "receive" subsystem. MR signals are characterized by an oscillating waveform where the signal at the coil is an oscillating change in voltage with frequencies between 40 to 80 megahertz. Similarly the noise in an MR signal is also oscillatory and over a much broader frequency range. Similar to a radio, weaker signals

require boosting by a process known as "receiver gain." This is accomplished through running the receive coil signals through a sensitive radiofrequency amplifier. This is an imperfect process so that the noise in the signal is often amplified more than the true signal, limiting its usefulness. In MR imaging, because we know the frequency of the expected signal, other processes can be used to increase signal. First the signal is digitized by an analog-to-digital convertor, and the digitized signal is then run through a Fourier transformer to identify the frequency content within the signal. Because we know the frequency of the expected signal, a "band pass" filter can be applied to remove noise. The receive bandwidth defines the range of frequencies of the signal given, which includes the fundamental frequency given by the Larmor equation, as well as any small shifts above and below the Larmor frequency resulting from imposed gradients. This range of frequencies is known as the "receive bandwidth." In an effort to optimize raw signal strength, one can employ a variety of surface coils—this is the best thing one can do to improve image quality.

Differential Diagnosis

- Enteric duplication cyst
- Lymphatic malformation
- Presacral teratoma
- Ovarian cyst
- Presacral meningocele
- Obstructed ectopic pelvic kidney

Variants

Cloacal malformation has a single perineal opening for the urinary, intestinal, and genital systems. This unusual malformation results from an arrest in embryogenesis, only occurs in girls, and has a high incidence of associated Müllerian abnormalities and hydrocolpos.

Persistent UG sinus has a single opening for the urinary and genital systems with a normal anus. Hydrocolpos and Müllerian abnormalities are also common with this abnormality. Vaginal atresia/aplasia is part of the Mayer-Rokitansky-Kuster-Hauser (MRKH) syndrome. Affected girls lack a normal uterus and the lower two-thirds of the vagina or the entire vagina. There are two types; the second group of MRKH patients may also have renal, otologic, vertebral, and cardiac anomalies. The ovaries and fallopian tubes are usually normal, so these patients may be asymptomatic and go undiagnosed until primary amenorrhea. McKusick-Kaufman syndrome is hydrometrocolpos together with postaxial polydactyly and congenital heart disease and is more common in the Amish.

Clinical Issues

The distended vagina may exert significant mass effect on and partially obstruct the adjacent ureters, bowel or lower extremity vasculature. Ultrasound-guided drainage of the vaginal fluid in a neonate can be performed to relieve symptoms from mass effect. Pyometrocolpos is infection of the fluid within the obstructed vagina and uterus. If the hydro- or pyometrocolpos is caused by an imperforate hymen, then surgical excision of the hymen will treat the obstruction and also allow drainage of the fluid. Percutaneous US-guided drainage of the infected fluid can help treat or prevent potentially life-threatening urinary tract infections or sepsis in infants with vaginal obstruction from more complex anomalies such as UG sinus or obstructed cloacal malformation. Depending on the cause of the hydrocolpos, diagnosis and/or definitive surgery may be delayed. With the onset of menarche, menstrual blood accumulates proximal to the obstruction and can move retrograde into the fallopian tubes and peritoneal cavity resulting in endometriosis. This may in part contribute to the increased incidence of ectopic pregnancy.

Key Points

- Symptoms and age at presentation vary with the cause.
- Can be diagnosed in a fetus, newborn, or at puberty.
- US and MRI are used to define anatomy of the reproductive and urinary tracts.
- Transverse vaginal septum or imperforate hymen are most common causes of vaginal and uterine obstruction.
- There is an association with renal, UG sinus and cloacal abnormalities.
- Pyometrocolpos can be lifethreating and requires drainage.

Further Reading

Blask AR, Sanders RC, Gearhart JP. Obstructed uterovaginal anomalies: demonstration with sonography. *Radiology.* 1991;*179*(1):79–83.

Blask AR, Sanders RC, Rock JA. Obstructed uterovaginal anomalies: demonstration with sonography. *Radiology.* 1991;*179*(1):84–88.

Larsen's Human Embryology. Fourth edition. Philadelphia, PA: Churchill, Livingstone, Elsivier; 2009:479–541.

Nazir Z, Rizvi RM, Qureshi RN, Khan ZS, Khan Z. Congenital vaginal obstructions: varied presentation and outcome. *Pediatr Surg Int.* 2006;*22*(9):749–753.

Stallion A. Vaginal obstruction. *Semin Pediatr Surg.* 2000;*9*(3): 128–134.

CHAPTER 57

Neonatal Adrenal Hemorrhage

Sudha P. Singh, MD

Definition

Neonatal adrenal hemorrhage refers to perinatal hemorrhage into the adrenal gland(s).

Clinical Features

Adrenal hemorrhage has been reported as early as 21 weeks gestation but is most often discovered in the third trimester or in the first week after birth.

Although most infants present during the first week of life, some present at 3 or 4 weeks of age. Seventy percent of the cases are right-sided and ten percent are bilateral. The clinical presentation is variable. Perinatal adrenal hemorrhage is of uncertain etiology but is typically associated with significant physical stress such as birth trauma, anoxia, sepsis, or coagulopathy. Infants of diabetic mothers or those that are large for gestational age are at greater risk than small or preterm infants. Adrenal hemorrhage may be detected incidentally during ultrasound (US). Signs and symptoms of adrenal hemorrhage include prolonged jaundice, anemia, dropping hematocrit, hypotension, and/or palpable flank mass. Scrotal hematoma has been reported in several infants with adrenal hemorrhage. Transient adrenal insufficiency can occur however most infants recover completely. Prolonged adrenal insufficiency occurs if more than 90 percent of the adrenal tissue is damaged.

Pathophysiology

The exact etiology is unclear. It is hypothesized that hypoxia, fluctuations in blood pressure, sepsis, or other forms of perinatal stress may lead to shunting of blood to vital organs leading to hemorrhagic infarction of the adrenals. Sometimes the glands are enlarged and echogenic but maintain their smooth contour suggesting congestion rather than obvious hemorrhage. Adrenal congestion and hemorrhage are thought to be part of a continuous spectrum. Another theory relates to the fact that neonatal adrenal glands are nearly twice the size of normal adult adrenal glands. As the cortex of the gland rapidly decreases in size in the perinatal period, there may be relatively increased potential space for hemorrhage.

Imaging Findings

- Acute hemorrhages may be diffusely echogenic or have a heterogeneous appearance, with both echogenic and anechoic foci (Fig. 57.1A)
- Large hemorrhages may obscure the entire gland with no normal adrenal tissue identified
- Large hemorrhages may have mass effect on the kidney and/or displace the kidney inferiorly
- Color Doppler imaging demonstrates a consistent lack of internal blood flow (particularly important in differentiating adrenal hematoma from adrenal neuroblastoma; (Fig. 57.1B)
- Small hemorrhages may be triangular or circular, effacing only a part of the adrenal gland or a limb of the adrenal gland
- Over time increasing internal liquefaction seen as increasing anechoic foci, usually proceeding from center to periphery
- Chronic hemorrhages may become echogenic and then calcify
- Posterior acoustic shadowing occurs with larger dystrophic calcifications
- Diagnosis of adrenal hemorrhages is based on the expected chronologic changes of decreasing size and evolving internal echo texture of the hemorrhage on US (Figs. 57.1C and 57.1D)

Imaging Strategy

Ultrasound is the modality of choice; CT and MRI may be helpful in atypical cases.

Imaging findings are always considered in the context of the perinatal clinical history. Adrenal hemorrhage should demonstrate lack of internal blood flow, chronological changes in internal architecture, and decreasing size with serial ultrasound examinations. Initially US may be performed at 3 to 5 days, then at 1- to 2-week intervals until the lesion resolves or nearly resolves and is stable. The rate at which these changes occur varies from patient to patient.

Demonstration of evolving blood products on MRI is of limited value as neuroblastoma, the main differential consideration, may also demonstrate internal hemorrhage.

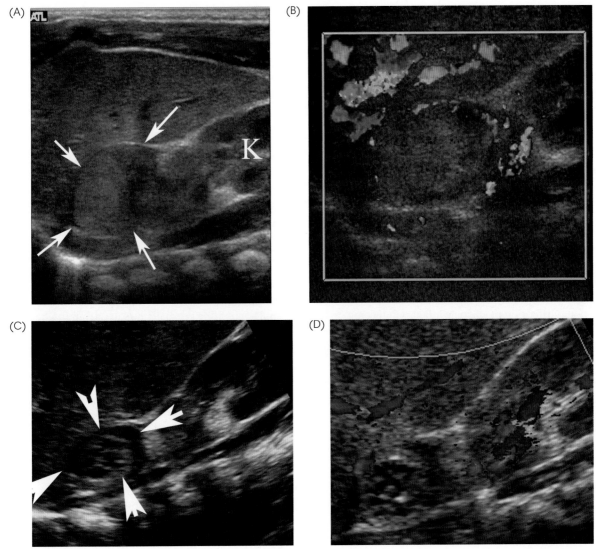

Figure 57.1. Sagittal US image (A) in a 1-day-old term infant with hypoplastic left lung and hypoxia demonstrates a moderately echogenic mass (white arrows) in the adrenal gland superior to the kidney (K). Ultrasound with color Doppler (B) shows lack of internal flow. Sagittal US 7 days later (C) shows interval decrease in size of the adrenal mass with multiple sonolucent foci (arrowheads) indicating breakdown of blood products. Ultrasound with color Doppler (D) shows no internal flow.

If a survey of the liver is positive for liver masses, then metastatic disease from adrenal neuroblastoma is likely. Skin metastasis may also be clinically evident in some cases of neonatal neuroblastoma.

Related Physics

The first-line choice for abdominal imaging of the newborn is US as it is portable, affords high resolution and does not carry the risks associated with ionizing radiation. Acoustic artifacts including through transmission enhancement and posterior acoustic shadowing are used to one's advantage in evaluating newborn adrenal lesions. Through transmission enhancement occurs when the US beam traverses a structure that is less attenuating than adjacent structures. This is most commonly seen with fluid-filled or cystic structures.

With early adrenal hemorrhage, ultrasound will show an echogenic or hypoechoic mass within the adrenal gland and a band of increased signal intensity in the tissues lying within the far field of the beam. Color Doppler will verify the cystic nature of the lesion by showing absence of internal flow. As the lesion ages, dense calcification may develop within the adrenal gland. This will produce the opposite effect of attenuating the beam at the foci of calcification thus creating a band of decreased signal in the far field, also known as "posterior acoustic shadowing."

Differential Diagnosis

- Neuroblastoma: the main differential diagnosis of an adrenal mass in a neonate. Congenital neuroblastoma may present as a solid or cystic adrenal mass.

A complex mass that does not show the expected chronologic involution associated with adrenal hemorrhage on serial US is likely neuroblastoma. The presence of elevated urine catecholamines supports this diagnosis.

- Renal duplication with upper pole hydronephrosis: an accompanying upper pole hydroureter confirms the diagnosis. A UPJ obstruction of the upper pole moiety would be more likely to be confused with an adrenal hemorrhage.
- Subdiaphragmatic congenital pulmonary airway malformation or sequestration: a small number of congenital pulmonary airway malformations (CPAM) are subdiaphragmatic. A normal adrenal gland is seen separate from the mass. The mass demonstrates internal flow on color Doppler imaging from a systemic arterial supply.
- Congenital adrenal hyperplasia (CAH): The diagnosis may be suspected on the basis of physical examination, virilization of a female infant, salt loosing crisis, or a positive family history. Imaging demonstrates bilateral adrenal gland enlargement that may be diffuse or nodular. A wrinkled or cerebriform appearance of the adrenal cortex has also been described. The diagnosis is made on the basis of genetic markers or blood and urine tests.
- Wolman's disease: this is a rare inborn error of metabolism that results in the deposition of lipids in multiple organs. The disease presents in the newborn period with rapidly progressive hepatosplenomegaly, failure to thrive, diarrhea, vomiting, and bilateral progressive enlargement of the adrenal glands. The adrenal glands may be normal at birth. As the adrenals enlarge they maintain their shape and develop punctate parenchymal calcifications. Adrenal cortical insufficiency may occur.

Variants

Adrenal hemorrhage does occur in older children as a result of trauma and is typically associated with other traumatic injuries. Large hematomas in the neonate may rupture the adrenal capsule allowing blood products to enter the peritoneal cavity or extend into the retroperitoneal space to the wall of the scrotum. Large intraperitoneal hemorrhages may extend via the processus vaginalis into the peritesticular space in the scrotum. Adrenal abscess may rarely present as a focal mass as a result of hematogenous seeding of an adrenal hematoma or the normal adrenal gland, in a neonate with septicemia or history or maternal infection.

Key Points

- Neonatal adrenal hemorrhage is a perinatal hemorrhage associated with an episode of physical stress, coagulopathy, or trauma.
- Large or term infants are affected more often than preterm infants.
- Serial US demonstrates progressive change in echotexture, constant lack of internal blood flow and progressive decrease in size (mainstay of diagnosis of neonatal adrenal hemorrhage and helps differentiate adrenal hemorrhage from congenital neuroblastoma).
- Hemorrhage is usually unilateral, but can be bilateral.
- Dystrophic calcifications may form in resolving adrenal hemorrhages.
- Large hematomas may extend beyond the capsule into the peritoneal cavity or into the retroperitoneum.
- Transient adrenal insufficiency is uncommon, permanent adrenal insufficiency is rare.

Further Reading

Deeg KH, Bettendorf U, Hofmann V. Differential diagnosis of neonatal adrenal haemorrhage and congenital neuroblastoma by colour Doppler sonography and power Doppler sonography. *Eur J Pediatr.* 1998;*157*(4):294–297.

Kawashima A, Sandler CM, Ernst RD, Takahashi N, Roubidoux MA, Goldman SM, Fishman EK, Dunnick NR. Imaging of nontraumatic hemorrhage of the adrenal gland. *Radiographics.* 1999;*19*(4),949–963.

Schwarzler P, Bernard JP, Senat MV, Ville Y. Prenatal diagnosis of fetal adrenal masses: differentiation between hemorrhage and solid tumor by color Doppler sonography. *Ultrasound Obstet Gynecol.* 1999;*13*(5):351–355.

Westra SJ, Zaninovic AC, Hall TR, Kangarloo H, Boechat MI. Imaging of the adrenal gland in children. *RadioGraphics.* 1994;*14*(6):1323–1340.

CHAPTER 58

Neuroblastoma

Marguerite T. Parisi, MD, MS Ed

Definition

Neuroblastoma is a malignant tumor of the sympathetic nervous system whose cell of origin is derived from primitive neural crest tissues.

Clinical Features

With an incidence of 10.5 cases per 1 million children less than 15 years of age, neuroblastoma is the second most common extracranial tumor of childhood and the most common solid tumor of infancy. Neuroblastoma accounts for 8 to 10 percent of all childhood cancers and for approximately 15 percent of cancer deaths in children. The clinical presentation of neuroblastoma is highly variable, ranging from an asymptomatic mass to tumors that cause critical illness as a result of local invasion, widely metastatic disease, or both. Clinical presentation is dependent upon the site of tumor origin, the extent of disease, and the presence of paraneoplastic syndromes. Abdominal distention, pain, or palpable mass are the most common complaints, but fever, irritability, malaise, weight loss, shortness of breath, and peripheral neurologic defect from spinal canal invasion (5 to 15 percent) also occur. Other less common presentations include:

- Opsoclonus-myoclonus: myotonic jerking, random eye movements, +/-cerebellar ataxia (1 to 3 percent)
- Horner syndrome: unilateral ptosis, myosis, and anhydrosis resulting from cervical or thoracic tumor
- "Raccoon eyes": periorbital swelling, proptosis, and ecchymoses resulting from periorbital disease
- Pepper syndrome: massive hepatic metastatic involvement with or without respiratory distress
- Kerner-Morrison syndrome: intractable diarrhea from tumor secretion of vasointestinal peptides
- Hutchinson syndrome: limping and irritability associated with bone and marrow metastases
- Neurocristopathy syndrome: neuroblastoma associated with congenital hypoventilation syndrome, Hirschsprung's disease or other neural crest disorders

Neuroblastoma can arise anywhere along the sympathetic chain. Approximately 65 percent of neuroblastomas arise in the retroperitoneum, the majority in the adrenal gland. Other primary tumor sites include the neck (5 percent), the posterior mediastinum (15 to 20 percent), and the pelvis (3 percent). In 1 percent of patients, the primary tumor is not detectable. Median age at diagnosis is 17 months. Over 50 percent of infants and 70 percent of older children with neuroblastoma have metastases at diagnosis. Disease dissemination occurs via lymphatic and hematogenous routes with bone, bone marrow, liver, lymph nodes, and skin being the most common sites of metastatic disease.

Anatomy and Physiology

Until recently, little was known about the genetic basis of neuroblastoma. Recent genetic associations have been identified and include:

- Anaplastic lymphoma kinase (ALK) oncogene accounts for most cases of hereditary neuroblastoma.
- Those with either sporadic or familial neuroblastoma have loss of function mutations in the homeobox gene PHOX2B.
- Alleles with single-nucleotide polymorphism within the putative genes FLJ22536 at chromosome band 6p22.3 and BARD1 at 2q35 are enriched in neuroblastoma patients.
- A copy-number variation at 1q21 is associated with neuroblastoma development.
- *Myc*-N oncogene located on the distal end of chromosome arm 2p is amplified in up to 35 percent of neuroblastomas and associated with rapidly progressive disease and poor outcome.
- Gains of all or parts of chromosome 17 or 17q occur in >60 percent of neuroblastomas.

These findings suggest that this cancer is influenced by common DNA variations in which neuroblastoma cells often suffer from extensive, nonrandom genetic damage at multiple genetic loci.

Imaging Features

Radiography:

- Soft-tissue mass and/or mass effect with calcifications detectable in 30 to 50 percent (Fig. 58.1A)
- Splaying or erosion of adjacent ribs in posterior mediastinal tumors (Fig. 58.2)
- Pedicle erosion from intraspinal extension in posterior mediastinal or retroperitoneal disease
- Lytic bone lesions (Fig.58.1B)
- Periostitis
- Metaphyseal lucent lines

US:

- Echogenic, heterogenous soft-tissue mass +/- necrosis or hemorrhage; increased vascularity on color Doppler
- Calcification: focal echogenic areas +/- posterior acoustic shadowing or diffuse increased echogenicity

CT:

- Typically large, heterogenous mass with calcifications in 80 to 90 percent (Fig. 58.3A-C)
- Mass often crosses midline and encases rather than displaces surrounding vessels
- Invasion into spinal canal and effectively excludes Wilms' tumor
- Hepatic metastases: focal hypoattenuating mass(es) or diffuse infiltration
- Nodal metastases: calcification (Fig. 58.5A)
- CT essential in detection of pulmonary and pleural metastases

MRI:

- Preferred modality to evaluate tumors adjacent to or invading the spinal canal (Fig. 58.4)
- Heterogeneous, variably enhancing, low T1 and high T2 signal intensity (SI)
- Calcifications may be difficult to detect
- Marrow infiltration: low T1, high T2 SI

Nuclear medicine:

- Tc-99m MDP-positive in most primary soft-tissue lesions (Fig. 58.3D)
- Osseous metastases: areas of increased or decreased radiotracer uptake in metaphyses of both the appendicular and axial skeleton, often symmetric (Fig. 58.5B-C)
- I-123 MIBG (Fig. 58.3E): high sensitivity (90 percent) and specificity (nearly 100 percent); uncomplicated normal biodistribution (expected uptake in salivary glands, heart, liver, urinary bladder) and lack of uptake in normal bone eases scan interpretation and improves rates of disease detection compared to anatomic imaging and bone scan; detects sites of both cortical bone and bone marrow involvement by neuroblastoma, unlike Tc-99m MDP bone scan which images only cortical bone; allows functional assessment to help differentiate active tumor from post-therapy change; when labeled with I-131 or I-125, can be used as a radiotherapeutic agent
- Somatostatin receptors imaging (e.g., Octreotide): present on neuroblastoma cells; imaging with

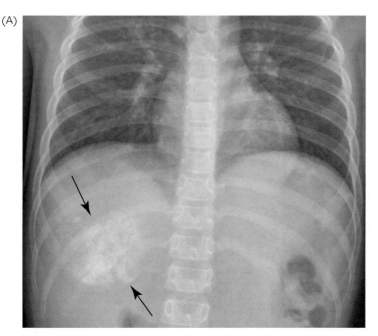
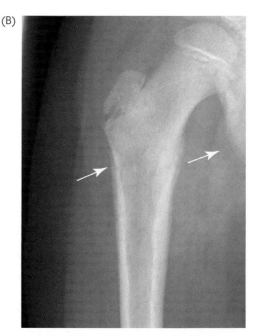

Figure 58.1. Frontal abdominal radiograph (A) in a 7-year-old with newly diagnosed neuroblastoma shows a calcified right-upper quadrant mass (white arrow). Frontal radiograph of the femur (B) shows a proximal metaphyseal lytic lesion (black arrow) with associated periosteal reaction making this stage 4.

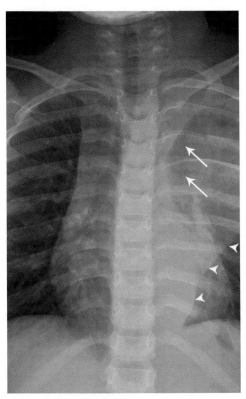

Figure 58.2. Frontal chest radiograph in a 5-year-old with stage 3 high-risk neuroblastoma shows a posterior mediastinal mass (arrowheads) with rib splaying (arrows).

Indium-111 label is sensitive but nonspecific; normal biodistribution with marked uptake in liver, spleen, kidneys, and gut may obscure tumor visualization; higher patient radiation dose than Tc-99m MDP, I-123 MIBG, and FDG-PET

- Radiolabeled monoclonal antibodies imaging: sensitive, specific; use as potential targeted radiotherapeutic agent but not readily available
- Fluoride-18 Fluorodeoxyglucose PET or PET/CT (FDG-PET): uptake in majority of primary tumors prior to chemo or radiation therapy; useful in the 10 percent of neuroblastomas that are poorly or non-MIBG-avid at diagnosis; should be used when disease involvement on CT or MRI appears more extensive than demonstrated on I-123 MIBG; or when MIBG-negative disease recurrence is suspected; role still debatable
- Other non-FDG-PET agents: C-11 epinephrine; C-11 hydroxyephedrine; 6-[F-18]fluorodopamine; 6-[F-18]fluoronorepinephrine; 6-[F18]fluorometaraminol; [F-18]fluoroiodobenzylguanidine; exploit catecholamine transport and storage systems that characterize adrenergic tissues and related tumors; expensive; not readily available; roles remain in evolution

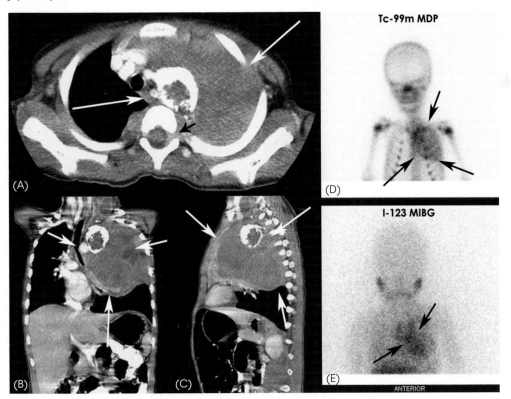

Figure 58.3. Axial (A), coronal (B), and sagittal (C) CT images of the chest in a 3-year-old girl with dyspnea demonstrate a large, calcified mass (white arrows) in the left thorax which causes tracheal displacement, encases vessels, and invades the spinal canal (black arrow), findings consistent with neuroblastoma. Anterior views of the head and chest from a nuclear medicine bone scan (D) and corresponding views from a I-123 MIBG scan (E) demonstrate abnormal radiotracer uptake in the primary mass in the left-upper thorax (black arrows). Uptake on I-123 MIBG scan confirms the diagnosis of neuroblastoma.

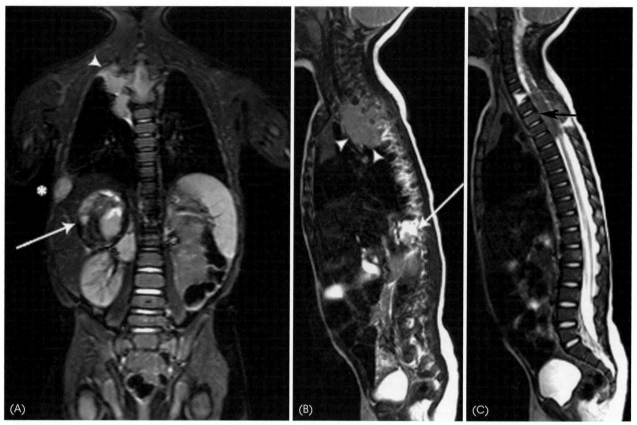

Figure 58.4. Coronal T1 (A) and sagittal T2 (B, C) images from an MRI of an 18-month-old with neuroblastoma who presented with progressive difficulty walking show a heterogeneous, hemorrhagic right adrenal mass (white arrow), with widely metastatic disease including a right paraspinal mass extending into the neural foramina and causing cord compression at T2 to T6 (arrowheads) and a right rib lesion (*). Increased signal within vertebral bodies at the T3 and L1 levels are indicative of marrow metastases (black arrow).

IMAGING PITFALLS: Neuroblastoma can spread along the retroperitoneum, invade the kidney, and mimic renal origin. In greater than 90% of cases, MIBG imaging can distinguish neuroblastoma from renal tumors which do not exhibit MIBG avidity (Fig. 58.6).

Imaging Strategy

The primary mass is often detected on US. Contrast-enhanced CT or MRI is used for further evaluation, to determine the organ of origin, and define local extent. A CT chest scan is required for detection of pleural metastases. Spinal MRI must be performed if the primary tumor extends into the spinal canal or if the patient presents with neurologic impairment/paralysis. Contrast-enhanced CT brain or MRI is recommended if the patient presents with "raccoon eyes," other appropriate clinical symptoms, or to elucidate sites of disease identified as part of the metastatic workup. For initial metastatic evaluation and response to therapeutic intervention, Tc99m MDP bone scan is performed. For serial follow-up, bone scan is performed if

tumor MIBG-negative. An I-123 MIBG scan is performed at diagnosis and in serial follow-up if primary tumor is MIBG-avid at diagnosis. In neuroblastoma FDG-PET imaging is reserved for patients who are MIBG-negative at diagnosis or following bone marrow transplant and for those who have either residual soft-tissue disease or are suspected of disease recurrence.

Related Physics

Neuroblastoma can be elegantly imaged with US to show its unique properties of vascular encasement, retroaortic extension, and lack of renal vein extension which will differentiate it from Wilms' tumor. This requires both gray-scale and Doppler techniques. Power Doppler is a method used to show low flow without directional information. In the case of neuroblastoma, power Doppler images will show some flow in the vascular tumor that surrounds the intensely flowing aorta, celiac, or superior mesenteric artery. With Wilms' there will be displacement of aorta and inferior vena cava posteriorly and contralaterally without retroaortic

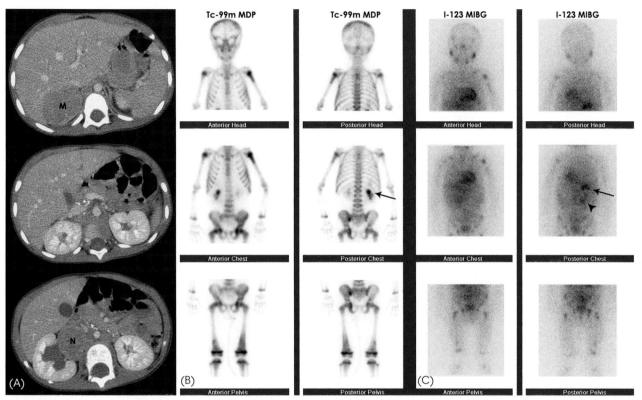

Figure 58.5. Axial CT (A) in a 3-year-old with newly diagnosed neuroblastoma demonstrates a right suprarenal mass (M), with scattered retroperitoneal calcifications and a nodal metastasis (N) in the renal hilum. Tc-99m MDP bone scan (B) and corresponding anterior and posterior views from a I-123 MIBG scan (C) show the primary mass (black arrow); the nodal mass is only depicted on MIBG scan (black arrow). Diffuse osseous disease is present, the full extent easier to depict on the MIBG scan (because there is no expected bone uptake in the absence of disease). This is particularly evident in the proximal femurs where symmetric disease adjacent to the normally radio-avid physeal plates makes detection on bone scan particularly difficult.

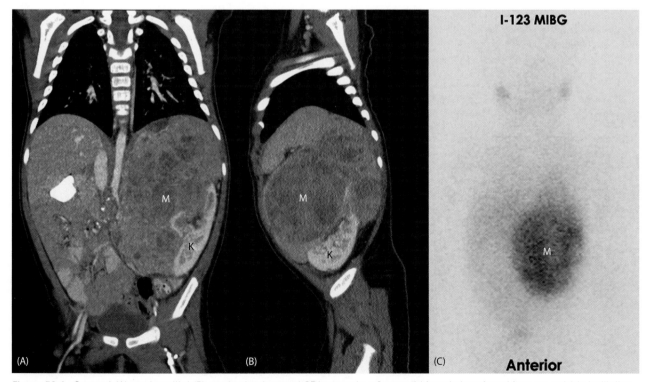

Figure 58.6. Coronal (A) and sagittal (B) contrast-enhanced CT images in a 1-year-old female transferred from an outside institution for evaluation of a "renal mass" demonstrate a large mass (M) with speckled calcification either arising from or invading the left kidney (K). I-123 MIBG image (C) shows marked uptake excluding Wilms' tumor and confirming a diagnosis of neuroblastoma.

extension. Doppler has the added advantage of ruling out renal vein extension in the cases of Wilms'. Power Doppler is easily adjusted by a single setting which adjusts transmit and receive gain, which allows for low flow (venous) and high flow (arterial) detection. Flow is displayed in a grade of yellow to orange to red for high to low flow.

Differential Diagnosis

- Adrenal hemorrhage (infants): decreased echogenicity and avascular on US; MIBG-negative
- Wilms' tumor (older child): renal origin; "claw" sign; displaces vessels; calcifications rare; invades renal vein, IVC; pulmonary metastases common; bone metastases rare; MIBG-negative
- Pheochromocytoma
- Adrenocortical carcinoma

Common Variants

Ganglioneuroblastoma and ganglioneuroma are also tumors that originate from primordial neural crest cells. They differ from neuroblastoma in their degree of cellular and extracellular maturation. Ganglioneuroblastoma, composed of both mature gangliocytes and immature neuroblasts, is intermediate between the highly malignant neuroblastoma and the more benign ganglioneuroma. Ganglioneuroma, composed of gangliocytes and mature stroma, presents in older children (median age of approximately 7 years), with a slight female predominance. It is radiologically difficult to distinguish neuroblastoma, ganglioneuroblastoma, and ganglioneuroma, as imaging features are very similar with one exception: metastases are rare in ganglioneuroma.

Clinical Issues

Approximately 85% of patients have elevated urinary catecholamine levels at diagnosis. Prognosis is highly variable and dependent upon patient age, stage, and the presence of biologic factors such as ploidy and MYC-N amplification. Treatment spans a wide gamut ranging from supportive care with no treatment (some stage 4s) to simple excision (stage 1) or intensive chemotherapy followed by autologous bone marrow transplant (stage 4). Given this, the ability to provide whole-body assessment of disease extent is crucial for accurate diagnosis, staging, and therapeutic response monitoring. Neuroblastoma is staged according to the International Neuroblastoma Staging System as follows:

Stage 1: localized tumor with complete gross resection. No regional lymph node involvement

Stage 2: localized tumor with incomplete gross resection or ipsilateral lymph node involvement

Stage 3: tumor crossing midline or tumor with contralateral lymph node involvement

Stage 4: tumor with distant metastases

Stage 4s: patients younger than 12 months of age with localized tumor and metastases confined to liver, skin, and/or bone marrow

Patients with stages 1, 2, or 4s disease typically have an excellent prognosis with overall 5-year survival ranging from 85 to 95 percent compared to 30 to 45% survival for those with stage 4 disease.

Key Points

- Protean disease with course and treatment determined by patient age, stage, and histology
- Many syndromic associations and presentations, including opsoclonus-myoclonus, "racoon eyes," and watery diarrhea, among others
- Large, calcified mass, which often crosses midline and encases rather than displaces vessels
- Spinal canal invasion excludes Wilms' tumor
- Over 90% of neuroblastomas MIBG-avid

Further Reading

Kushner BH. Neuroblastoma: A disease requiring a multitude of imaging studies. *J Nucl Med.* 2004; *45*(7):1172–1188.

Lonergan GJ, Schwab CM, Suarez ES, Carlson CL. Neuroblastoma, ganglioneuroblastoma, and ganglioneuroma: radiologic-pathologic correlation. *Radiographics.* 2002;*22*(4):911–934.

Maris JM. Recent advances in neuroblastoma. *N Engl J Med.* 2010;*362*(23):2202–2211.

Park JR, Eggert A, Caron H. Neuroblastoma: biology, prognosis, and treatment. *Hematol Oncol Clin North Am.* 2010;*24*(1):65–86.

Rosenfield NS, Leonidas JC, Barwick KW. Aggressive neuroblastoma simulating Wilms tumor. *Radiology.* 1988;*166*(1): 165–167.

Sharp SE, Gelfand MJ, Shulkin BL. Pediatrics: diagnosis of neuroblastoma. *Semin Nucl Med.* 2011;*41*(5):345–353.

Sharp SE, Shulkin BL, Gelfand MJ, Salisbury S, Furman WL. 123I-MIBG scintigraphy and 18F-FDG PET in neuroblastoma. *J Nucl Med.* 2009;*50*(8):1237–43.

CHAPTER 59

Genitourinary Rhabdomyosarcoma

Jamie L. Coleman, MD

Definition

Rhabdomyosarcoma (RMS) is a soft-tissue malignancy arising in the male or female genitourinary (GU) tract including the bladder, prostate, paratesticular tissues, vagina, or cervix/uterus.

Clinical Features

Accounting for 5 to 8 percent of childhood cancers, RMS is the most common soft-tissue tumor of childhood. Sites of origin are head and neck region (35 to 40 percent), GU tract (25 percent), extremities (20 percent), and other sites. The clinical presentation of RMS depends largely on the location of the tumor. Tumors arising in the bladder may cause hematuria and urinary obstruction. In boys, prostatic tumors may grow quite large and result in urinary symptoms such as obstruction, frequency, or both, as well as constipation from mass effect on the rectosigmoid colon. In the paratesticular soft tissues, a painless mass or swelling is often noted. Young girls with vaginal tumors may present with a mucosanguineous discharge or a polypoid mass protruding from the vagina. Cervical/uterine tumors are more common in adolescents. There is a better prognosis overall with tumors arising in the vagina/testes than prostate/bladder.

Anatomy and Physiology

Rhabdomyosarcoma arises from immature precursor cells of striated skeletal muscle that can be present anywhere in the body. It is a small round blue cell tumor of childhood along with Ewing sarcoma, neuroblastoma, and lymphoma. Most cases of GU RMS are sporadic, but there is an association with inherited syndromes such as Li-Fraumeni syndrome, Costello syndrome, neurofibromatosis type 1, and Beckwith-Wiedemann syndrome. In general, the precise etiology and risk factors are unclear.

Imaging Findings

Radiography:
- Mass or low intestinal obstruction

US:
- Heterogenous pelvic mass with flow on color Doppler
- "Bunch of grapes": sarcoma botryoides (protruding from introitus in female)
- Hydroureteronephrosis and bladder distension
- Hyperemic scrotal mass (extratesticular tumor)

CT/MRI:
- Heterogeneous enhancement with areas of necrosis (Figs. 59.1, 59.2)
- Center of mass in prostate/bladder base or vagina (Fig. 59.3)

F-18 FDG-PET:
- FDG avidity with areas of necrosis (Fig. 59.4)

Imaging Strategy

Depending on the location, US is often the best first test. If the mass is large or attached to the bladder, a complete US assessment would include evaluation of the kidneys to exclude hydronephrosis. Contrast-enhanced CT can yield significant information about the location, size, and extent of a tumor, associated regional or distant adenopathy and is the modality of choice for detecting pulmonary metastases. Multiplanar reconstructions in the coronal and sagittal plane are often helpful. For tumor evaluation MRI is superior to CT because of its superior soft-tissue contrast, multiplanar capabilities, and lack of ionizing radiation. The detail available on MRI may best depict bladder invasion in tumors of prostatic origin as well as invasion into adjacent structures and will allow the detection of adenopathy. FDG-PET imaging is helpful in assessing the metabolic activity and extent of the primary tumor as well as evaluating metastatic disease and in therapy follow-up.

Related Physics

Sarcoma botryoides is characterized by multiple cystic lesions within soft tissue of the pelvis, likened to a "bunch of grapes." Imaging such a mass with US can be a challenge in the presence of inadequate transducer designs that incorporate large elevational image thickness. Similar to slice thickness in CT or MRI, the elevational image thickness represents the beam thickness. As with CT and MRI, a thickness that exceeds the Z-axis diameter of the lesion will cause partial volume effects, which include diminution of image contrast between the lesion and surrounding structures and the possibility of places artifactual echoes inside anechoic structures. Modern transducer configurations allow for Z-axis beam focusing in two-dimensional arrays.

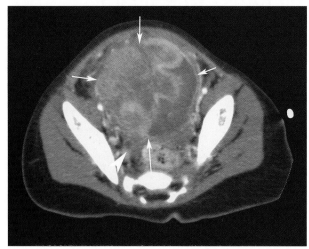

Figure 59.1. Axial contrast-enhanced CT image in a 2-year-old girl with hematuria shows an irregular lobular enhancing mass within the bladder (arrows) with wall thickening, large feeding vessels, and the mildly dilated distal right ureter (arrowhead). Pathology was embryonal rhabdomyosarcoma of the botryoid type.

Differential Diagnosis
- Extraosseous Ewing sarcoma
- Nonrhabdomyomatous sarcoma
- Neuroblastoma
- Lymphoma
- Epididymoorchitis (paratesticular mass)

Common Variants
- Alveolar RMS
- Sarcoma botryoides

Clinical Issues
Significant functional morbidity often complicates en bloc resection of large pelvic tumors, because operative

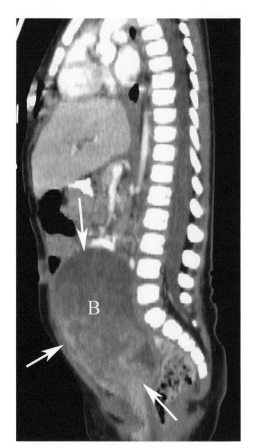

Figure 59.3. Sagittal reconstruction in a 2-year-old girl with hematuria demonstrates the lobular mass (arrows) within the bladder (B).

intervention may require complete pelvic exenteration and creation of a diverting ileostomy and colostomy. For this reason preoperative chemotherapy is often employed to debulk the tumor for easier surgical resection. The surgical approach to paratesticular tumors consists of radical

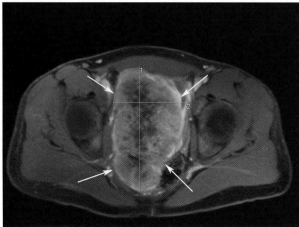

Figure 59.2. Axial contrast-enhanced T1 MR image with fat suppression in a 17-year-old male with pelvic discomfort and urinary retention shows a large, enhancing, heterogeneous, and centrally necrotic mass deep in the pelvis, suspected to arise from the prostate (arrows).

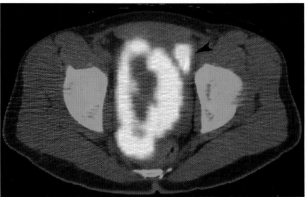

Figure 59.4. Axial fused F-18 FDG-PET CT image suppression in a 17-year-old male with pelvic discomfort and urinary retention shows intense FDG avidity in the periphery of the tumor with central photopenia consistent with necrosis seen on MR. A portion of the displaced urinary bladder containing excreted urine is seen anteriorly and to the left (arrowhead). Transrectal biopsy confirmed prostatic rhabdomyosarcoma, embryonal subtype.

inguinal orchiectomy and resection of the spermatic cord. Enlarged or suspicious lymph nodes identified on imaging or at the time of surgery must be sampled or removed as these directly impact staging and prognosis. Radiation therapy is an integral part of therapy for higher stages.

Key Points

- Small round blue cell tumor of childhood
- GU tract is second most common primary site of rhabdomyosarcoma
- Two main types: embryonal (80%) and alveolar (20%)
- Favorable sites are vagina and testes
- US is the first-line test for assessment of tumor and hydroureteronephrosis from bladder outlet obstruction

Further Reading

Kaste SC, McCarville MB. Imaging pediatric abdominal tumors. *Seminars in Roentgenology.* 2008;*43*(1):50–59.

Mak CW, Chou CK, Su CC, Huan SK, Chang JM. Ultrasound diagnosis of paratesticular rhabdomyosarcoma. *British Journal of Radiology.* 2004;*77*(915):250–252.

Stehr M. Pediatric urologic rhabdomyosarcoma. *Current Opinion in Urology.* 2009;*19*(4):402–406.

Van Rijn RR, Wilde JC, Bras J, Oldenburger F, McHugh KM, Merks JH. Imaging findings in noncraniofacial childhood rhabdomysarcoma. *Pediatric Radiology.* 2008;*38*(6):617–634.

CHAPTER 60

Sacrococcygeal Teratoma

Geetika Khanna, MD, MS

Definition

Sacrococcygeal teratoma (SCT) is a tumor arising from the pericoccygeal tissues composed of all three germ cell layers (ectoderm, mesoderm, and endoderm).

Clinical Features

Sacrococcygeal teratoma is the most common germ cell tumor in children and the most common solid tumor in neonates. With the increased use of prenatal ultrasound (US), most SCTs are discovered during routine obstetric screening, typically during the second trimester. Fetal SCTs can cause polyhydramnios, premature labor, dystocia, tumor hemorrhage/rupture, obstructive uropathy, and fetal hydrops. In the newborn, SCT presents as a large exophytic pelvic mass. If the teratoma is predominantly intrapelvic in location it may present with mild swelling of the buttock region, constipation secondary to mass effect on the rectum, or pelvic masses that are palpable on rectal examination. Sacrococcygeal teratomas are 3 to 4 times more common in females than in males.

Anatomy and Physiology

Sacrococcygeal teratomas are thought to develop from the totipotential residual cells of Hensen's node, a primitive streak in the coccygeal region. Normally the primitive streak degenerates, but remnants may remain in the sacrococcygeal region and develop into teratomas. A positive family history of twins in many patients leads some to believe that SCT may be a form of incomplete twinning. As the lesions are present in a developing fetus, mass effect may adversely affect the development of surrounding structures with anterior displacement of the anus, anorectal malformation, bladder outlet obstruction, obstructive nephropathy, sacral anomalies, and intraspinal invasion, causing neurologic deficits. Solid SCT can be highly vascular with intratumoral shunting that can result in fetal hydrops, a poor prognostic sign. Based on the presence or absence of malignant components, SCTs are classified as mature or immature. Immature teratomas tend to be bulkier and more solid than their mature counterparts, are more likely to recur locally and have malignant degeneration. Immature teratomas can also

contain foci of endodermal sinus tumors and less often choriocarcinoma.

Imaging Findings

- Midline mass extending from the sacrococcygeal region
- Coccyx rarely involved unless the tumor is malignant
- Ranges from 1 to 30 centimeters (average 8 cm; Fig. 60.1)
- Heterogeneous with variable cystic and solid components
- Calcification/ossification (up to 50%)
- Four main types:
  - Type 1: predominantly external with only a minimal presacral component
  - Type 2: external with significant intrapelvic extension (Fig. 60.2)
  - Type 3: minimal perineal bulging but mostly intrapelvic (Fig. 60.3)
  - Type 4: presacral with no external component
- US: complex mass with solid and cystic areas and focal areas of increased echogenicity that may represent calcifications and/or fat within the tumor
- CT: solid portions enhanced; fatty components well-demonstrated

Imaging Strategy

Prenatal US may demonstrate a mass in the sacrococcygeal region. The fetal spine should be meticulously evaluated to rule out spinal dysraphism, as a meningomyelocele is the primary differential. The next step in imaging is fetal MRI to confirm the presence of a mass, characterize its internal components (cystic/solid), evaluate its extent, and identify associated fetal anomalies. If SCT is confirmed, serial US should be performed to evaluate growth and identify findings that suggest poor prognosis, such as fetal hydrops, placentomegaly, and polyhydramnios. Plain radiography will identify tumor-related calcification and associated sacral anomalies in the newborn. To determine the degree of intrapelvic extension (or type), CT or MRI of the pelvis is required; however, MRI is the preferred modality to rule out intraspinal extension. Bladder catheter and rectal tube may be helpful to

(A)

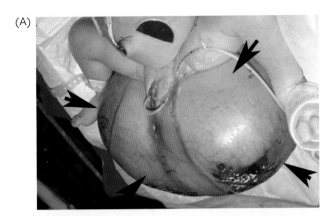

(B)

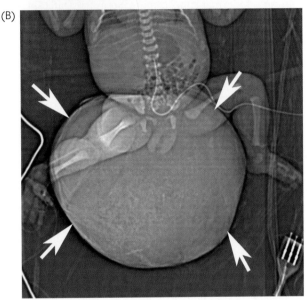

Figure 60.1. Photograph (A) and CT topogram (B) of a baby born with a large buttock mass (arrows) show a large SCT causing marked abduction of the lower extremities.

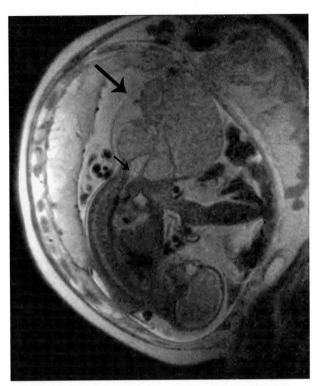

Figure 60.2. Sagittal HASTE MR image of a fetus following US detection of pelvic mass shows a large predominantly solid mass protruding externally from the pelvis (large arrow) with a small intrapelvic component (small arrow) consistent with a type 2 SCT.

The displaced tissues will be "misregistered" more deeply in the image because of a delay in transmission and return of sound through the slower fatty medium.

provide landmarks for imaging especially if the mass is large. Chest CT is performed for malignant lesions for staging.

Related Physics

Sacrococcygeal teratoma is characterized by multiple tissue types that can often be differentiated with US. This is accomplished by taking advantage of various US artifacts including reverberation, through-transmission enhancement, interface displacement resulting from sound speed differences, shadowing, and Rayleigh scattering. The cystic components can create reverberation or enhancement depending on cyst size relative to wavelength used. Reverberation occurs in very small cystic structures where the size is near the wavelength of the sound beam (1 to 2 mm). When cysts are larger than this, through-transmission enhancement is more common. With fatty components, there are large speed differences between fat and surrounding soft tissues (1490 m/s vs. 1540 m/s, respectively) which can displace tissues deep to the fat as a result of deceleration of sound within the fat.

Differential Diagnosis

Cystic SCT:

- Meningocele (typically more superior to the sacrococcygeal region, always associated with sacral dysraphism, and lack the septations seen with cystic teratomas)
- Dermoid cyst (can have fat and calcification)
- Enteric duplication cyst (can occur in the presacral space as well-marginated cystic lesions that share a wall with the rectum; lumen of duplication cyst may communicate with the rectal lumen
- Lymphatic malformation

Solid SCT:

- Ewings sarcoma
- Rhabdomyosarcoma
- Neurogenic tumors such as neuroblastoma and peripheral nerve sheath tumors

Common Variants

Sacrococcygeal teratoma can occur as part of Currarino's triad ("ASP triad": *a*norectal malformation, *s*acrococcygeal osseous defect, and *p*resacral mass).

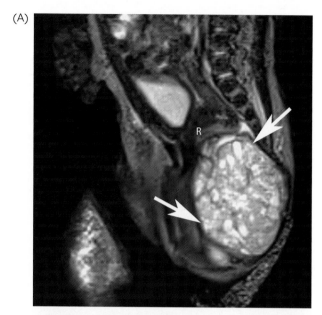

(A)

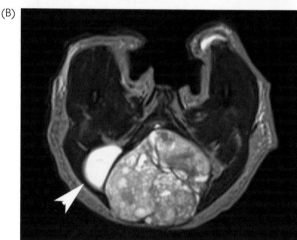

(B)

Figure 60.3. Sagittal (A) and axial (B) T2 MR images in a newborn girl with bulging perineum show a mass inferior to the spine with a large presacral component (arrows) displacing the rectum (R) anteriorly. A small portion of the mass protrudes into the gluteal region (arrowhead) consistent with a type 3 SCT.

Clinical Issues

When discovered prenatally, SCT has a significantly worse prognosis. Mortality rate of SCT detected in the fetus is almost 50 percent, in contrast to 5 percent when detected in the neonatal period. Fetal teratomas can result in fetal demise secondary to fetal hydrops, premature labor, intratumoral hemorrhage, and dystocia. In the postnatal period, the main treatment for a benign SCT is complete surgical resection and coccygectomy. If the coccyx is not resected, approximately one-third of these tumors can recur. Malignant SCT requires surgical resection and multiagent chemotherapy. Poor prognostic factors for tumor recurrence/malignant transformation include older age at diagnosis, types 3 and 4 (as they are more likely to be diagnosed in older children), and mixed malignant teratomas/endodermal sinus tumors. Serum alphafetoprotein levels are positive in teratoma and useful to monitor tumor activity.

Key Points

- The sacrococcygeal region is the most common location of teratomas in the newborn.
- The lesion is most commonly solid/cystic arising inferior to the coccyx with variable degrees of intrapelvic and extrapelvic extension.
- Fetal SCT requires close US surveillance to detect complications such as polyhydramnios, placentomegaly, and fetal hydrops.

Further Reading

Hedrick HL, Flake AW, Crombleholme TM, et al. Sacrococcygeal teratoma: prenatal assessment, fetal intervention, and outcome. *J Pediatr Surg.* 2004;39(3):430–438.

Keslar PJ, Buck JL, Suarez ES. Germ cell tumors of the sacrococcygeal region: radiologic-pathologic correlation. *Radiographics.* 1994;14(3):607–620.

Kocaoglu M, Frush DP. Pediatric presacral masses. *Radiographics.* 2006;26(3):833–857.

Woodward PJ, Sohaey R, Kennedy A, Koeller KK. From the archives of the AFIP: a comprehensive review of fetal tumors with pathologic correlation. *Radiographics.* 2005;25(1):215–242.

CHAPTER 61

Ovarian Torsion

Geetika Khanna, MD, MS

Definition

Ovarian torsion refers to partial or complete twisting of the ovarian vascular pedicle resulting in a compromise of its blood supply. Adnexal torsion refers to torsion of the ovary, the fallopian tube, or both structures together.

Clinical Features

Symptoms of adnexal torsion in children are often nonspecific such as abdominal pain, nausea, and vomiting. If torsion has advanced to ovarian infarction, fever and peritonitis may be present. Neonates present differently related to limitations in assessing their pain. Presenting features are often demonstrated on prenatal imaging, followed by palpable mass and feeding intolerance.

Anatomy and Physiology

Ovarian torsion has a bimodal distribution at < 1 year of age and 11 to 18 years. In contrast to adult women, ovarian torsion in children is most often associated with normal ovaries, followed by an ovarian cyst or a benign tumor. Proposed etiologies for torsion of normal ovaries in children include: congenitally long ligaments, laxity of the mesovarium, sudden changes of intraabdominal pressure related to exercise, and spasm of the fallopian tube. Adnexal masses can predispose the ovary to twist on its vascular pedicle. The most commonly identified benign tumor in torsed ovaries is a mature teratoma. Twisting of the adnexal pedicle obstructs the lymphatic drainage resulting in enlargement of the ovary. This is followed by obstruction of the venous drainage resulting in hemorrhagic infarction. Finally, the arterial supply is obstructed resulting in necrosis.

Imaging Findings

The single most important criterion for diagnosis of ovarian torsion is ovarian size. Ovarian enlargement greater than 5 centimeters has a reported sensitivity of 83 percent. An adnexal volume < 20 milliliters is strong evidence against a diagnosis of ovarian torsion. The torsed ovary is larger in size compared to the normal contralateral ovary, with an average adnexal ratio of 12 to 15 times (Fig. 61.1A). Edema of the torsed ovary can displace the ovarian follicles

to the periphery ("string-of-pearls" sign) and fluid-debris levels may be present in the follicles (Fig. 61.1B). Doppler evaluation is neither sensitive nor specific for the diagnosis of ovarian torsion. Flow may not be detected in normal pediatric ovaries. Flow, especially arterial flow, may be present in a torsed ovary if the torsion is intermittent or early/partial. Typical CT findings of ovarian torsion are a well-defined adnexal mass, deviation of the uterus to the involved side, and free fluid in the pelvis (Fig. 61.2A). The enlarged adnexa may be midline in position, often located in the pouch of Douglas behind the uterus (Fig. 61.2B).

Imaging Strategy

Pelvic ultrasound (US) is the imaging modality of choice for evaluation of ovarian torsion. This is often limited to the transabdominal approach in the pediatric patient. The US should include both gray-scale and Doppler evaluation, keeping in mind that the gray-scale findings are most important in making a diagnosis of ovarian torsion.

Related Physics

Transducer selection is the single most important factor in obtaining high-resolution imaging of the female genitourinary system. An array of probes is available for this diagnosis and includes extracorporeal and transvaginal (intracavitary) probes. Extracorporeal probes use the full bladder as an "acoustic window," the principal being that the full bladder presents a minimally attenuating path to the uterus and ovaries. The choice of extracorporeal probe is dictated by body habitus whereby larger patients must be scanned with lower frequency, to the detriment of image resolution. These probes are available in a range of 2 to 9 megahertz. Where clinically appropriate, transvaginal probes are optimal in that they are not dependent on body habitus, and by eliminating multiple attenuating layers from the transmission path, higher-spatial-resolution images are generated. This allows one to use higher-frequency probes as lesser depth of penetration is required. Transvaginal probes are available in a frequency range of 8 to 15 megahertz and optimize both B-mode and color Doppler imaging. The latter facilitates discrimination from other pathologies such as ectopic pregnancy.

(A)

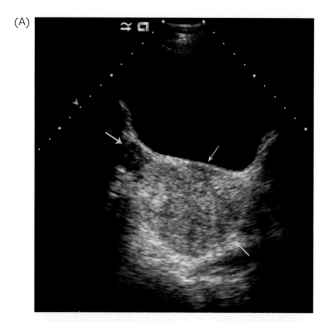

(B)

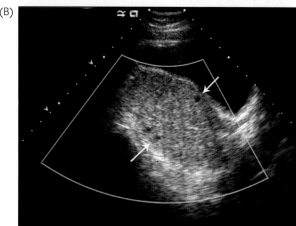

Figure 61.1. Transverse gray-scale US image (A) in a child with abdominal pain shows a large well-circumscribed pelvic mass in the midline (thin arrows), with a normal appearing right ovary (thick arrow). Sagittal US image with color Doppler (B) shows lack of flow in the mass with "string of pearls" (arrows).

(A)

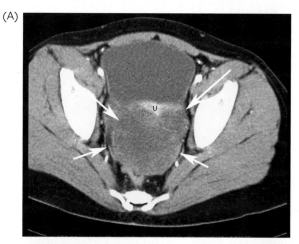

(B)

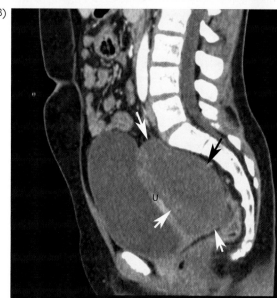

Figure 61.2. Axial contrast-enhanced CT image (A) in an 11-year-old girl with 2 weeks of abdominal pain, nausea, and vomiting shows a well-circumscribed midline pelvic mass (arrows) situated behind the uterus (U). Sagittal reconstructed image (B) confirms the location of the mass (arrows) in the pouch of Douglas (U: uterus).

Differential Diagnosis

- Hemorrhagic ovarian cyst: blood products in the cyst can have a variable appearance including a reticular pattern, echogenic retracting clot, or fluid-fluid level. Clinical evaluation is important in differentiating this from ovarian torsion.

Common Variants

Antenatal ovarian torsion can result in autoamputation of the ovary, which may then present as a wandering cyst with a fluid-fluid level or calcified mass in the abdominal cavity.

Clinical Issues

A conservative surgical approach with ovarian detorsion is now established as the treatment of choice. Follow-up

US, performed about 6 weeks postoperatively, can assist in excluding underlying cyst or tumor after the ovarian edema has resolved. Oophoropexy to prevent future episodes of torsion remains a controversial topic.

Key Points

- Ovarian torsion has a bimodal distribution in children: < 1 year of age and 11 to 18 years of age.
- The most constant finding in ovarian torsion is an enlarged ovary.
- Doppler evaluation is neither sensitive nor specific in making this diagnosis.
- Adnexal masses predispose the ovary to torse, though ovarian torsion in children is most often associated with normal ovaries.

Further Reading

Chang HC, Bhatt S, Dogra VS. Pearls and pitfalls in diagnosis of ovarian torsion. *Radiographics*. 2008;28(5):1355–1368.

Hiller N, Appelbaum L, Simanovsky N, Lev-Sagi A, Aharoni D, Sella T. CT features of adnexal torsion. *AJR Am J Roentgenol*. 2007;189(1):124–129.

Linam LE, Darolia R, Naffaa LN, Breech LL, O'hara SM, Hillard PJ, Huppert JS. US findings of ad exam torsion in children and adolescents: size really does matter. *Pediatr Radiol*. 2007;37(10):1013–1019.

Servaes S, Zurakowski D, Laufer MR, Feins N, Chow JS. Sonographic findings of ovarian torsion in children. *Pediatr Radiol*. 2007;37(5):446–451.

CHAPTER 62

Epididymitis-Epididymoorchitis

Himabindu Mikkilineni, MD and Pinar Karakas, MD

Definition

Epididymitis is defined as inflammation of the epididymis, and epididymoorchitis involves both the epididymis and testis together. These conditions may occur with or without infection.

Clinical Features

These entities are common in childhood and account for up to two-thirds of all cases of acute scrotum. In prepubertal children the most common cause of epididymitis is idiopathic. There is a bimodal distribution: under 2 years of age and over 6 years of age. If bacteria are detected, the most common causes are E. coli and Proteus Mirabilis. In postpubertal sexually active boys, infection is the most common cause of epididymitis. Chlamydia and gonorrhea are the most common organisms. Other causes, although not frequent, include systemic diseases such as serositis (Kawasaki disease) and vasculitis (Henoch Schonlein purpura). Epididymitis can also be reactive and induced by trauma, torsion of the appendix, or surgical manipulation of the genitourinary (GU) tract. Recurrent chemical or infectious epididymitis can be seen in patients with underlying functional and anatomic abnormalities of the GU tract. Patients present with acute scrotal pain, swelling, and redness. The pain is usually relieved by elevating the testicles above the symphysis pubis, which is known as the Prehn sign. The cremasteric reflex is preserved. In contrast, the Prehn sign and cremasteric reflex are usually absent in testicular torsion. Patients may also have fever and dysuria. If the cause is infectious, laboratory tests can reveal leukocytosis, bacteriuria, and elevated C-reactive protein (CRP).

Anatomy and Physiology

With infectious etiologies, bacteria typically ascend from the urethra to the vas deferens and lymphatics of the spermatic cord and then to the epididymis. Less commonly, the bacteria spread directly by the hematogenous route. Inflammation usually begins as epididymitis in the epididymal tail and subsequently spreads to the body and head. In about 20% of cases, the infection spreads directly to the testis causing associated orchitis. Congenital lower GU tract structural and functional anomalies can result in retrograde urine reflux causing infectious or chemical epididymitis.

These anomalies include meatal stenosis in hypospadias, urethral stenosis, posterior urethral valves, ectopic ureter, vesicoureteral reflux, rectourethral fistula in an imperforate anus, and neurogenic bladder in meningomyelocele. The testicular appendages are embryonic remnants of the mesonephric and paramesonephric ducts and consist of sessile vascularized connective tissue prone to torsion. When torsed, they usually cause reactive epididymitis and hydrocele. A torsed appendix can be seen as a nodule of the upper scrotum with bluish skin discoloration ("blue-dot" sign).

Imaging Findings

- Enlargement of the epididymis (Fig. 62.1A)
- Increased vascularity on color Doppler (Fig. 62.1B)
- Hypoechoic with areas of hemorrhage causing heterogeneity or increased echogenicity
- With orchitis, the testis will also appear enlarged with increased vascularity and either decreased or heterogeneous echogenicity (Fig. 62.2A)
- Spectral analysis of orchitis shows a low-resistance waveform with resistive indices (RIs) below 0.5 (a normal RI of the testis is rarely less than 0.5; Fig. 62.2B)
- Torsed appendix shows a round extratesticular mass with increased heterogeneous echogenicity which changes its appearance with time (Fig. 62.3A)
- Scrotal wall thickening and reactive hydrocele which may contain debris and septations (Fig. 62.3B)
- Increased vascularity of the testis and epididymis in epididymoorchitis can appear similar to reactive inflammation and increased perfusion that occurs after detorsion
- Heterogeneous appearance of the testis can mimic infiltrative malignancies such as leukemia or lymphoma

Imaging Strategy

In a patient with acute scrotal pain, the imaging modality of choice would be ultrasound (US) with a high-frequency linear transducer and color Doppler. The testis, epididymis, and spermatic cord should all be carefully evaluated with comparison to the contralateral side. In prepubescent boys, evaluation of the kidneys and bladder should be considered because of the associated incidence of GU abnormalities in this age group. Some institutions may also use scintigraphy as

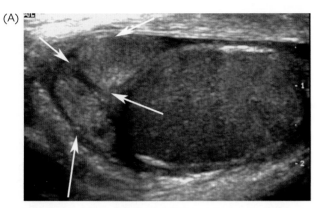

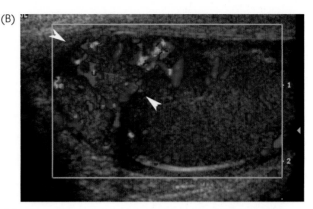

Figure 62.1. Sagittal US image (A) in an 8-year-old male with scrotal pain, swelling, and redness shows an enlarged epididymis (arrows). Ultrasound image with color Doppler (B) shows marked increase in vascularity of the epididymis (arrowheads) with normal testicular flow.

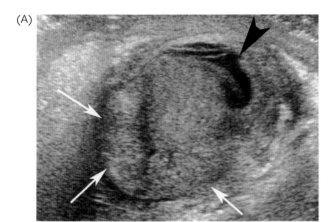

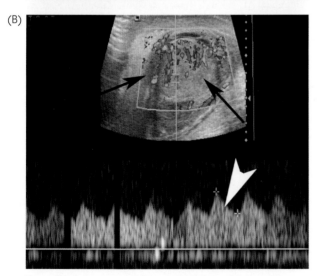

Figure 62.2. Transverse US image (A) in an 11-year-old male with scrotal swelling and pain shows an enlarged epididymal head and body (white arrows) with a small hydrocele (black arrowhead). Transverse color Doppler image (B) shows increased blood flow to the epididymis and testis (black arrows) with low-resistance waveform resulting from hyperemia (white arrowhead).

an adjunct study. Scintigraphy would show increased activity on perfusion and blood pool images on the affected side.

Related Physics

Epididymoorchitis must be differentiated from testicular torsion and US will show this distinction through subtle differences in flow between the two sides. Scrotal thickening may hinder the transmission of sound into the testis by a process called acoustic impedence where there is a large difference in density between the two tissues. As sound propagates through the scrotum and encounters the testis, sound reflection may occur, where the strength of reflection is characterized by the reflection coefficient. This coefficient is in turn related to acoustic impedance, which is a product of sound speed and tissue density. Sound interacts with the tunica albuginea through specular reflection whereas it interacts with the testicular parenchyma by diffuse reflection, giving rise to the characteristic speckled pattern in the testis. Sound incident on the tunica will reflect according to Snell's law, which states that the angle of incidence on the surface is equal to the angle of reflection off the surface. When sound is incident normal to the surface the reflected wave is back scattered at 180 degrees, whereas all other incident sound will be reflected at an oblique angle given by Snell's law. Any sound transmitted into the tissues at an oblique angle will bend off its true path again following Snell's law.

Differential Diagnosis
- Testicular torsion
- Testicular appendage torsion
- Acute idiopathic scrotal edema
- Testicular trauma
- Testicular neoplasm

Common Variants

Primary orchitis is rare and can occur without associated epididymitis. It is most often caused by mumps and can be bilateral.

(A)
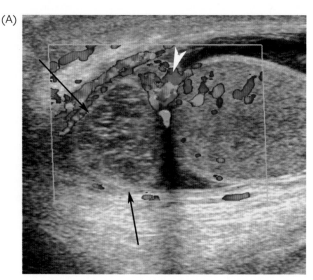

(B)
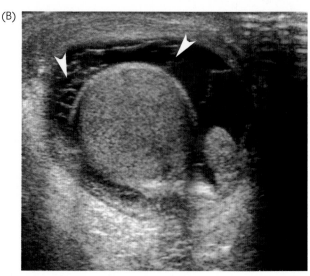

Figure 62.3. Transverse US image (A) in a 7-year-old boy with left scrotal pain shows a torsed appendix (black arrows) which appears as a round complex echogenic structure without blood flow adjacent to the prominent hyperemic epididymal head (arrowhead). Transverse US image (B) shows a complex hydrocele with septations (white arrowheads).

Clinical Issues

Treatment includes nonsteroidal anti-inflammatory drugs for pain relief and antibiotics only if the urine culture is positive. With prompt treatment, most patients' symptoms resolve quickly. A follow-up US may be indicated if an underlying tumor cannot be excluded, or to exclude an abscess if the patient's clinical presentation worsens. Prepubescent boys with recurrent epididymitis may also be referred to urology because of the high associated incidence of GU abnormalities.

Key Points

- Prepubertal boys: cause is usually idiopathic
- Postpubertal sexually active boys: cause is usually infectious
- Findings include enlarged epididymis and testis with increased vascularity
- Important to differentiate from testicular detorsion, correlation to clinical history and timing of pain will be helpful

Further Reading

Aso C, Enriquez G, Fite M, Toran N, Piro C, Piqueras J, Lucaya J. Gray-scale and color Doppler sonography of scrotal disorders in children: an update. *Radiographics*. 2005;25(5):1197–1214.

Baldisserotto M. Scrotal emergencies. *Pediatr Radiol*. 2009;39(5):516–521.

Dogra V, Bhatt S. Acute painful scrotum. *Radiol Clin N Am*. 2004;42(2):349–363.

Graumann LA, Dietz HG, Stehr M. Urinalysis in children with epididymitis. *Eur J Pediatr Surg*. 2010;20(4):247–249. Epub 2010 May 3.

Wittenberg AF, Tobias T, Rzeszotarski M, Minotti AJ. Sonography of the acute scrotum: the four T's of testicular imaging. *Curr Probl Diagn Radiol*. 2006;35(1):12–21.

CHAPTER 63

Testicular Torsion

Himabindu Mikkilineni, MD and Pinar Karakas, MD

Definition

Testicular torsion is the result of twisting of the spermatic cord, which in turn impairs the blood supply to the testicle and epididymis.

Clinical Features

Testicular torsion most commonly occurs in adolescent males between the ages of 12 to 18 years. Patients present with acute scrotal pain. Classic physical exam findings include scrotal swelling, diffuse tenderness and erythema, an abnormally high and horizontal position of the testis, and an absent ipsilateral cremasteric reflex. Absence of the ipsilateral cremasteric reflex is the most important clinical exam finding and can be tested by pinching the inner thigh.

Anatomy and Physiology

The testicular artery and deferential artery are located within the spermatic cord and have multiple and variable anastomotic channels. The testicular artery, which arises from the aorta, is the main blood flow to the testis and is the main artery affected in testicular torsion. The deferential artery arises from the superior vesicle artery and supplies the epididymis. The cremasteric artery arises from the inferior epigastric artery and supplies the epididymis, vas deferens, and peritesticular tissues. Pudendal artery branches supply the scrotal wall. Testicular torsion can be categorized as intravaginal, which is the most common type, extravaginal, or mesorchial. Normally, the tunica vaginalis attaches to the posterolateral surface of the testis (Fig. 63.1A). Predisposition to intravaginal testicular torsion occurs when the tunica vaginalis surrounds the entire testis and epididymis and prevents their fixation to the scrotal wall resulting in free mobility of the testis (Fig. 63.1B). This abnormality is also known as "bell-clapper" deformity and is bilateral in 12 percent of patients.

Imaging Findings

US:
- Normal in early torsion which is a strong predictor of viability (Fig. 63.2)
- Enlarged, hypoechoic, and/or heterogeneous in late torsion (Fig. 63.3)
- Scrotal edema and reactive hydrocele

Color Doppler:
- No flow if the degree of spermatic cord rotation is severe (Fig. 63.4)
- Normal blood flow if the cord rotation is less severe (normal prepubertal blood flow shows a high-resistance waveform, and diastolic flow may not be detectable; in postpubertal males, normally there is a low-resistance waveform with an average resistive index (RI) of 0.62 and range of 0.48 to 0.75)
- With partial torsion, the testis may show either high-resistance flow with absent or reversed diastolic flow ordampened arterial flow with a "tardus parvus" pattern (Fig. 63.5)
- Occasionally regional variations of the blood flow within an incompletely torsed testis
- Epididymis enlarged, especially in cases of partial or intermittent torsion, and avascular
- Epididymis infrequently hypervascular as an early finding or in the case of recent detorsion
- "Whirlpool" sign: direct visualization of a twist within the spermatic cord (high specificity; Fig. 63.6)"

IMAGING PITFALL: One should be careful not to confuse capsular flow for peripheral testicular parenchymal flow.

Imaging Strategy

In a male with acute scrotal pain and concern for testicular torsion, US using a high-frequency linear transducer with color Doppler and spectral analysis is the imaging modality of choice. The testis, epididymis, and spermatic cord should all be carefully evaluated and compared to the contralateral side. Some institutions may also use scintigraphy as an adjunct study.

Related Physics

Doppler has largely replaced nuclear medicine imaging for the diagnosis of testicular torsion. Ultrasound is superior in that it provides both exquisite gray scale and clinically useful Doppler flow information. In addition it is fast, accessible, does not use ionizing radiation, and with meticulous Doppler technique has a high sensitivity and specificity for

(A)

(B)

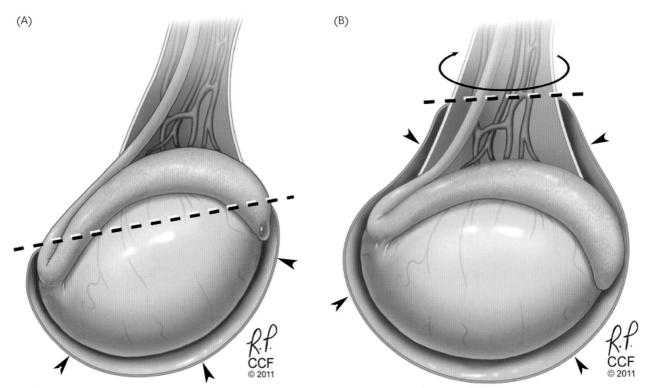

Figure 63.1. The bell-clapper deformity predisposing to intravaginal torsion. (A) Normal tunica investment (arrowheads) allows the remainder of the testis to attach to the scrotum along a broad base (dotted line). (B) In the bell-clapper deformity, the tunica (arrowheads) wraps almost completely around the testis leaving little room for scrotal fixation, making it prone to twist within the tunica.

the diagnosis. Doppler theory makes use of the phenomenon that moving objects will alter acoustic wavelengths in a predictable manner in which objects moving away from the source will lengthen the wavelength whereas objects moving toward the source will shorten the wavelength. Because wavelength and frequency are related, medical US units detect change in wavelength by detecting changes in frequency. This phenomenon is known as the Doppler shift frequency. When examining the testis, one must detect low-velocity arterial and venous flow and settings must be optimized to show flow where flow is indeed present. Range gating is a tool on the US platform that allows the

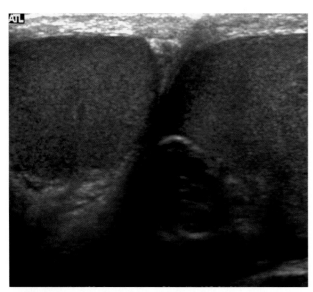

Figure 63.2. Transverse gray-scale US images in a 10-year-old boy with left scrotal pain and swelling for a few hours show homogeneous echogenicity.

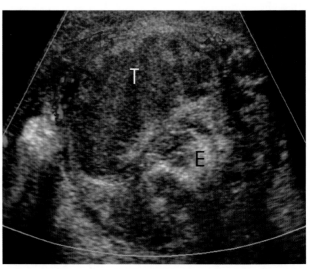

Figure 63.3. Transverse US image in a 14-year-old boy with a 2-day history of right scrotal pain shows heterogeneous/hypoechoic appearance of the testis (T) with enlargement and heterogeneity of the epididymis (E). This is a case of missed torsion and the testis was necrotic during surgery.

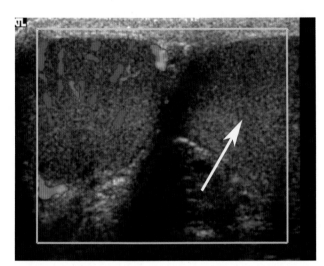

Figure 63.4. Ultrasound with color Doppler in a 10-year-old boy with left scrotal pain and swelling shows asymmetric, absent flow to the left testis (arrow).

permits Doppler to not only quantify the magnitude of flow but also its origin.

Differential Diagnosis
- Epididymoorchitis
- Torsion of testicular appendage
- Acute idiopathic scrotal edema
- Testicular trauma
- Testicular tumor

Common Variants
Extravaginal torsion is a phenomenon in newborns in which the testis has torsed before descent in utero. Most often there is irreversible ischemia at birth. The diagnosis of torsion of an undescended testis can be difficult because it can mimic different clinical conditions depending on the location. Most commonly, an undescended testis would be located in the inguinal canal and its torsion may mimic an incarcerated inguinal hernia. Mesorchial testicular torsion is extremely rare and is related to an abnormally narrow mesenteric (mesorchium) attachment allowing increased testicular mobility.

user to select a depth at which Doppler shift frequencies will be detected. As one is looking for presence or absence of flow anywhere in the testis, the range gate can be opened up to include the entire testis. Spectral analysis is a tool that provides a graphic depiction of the range of velocities present within the range gate. Spectral allows one to compare sides where there may be increased or decreased flow on the abnormal side. Doppler can be performed as continuous-wave or pulsed-wave, where the former is used in obstetrical imaging and the latter in vascular imaging. Continuous-wave can be difficult to interpret as there may be misregistration of the source of the signal. Unlike continuous-wave, pulsed Doppler uses a fixed-length pulse waveform from which frequency shifts are elicited. This

Clinical Issues
Testicular torsion is a surgical emergency. Treatment depends on the viability of the testis and may include either detorsion and orchiopexy or oorchiectomy. Early detection and treatment is critical because viability significantly drops after 6 hours and approaches 0 percent at 24 hours. Because the bell-clapper deformity can be bilateral, patients

(A)

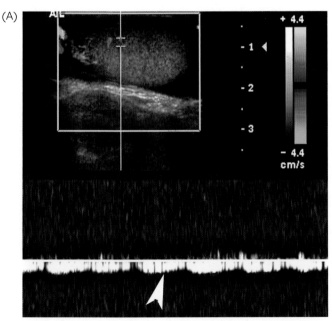

(B)

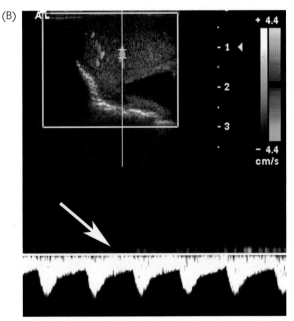

Figure 63.5. Color Doppler US of the right (A) and left (B) testes in an 11 year old boy with right scrotal swelling and pain shows a dampened "parvus tardus" waveform on the right (arrowhead) and normal flow on the left (arrow).

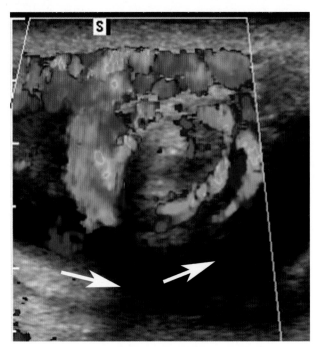

Figure 63.6. Transverse US with color Doppler of the right epididymis in a 12-year-old male with right scrotal pain shows the positive whirlpool sign (arrows) indicating incomplete torsion.

will undergo prophylactic orchiopexy of the contralateral testis at the time of surgery.

Key Points

- Due to twisting of the spermatic cord with impaired blood supply.
- Presents diagnostic challenge with variable appearance of testis and epididymis depending on the extent of ischemia and duration of the torsion.
- Lack of blood flow or asymmetric blood flow are the key findings.
- Direct visualization of twist in spermatic cord is the most specific finding.
- Is a surgical emergency, and a delay in treatment can cause irreversible ischemia.

Further Reading

Arce JD, Cortes M, Vargas JC. Sonographic diagnosis of acute spermatic cord torsion. *Pediatr Radiol*. 2002;*32*(7):485–491.

Aso C, Enríquez G, Fité M, Torán N, Piró C, Piqueras J, Lucaya J. Gray-scale and color Doppler sonography of scrotal disorders in children: an update. *Radiographics*. 2005;*25*(5):1197–1214.

Baldisserotto M. Scrotal emergencies. *Pediatr Radiol*. 2009;*39*(5):516–521. PMID: 19189096.

Dogra VS, Rubens DJ, Gottlieb RH, Bhatt S. Torsion and beyond: new twists in spectral Doppler evaluation of the scrotum. *J Ultrasound Med*. 2004;*23*(8):1077–1085.

Karmazyn B, Steinberg R, Kornreich L, Freud E, Grozovski S, Schwarz M. Clinical and sonographic criteria of acute scrotum in children: a retrospective study of 172 boys. *Pediatr Radiol*. 2005;*35*(3):302–310.

Nussbaum Blask AR, Rushton HG. Sonographic appearance of the epididymis in pediatric testicular torsion. *Am J Roentgenol*. 2006;*187*(6):1627–1635.

Vijayaraghavan SB. Sonographic differential diagnosis of acute scrotum: real time whirlpool sign, a key sign of torsion. *J Ultrasound Med*. 2006;*25*(5):563–574.

CHAPTER 64

Pyelonephritis

Kailyn Kwong Hing, MD and Paul Babyn, MD

Definition

Pyelonephritis (PN) is an inflammatory condition of the renal parenchyma and its pelvic urothelial lining commonly resulting from bacterial infection. There are many forms of pyelonephritis including acute, chronic, emphysematous, and xanthogranulomatous pyelonephritis. Acute PN (APN) is also known as an upper urinary tract infection (UTI). Chronic PN consists of recurrent or persistent infection leading to renal injury. Emphysematous PN is a severe necrotizing infection of the renal parenchyma causing gas formation in the urinary tract. Xanthogranulomatous PN (XGPN) is a chronic infection leading to a suppurative granulomatous infection.

Clinical Features

High fever and irritability are the most common findings in children with PN, but are nonspecific. Other signs and symptoms associated with UTI include nausea, vomiting, flank or abdominal pain, and hematuria. Older children are more likely to present with lower tract signs such as low-grade fever, dysuria, frequency, and suprapubic pain. Patients with chronic PN may have failure to thrive. Associations with vaginitis, ureterocele, fungal disease, anatomic abnormalities of the urinary tract, vesicoureteric reflux (VUR), and ureteropelvic junction obstruction (UPJ) have been noted. Urine cultures that show growth of gram-negative bacteria are indicative of a UTI either of the upper or lower tract. Urinalysis with the presence of white blood cells is a sensitive but nonspecific laboratory sign for UTI. Antibiotics are given dependent on urine cultures. Timely recognition and treatment are essential to prevent long-term consequences particularly in young children because risk of renal damage is greatest in infants and young children (< 5 years of age).

Anatomy and Physiology

In neonates and immunocompromised patients, bacteremia is a frequent source of infection. After the newborn period PN is more likely the cause of bacteremia, rather than a secondary result. Overall, one-third of infections are ascending in origin, originating in the bladder and ascending through urinary tract to the kidneys. Any organism that enters the urinary tract may be the source of infection. Most infectious organisms are perineal contaminants, predominantly Escherichia coli (E. coli). The fimbriae of E.coli aid in attachment of this bacteria to urothelium. Even in the setting of normal urine flow, the attachment increases the odds for development of infection. Vesicouerteric reflux represents one important host factor that increases the risk of ascending infection and delivery of bacteria to the renal parenchyma. Vesicouerteric reflux alone causes little renal damage. The higher the grade of reflux in combination with parenchymal infection, the more likely the patient will undergo renal scarring following acute PN. Low toll-like receptor 4 (TLR4) expression levels have been observed in children with asymptomatic bacteriuria. The TLR4 controls the innate immune response to E. Coli. Thus TLR4 promoter variants may influence TLR4 expression and immune response in eliminating pathogens. This may contribute to increased susceptibility to UTI and PN.

Imaging Findings

US:

- Abnormal echogenicity, increased, decreased, or heterogeneous (Fig. 64.1A)
- Zonal decrease or absence of blood flow of the renal parenchyma on power or color Doppler US (Fig. 64.1B)
- Diffuse or local parenchymal swelling
- Loss of corticomedullary differentiation
- Perinephric fluid or phlegmon

CT:

- Round area of decreased enhancement, may have mass effect or expand the cortical contour (Fig. 64.2A)
- Perinephric fat stranding, phlegmon, or abscess may be seen (Fig. 64.2B)
- Wedge-shaped poorly enhancing region extending from renal sinus to periphery; may be multiple (striated nephrogram; Figs. 64.3, 64.4)
- Loss of renal volume in cases of chronic PN

Dimercaptosuccinic acid scintigraphy (DMSA):

- PN: vague area of photopenia without volume loss (Fig. 64.5)

(A)
(B)

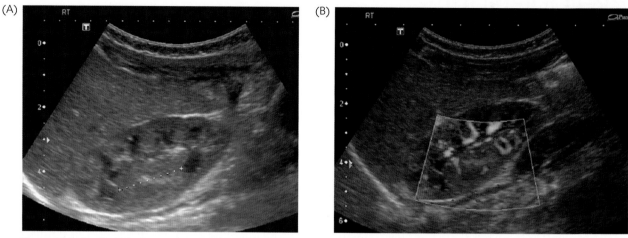

Figure 64.1. Sagittal US (A) in a 6-week-old infant with high fever shows a focal area of increased echogenicity and loss of the normal corticomedullary differentiation within the posterior aspect of the right kidney (calipers). Sagittal US with power Doppler (B) shows decreased blood flow in this region of the right kidney. Decreased perfusion is consistent with an area of focal PN (also known as lobar nephronia).

(A)
(B)

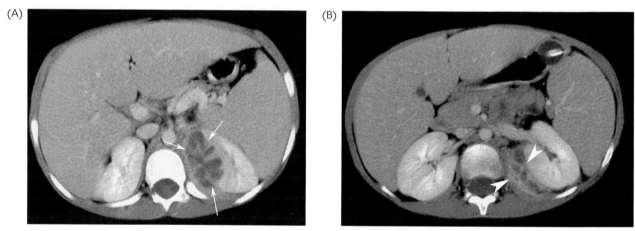

Figure 64.2. Axial contrast-enhanced CT image (A) in a 7-year-old male with glycogen storage disease presenting with a 14-day history of fever shows a renal abscess involving the left kidney (arrows). Adjacent axial image (B) shows extension to the perinephric and posterior pararenal space (arrowheads). The appearance is somewhat suggestive of XGPN given the septation.

- Renal scarring: a triangular, well-demarcated photopenic focus with volume loss

MRI:

- Decrease or loss of corticomedullary differentiation
- Areas of striated or nonenhancement after contrast administration
- Perinephric collections
- Loss of renal volume in cases of chronic PN

Imaging Strategy

There is currently no recommended imaging algorithm for PN. Given the nonspecific presentation, PN may be discovered when imaging is performed for other conditions. The presence of UTI can be determined with a positive urine culture obtained from a clean-catch specimen or after sterile catheterization. Imaging studies are infrequently needed to confirm a diagnosis but are commonly used to assess for

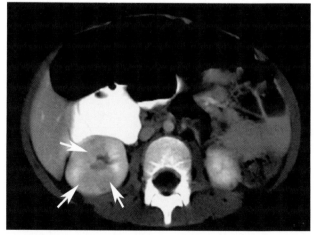

Figure 64.3. Axial contrast-enhanced CT image in a 2-year-old female with a history of abdominal pain and fever shows heterogeneous contrast enhancement of the kidneys with low-density focal areas within the right-lower pole anteriorly and posteriorly in keeping with unsuspected PN (arrows).

(A)

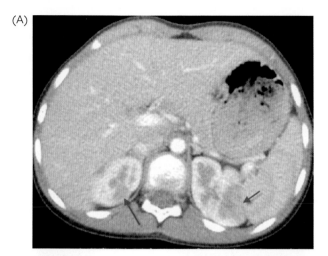

(B)

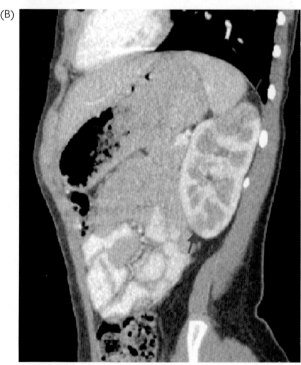

Figure 64.4. Axial contrast-enhanced CT image (A) in a 10-year-old male with recurrent abdominal pain shows decreased attenuation in the parenchyma of both kidneys in keeping with bilateral PN not identified on ultrasound. Sagittal reconstructed image of the left kidney (B) shows the upper and lower pole changes (arrows).

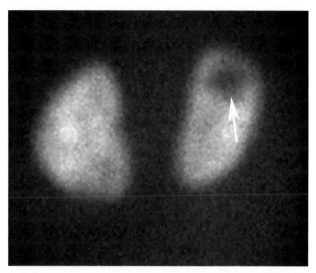

Figure 64.5. A DMSA scan in a 2-year-old female with a history of abdominal pain and fever shows a focal round photopenic area in the lower pole of the right kidney surrounded by normal parenchyma and without volume loss consistent with PN and/or possible abscess (arrow).

renal changes and scarring. Recently, the role for DMSA is less clear as normal scans do not rule out VUR though abnormal scans have high correlation with VUR. DMSA should not be used as a replacement for voiding cystoure-thrography (VCUG) in evaluation of children with febrile

variations or anomalies of the urinary tract, renal scarring, and VUR (Fig. 64.6). Renal US and/or DMSA renal cortical scintigraphy may be used to detect PN. Gray-scale US has a low sensitivity for PN, but is sensitive in the detection of many anatomic variants or abnormalities. Power Doppler increases specificity and sensitivity to 90 percent in children with APN. Positive signs for PN include hypoperfusion and decreased or absent flow compared with normal adjacent parenchyma. The American Association of Pediatrics (AAP) formerly recommended the use of Tc-99m DMSA scintigraphy for imaging the progression of inflammatory

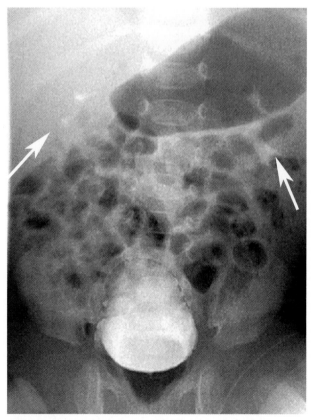

Figure 64.6. Frontal image from VCUG in a 6-week-old infant with high fever shows Grade II VUR bilaterally (arrows).

UTI as its use alone would result in failure to diagnose a considerable number of cases of VUR in infants. DMSA use in predicting long-term renal impairment with abnormal scan findings remains controversial. VCUG is usually performed after the patient is on antibiotics. VUR can also be detected via radionuclide cystogram (RNC). Like VCUG, RNC also requires bladder catheterization, however VCUG offers better anatomic detail. Even so, VCUG is an invasive procedure with several drawbacks such as radiation exposure and possible dysuria, hematuria, and perineal discomfort. The AAP 2011 practice guidelines for the diagnosis and management of the first febrile UTI in 2- to 24-month-old old children recommends renal and bladder US. For the first febrile UTI, VCUG is only indicated if US is abnormal with findings suggestive of high-grade VUR such as hydronephrosis, scarring, obstructive uropathy or other atypical findings. After the second febrile UTI, VCUG is also recommended. Ultrasound and VCUG have proven effective when used together in the identification of anatomic anomalies that increase the likelihood of UTI recurrence as well as renal scarring. DMSA may be reserved for assessing differential renal function and degree of renal parenchymal scarring in children with coexisting VUR or obstruction that may require surgical intervention. After 2 days of initial antibiotic therapy, if the patient with a febrile UTI is not responding clinically, the patient may undergo imaging reevaluation with US to look for signs of a renal abscess or PN, and VCUG would be added to assess for reflux. Imaging after the resolution of PN is based on urologist or pediatrician preference. However, to exclude renal scarring, a follow-up study for confirmation should be done at least 6 months after the acute infection. Follow-up studies performed prior to 6 months may detect residual renal edema and resolving infection. CT scans are more sensitive than US for detecting PN but are used infrequently because of the associated radiation exposure. The absence of ionizing radiation in MRU is advantageous when compared to CT and DMSA. MRU can provide anatomic and functional information and assess renal perfusion, but it is relatively expensive and typically requires IV contrast, bladder catheterization, and in some cases sedation.

Related Physics

Ultrasound is used in PN to evaluate for underlying structural anomalies, calcifications, and decreased flow resulting from interstitial edema. When using US it is important to choose the appropriate transducer type, shape, and frequency. With small children high-frequency linear-array transducers can be used because of lesser tissue thickness. In addition to providing superior axial resolution, these provide uniform lateral resolution across the image and at all depths. In larger children, phased-array transducers of lower frequency sacrifice axial and lateral resolution. The axial resolution degradation is results from the longer sound wave packet created at lower freqency. The lateral resolution degradation results from divergence of scan lines related to the phased array architecture of the image. As the lines diverge from the transducer face, lateral resolution will deteriorate with depth.

Differential Diagnosis

- Ureteral obstruction
- Renal infarction
- Perinephric abscess
- Renal cyst
- Ureteropelvic junction obstruction: chronic with acute trauma, or intermittently acute resulting from crossing vessel
- Wilms' tumor

Common Variants

XGPN:

- Rare and may follow obstruction from calculi, stricture, or a tumor
- Characterized by the presence of lipid-laden foamy macrophages, also known as xanthoma cells
- Associated with chronic granulomatous disease, pyonephrosis, leukocytosis, nephromegaly, and diabetes mellitus
- Tumefactive inflammation with dilated debris-filled collecting system and large obstructing calculi are common
- Most often unilateral
- Foci of parenchymal necrosis do not enhance and xanthomatous tissue does not enhance
- Septations extending centrally (Fig. 64.2)
- Extensions of the process into the perirenal space or adjacent structures, with perinephric abscess or fistula to the mesentery, psoas or body

Emphysematous PN:

- Rare condition which mainly affects diabetics
- May be found in association with renal stones, renal calculi, malnourishment, and diabetic ketoacidosis
- On US and CT there is inflammation with intraparenchymal gas and extension into the perinephric space

Clinical Issues

There is a greater incidence of PN in girls than in boys after the first 3 postnatal months and a high prevalence in febrile infants. The rate in circumcised boys is low and studies suggest that the rate is 4 to 20 times higher in uncircumcised boys. The frequency of APN tends to decrease with age in boys and increase with age in girls. PN can lead to irreversible scarring, hypertension, and chronic renal failure. Thus, it is important to differentiate children with less serious lower UTI from those with PN. By imaging alone, it is difficult to know whether the first documented UTI is in fact the first UTI. Younger children are at the greatest risk for renal scarring and repeated infections can lead to additional renal scarring. The most important risk factor in developing PN and renal complications is VUR. Patients with positive DMSA do not always present with VUR, however, if VUR is present at the time of investigation, 80 to 90 percent of patients will be found to have a positive DMSA according to the AAP.

Key Points

- VUR coexists in one-third of children with PN.
- Higher grades of VUR increase risk of renal scarring following PN.
- VCUG is the reference method for detecting VUR.
- US aids in detecting anatomic abnormalities that predispose young children to PN, as well as diagnosing PN and assessing infection resolution and subsequent renal growth.
- DMSA is not recommended as a replacement for VCUG for VUR.

Further Reading

Mantadakis E, et al. Acute Tc-99m DMSA scan for identifying dilating vesicoureteral reflux in children: a meta-analysis. *Pediatrics.* 2011; *128*:e169–e179.

Montini G, Tullus K, Hewitt I. Febrile urinary tract infections in children. *N Engl J Med.* 2011;365(3):239–250.

Shaikh N, Ewing AL, Bhatnagar S, Hoberman A. Risk of renal scarring in children with a first urinary tract infection: a systematic review. *Pediatrics.* 2010;*126*:1084–1091.

Slovis TL, ed. *Caffey's Pediatric Diagnostic Imaging.* Eleventh edition. Philadelphia, PA: Mosby Elsevier; 2008.

Smith EA. Pyelonephritis, renal scarring, and reflux nephropathy: a pediatric urologist's perspective. *Pediatric Radiology.* 2008;*38*: S76–S82.

Subcommittee on Urinary Tract Infection, Steering Committee on Quality Improvement and Management. Urinary tract infection: clinical practice guideline for the diagnosis and management of the initial UTI in febrile infants and children 2 to 24 Months. *Pediatrics.* 2011;128:595–609.

CHAPTER 65

The Exstrophy-Epispadias Complex

Heather McCaffrey, MD, Jeffrey C. Hellinger, MD, and Monica Epelman, MD

Definition

The exstrophy-epispadias complex (EEC) comprises a spectrum of congenital abnormalities involving the genito-urinary (GU), gastrointestinal (GI), and/or the musculoskeletal (MSK) systems, ranging in severity from epispadias to bladder exstrophy and exstrophy of the cloaca. Depending on the degree of complexity, EEC may affect the pelvis, spine, extremities, abdominal wall, pelvic floor, genitalia, and anus. Across the EEC complex, all conditions affect pelvic ring, infraumbilical abdomen, and the genitals. In short, all have pubic symphysis diastasis ranging from minimal in epispadias to severe in cloacal exstrophy.

Clinical Features

Exstrophy-epispadias complex is most common in Caucasians, in infants born to younger mothers, and multiparous women. Classic bladder exstrophy (CBE) is the most common form of the EEC; the incidence of bladder exstrophy is 3.3 per 100,000 live births. The male to female ratio in CBE is 2.3:1. Maternal tobacco exposure is associated with the more severe forms of cloacal exstrophy (CE). There is evidence to suggest an increased risk for EEC in pregnancies that utilize assisted reproductive technologies. Patients with epispadias and classic exstrophy are usually term infants. In contrast, patients with cloacal exstrophy are often preterm.

Epispadias

Epispadias primarily affects the genitalia and pubic symphysis. In males the phallus is short and broad with a dorsal chordee (curvature of the phallus upward or cephalad). The glans is open along the dorsal surface and flat (shaped like a spade). The dorsal foreskin is absent. The urethral meatus is located along the dorsal penile shaft, between the peno-pubic angle and the proximal glans. In females the clitoris is bifid with superiorly divergent labia. The distal and dorsal aspect of the urethra is open with a patulous bladder neck, allowing the possibility of visualization of the bladder. Prolapse of bladder mucosa has been noted. The pubic symphysis is usually diastatic with divergent distal rectus abdominis muscles.

Classic Bladder Exstrophy

CBE presents with an open, everted bladder on the infraumbilical abdomen, with bladder mucosa exposed through a triangular-shaped fascial defect. The umbilicus is low-set, located on the upper edge of the bladder plate. Rectus abdominis muscles diverge and attach to diastatic pubic bones. Indirect inguinal hernias are common secondary to wide inguinal rings and short inguinal canals. In males, genital features of epispadias are also present as described above. The urethral and bladder plate are in continuity along the lower abdominal wall and onto the dorsal surface of the penis. The verumontanum and prostatic ducts are present and visible along the prostatic urethral plate. Females also have the same genital features of epispadias, and the open urethral plate is in continuity with the bladder plate. There is anterior displacement of the vagina. In both sexes, the anus is displaced anteriorly but has a normal sphincteric mechanism. The pubic symphysis is widely diastatic with distally divergent rectus abdominis muscles, which is the result of outward rotation of the innominate bones. There is outward and downward rotation of the anterior pelvic ring ultimately resulting in the classic waddling gait.

Cloacal Exstrophy

In cloacal exstrophy, the bladder is widely open on the infraumbilical abdominal wall and separated into two distinct halves; usually, the cecum or foreshortened hindgut is present in between both halves of the bladder. Most patients (70 to 90 percent) have an associated omphalocele. The terminal ileum may also prolapse resulting in the "trunk sign" (soft-tissue structure shaped like an elephant's trunk protruding from below the umbilical cord, representing prolapsed ileum between the two bladder halves). In males the phallus is small and bifid, with a hemi-glans caudal to each hemi-bladder. Females have a bifid clitoris and two vaginas. The pelvic ring has a similar configuration to classic bladder exstrophy. Sixty-five percent of these patients can have major deformities of the lower extremity, such as clubfoot. Eighty percent have vertebral anomalies and ninety-five percent have myelodysplasia including occult spinal dysraphism and cord tethering.

Anatomy and Physiology

A definite cause of EEC has not yet been elucidated, but it is hypothesized that early in fetal development there is an abnormal overdevelopment of the cloacal membrane, which causes failure of the medial migration of mesenchyme between the ectodermal and endodermal layers of the lower abdominal wall preventing proper lower abdominal wall development. This phenomenon makes the cloacal membrane unstable and prone to early rupture (before it migrates into its normal caudal location). The severity along the EEC spectrum is determined by the time when this premature rupture occured. When rupture occurs after complete separation of the GU and GI tracts, CBE results. When rupture occurs prior to the descent of the urorectal septum, externalization of the lower urinary tract and distal GI tract occurs, causing cloacal exstrophy. (Note: this is different from cloacal malformations, which have no abdominal wall defect). In epispadias, there is normal bladder formation, however, urethral tubularization is incomplete.

Imaging Findings

Prenatal US and fetal MRI findings suggestive of EEC:

- Repeated failure to visualize the bladder (Fig. 65.1)
- Absence of bladder filling
- Lower abdominal wall mass increasing in size as intra-abdominal contents grow
- Low-set umbilicus
- Abnormal/diminutive genitalia
- Increased pelvic diameter/pubic bone diastasis

Prenatal US and fetal MRI findings more suggestive of cloacal exstrophy include:

- Low abdominal wall defect
- Herniation of bowel between two halves of bladder
- Limb abnormalities
- Myelomeningocele and vertebral anomalies

Postnatal evaluations:

- US similar to prenatal US
- VCUG may show abnormal course of urethral drainage, abnormal bladder capacitance, an abnormal bladder neck, and vesicoureteral reflux
- Radiographs may show an inferiorly placed pelvis, a wide pubic diameter, a splayed symphysis pubis, and externally rotated sacroiliac joints (Fig. 65.2)
- CT and MRI provide more detailed assessment of US and radiographic findings; in addition they may demonstrate a flatter pelvic floor, more laterally placed levator ani fibers, an anteriorly placed anus, and shorter anterior corporal bodies (Fig. 65.3)

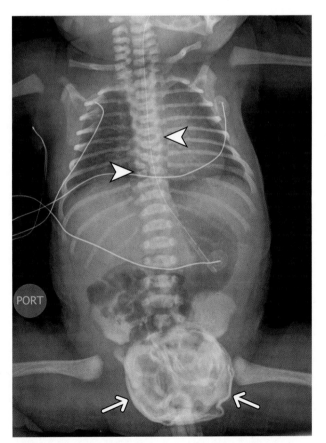

Figure 65.2. Frontal radiograph in a newborn with cloacal exstrophy shows soft-tissue density projecting over the pelvis and lower abdomen consistent with a low abdominal wall defect (arrows) with externalized GI and GU contents. Note multiple vertebral fusion and segmentation anomalies (arrowheads) and hyperabduction of the hips. The splayed pubic bones are obscured by the abdominal wall defect.

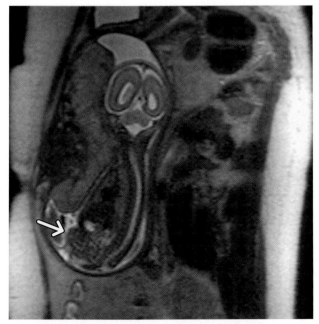

Figure 65.1. Sagittal T2 MR image in a fetus shows a low abdominal wall defect (arrow) and nonvisualization of the bladder because of cloacal exstrophy.

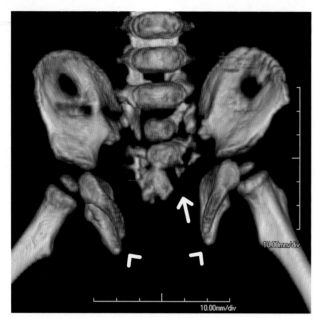

Figure 65.3. Coronal volume-rendered CT image of the bony pelvis in an 18-month-old with cloacal exstrophy shows severe pubic diastasis (arrowheads) and sacral spine dysraphism (arrow).

Imaging Strategy

Most often EEC is detected on screening fetal US. Fetal MRI may be obtained for further characterization and screening of other anatomical systems. For postnatal imaging of patients with EEC, diagnostic algorithms may utilize US, VCUG, radiographs, MRI and CT. Baseline renal US should be obtained when the clinical diagnosis along the spectrum of EEC has been made (increased bladder pressure after surgical closure can lead to hydronephrosis with subsequent upper tract deterioration; knowledge of existing hydronephrosis is helpful in following patients postoperatively). When cloacal exstrophy has been diagnosed, spinal US or MRI should be performed to assess for spinal dysraphism and detection of occult spinal cord anomalies (that could lead to cord tethering as the patient grows). In patients with epispadias, VCUG is useful to evaluate the bladder neck and proximal urethra (VCUG is performed in nearly all patients with bladder exstrophy to exclude vesicoureteral reflux and assess bladder capacity in preparation for bladder neck reconstruction and continence surgery). Radiographs may be obtained for assessment or screening of axial and appendicular skeleton and are useful in preoperative osteotomy planning. For greater characterization of the abdominal wall, viscera, spine, spinal canal, or musculoskeletal system, MRI or CT should be considered.

Related Physics

When performing US for exstrophy of the bladder it is important for sound to be effectively produced and transmitted from the transducer into the bladder. This requires

sophisticated engineering in transducer construction. Included in this are electronics design, proper matching layer technology and backing layer technology. More now than ever before, electronics are being miniaturized and incorporated into the transducer head to minimize signal loss and aid in low-signal amplification. Materials technology has helped to develop coating on the transducer face that limits sound loss as the wavefront moves from the crystals into the soft tissues. Lastly, effective backing layers on the transducer help to propel sound that was originally moving away from the tissues.

Differential Diagnosis

- Patent urachus
- Omphalocele
- Gastroschisis
- Persistent cloaca/cloacal malformation

Common Variants

- Superior vesical fissure
- Pseudoexstrophy
- Duplicate exstrophy
- Covered exstrophy
- OEIS (omphalocele-exstrophy-imperforate anus-spinal defects) complex

Exstrophy variants all have a widely diastatic pubic symphysis with distally divergent rectus abdominis muscles. A low or elongated umbilicus is common. There may be a small bladder opening or patch of isolated bladder mucosa as in superior vesical fissure.

The OEIS complex refers to the most severe form in the epispadias-exstrophy sequence. Features include an omphalocele; imperforate anus or anal atresia; spinal dysraphism with incomplete development of lumbosacral vertebrae; and exstrophy of a common cloaca that receives ureters, ileum, and a rudimentary hindgut. There is also failure of fusion of the genital tubercles and pubic rami, epispadias in males, and mullerian duct anomalies in females, with an associated wide range of urinary tract anomalies.

Clinical Issues

Patients with EEC have increased sensitization to latex antigen. Seventy percent of patients with CBE are sensitized to the antigen (based on serum elevation of IgE antibody to latex), though thirty percent have symptoms of latex allergy. As radiologic tests and surgical procedures generate increased exposure to latex antigen, patients should be approached with full latex precautions. Definitive treatment for EEC ranges from chordee repair and urethral reconstruction in epispadias to complex, multidisciplinary primary or multistage surgical corrections in CBE and cloacal exstrophy. In addition to genitalia and urethral reconstructions,

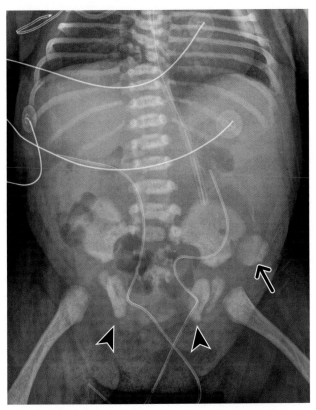

Figure 65.4. Abdominal radiograph in a newborn with cloacal exstrophy following initial bladder closure demonstrates the diastasis of the symphysis pubis (arrowheads) and an enteric ostomy in the left-lower quadrant (arrow).

the exstrophy repairs also require abdominal wall, bladder, and/or GI tract reconstructions with or without diversion (urinary or intestinal). Pelvic osteotomies may be required to facilitate closure (Fig. 65.4).

Additional Issues

- Antibiotic therapy is initiated for all exstrophy patients immediately after delivery and continued through the peri- and postoperative periods.
- Renal US monitoring is required in postoperative exstrophy patients (reconstructed or diverted) to assess for obstruction or renal dysfunction.

- Short-gut syndrome will develop in nearly all postoperative exstrophy patients.
- Spinal cord tethering is seen in up to 33 percent of postoperative (neurosurgical) symptomatic exstrophy patients.

Key Points

- Spectrum of congenital anomalies of GU, GI and MSK systems
- Includes epispadias, classic bladder exstrophy, and cloacal exstrophy
- Pubic symphysis diastasis occurs along the entire EEC complex
- Prenatal US diagnosis
- Full latex precautions

Further Reading

Ebert AK, Reutter H, Ludwig M, et al. The exstrophy-epispadias complex. *Orphanet J Rare Dis.* 2009;4:23.

Eeg KR, Khoury AE. The exstrophy-epispadias complex. *Curr Urol Rep.* 2008;9:158–164.

Gearhart JP, Mathews R. Exstrophy-epispadias complex. In: Wein AJ, Kavoussi LR, Novick AC, et al., eds. *Campbell-Walsh Urology.* Philadelphia, PA: Saunders Elsevier; 2007: 3497–3553.

Grady RW, Mitchell ME. Surgical techniques for one-stage reconstruction of the exstrophy-epispadias complex. In: Wein AJ, Kavoussi LR, Novick AC, et al., eds. *Campbell-Walsh Urology.* Philadelphia, PA: Saunders Elsevier; 2007:3554–3572.

Halachmi S, Farhat W, Konen O, et al. Pelvic floor magnetic resonance imaging after neonatal single stage reconstruction in male patients with classic bladder exstrophy. *J Urol.* 2003;*170*:1505–1509.

Meglin AJ, Balotin RJ, Jelinek JS, Fishman EK, Jeffs RD, Ghaed V. Cloacal exstrophy: radiologic findings in 13 patients. *AJR Am J Roentgenol.* 1990;*155*(6):1267–1272.

Moore KL, Persaud TVN. *Before We Are Born.* Seventh edition. Philadelphia, PA: Saunders Elsevier; 2008.

Woodhouse CR, North AC, Gearhart JP. Standing the test of time: long-term outcome of reconstruction of the exstrophy bladder. *World J Urol.* 2006;*24*(3):244–249.

Musculoskeletal

CHAPTER 66

Pediatric Fractures

Adam Delavan, MD and Laura Z. Fenton, MD

Definition

Common pediatric fractures include a spectrum of longitudinal compression (bowing, buckle, and greenstick), physeal (Salter-Harris types), stress, toddler, and elbow (supracondylar, lateral condyle, and medial epicondyle avulsion).

Clinical Features

Accidental pediatric trauma is the most common reason for a child to seek emergency medical care. Most pediatric fractures present with a history of known trauma, acute pain, swelling, decreased range of motion, or inability to bear weight. Bowing fractures often present with decreased range of forearm pronation and supination. Subacute or more indolent fractures such as stress or toddler fractures may present with refusal to use the affected extremity.

Anatomy and Physiology

The pediatric skeleton is anatomically different from the adult because of the presence of the physis (growth plate, epiphyseal plate), thus common pediatric fractures are quite different from adult fractures. In addition, pediatric bone is relatively elastic compared to adult bone, therefore absorption of longitudinal force transferred along the length of the bone leads to a unique spectrum of fractures: bowing, buckle, and greenstick. Prior to fusing, the cartilaginous physes are sites of longitudinal bone growth, but are also sites of relative bone weakness and therefore prone to fracture. The pediatric joint capsule and ligaments are 2 to 5 times stronger than the physis. Therefore, forces that produce a sprain or dislocation in the adult are more likely to cause a physeal fracture in the child. Normally, bone resorption (osteoclastic activity) and new bone formation (osteoblastic activity) are in balance. Repetitive stress causes multiple microfractures, stimulating osteoclastic activity, creating regions of relative weakness (stress fracture) predisposed to a complete fracture.

Elbow cartilaginous-osseous anatomy is complex. Six ossification centers develop in an orderly sequence (Fig. 66.1). The mnemonic "CRITOE" is useful to remember the order: *C*apitellum (1 to 2 years of age), *R*adial head (2 to 4 years), *I*nternal (medial) epicondyle (4 to 6 years), *T*rochlea (8 to 11 years), *O*lecranon (9 to 11 years) and *E*xternal (lateral)

epicondyle (10 to 11 years). The ossification centers are usually ovoid and smooth with the exception of the trochlea, which can be fragmented and irregular. Knowledge of this ossification sequence is especially helpful in medial epicondyle avulsion.

Imaging Findings

Longitudinal compression fractures—bowing, buckle, and greenstick:

- Pediatric bones tend to bow, buckle, then break.
- Bowing fracture often subtle with no fracture line and minimal healing reaction, therefore comparison radiographs of the contralateral extremity may

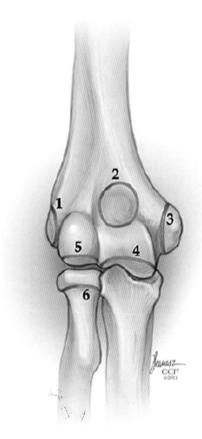

Figure 66.1. CRITOE: order of elbow ossification. **C**apitellum(5), **R**adial head (6), **I**nternal (medial) **E**picondyle(3), **T**rochlea(4), **O**lecranon(2), and **E**xternal (lateral) epicondyle(1).

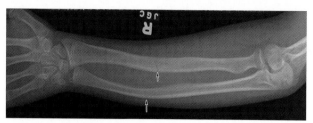

Figure 66.2. Frontal radiograph of the forearm shows medial bowing of the ulna (bowing fracture) (white arrow) and incomplete cortical break in the mid-shaft of the radius (greenstick) (black arrow).

assist in diagnosis; most common in radius, ulna, and fibula and often coexists with a fracture in the companion bone (Fig. 66.2).

- Buckle fracture (aka torus fracture) shows characteristic subtle cortical buckling in the metaphysis of long bones where the cortex is thinnest; most common location is dorsal distal radius (Fig. 66.3); distal cortex of normal long bones should always have smooth and continuous contour without notch or abrupt angle.

- Greenstick is caused by increased axial load on bone, breaking the convex cortex, while the concave cortex remains intact resembling a green tree branch; often coexists with a buckle or bowing fracture in the forearm or leg companion bone.

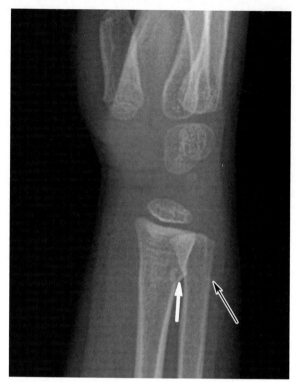

Figure 66.3. Oblique lateral radiograph of the distal forearm shows cortical buckle fractures of the dorsal distal radial (white arrow) and ulnar (black arrow) metaphyses.

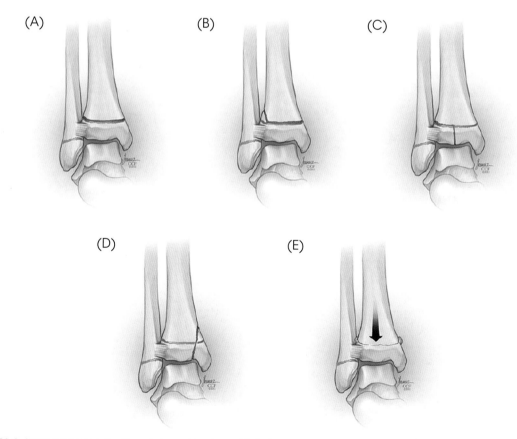

Figure 66.4. Salter-Harris classification of physeal fractures. (A) Salter I; (B) Salter II; (C) Salter III; (D) Salter IV; (E) Salter V.

Table 66.1 – Salter-Harris classification of physeal fractures

SALTER-HARRIS	ANATOMY	CLASSIC EXAMPLES	PROGNOSIS
I (Fig. 66.5)	Physis	Wrist; Slipped capital femoral epiphysis (SCFE); apophyseal avulsion	Excellent
II (Fig. 66.6)	Physis and metaphysis	Proximal and middle phalanges	Excellent
III (Fig. 66.7)	Physis and epiphysis; intra-articular	Juvenile Tillaux	Good
IV (Fig. 66.8)	All three components; intra-articular	Triplane (tibia)	Fair (growth arrest, osteoarthritis)
V	Crush through physis		Poor (premature physeal fusion/ growth arrest)

Physeal fractures:

- Salter-Harris classification applies to fractures involving the physis and is both descriptive and prognostic (Fig. 66.4)
- Approximately 20% of pediatric fractures involve the physes
- Physeal widening, lucent fracture line with or without displacement, and soft-tissue swelling
- Higher Salter-Harris classification associated with increased incidence of premature physeal fusion and growth disturbance resulting from injury to the vascular supply (Table 66.1).

Stress fractures:

- Repetitive stress on normal bone
- Most common in toddlers (tibia and tarsal bones) and young athletes (location depending on involved sport, tibia most common)
- Occult on initial radiographs in 85%
- Cortical thickening or irregularity, periosteal reaction, and sclerotic bands (Fig. 66.9)
- Nuclear bone scan and MRI are nearly 100% sensitive, demonstrating radiotracer uptake at the fracture site and low T1 and T2 intensity fracture line and/or focal marrow edema, respectively

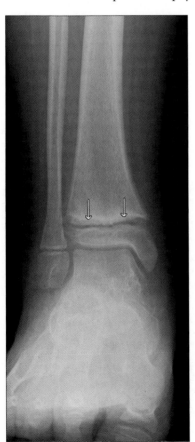

Figure 66.5. Frontal radiograph of the ankle shows physeal widening (white arrows) and metaphyseal sclerosis of the tibia consistent with Salter-Harris type I fracture.

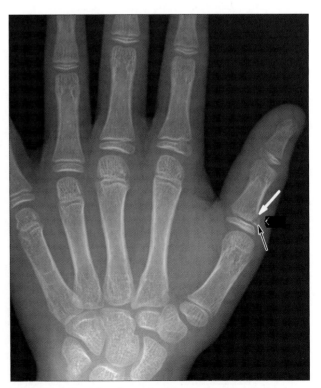

Figure 66.6. Frontal radiograph of the proximal first phalanx shows minimal physeal widening (white arrow) and metaphyseal fracture with a small Thurston-Holland fragment (black arrow) consistent with Salter-Harris type II fracture.

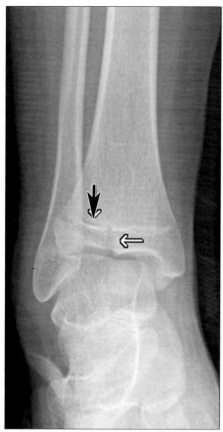

Figure 66.7. Frontal radiograph of the ankle shows a vertical fracture through the distal tibial epiphysis (white arrow) with widening of the unfused lateral physis (black arrow) consistent with Salter-Harris type III (juvenile Tillaux) fracture.

Toddler fractures:
- Between 9 months and 3 years following pivot/rotational force, often presenting with refusal to bear weight
- Nondisplaced oblique fracture through the tibial diaphysis (Fig. 66.10); may be subtle or occult on initial radiographs
- Follow-up radiographs in 7 to 10 days show healing response, confirming a fracture in initially occult cases
- Bone scan/MRI very sensitive showing diffuse uptake in the affected tibial diaphysis.

Elbow fractures—supracondylar, lateral condyle, and medial epicondyle avulsion:
- Effusion: visualization of the posterior fat pad (anterior is normally seen); 85% association with a fracture.
- Radiographic lines (Fig. 66.11) aid in interpreting elbow radiographs.
- Supracondylar fracture is the most common fracture of the pediatric elbow, caused by a fall on an outstretched hand (FOOSH); area between the coronoid and olecranon fossae is very thin and susceptible to fracture; elbow joint effusion, abnormal anterior humeral line resulting from dorsal displacement of the distal humerus, subtle fracture (Fig. 66.12).
- Lateral condyle fracture is the second most common fracture of the pediatric elbow; Salter-Harris type II or IV fractures, separating a small fragment of distal

(A)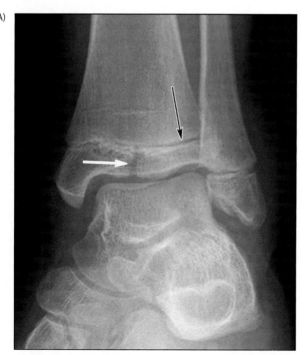

(B)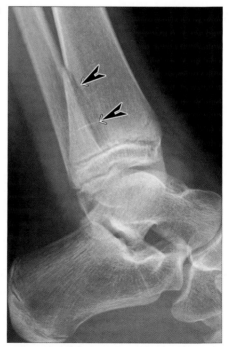

Figure 66.8. Oblique (A) and lateral (B) radiographs of the ankle show a distal tibial epiphyseal fracture in the sagittal plane (white arrow), widening of the lateral distal tibial physis in the horizontal plane (black arrow), and a distal tibial metaphyseal fracture in the coronal plane (arrowheads) consistent with Salter-Harris type IV (triplane) fracture.

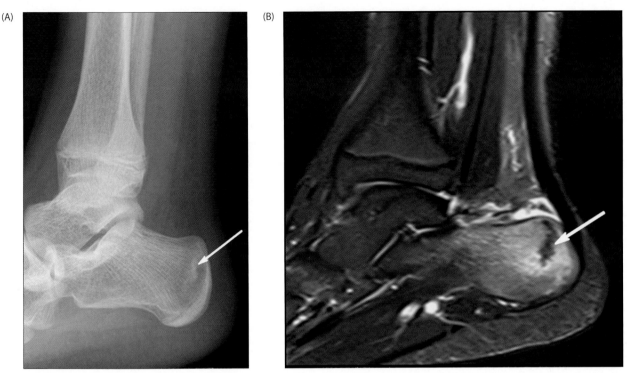

Figure 66.9. Lateral radiograph (A) of the calcaneus at 7 days after injury shows healing response with a sclerotic band (arrow). Fluid-sensitive MR image (B) shows hypointense fracture line (arrow) and marrow edema consistent with stress fracture.

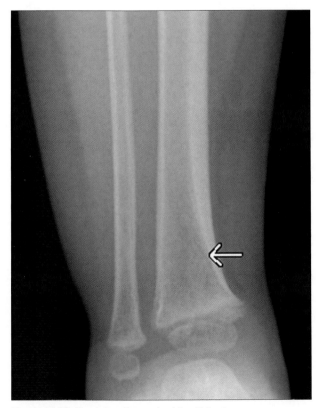

Figure 66.10. Frontal radiograph of the tibia shows a nondisplaced oblique fracture (arrow) through the distal tibial diaphysis consistent with toddler fracture.

humeral metaphysis and variable amount of unossified/ossifying epiphysis; elbow joint effusion and fracture line, with only a small sliver of bone separated from the lateral distal humeral metaphysis (Fig. 66.13), as the majority of the fracture is through the unossified/ossifying distal humeral epiphysis; MRI can better define extension into epiphysis.

■ Medial epicondyle apophysis may be avulsed from pull of the flexor pronator tendon; range of injuries from separation of the epicondyle to complete dislocation and/or intra-articular entrapment; best seen on frontal radiograph; need fixation if separation more than 3 millimeters; entrapped medial epicondyle should not be mistaken for the trochlear ossification center (Fig. 66.14).

Imaging Strategy

Frontal and lateral radiographs of the affected bones including the adjacent joints are diagnostic for most pediatric fractures. Oblique views are helpful in the forearm, elbow, hand, foot, and leg. Comparison views of the contralateral side are reserved for sites of complex anatomy (elbow) or subtle fractures (bowing and Salter-Harris type I). Soft tissues should be evaluated for localized or general swelling. CT is helpful for complex fractures, MRI or bone scan for occult fractures, and MRI for fractures through unossified cartilage. Fractures involving the knee or ankle physis should be followed for premature physeal fusion and growth disturbance.

(A)

(B)

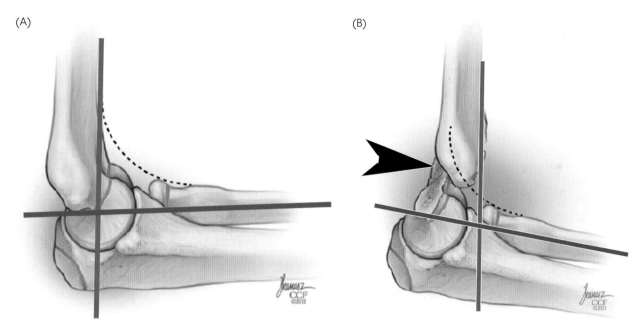

Figure 66.11. A. Normal radiographic lines of the elbow. B. Disruption of the normal lines from angulation in supracondylar fracture (arrowhead) (anterior humeral line (red line); radiocapitellar line (blue line); normal arc (black, dotted line)).

> **IMAGING PITFALL:** It is important not to miss an additional fracture after one is identified, always examine all imaged bones.

Related Physics

CT is more sensitive in detecting subtle fractures than plain radiography and the high effective atomic number

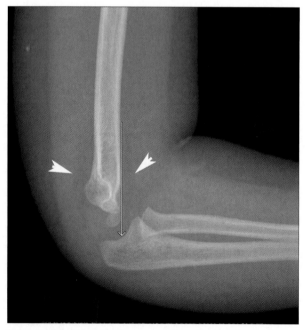

Figure 66.12. Lateral radiograph of the elbow shows a joint effusion with anterior and posterior fat pad displacement (arrowheads) and abnormal anterior humeral line (line), without visible fracture line in a supracondylar fracture.

of calcified bone makes it possible to image at very low dose. Fracture detection requires high-spatial-resolution imaging or many line pairs detectable per millimeter. High-resolution imaging is best achieved with thin collimation, small focal spot, high-resolution kernel, and small field of view (FOV). Thin collimation engages the smallest detector elements within a multirow CT and this allows for very fine localization of projections within the human body. When the small focal spot is engaged, photons emanate from the source in a manner akin to a point source, which potentiates higher spatial resolution. Using a high-resolution kernel allows one to visualize high-spatial-frequency structures (small high-attenuation objects that lie adjacent to each other) imaged by the thin collimation and small focal spot. Finally, this information is optimally appreciated when the mosaic CT image is reconstructed using small pixels. One controls this by choosing the smallest possible field of view to include the region of interest (pixel size= FOV/512). Wide window width and level are usually employed to visualize the broad range of CT values in an orthopedic image. To this end, it is recommended that images are viewed with a width/level setting of 1000/~200 Hounsfield Units (HU). Multiplanar reformating allows visualization of fractures in their optimal plane. Three-dimensional reconstruction using volume-rendering techniques may be requested for presurgical planning.

Differential Diagnosis

- Pathologic fracture: fracture from normal stress on abnormal bone, with underlying neoplasm

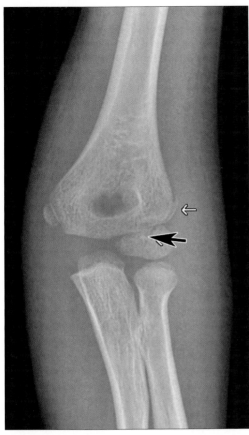

Figure 66.13. Frontal radiograph of the elbow shows a sliver of bone separated from the lateral condyle (white arrow) and fracture line (black arrow) crossing the physis and capitellum consistent with lateral condyle fracture (Salter-Harris type IV).

- Insufficiency fracture: fracture from normal stress on abnormal bone, excluding underlying neoplasm; etiologies include osteogenesis imperfecta, rickets, renal osteodystrophy, steroid administration, or disuse osteopenia (prolonged immobilization)
- Infection: Soft-tissue swelling and fat plane obliteration; variable appearance in bone, including focal lucency, cortical disruption, permeative destruction, and physeal widening
- Neoplasm: aggressive periosteal reaction, cortical disruption, soft-tissue mass, chondroid or osteoid matrix

Common Variants

If multiple fractures occur over time, consider bone weakness as in osteogenesis imperfecta. If fractures are of different ages or no correlating trauma, consider child abuse.

Clinical Issues

Bowing, buckle and greenstick fractures generally heal completely with immobilization. Salter-Harris type fractures are treated based on degree of displacement and angulation. With satisfactory reduction, conservative treatment with immobilization yields adequate healing in the majority. Types III to V are at risk of vascular injury. Complications include premature physeal fusion that can lead to growth arrest. Entrapped periosteum or perichondrium may delay or prevent healing. Stress fracture treatment includes rest

(A)

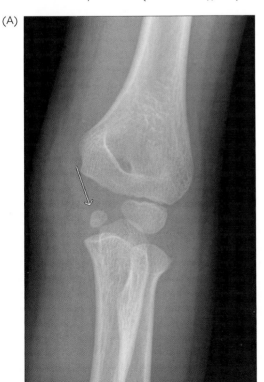

(B)

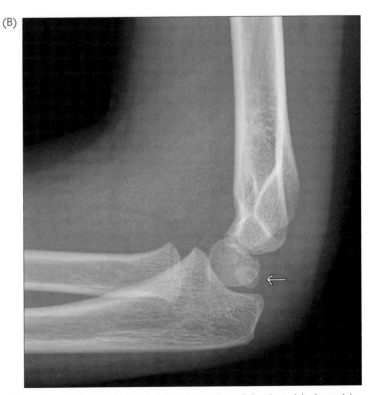

Figure 66.14. Frontal (A) and lateral (B) radiographs of the elbow show entrapment of a displaced medial epicondyle (arrow) in the elbow joint.

and activity reduction. The most common supracondylar fracture complication is cubitus varus deformity.

Key Points

- Radiographs first; 7- to 10-day follow-up radiographs; MRI or bone scan for suspected occult fractures
- Distal cortex of normal long bones always has smooth and continuous contour without notch or abrupt angle
- Physes are weakest part of the growing skeleton predisposing to Salter-Harris I to V (type II most common)
- Comparison views can assist with complex anatomy (elbow) or subtle fractures (bowing and Salter-Harris type I).
- Stress fractures result from abnormal stress on normal bone; ensure no underlying neoplasm or decreased bone density to exclude pathologic or insufficiency fracture
- Elbow joint effusion 85% chance of fracture in trauma
- If the anterior humeral line intersects the anterior third of the capitellum on a true lateral view, suspect a supracondylar fracture
- CRITOE mnemonic describes the order of elbow ossification centers and aids in diagnosing medial epicondyle avulsion fractures; if an ossification center is present in the trochlear position without a medial epicondyle ossification center, suspect a displaced and entrapped medial epicondyle

Further Reading

Beaty JH, Kasser JR. The elbow region: general concepts in the pediatric patient. supracondylar fractures of the distal humerus. In: Beaty JH, Kasser JR, eds. *Rockwood and Wilkins' Fractures in Children.* Sixth edition. Philadelphia, PA: Lippincott Williams and Wilkins; 2006:529–551, 628–642.

Benton C, Anton CG. Musculoskeletal trauma. In: Donnelly LF, Jones BV, O'Hara SM, et al., eds. *Diagnostic Imaging: Pediatrics.* Salt Lake City, UT: Amirsys; 2005:6-6–6-9, 6-18–6-33.

Pudas T, Hurme T, Mattila K, Svedström E. Magnetic resonance imaging in pediatric elbow fractures. *Acta Radiol.* 2005;46(6):636–644.

Rathjen KE, Birch JG. Physeal injuries and growth disturbances. In: Beaty JH, Kasser JR., eds. *Rockwood and Wilkins' Fractures in Children.* Sixth edition. Philadelphia, PA: Lippincott Williams and Wilkins; 2006:99–119.

Strouse PJ. Skeletal trauma. In: Slovis TL, Adler BH, Bloom DA, et al., eds. *Caffey's Pediatric Diagnostic Imaging.* Eleventh edition. Philadelphia, PA: Mosby; 2008:2778–2782, 2786–2792, 2803–2804, 2833–2836.

CHAPTER 67

Osteomyelitis and Chronic Recurrent Multifocal Osteomyelitis

Mahesh Thapa, MD and Sumit Pruthi, MD

Osteomyelitis

Definition
Osteomyelitis is infection of cortical bone and bone marrow.

Clinical Features
Osteomyelitis is most common in childhood and boys are affected more than girls. Clinical presentation can be nonspecific. The child may refuse to bear weight or may limp. Back pain and neurological changes may indicate vertebral or spinal canal infection. Laboratory changes include elevated erythrocyte sedimentation rate (ESR) and leukocytosis. *Staphylococcus aureus* is the most common organism to cause osteomyelitis. Tuberculosis (TB) is rarely seen in developed countries, but continues to be prevalent in third-world nations. Fungal osteomyelitis (typically Aspergillus) may occur in immunocompromised children. The most commonly involved sites in decreasing order of frequency are the metaphysis of the distal femur, proximal tibia, distal humerus, distal radius, proximal femur, and proximal humerus.

Anatomy and Physiology
The usual route of inoculation is hematogenenous, but direct spread from an adjacent structure is sometimes seen. Hematogenous infection usually begins at the metaphysis because of its rich blood supply and slow flow within the venous channels. There is also diminished phagocytic activity near the metaphysis. In infants less than 1 year old, transphyseal bridging vessels facilitate spread of infection to the epiphysis and joint space. From 1 year of age until the physis is closed, extension of infection into the joint space is uncommon, because circulatory connection between the metaphysis and epiphysis is interupted. Physeal closure reestablishes vascular connection, and the joint cavity once again is susceptible to infection. Acute infection elicits an inflammatory response leading to exudate formation, increased intraosseous pressure, blood stasis, thrombosis, and subsequent bone necrosis. Findings include cortical destruction, periosteal elevation and spread of infection into the contiguous soft tissues. Subacute infection is often localized either by the low virulence of the organism or increased host resistance. Chronic infection generally results either from untreated acute infection or ongoing low-grade infection. There is extensive bony sclerosis, often resulting in formation of sequestrum (necrotic bone), involucrum (thick periosteal bone formation surrounding a sequestrum), and cloaca (connection between marrow and periosteum) or sinus (connection between marrow and skin) formation. Because of rapid decompression of the exudate in neonates, sequestrum is uncommon, however, periosteal elevation is more pronounced compared to adults because of loose attachment of the periosteum to bone.

Imaging Findings
Radiography:
- Lytic lesion near metaphysis (Fig 67.1)
- Loss of soft-tissue planes and soft-tissue swelling in the early stages
- Cortical destruction: loss of 30 to 50 percent of bone mineralization is required for changes to be apparent on XR, usually occuring after 7 to 10 days
- Periosteal elevation
- Sensitivity of 43 to 75 percent and specificity of 75 to 83 percent

US:
- Periosteal elevation
- Soft-tissue swelling, fluid, or abscess
- Can guide percutaneous drainage of the fluid collections associated with infection, both for diagnostic and therapeutic purposes

Bone scintigraphy
- Elevated blood flow and abnormal increased deposition of tracer at the site of infection
- Nonspecific and may not enable confident differentiation between infection, neoplasm, and trauma
- Initial false-negative exams secondary to relative ischemia from vascular compression and thrombosis or decreased conspicuity of subtle abnormal uptake at the metaphysis due to adjacent physis that shows high uptake

CT:
- Intraosseous gas
- Cortical erosion or destruction
- Tiny foreign bodies

- Involucrum/sequestrum formation in chronic disease
- Contrast-enhanced CT: extent of soft-tissue involvement or presence of abscesses

MRI:

- Features parallel the ongoing pathological process
- Low T1 and high T2 and short tau inversion recovery (STIR) signal intensity (SI): marrow edema and inflammatory infiltrate
- Because of normal conversion of hematopoietic marrow to fatty marrow, marrow normally bright on fluid-sensitive sequences and can be confusing
- T1 is ideal sequence to assess marrow as it better delineates normal marrow morphology
- Cortical destruction, periosteal elevation and spread of infection into contiguous soft-tissue structures causing cellulitis, myositis, phlegmon, soft-tissue abscesses and associated sinus tracts.
- Periosteal reaction, sequestra, or involucra identified on MRI as focal hypointense regions on all imaging sequences
- GRE will exaggerate mineralization through susceptibility artifact
- Contrast-enhanced images defines extent of soft-tissue abscesses and differentiates viable from non-viable tissue

Imaging Algorithm

Imaging may be used to confirm clinical suspicion of infection, assess the extent of involvement, evaluate for associated complications such as an abscess, help guide drainage or biopsy for diagnostic and therapeutic purposes, and to

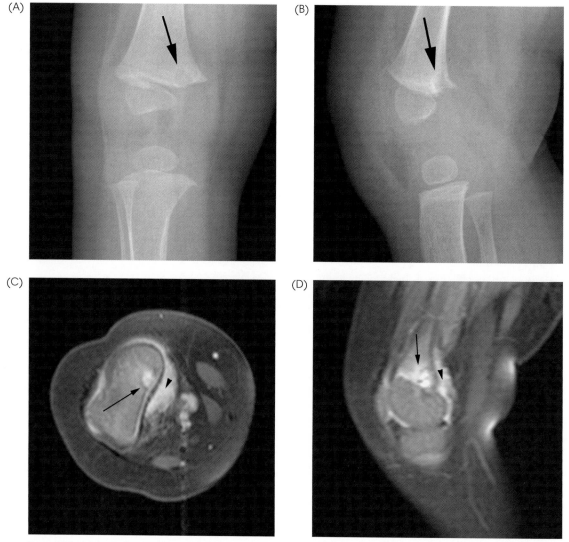

Figure 67.1. Frontal (A) and lateral (B) radiographs of the right knee in a 14-month-old boy with refusal to bear weight demonstrate a relatively well-defined lucency in the distal medial femoral metaphysis (arrow). Axial (C) and sagittal (D) T1 MR images with fat suppression through the same area reveal enhancing osteomyelitis (arrow) with extension to the adjacent periosteum and soft tissues (arrowhead). This patient was proven to have acute bacterial osteomyelitis.

assess response to therapy. Conventional radiography is usually the initial imaging modality. Although often negative, radiographs may provide guidance for further imaging and exclude other entities such as fractures or tumors. Ultrasound can assess for abscess or fluid collection and guide percutaneous drainage. Scintigraphy is less expensive than MRI and rarely requires sedation. Imaging can be performed more than once with the option of performing delayed imaging (24 hours after the injection) to improve detection of subtle lesions. Scintigraphy can also detect multiple foci of disease. The capacity to image the entire skeleton can be crucial in infants and neonates, in whom localizing signs are generally poor and often nonspecific. CT scan can provide excellent cortical detail and can be used to guide biopsy and drainage of deep-seated pelvic abscesses. The biggest disadvantage of CT is the associated radiation dose. Therefore, it should be used sparingly and tailored to answer specific clinical questions. Although costly and often requiring sedation, MRI is the best imaging tool to diagnose, assess response to therapy, and follow up cases of suspected or known osteomyelitis. Additionally, MRI can reliably differentiate acute from chronic infection and has excellent soft-tissue contrast and inherent multiplanar capabilities. The basic imaging protocol consists of: T1, T2 with fat suppression, and STIR performed in orthogonal planes. Although the use of intravenous gadolinium for osteomyelitis is still debatable, fat-suppressed contrast-enhanced T1 MR images have become a routine part of the diagnostic evaluation for osteomyelitis at various centers. Intravenous contrast may not be helpful in differentiating infection from noninfectious inflammatory conditions.

Clinical Issues

Early diagnosis of osteomyelitis can avoid consequences such as sepsis, chronic infection, and growth arrest.

Key Points

- Osteomyelitis is a hematogenous infection that usually begins at the metaphysis.
- Chronic infection generally results either from untreated acute infection or ongoing low-grade infection.
- Conventional radiography is usually the initial imaging modality.
- Although often negative, radiographs may provide guidance for further imaging and exclude other entities such as fractures or tumors.
- CT is best for small foci of intraosseous gas, cortical erosion/destruction, tiny foreign bodies, and involucrum/sequestrum formation in chronic cases.
- Contrast-enhanced MRI delineates normal from abnormal marrow and defines the extent of soft-tissue abscesses.

Chronic Recurrent Multifocal Osteomyelitis (CRMO)

Definition

A rare inflammatory disorder of unknown etiology that is noninfectious and clinically distinct from bacterial osteomyelitis.

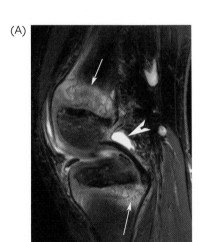
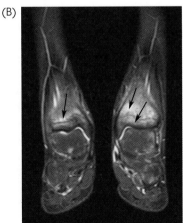
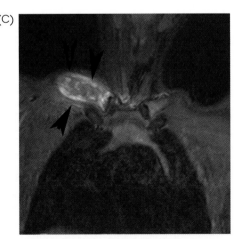

Figure 67.2. Sagittal T2 MR image with fat suppression (A) of the knee in a 9-year-old male with ankle, knee, and right clavicular pain, relapsing over several months shows edema (white arrows) in the distal femoral and proximal tibial metaphysis with a small joint effusion (arrowhead). Coronal STIR MR image of the ankles (B) shows edema (black arrows) in the metaphysis and epiphysis of both distal tibias. Coronal STIR MR image of the right clavicle (C) shows extensive edema (arrowheads) of the medial clavicle and surrounding periosteum/soft tissue. Biopsy showed no evidence of bacterial infection and confirmed diagnosis of CRMO.

Clinical Features

Primarily seen in the pediatric population, CRMO has a strong female predominance. This entity presents with bone lesions at several sites in the body, usually waxing and waning in severity over time. Tubular bones are most commonly affected, with the spine, clavicle, and pelvis less commonly affected. Multifocal disease is the norm, although in rare cases, a single site may be involved. The patient presents with pain, swelling, and erythema over the affected region, and skin lesions such as marked acne, psoriasis, and palmoplantar pustulosis may be present. As a result, this entity may represent a variant of SAPHO syndrome (synovitis, acne, pustulosis, hyperostosis, and osteitis), a disease traditionally thought of as exclusive to the adult population, consisting of inflammatory bony lesions and skin eruptions. There is ongoing debate as to whether CRMO and SAPHO are separate entities or two different points of the same continuum.

Anatomy and Physiology

Although often seen in association with other autoimmune disorders, serological tests for rheumatoid factor, antinuclear antibodies, and HLA-B27 are usually negative. Histopathology, laboratory findings, and bacterial culture are also usually negative or inconclusive. As a result, the diagnosis is one of exclusion, after more common entities such as infection and tumor have been ruled out.

Imaging Findings

Radiography:

- Foci of lytic destruction adjacent to the growth plate
- Defined sclerotic rim demarcating lesion from normal bone
- No periosteal reaction or soft-tissue swelling
- No sequestrum

MRI:

- More extensive involvement than XR and additional lesions detected
- No abscess or sinus track
- MRI can guide biopsy
- Eccentric areas of low T1 and high STIR SI in metaphysis and extending to the growth plate (Fig 67.1)
- Rare epiphyseal involvement (Fig 67.2b)
- Can rarely spread to the diaphysis
- Lesions evolve and heal over time, with sclerosis and resolution of abnormal STIR SI
- Sequela can be well-defined area of metaphyseal sclerosis, which can be difficult to differentiate from subacute osteomyelitis or Brodie abscess
- Spine: lytic phase shows decreased T1 and increased T2 SI with endplate erosion and either no disc involvement or partial disc involvement and avid enhancement; chronic, sclerotic phase shows low T1 and T2 SI without enhancement

- Multifocal involvement of the spine usually skips vertebral bodies, with predominantly anterior vertebral involvement and does not cross the disc
- Vertebra plana: can be difficult to distinguish from Langerhans cell histiocytosis or other tumors
- Clavicle: lytic medullary lesion in medial clavicle with laminated periosteal reaction on XR; homogenous low T1 and high STIR SI with bone expansion with extension to surrounding soft tissues; contrast enhancement within clavicle and surrounding tissue; no fluid collection or abscess; difficult to differentiate from chronic infection or malignancy; heals with hyperostosis (fig 67.2c)

Bone scintigraphy:

- Defines full extent of disease

Imaging Algorithm

Radiography is the first-line imaging modality. Bone scintigraphy or whole body MRI can define the full extent of disease. Specific lesions can be best defined with MRI.

Differential Diagnosis

- Osteomyelitis
- Leukemia
- Rickets

Related Physics

When osteomyelitis or CRMO involves a long bone, patient positioning can be challenging. It is important to have the region of interest centered as closely as possible to the center of the bore of the magnet—the so-called "sweet spot." In the pediatric patient this can often be achieved by asking the patient to slide to the side of the table allowing the limb of interest to fall at the center of the bore. The technologist must also place the limb so that it lies colinear to the long axis. Unlike for adults, children will rarely lie for extended periods of time with the arm above the head without moving. For this reason, the "prone Superman" position is impractical and will lead to multiple repeated sequences and unnecessary prolongation of the study. For wrist and elbow imaging, the arm is best placed at the patient's side. The technologist must therefore compensate for the extra volume of tissue that will be included in the phase encoding steps on coronal imaging (from the adjacent body). This is done by adding phase oversampling or increasing the imaging field of view and including the body in the image.

Clinical Issues

The following criteria are recommended for a diagnosis of CRMO: (1) multifocal (two or more) bone lesions, clinically or radiographically diagnosed; (2) a prolonged course (over 6 months) characterized by varying activity of disease and with most patients being healthy between recurrent attacks of pain, swelling, and tenderness; (3) lack of response to antimicrobial therapy given for at least 1 month; (4) typical radiographic lytic regions surrounded by sclerosis with increased uptake on bone scan; (5) lack of an identifiable organism; (6) no abscess, fistula, or sequestrum formation; (7) atypical site for classical bacterial osteomyelitis such as clavicles and multiple sites; (8) non-specific histopathologic findings and laboratory results compatible with osteomyelitis; and (9) (sometimes) acne and palmoplantar pustulosis. Additionally, symmetry of the lesions has been reported as a helpful feature.

Key Points

- Metaphysis of long bones is the most common area of involvement.
- CRMO can also be seen in the clavicles, spine, and pelvis.
- Diagnosis is through exclusion; all suspected lesions should be biopsied.
- Abscess and sinus tract formation are not present in CRMO.
- CRMO can cause vertebra plana.

Further Reading

Jurik AG. Chronic recurrent multifocal osteomyelitis. *Seminars in Musculoskeletal Radiology.* 2004;8(3):243–253.

Kan JH. Major pitfalls in musculoskeletal imaging-MR. *Pediatr Radiol.* 2008;38(Suppl 2):S251–S255.

Pruthi P, Thapa M. Infectious and inflammatory disorders. *Magn Reson Imaging Clin N Am.* 2009;17:423–438.

Schmit P, Glorion C. Osteomyelitis in infants and children. *European Radiology.* 2004;14:L44–L54.

CHAPTER 68

Ewing's Sarcoma

Siobhan McGrane, MD and Nabile M. Safdar, MD

Definition

Ewing's sarcoma of bone is an aggressive small round blue cell tumor of childhood, which can present with signs and symptoms suggesting osteomyelitis or systemic inflammation.

Clinical Features

Ewing's is the second most common primary malignant bone tumor in children, most common between 10 to 20 years (median age 15 years). It is rare in African-American and Asian-American populations. Male to female ratio is 1.5:1. Bone pain can be intermittent over several weeks or months. Swelling, palpable mass, weight loss, and pathologic fracture are less common complaints. On physical examination an enlarged, tender bony prominence or a palpable soft-tissue mass, which may feel warm or appear erythematous, may be apparent. Intermittent fevers, elevated erythrocyte sedimentation rate (ESR), raised white blood count (WBC), and anemia can mimic osteomyelitis.

Anatomy and Physiology

Ewing's sarcoma of the bone affects the axial and appendicular skeleton with equal frequency, with the central axis the primary affected site in 45 percent. It is usually located within the metaphysis (59 percent) or the diaphysis (35 percent) of a single long bone. The primary sites of bone disease are lower extremity (femur), pelvis, chest wall, upper extremity, spine, and skull, in decreasing order of frequency. Tumor generally arises from the medullary canal, however can originate in the subperiosteal space or extraosseous soft tissues. There may be large adjacent soft-tissue masses and cortical destruction. Hematogenous and local spread through the system of Haversian canals are both common. Microscopically Ewing's consists of densely packed uniform "small round blue cells" in sheets and their glycogen constituent causes a positive reaction to the periodic acid-schiff (PAS) stain; cells are CD99- positive (MIC2-positive).

Imaging Findings

Radiography:
- Wide zone of transition (Fig. 68.1A)
- Permeative or moth-eaten destruction

- Aggressive periosteal reaction: Codman's triangle, perpendicular (hair-on-end) or lamellar (onion skin) (Fig. 68.1B)
- Soft-tissue mass
- Cortical saucerization: resulting from subperiosteal tumor extension
- Cortical destruction
- Sclerosis (40 percent purely or mixed sclerotic)

CT/MRI:
- Medullary and cortical destruction
- Marrow edema
- Large soft-tissue mass +/- necrosis or hemorrhage (Fig. 68.2A)
- Skip lesions/metastases (Fig. 68.2B)

Imaging Strategy

Conventional radiographs in two planes are the initial investigation of choice. Contrast-enhanced MRI of the whole bone including adjacent joints is the best modality for local staging. In the pelvis, this includes the sacroiliac joint and sacrum. Use of CT is reserved for cases in which there is diagnostic doubt or for guiding intervention in the form of biopsy, although ultrasound (US) can also guide biopsy in some cases. Chest radiographs, CT of the thorax, and bone scintigraphy are typically performed to assess for distant metastasis.

Difficulties arise in post-therapy follow-up imaging when fibrosis and soft-tissue edema can appear identical to residual or recurrent tumor. Techniques such as dynamic enhanced MRI, PET/CT and PET in conjunction with MRI can be helpful in these diagnostic dilemmas.

Related Physics

Each MRI sequence includes three orthogonal axes, referred to as slice-select (z-axis) and phase and frequency (x and y). The slice-select direction is defined by the desired imaging plane. The phase direction is the most time-consuming and is therefore chosen as the smallest distance (anteroposterior or left-to-right direction). The frequency direction is not time-consuming and is chosen by default following the choice of phase. One caveat is that the phase direction is most susceptible to artifact from patient motion (fidgeting or respirations) and vascular motion (pulsatility). If the

(A)

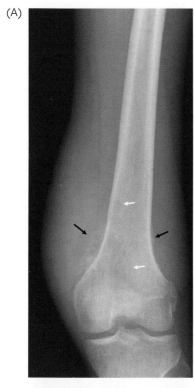

(B)

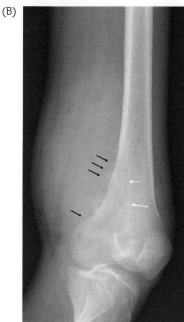

Figure 68.1. Frontal (A) and lateral (B) radiographs of the distal femur in a 16-year-old with leg pain demonstrate areas of periosteal reaction (black arrows) and bone destruction (white arrows) with a wide area of transition.

(A)

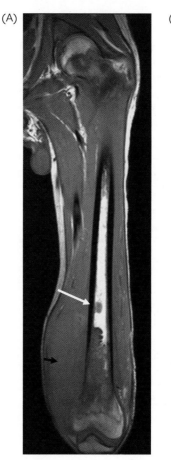

(B)

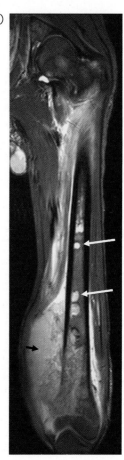

Figure 68.2. Coronal T1 MR image (A) in a teen with knee pain demonstrates a large soft-tissue mass (black arrow) and a skip lesion (white arrow). Coronal contrast-enhanced T1 MR image with fat suppression (B) demonstrates diffuse enhancement of the large soft-tissue mass (black arrow) and multiple skip lesions (white arrows).

region of interest (ROI) falls within artifact caused in the phase direction, phase and frequency can be "swapped" and the sequence repeated. It is important to recognize that ALL TISSUE in the phase direction is included in the phase encoding steps, regardless of chosen field of view (FOV); if one chooses a FOV that only includes the ROI, aliasing of structures outside the FOV will be superimposed on the ROI. When performing coronal images of a lower extremity, one can either choose a FOV large enough to include both legs, or decrease the FOV to cover the ROI and apply "phase oversampling" to electronically add phase encoding steps outside the ROI. Both measures will eliminate aliasing or "wrap."

Differential Diagnosis

- Osteosarcoma
- Primitive neuroectodermal tumor (PNET)
- Osteomyelitis
- Metastases

Common Variants

The small round blue cell tumor includes the Ewing's family of tumors, which in turn includes PNET, Askin's tumor (chest wall) and extraosseous Ewing's sarcoma. These commonly share a specific chromosomal translocation t(11:22) (q24;q12).

Clinical Issues

Bone metastases can present as skip lesions in the same bone or as distant metastases. Between 20 to 25 percent of patients are diagnosed with metastatic disease at presentation (10 percent lung, 10 percent bones/bone marrow, 5 percent combinations or others). Poor prognostic factors at presentation are large tumor size/volume, axial location, older age (> 15 years) and elevated serum LDH. Other poor prognostic factors include a poor response to preoperative chemotherapy. Needle biopsies should always be planned in consultation with the appropriate surgical service.

Key Points

- Ewing's sarcoma is the second most common primary malignant bone tumor in children.
- Common sites of metastasis are lung and bone.
- MRI is modality of choice for evaluation of the entire affected bone.
- Initial workup includes chest CT and bone scintigraphy.
- Needle biopsies should always be planned in consultation with the appropriate surgical service.

Further Reading

Baraga JJ, Amrami KK, Swee RG, Wold L, Unni KK. Radiographic features of Ewing's sarcoma of the bones of the hands and feet. *Skeletal Radiology*. 2001;*30*(3):121–126.

Hogendoorn PCW, On behalf of the ESMO/EUROBONET Working Group, Writing Committee, et al. Bone sarcomas: ESMO clinical practice guidelines for diagnosis, treatment and follow-up. *Annals of Oncology*. 2010;*21*(Supplement 5):v204–v213.

Ludwig JA. Ewing sarcoma: historical perspectives, current state-of-the-art, and opportunities for targeted therapy in the future. *Curr Opin Oncol*. 2008;*20*(4):412–418.

Mar WA, Taljanovic MS, Bagatell R, et al. Update on imaging and treatment of Ewing sarcoma family tumors. *Journal of Computer Assisted Tomography*. 2008;*32*(1):108–118.

CHAPTER 69

Osteosarcoma (aka Osteogenic Sarcoma)

Gerald Behr, MD

Definition

Osteosarcoma is a malignant neoplasm with a propensity to produce varying degrees of osteoid matrix and represents the most common malignant primary bone tumor in children and young adults.

Clinical Features

Osteosarcoma is most commonly a disease of the young, affecting males more frequently than females by an average 3:2 ratio, most often during the second decade of life. Parosteal osteosarcoma, the most common surface osteosarcoma, is a notable exception, usually presenting during the third and fourth decade. Thirty percent of osteosarcomas occur in patients over 40 years of age; these are typically secondary, related to prior radiation therapy, Paget's disease, or less commonly, osteonecrosis, chronic infection or even fibrous dysplaisa. Although usually sporadic, studies have reported that alteration of the retinoblastoma gene (Rb) predisposes to the formation of osteosarcoma. Classically, patients present with deep-seated and intermittent pain, persisting for weeks to months and finally becoming unremitting. Eighty-five percent of patients present with pain during activity and nearly one-half attribute their pain to minor trauma. This is a departure from the typical presentation of a primary malignant bone neoplasm which is usually most painful during rest, particularly at night. As such, the clinical presentation of the osteosarcoma may be strikingly similar to the more common benign musculoskelatal disorders, a phenomenon which may lead to delayed diagnosis. In fact, pain from a localized osteosarcoma may subside after refraining from physical activity, further giving false reassurance to both patient and physician. Osteosarcoma may also come to medical attention as an incidental finding during radiographic evaluation for another reason such as trauma. As with many osseous lesions, the structural weakening of the underlying bone suggests that many of these "incidental" osteosarcomas were actually imaged because of pathologic fracture that may not have occurred given the same degree of trauma to normal bone matrix. Initial presentation with pathologic fracture represents about 5 to 10 percent of cases and portends a worse prognosis, perhaps as a result of local contamination by neoplastic cells. On examination, there may be a palpable, tender mass, but this is variable. Edema and warmth may be noted. Telangiectatic osteosarcomas may present with a localized bruit. Conspicuously absent are weight loss, fever, and fatigue. LDH, alkaline phophatase, and ESR may be elevated.

Anatomy

Osteosarcomas typically arise in the metaphyses of the long bones of the appendicular skeleton. Only 9 percent occur in the diaphysis and occurence in the epiphysis is extremely rare although tumors may cross the physis to secondarily involve the epiphysis. Most osteosarcomas occur in the distal femur or proximal tibia. The next most common sites are the proximal humerus and middle and proximal femur. Metastases are seen at the time of diagnosis in 15 percent, of which 97 percent involve the lungs. Osteosarcomas may be classified into intramedullary type and the less common surface types. The intramedullary (or "classic" osteosarcoma) subtypes are currently defined by their histology and include chondroblastic, osteoblastic, telangiectactic, round cell, fibroblastic or malignant fibrous histiocytoma-like tumors. The three most common tissue components of the tumor matrix are osteoblastic, chondroblastic, and fibroblastic. The surface osteosarcomas are divided into parosteal, periosteal, and the extremely rare intracortical types.

Parosteal and periosteal osteosarcoma tend to be less aggressive than medullary tumors. Periosteal osteosarcoma tends to arise in the diaphysis of a long bone, in contradistinction to parosteal osteosarcoma and intramedullary varieties, which are metaphyseal in origin. Rarely, osteosarcomas may arise from soft tissue without any apparent connection with an adjacent bone, including the deep soft tissues of the thigh, upper extremity, and retroperitoneum in decreasing order of incidence.

Imaging Findings

Intramedullary (Classic) Osteosarcoma

High-Grade (75%)
  Radiography:
  - Large, intraosseous lesion
  - Frequent soft-tissue extension
  - Three radiographic patterns: osteoblastic, osteolytic, and mixed

- Disorganized osteoid matrix characterized by fluffy, cloudlike opacities mixed with lucencies giving a mixed sclerotic/lucent appearance (Fig. 69.1)
- Fibroblastic subtype completely lytic
- Cortical breech without expanding cortical contours
- Aggressive periosteal reaction: Codman triangle, "sunburst," laminated, or "hair-on-end" (Fig. 69.2)

CT:

- Highlights the ostoid proliferation (Fig. 69.3)
- Aggressive periosteal reaction
- Soft-tissue mass
- Lung metastases

MRI:

- Low T1 and high T2 SI
- Perilesional edema can falsely suggest greater tumor extent
- Intralesional fluid SI may signify necrosis
- Tumor hemorrhage: high T1 SI
- Regions of low SI typical, reflecting mineralized matrix (Fig. 69.4)
- Aggressive sunburst periosteal reaction (Fig. 69.5)

Telangiectatic Osteosarcoma

- Cystic or multilocular lesion mimicking aneuysmal bone cyst (ABC), unicameral bone cyst, or giant cell tumor as it expands rather than destroys bone
- Little or no periosteal reaction
- Moth-eaten, lytic lesionwith periosteal reaction and a wide zone of transition (rare)
- Fluid-fluid levels (DDx ABC)
- Thick, peripheral enhancing nodular tissue*
- Intralesional mineralization, which may be seen best on CT*
- Cortical destruction with an infiltrative margin lacking a capsule*

Low-Grade (Well-Differentiated) Central Osteosarcoma (LGOS)

- Most often lytic with coarsened trabeculation
- Mimics fibrous dysplasia
- Differential includes ossifying fibroma, nonossifying fibroma, and fibroxanthoma

Small Cell Osteosarcoma

- Permeative appearance may also be seen with small cell osteosarcoma
- Cortical breakthrough
- Aggressive periosteal reaction
- Soft-tissue mass
- Osteoid matrix can be subtle and, at times, only appreciated on CT

*May be distinguishing features for telangiectatic osteosarcoma vs. ABC

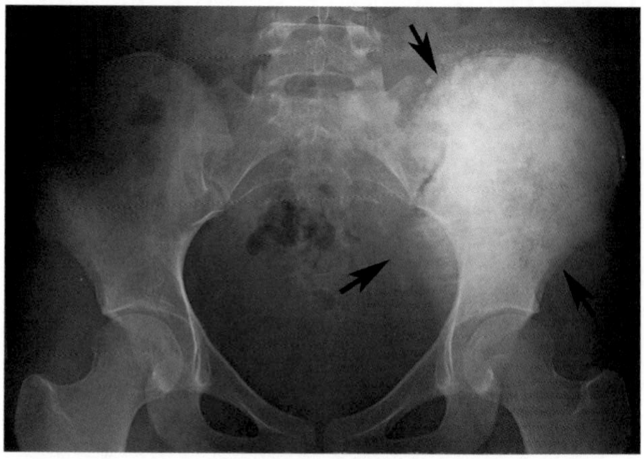

Figure 69.1. Frontal radiograph of the pelvis in a 16-year-old girl who was complaining of left hip pain shows robust osteoid matrix in the left iliac wing (black arrows).

Parosteal Osteosarcoma

- Sessile, densely sclerotic, lobulated mass (cauliflower-like appearance) involving or appearing adjacent to the cortex
- Radiolucent line at its attachment to the cortex, representing nonmineralized, thickened periosteum although not a constant finding

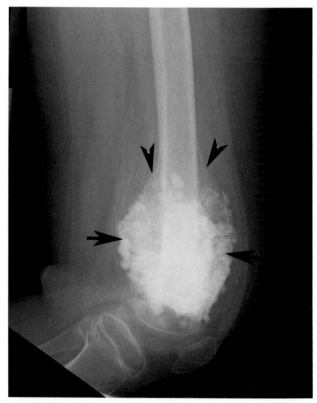

Figure 69.2. Lateral radiograph of the knee in a 9-year-old girl with knee pain shows cloud-like opacities (black arrows) typical for osteoid matrix as well as aggressive periosteal reaction and Codman's triangle (arrowhead).

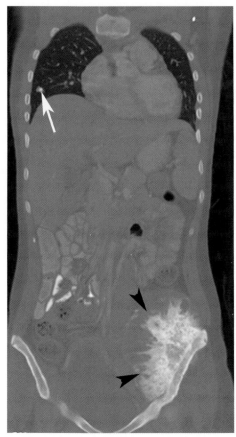

Figure 69.3. Coronal reconstruction from a noncontrast CT in a 16-year-old girl who was complaining of left hip pain shows the sunburst periosteal reaction (black arrowheads) and one calcified pulmonary metastasis (white arrow).

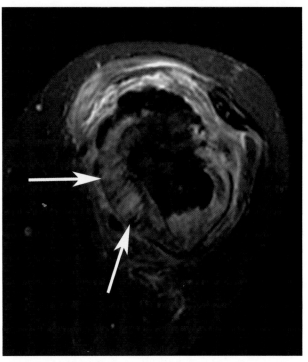

Figure 69.4. Axial T2 MR image of the knee with fat suppression in a 9-year-old girl with knee pain demonstrates classic "sunburst spiculation" type of periosteal reaction (arrows) as multiple radiating hypointense lines arising from the cortex and central low-signal osteoid.

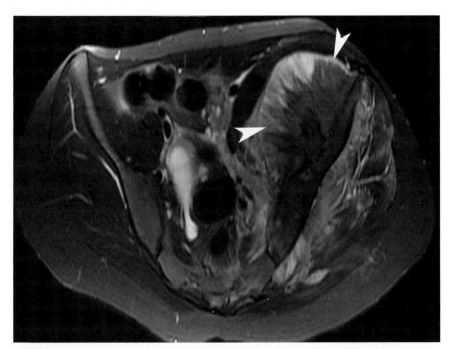

Figure 69.5. Axial T2 MR image with fat suppression in a 16-year-old girl who was complaining of left hip pain demonstrates the dramatic sunburst pattern (arrowheads) involving the left ilium medially and the soft-tissue extent on both sides of the bone.

- Radiologic overlap with myositis ossificans (myositis ossificans ossification peripheral whereas parosteal osterosarcoma is central, known as "reverse zoning")
- Cartilage cap (rare) without continuity of medullary cavity

Periosteal Osteosarcoma
- Arises from deep periosteum of diaphysis
- Thickened, scalloped, or irregular cortex
- Perpendicular spiculated or solid periosteal reaction
- Soft-tissue mass arising from cortex
- Broad base as seen on cross-sectional studies
- Prominent regions of low T1 and very high T2 SI, reflecting chondroblastic histology

Soft Tissue Osteosarcoma (4%)
- Also known as extraskeletal osteosarcoma or simply soft-tissue osteosarcoma
- Mass with osteoid matrix
- Lower extremities and pelvis
- "Fluffy" densities and may mimic myositis ossificans
- "Reverse zoning" phenomenon

Imaging Strategy

Radiography is the first modality to characterize the zone of transition and matrix. MRI will assess the true extent of the lesion which can be far greater than suggested by XR. CT more eloquently shows the aggressive periosteal reaction, cortical destruction and ostoid proliferation. It is important to define anatomic relationships, presence of skip lesions, epiphyseal or articular involvement, soft-tissue extension and involvement of structures such as neurovascular bundles. To select an appropriate site for biopsy, MRI can be used. Chest CT is necessary to rule out pulmonary metastases and technetium-99m MDP bone scintigraphy to exclude nonpulmonary metastases. Follow-up chest CT for the first 2 years following therapy is typically performed as 80 percent of relapses occur in the lungs exclusively. The remainder recur in the bones, therefore a follow-up radionuclide bone scan is also typically performed.

Related Physics

High-resolution technology is usually required for bone radiography especially for the evaluation of subtle changes in trabecular pattern. Requirements include dual focus X-ray tube, adequate filtration, manual collimation capability, automatic exposure control, appropriate grid, and in select cases compensation filters. Small focal spot radiography is always preferred for evaluation of subtle changes in trabecular pattern (0.6 mm is upper limit for an adequate small focal spot). Added aluminum filtration is recommended in order to minimize entrance skin exposure (ESE). Federal minimum is 2.9 millimeters aluminum at

80 kVp; many large academic centers use 3.2 to 3.4 millimeters. Added filtration is determined by a physicist in conjunction with a field service engineer and is a permanent adjustment to the machine. Automatic collimation defaults to the cassette size, which for small children is still too large, so that manual collimation must also be applied. Ideally, the extremity should be aligned with the long axis of the cassette to maximize manual collimation capabilities. Automatic exposure control is used with "in the Bucky" radiography, which employs phototimers to control exposure time but it is at the expense of higher ESE than table-top; typically larger children who can hold still will be imaged this way. "In the Bucky" radiography makes use of the antiscatter grid (with the associated Bucky factor of 3 to 5) thus raising the ESE by a factor of 3 to 5 when compared to table-top. The up side is that much lower scatter images are produced. Most of these adjustments, except for filtration and grid, can be easily made by the technologist at the console.

Differential Diagnosis

Classic high-grade intramedullary osteosarcomas:
- Osteomyelitis
- Aggressive osteoblastoma
- Lymphoma
- Ewing's Sarcoma

Telangiectatic osteosarcoma:
- Aneuysmal bone cyst
- Giant cell tumor
- Unicameral bone cyst

Low-grade medullary osteosarcoma (rare):
- Fibrous dysplasia
- Ossifying fibroma
- Nonossifying fibroma
- Fibroxanthoma

Parosteal osteosarcoma:
- Myositis ossificans
- Osteochondroma

Periosteal osteosarcoma:
- Ewing's sarcoma

Key Points
- Most common primary malignant tumor of bone in children and young adults
- Can mimic sports-related injury causing a delay in diagnosis
- Radiography (possibly CT) needed to characterize matrix
- Aggressive periosteal reaction: Codman's triangle, hair-on-end, or sunburst
- MRI for lesion extent and preoperative planning
- 15% present with metastases, of which 97% are in lungs

Further Reading

Beall DP, Ly J, Bell JP. Pediatric extraskeletal osteosarcoma. *Pediatr Radiol.* 2008; *38*(5):579–582.

Murphey MD, et al. The Many faces of osteosarcoma—from the archives of the AFIP; *Radiographics.* 1997;*17*:1205–1231.

Kim HJ, Chalmers PN, Morris CD. Pediatric osteogenic sarcoma. *Curr Opin Pediatr.* 2010;*22*(1):61–66.

Murphey MD, Jaovisidha SW, Temple HT, *et al.* Telangiectatic osteosarcoma: radiologic-pathologic comparison, *Radiology.* 2003;*229*(2):545–553.

Suresh S, Saifuddin A. Radiological appearances of appendicular osteosarcoma: a comprehensive pictorial review. *Clin Radiol.* 2007;*62*(4):314–323.

CHAPTER 70

Leukemia

Paul Guillerman, MD

Definition

The leukemias are a heterogeneous group of hematologic malignancies that arise from bone marrow precursors of lymphoid, myeloid, monocytic, erythroid, or megakaryocytic cell lineages. Nearly all childhood leukemia is acute and is classified by the World Health Organization (WHO) according to morphology, immunophenotype, cytogenetics, and specific gene mutations.

Clinical Features

Acute lymphoblastic leukemia (ALL; 75 percent) and acute myeloid leukemia (AML; 20 percent) are the most common and leukemia is the most common childhood cancer with a peak incidence at 2 to 3 years of age. An increased risk of leukemia is associated with certain genetic disorders, including trisomy 21, neurofibromatosis type 1, and ataxia-telangiectasia. Prenatal or postnatal radiation exposure have been reported to increase the risk of leukemia, although the magnitude of risk is uncertain. Fever, bleeding, lethargy, and pallor are common at presentation. Over one-third of children with leukemia present with limping, bone pain, arthralgia, or other musculoskeletal complaints. Hepatosplenomegaly, lymphadenopathy, or thymic enlargement can also be noted.

Anatomy and Physiology

The presenting symptoms and signs primarily reflect the impact of bone marrow infiltration with leukemic cells and suppression of normal hematopoiesis. Organomegaly and lymph node enlargement are the result of extramedullary leukemic cell infiltration.

Imaging Findings

Radiography (40 percent have some abnormality):
- Transverse lucent metaphyseal bands ("leukemic lines"): disturbed endosteal mineralization adjacent to the zone of provisional calcification; most conspicuous at sites of rapid skeletal growth such as the distal femur, proximal tibia, and proximal humerus and usually resolve quickly with treatment (Fig. 70.1)
- Diffuse demineralization, especially from steroid exposure
- Insufficiency fractures, including vertebral compression fractures
- Subperiosteal resorption of the medial cortex of the proximal humerus (common)
- Permeative or geographic lytic bone lesions (less common)
- Acute bone infarction secondary to marrow infiltration
- Bone sclerosis and osteonecrosis may develop after therapy

Bone scintigraphy
- Symmetric increased uptake in the metadiaphyses of the lower limbs
- Diffuse increased uptake in a "superscan" pattern
- Focal increased uptake at sites of cortical bone destruction (Fig. 70.2)
- Photopenic areas: vascular compromise or avascular necrosis secondary to leukemic marrow infiltration

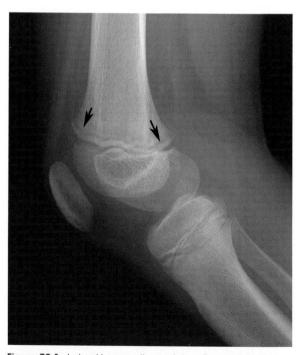

Figure 70.1. Lateral knee radiograph in a 7-year-old with ALL demonstrates a characteristic transverse lucent band ("leukemic line") (arrows) adjacent to the dense provisional zone of ossification along the distal femoral metaphysis.

(A)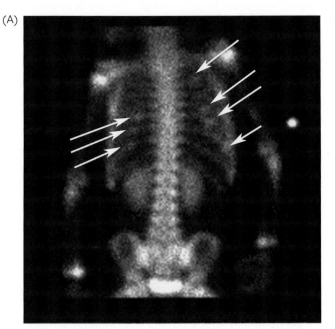

(B)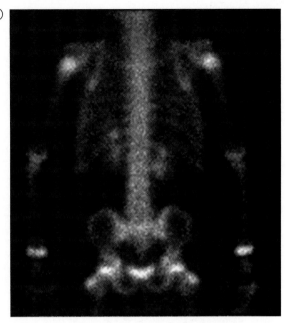

Figure 70.2. Technetium-99m MDP bone scan (A) in a 3-year-old with ALL shows diffuse increased radiopharmaceutical uptake in the skeleton, with more focal intense uptake in several ribs (arrows). Bone scan (B) in a 3-year-old without leukemia shows physiologic uptake.

MRI:

- Low T1, high T2, and STIR signal intensity (SI) (Fig. 70.3)
- Epiphyseal ossification centers: highest specificity and early involvement
- Following chemotherapy, residual leukemia, hematopoietic marrow regeneration (particularly in response to granulocyte colony stimulating factor (G-CSF) or granulocyte-macrophage colony stimulating factor (GM-CSF) therapy), marrow iron overload from transfusional hemosiderosis, and marrow fibrosis can all show decreased SI; marrow biopsy needed to differentiate
- Leukemia relapse may be observed on MRI several weeks before detection by iliac bone marrow biopsy; appears as well-defined nodules of low T1, high T2, and STIR SI

Imaging Strategy

In contrast to lymphoma and solid tumors, leukemia is a disseminated hematologic malignancy in which there is no current routine role of imaging in risk stratification, therapeutic response, or relapse surveillance. However, imaging studies are often requested to evaluate nonspecific musculoskeletal system complaints, in which imaging findings may suggest leukemia. Radiographic examination of symptomatic regions may be performed as first line. Nuclear scintigraphy or MRI may be used to help define the extent of disease and to help narrow the differential diagnosis and assess for secondary pathology such as pathologic fracture, osteomyelitis, or bone infarction. Conventional T1 and

fat-saturated T2 or STIR images are usually sufficient to suggest the diagnosis of leukemia. Contrast-enhanced T1 may be useful for identifying acute bone infarcts or areas of relative underperfusion and clarifying unclear findings on unenhanced sequences. Because of superior depiction of the symmetry and longitudinal pattern of marrow signal intensity, coronal and sagittal imaging planes are generally preferable to axial for evaluating the marrow. Fast whole-body MRI techniques, including single-shot sequences, parallel acquisition strategies, and multichannel systems with multiarray coils, permit rapid global assessment of the marrow; chemical shift and diffusion-weighted MRI techniques detect subtle differences in marrow composition, but their role in assessment of childhood leukemia is undefined.

Related Physics

Imaging disease processes that involve large body parts, or even the entire body, can be technically challenging and MRI is becoming the first-line imaging technique for some of these cases. Challenges include time, coil selection, patient positioning, and competing desires of high resolution as well as large volume of coverage. Marrow infiltrative disorders will appear throughout the widely distributed pediatric marrow and therefore one must include the entire body in surveillance studies. Sequences that offer high free-water conspicuity, such as short tau inversion recovery, are best performed in the coronal plane that allows the fewest "slices" over the largest volume of interest. A body phased array coil is chosen and is often coupled with the spine coil to optimize signal-to-noise and the field of view chosen approaches the z-axis limits of the

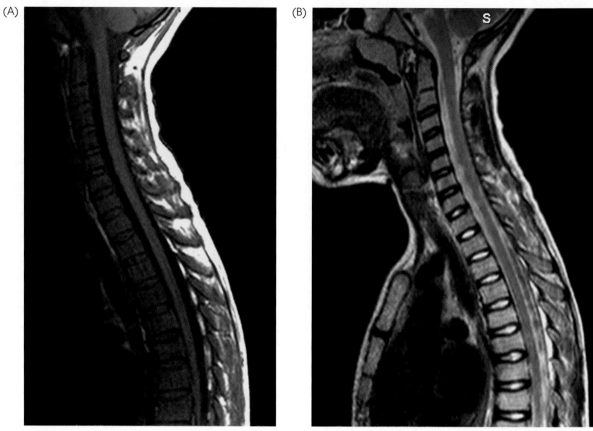

Figure 70.3. Sagittal T1 MR image of the cervical spine (A) in a 9-year-old with ALL reveals diffusely abnormally low SI. Sagittal T2 MR image (B) shows diffusely high SI.

coil. Although signal can be enriched through increasing slice thickness and signal excitations, the tradeoff for large field-of-view imaging is resolution. Any suspect areas on the coronal surveillance study can then be imaged in detail with surface coil and dedicated smaller parts techniques. One challenge with whole-body imaging is the need for multiple imaging "stations" whereby the coil and table must be moved several times during the study (depending on patient height).

Differential Diagnosis

Transverse lucent metaphyseal bands:
- TORCH infections (toxoplasmosis, other, rubella, cytomegalovirus, herpes simplex and HIV)
- Scurvy
- Systemic stress

Diffuse demineralization
- Steroid therapy
- Endocrinopathies
- Malabsorption syndromes
- Immobilization
- Osteogenesis imperfecta
- Homocysteinuria
- Juvenile idiopathic osteoporosis

Marrow infiltration on MRI:
- Lymphoma
- Metastatic neuroblastoma, rhabdomyosarcoma, Ewing's sarcoma (Fig. 70.4)
- Myelodysplastic/myeloproliferative syndromes
- Red marrow hyperplasia (hemolytic anemia, high-altitude residence, hematopoietic growth factor treatment)

Common Variants

Many childhood leukemia cases present with nonspecific bone or joint pain without leukocytosis or leukemic blasts on peripheral blood smear. This so-called "aleukemic" or "subleukemic" leukemia can masquerade clinically as osteomyelitis or arthritis and prompt referral for musculoskeletal MRI. Recognition of diffuse bone marrow infiltration, including the epiphyses, on MRI suggests the diagnosis of leukemia.

Clinical Issues

With contemporary pediatric risk-adapted therapy, the 5-year survival rate is nearly 90 percent for ALL and nearly 60 percent for AML. High initial leukocyte count and

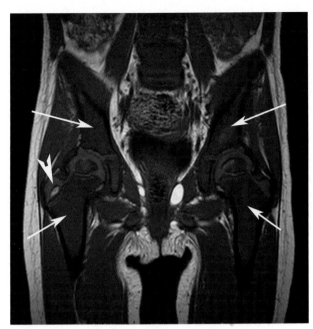

Figure 70.4. Coronal T1 MR image in a 3-year-old with metastatic neuroblastoma shows diffuse low SI throughout the marrow (arrows) including the epiphyses; the right greater trochanter shows normal fat SI and has been spared (arrowhead).

infancy are associated with poorer prognosis. Osteonecrosis and severe bone mineral density deficits are increasingly recognized toxicities in childhood leukemia survivors, especially those with a history of allogeneic bone marrow transplantation or prolonged corticosteroid treatment. Osteonecrosis can be debilitating if there is involvement of weight-bearing articular surfaces, and bone mineral density deficits can lead to insufficiency fractures and thoracic kyphosis with loss of height.

Key Points

- Widespread low T1, high T2, and STIR SI in marrow
- Early replacement of epiphyseal fat (high specificity)
- Can be mimicked by diffuse infiltration of the marrow by metastatic disease, myelodysplastic/myeloproliferative syndromes, and conditions associated with red marrow hyperplasia
- Five-year survival rate for ALL approximately 90%, AML approximately 60%
- Imaging helpful with nonspecific bone pain and for treatment-related complications
- Osteonecrosis is the most debilitating treatment-related complication in survivors

Further Reading

Bernard EJ, Nicholls WD, Howman-Giles RB, Kellie SJ, Uren RF. Patterns of abnormality on bone scans in acute childhood leukemia. *J Nucl Med.* 1998;39(11):1983–1986.

Guillerman RP. Normal and abnormal bone marrow. In: Slovis T, ed. *Caffey's Pediatric Diagnostic Imaging*, Eleventhth edition. Philadelphia, PA: Elsevier; 2008;2970–2996.

Kan JH, Hernanz-Schulman M, Frangoul HA, Connolly SA. MRI diagnosis of bone marrow relapse in children with ALL. *Pediatr Radiol.* 2008;38(1):76–81.

Sinigaglia R, Gigante C, Bisinella G, Varotto S, Zanesco L, Turra S. Musculoskeletal manifestations in pediatric acute leukemia. *J Pediatr Orthop.* 2008;28(1):20–28.

Smith MA, Seibel NL, Altekruse SF, et al. Outcomes for children and adolescents with cancer: challenges for the twenty-first century. *J Clin Oncol.* 2010;28(15):2625–2634.

Swerdlow SH, *Campo* E, Harris NL, et al., eds. *WHO Classification of Tumours of Haematopoietic and Lymphoid Tissues.* Fourth edition. Lyon, France: International Agency for Research on Cancer; 2008.

CHAPTER 71

Osteoid Osteoma

Sudha Pradumna Singh, MD

Definition

Osteoid osteoma is a benign bone-forming neoplasm of unknown etiology.

Clinical Features

Males are affected twice as often as females. Most patients are Caucasian. Age range varies from 19 months to 56 years (80 percent are between 5 to 25 years). The tumor can involve any bone, but predominantly involves the appendicular skeleton. The femur is the most common site (39 percent), followed by the tibia (23 percent). Twelve percent of tumors are found in the spine, especially lumbar, mainly involving the posterior elements. The hip is the most common site of intra-articular lesions. Although most lesions of the long bones are cortically based, intra-articular lesions are more likely to be located in cancellous bone and have less surrounding sclerosis. Patients most commonly present with chronic pain that increases in severity with time. The pain may be at the site of the lesion, distant, or referred to a local joint. The classic presentation is pain that is worse at night and is relieved by small doses of salicylates or nonsteroidal anti-inflammatories. The lesions are hypervascular and vasodilators usually increase pain. Spinal lesions may cause painful scoliosis, concave to the side of the lesion. Painless lesions may manifest with swelling, deformity, mass, or limp. Intra-articular lesions may present with nonspecific symptoms such as joint effusion, osteoarthritis, or synovitis. There is often regional muscle atrophy, possibly resulting from disuse. Soft-tissue swelling may be the dominant finding with lesions in the hands and feet.

Anatomy and Physiology

The tumor is also known as the nidus or core. It varies in size from 0.3 to 2 centimeters. It is composed of bone in varying stages of maturity within a very vascular connective tissue stroma. Mineralization is the densest at the center of the nidus. A fusiform sclerosis typically surrounds cortical lesions. There are two classification schemes for osteoid osteoma, both of which are based on location of the tumor or nidus in the bone on imaging examinations. The most commonly used classification divides the tumors into cortical, medullary or cancellous, and subperiosteal. Cortical osteoid osteomas are the most common and subperiosteal the least common. The second, more recently proposed scheme, divides the tumors into subperiosteal, intracortical, endosteal or intramedullary based on the location of the nidus on CT or MR imaging.

Imaging Findings

Radiography:

- Nidus 0.3 to 2 centimeters in diameter
- Varying degrees of mineralization (lucent to sclerotic)
- May resemble a sequestrum (sclerotic center, lucent periphery)
- Diaphyseal or metaphyseal lesions show variable degree of surrounding endosteal and cortical thickening and sclerosis (Fig. 71.1)
- Nidus near physis may cause growth disturbance/ bowing
- Scoliosis: degree of sclerosis depends on site of tumor; absent or minimal in medullary lesions and marked in cortical, endosteal, or subperiosteal lesions
- Painful scoliosis: posterior element lesions often lack sclerosis
- Intra-articular lesions have minimal or absent sclerosis, which may even be relatively distant from the tumor site

CT:

- Nidus is round or oval well-defined hypodense focus (Figs. 71.2, 71.3)
- Variable central hyperdensity representing the mineralized osteoid (Fig. 71.4)
- Dynamic postcontrast CT shows enhancement of the vascular nidus
- Variable degree of surrounding sclerosis and cortical thickening

MRI:

- Low to intermediate T1, variable T2 signal intensity (SI), depending on degree of mineralization
- Regional bone marrow edema (Fig. 71.5)
- Adjacent soft-tissue edema
- Joint effusion with intra-articular lesions
- Intense enhancement of the nidus

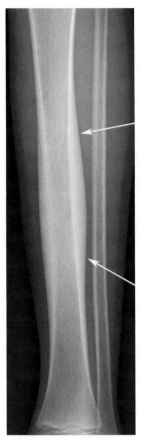

Figure 71.1. Frontal radiograph of the tibia/fibula in an 8-year-old girl with night pain and worsening limp for 1 year demonstrates cortical thickening or thick dense periosteal reaction (arrows) in the mid-diaphysis of the tibia. The nidus is obscured by the significant periosteal reaction.

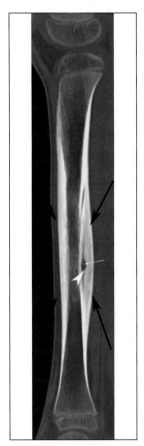

Figure 71.2. Sagittal CT reformation of the tibia and fibula in an 8-year-old girl with night pain and worsening limp for 1 year shows periosteal reaction (black arrows) along the mid-diaphysis of the tibia and a central well-circumscribed lucency (arrowhead) is visualized. A small hyperdense focus in the center of this lucency (small white arrow) represents the matrix in the nidus.

Bone scintigraphy:
- Intense uptake on Tc 99m MDP images at the site of the tumor (Fig. 71.6)
- Focal uptake on both immediate and delayed images
- SPECT may be useful in areas of complex anatomy
- Scintigraphic double-density sign: a small central focus of intense uptake superimposed on a larger area of increased uptake

Imaging Strategy

Radiography is the first imaging modality. Bone scintigraphy may demonstrate the tumor before radiographic findings are apparent. Although nonspecific, the double-density sign may suggest the diagnosis of osteoid osteoma and direct focused cross-sectional imaging. Bone scintigraphy may play an important role in preoperative localization of the nidus, intraoperative and postoperative confirmation

of the complete removal of the nidus. For precise localization of the nidus prior to therapy, CT is currently considered the ultimate diagnostic tool. Thin-section (2 mm) axial images, obtained with a bone algorithm accompanied by multiplanar reformations and viewed at bone window settings best depict the nidus. MRI may fail to adequately demonstrate a small, heavily ossified nidus. Recent MRI techniques that optimize spatial resolution and contrast enhancement have demonstrated promise.

Related Physics

An excellent second-line tool in the workup of osteoid osteoma is Tc-99m MDP bone scintigraphy. A gamma scintillation camera is most commonly used for standard bone scan. Its features include collimator type, acquisition

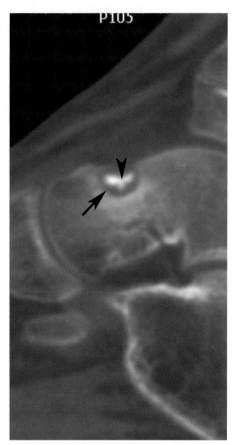

Figure 71.3. CT sagittal reformation through the talus in an 11-year-old female athlete with a 7-month history of ankle and foot pain and MRI showing edema in the talus shows a well-circumscribed lucent nidus (arrow) with central calcification (arrowhead). Mild surrounding sclerosis is seen.

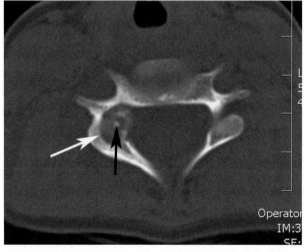

Figure 71.4. Axial CT image of the cervical spine in a 5-year-old male presenting with 9 months of neck pain that wakes him at night and settles with salicylates demonstrates a lucent lesion (white arrow) with central calcified nidus (black arrow) and surrounding sclerosis of the right facet.

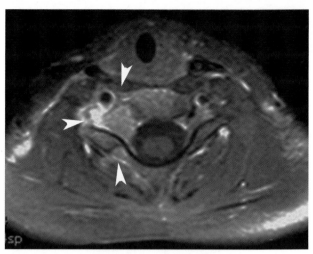

Figure 71.5. Axial T2 MR image of the cervical spine in a 5-year-old male presenting with 9 months of neck pain that wakes him at night and settles with salicylates demonstrates significant edema (white arrowheads) in the right facet and surrounding soft tissues but fails to demonstrate the nidus.

vmodes, measures of camera performance, and clinical imaging protocols. There are three types of collimator: parallel hole; pinhole; and specialized collimators. Parallel collimators are often used to image a large region of interest, such as the entire extremity in a child. A pinhole collimator is most often used for a small structure such as the proximal femoral metaphyseal cortex, a common site for osteoid osteoma. Specialized collimators include diverging and converging nonparallel-hole collimators, which result in image magnification and minification, respectively. Imaging acquisition modes include static, dynamic, and cardiac-gated acquisition. It is important to have a qualified medical physicist to evaluate the camera's performance on at least an annual basis. Tests that should be considered when evaluating a camera include uniformity, spatial resolution, energy resolution, spatial linearity, sensitivity, count rate performance and dead time. Dedicated imaging protocols have been developed for every organ system and clinical indication in pediatrics and adult medicine. The correct choice of protocol will maximize the diagnostic yield.

Differential Diagnosis

Cortical nidus:
- Brodie's abscess or chronic osteomyelitis
- Stress fracture
- Early stages of malignant tumor such as osteosarcoma
- Osteoblastoma

Intra-articular lesion:
- Arthritis: inflammatory, rheumatoid, septic, etc.
- Legg-Calvé-Perthes disease

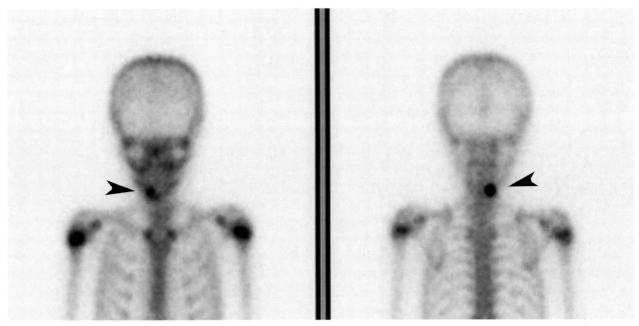

Figure 71.6. Frontal image from bone scintigraphy in a 5-year-old male presenting with 9 months of neck pain that wakes him at night and settles with salicylates shows intense uptake (black arrowheads) in the right half of C6.

Clinical Issues

Complete excision or radiofrequency ablation of the nidus leads to immediate cessation of the symptoms. This can be performed by the radiologist, using CT guidance under general anesthetic. Persistent symptoms may indicate incomplete excision of the nidus or a second lesion.

Key Points

- Osteoid osteoma is a benign bone tumor.
- Osteoid osteoma predominantly affects the appendicular skeleton, most often the femur.
- Intense reactive new bone formation is usually perilesional but may be distant with intra-articular tumors.

- CT is the modality of choice for visualization and identification of the nidus and can be used for imaging-guided radiofrequency ablation.
- Incomplete removal of the nidus may lead to continued symptoms.

Further Reading

Chai JW et al. Radiographic diagnosis of osteoid osteoma: from simple to challenging findings. *Radiographics.* 2010;*30*:737–749.

Kransdorf MJ, Stull MA, Gilkey FW, Moser, RP Jr. From the Archives of the AFIP: osteoid osteoma. *Radiographics.* 1991;*11*:671–696.

Liu PT et al. Imaging of osteoid osteoma with dynamic gadolinium-enhanced MR imaging. *Radiology.* 2003; *227*:691–700.

Nawaz Khan A. Emedicine—Osteoid Osteoma Radiology.

CHAPTER 72

Developmental Dysplasia of the Hip

Scott Dorfman, MD

Definition

Developmental dysplasia of the hip (DDH) is a spectrum of abnormalities that includes ligamentous laxity, subluxation, and dislocation of the hips with underdevelopment of the acetabulum. Developmental dysplasia of the hip can develop prenatally or postnatally and can improve or worsen in the first few months of life.

Clinical Features

The incidence of developmental dysplasia is 0.3 to 2 percent of live births with a female predominance. Developmental dysplasia of the hip affects the left hip more than the right and is bilateral in 25 percent. Risk factors include breech presentation, oligohydramnios, and positive family history. The diagnosis is typically first suspected during screening physical examination that reveals a hip click or clunk elicited with the Ortolani or Barlow maneuver. Asymmetric thigh skin folds are suggestive but less specific. Imaging is usually performed for further evaluation.

Anatomy and Physiology

Abnormal flexion of the hips in utero is thought to result in abnormal acetabular development. This is most common with breech presentation or conditions that increase uterine packing, such as oligohydramnios or multiple gestations, that can result in hyperflexion of the hips during development and subsequent subluxation and acetabular dysplasia. Developmental dysplasia of the hip is associated with other conditions that can arise from fetal movement restriction and compression such as club feet, torticollis, and molding deformity of the skull.

Imaging Findings

Graf and Harcke Ultrasound (US) Method

Hip US study consists of both a morphologic approach and a dynamic evaluation. Acetabular anatomy is assessed by the Graf technique imaging in the coronal plane through the mid-acetabulum. This approach classifies DDH into one of four main categories from acetabular immaturity to severe dysplasia based on measurements of the osseous

acetabular roof (the α angle) and the cartilaginous acetabular roof (the ß angle). Harcke developed a dynamic scanning technique that images during stress maneuvers used in the physical examination. A combination of these two techniques is called the standard minimum hip examination. A 7.5 to 15 megahertz linear-array transducer is typically used and each component of the examination is defined by the position of the transducer followed by the position of the hip.

Coronal View

The transducer is centered posterior to the femoral head, over the cartilage gap between the ischium and ilium while the femur is pushed downward, a maneuver that mimics the Barlow test. Key landmarks for this view include visualization of the iliac line, the osseous acetabular roof, and the sharp superolateral margin (Fig. 72.1).

- Normal femoral head coverage of at least 50 percent; femoral head coverage is assessed by extending the iliac line through the cartilaginous femoral head (Fig. 72.2A)
- Normal alpha angle is 60 degrees or greater and is formed by the junction of the line along the osseous acetabular roof and the iliac line; α angle is used to determine Graf hip type
- ß angle represents the junction of the iliac line with a line drawn along the cartilaginous acetabular roof
- With acetabular dysplasia, the lateral margin of the osseous acetabulum can be rounded or flattened, instead of the normal sharp and angular margin
- Shallow acetabulum in subluxation with less than 50 percent coverage (Fig. 72.2B)
- Femoral epiphysis moves craniad and toward the transducer in dislocation (Fig. 72.3)

Transverse View

With the transducer held in a transverse or axial position, relative to the pelvis, the hip is evaluated both in 90 degrees of flexion and in a neutral position. While the hip is flexed, it is passively moved between abduction and adduction to assess stability. Stress can also be applied during adduction, the US equivalent of the Barlow test. If already dislocated, the femoral head can be seen to relocate while in abduction,

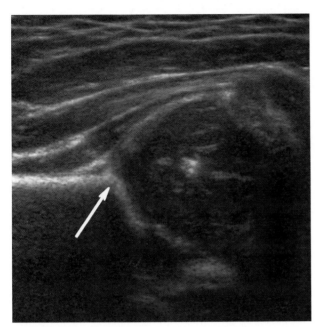

Figure 72.1. Coronal US image of a normal hip shows a sharp superolateral angle (arrow).

the US equivalent of the Ortolani test. With the hip in a neutral position, the location of the femoral head relative to the triradiate cartilage is also assessed.

Imaging Strategies

Hip US is the imaging study of choice in an infant 6 months or younger when DDH is suspected by clinical findings or as a screening examination in patients who are at higher

risk for the condition. Ultrasound permits direct visualization of cartilage and other soft tissues that are otherwise not visualized on plain films in the first few months of life. Hip US can evaluate acetabular development as well as femoral head position relative to the acetabulum. A dynamic study can assess for subluxable or dislocatable hips and can identify ligamentous laxity and reducibility. Ossification of the femoral epiphysis precludes US after 4 to 5 months of age at which time radiography is preferred. Hip position in spica cast can be confirmed with MRI or low-dose CT without sedation following operative reduction.

Related Physics

Ultrasound should be used to initially evaluate DDH prior to ossification of the proximal femoral epiphyses. Advanced DDH in an older infant is evaluated with radiography to determine angles and to follow after nonoperative or surgical correction. For DDH, radiographs must show the architecture of the entire hip including soft tissues in relation to the bones, however trabecular detail is not as important. Radiographic techniques should be designed to optimize subject contrast; lower kVp (50 to 60) will be optimal. In order to properly evaluate images, the workstation should have appropriate light output measured as luminance, sufficiently large matrix size (~1536 x 2048 or 3 M pixel), be calibrated for gray-scale integrity with a ratio of 500:1 or better, and have periodic control measures taken. The pictoral archive and communication system (PACS) hanging protocols should include tools to measure the acetabular angles from the frontal projection.

(A)

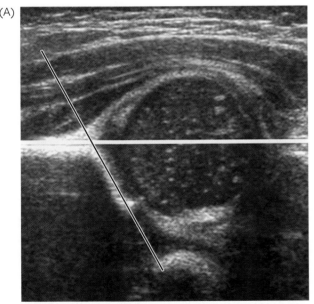

(B)

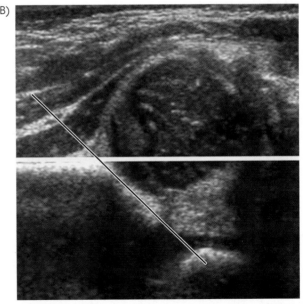

Figure 72.2. Coronal US image of a normal hip (A) shows the horizontal line (line) along the length of the iliac bone under which there should be at least 50 percent of the cartilaginous epiphysis. The black line runs along the lie of the acetabular roof. The normal angle (alpha) between these measures less than 60 degrees. Coronal US image in a dysplatic hip (B) shows less than 50 percent coverage and an alpha angle between the white and black lines of much less than 60 degrees.

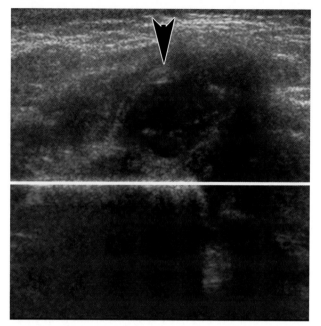

Figure 72.3. Coronal US image in a dislocated hip shows no alpha angle and no coverage of the epiphysis (arrowhead), which is displaced superficially toward the probe.

Differential Diagnosis

Teratologic hip dysplasia: (infants born with dislocated hip and often severe hip and pelvic changes at birth; not considered part of the spectrum of DDH)

- Neuromuscular disorder
- Arthrogryposis
- Myelomeningocele

Common Variants

Physiologic immaturity, which is caused by the maternal hormone relaxin in the first few weeks of life, is a normal variant and unless persistent after 4 weeks of age, should not be considered part of the DDH spectrum.

Clinical Issues

Ultrasound is utilized both as a screening and diagnostic tool as well as a guide during therapy. In a patient with an abnormal physical examination because of mild ligamentous laxity, or with a risk factor but normal physical examination, screening US should not be performed before 4 weeks to eliminate any unnecessary imaging in the setting of physiologic immaturity or laxity that requires no intervention. Hip subluxation/dislocation is treated with immobilization in a soft (Pavlik) harness with flexion-abduction and external rotation of the hips to ensure a normal relationship between the femoral head and acetabulum. Irreducible dislocations or delayed presentation of the condition after 6 months may necessitate surgical intervention. Follow-up imaging in patients treated with Pavlik harness can be performed with serial US while the patient is left in the harness. No stress maneuvers should be performed during treatment except passive abduction and adduction of the hips. The purpose of subsequent US is to confirm femoral head position and to document the morphology of the acetabulum. The α angle and femoral head coverage improve over time.

Treatment carries a low risk of avascular necrosis of the femoral head.

Key Points

- Development dysplasia of the hips (DDH) is a spectrum of abnormalities.
- Conditions that cause limited fetal motion or constraint carry a higher risk for DDH.
- Early detection and treatment of DDH lead to the best outcomes.
- US is the modality of choice for both diagnosis and follow-up, as it allows direct visualization of the cartilaginous femoral head and acetabulum.

Further Reading

American College of Radiology. ACR Appropriateness Criteria. Developmental Dysplasia of the Hip—Child. Effective October 1, 2010.

DiPietro MA, Harcke HT. Developmental dysplasia of the hip. In: Slovis TL, ed. *Caffey's Pediatric Diagnostic Imaging*. Vol. 2. Eleventh edition. Mosby; 2007:3049–3066.

Torres MFL, DiPietro MA. Developmental dysplasia of the hip. *Ultrasound Clinics.* 2009;4(4):445–455.

Chapter 14. Developmental dysplasia of the hip. In: *Musculoskeletal System and Vascular Imaging.* 628–636.

CHAPTER 73

Legg-Calvé-Perthes Disease

Tracey Mehlman, MD and Pinar Karakas, MD

Definition

Legg-Calvé-Perthes disease (LCPD), or Perthes disease is an idiopathic avascular necrosis (AVN) of the proximal femoral epiphysis which impairs endochondral ossification of the femoral head.

Clinical Features

There is a male predominance of 4:1 and LCPD is more common in Caucasians. The typical age group is 5 to 8 years old although the disease presents slightly earlier in females. Bilateral disease is noted in about 10 to 15 percent of patients with asynchronous presentation. The initial insult in LCPD is usually asymptomatic, however patients can present with a painless limp or with pain in the groin, hip, or ipsilateral knee, often present only during physical activity. There can be decreased range of motion with internal rotation and hip abduction. In addition, the ipsilateral thigh may demonstrate muscle atrophy.

Anatomy and Physiology

The cause of LCPD is insufficiency of the capital epiphyseal blood supply, either venous or arterial, with the physis acting as a barrier. Infarction leads to trabecular fracture with collapse of the femoral head and injury to the growth plate. The resultant deformity is one of the leading causes of premature osteoarthritis. The etiology remains controversial with many factors such as trauma, infection, or congenital factors having possible associations. More common causes of avascular necrosis such as leukemia, corticosteroid administration, Gaucher's or sickle cell disease or vasculitis must be excluded.

Imaging Findings

Avascular phase:

- XR: ossified epiphysis smaller and denser with surrounding osteopenia: interruption of endochondral ossification
- XR: joint space widening: articular cartilage receives nutrients through the synovial fluid and continues to grow
- MR: early marrow edema, synovial thickening and joint effusion

- Dynamic contrast-enhanced MRI with subtraction: decreased or absent perfusion of the femoral head (Fig. 73.1).
- Bone scintigraphy: decreased or absent perfusion

Revascularization:

- Fragmentation and even full resorption of the epiphysis
- "Crescent sign": subchondral fracture seen as linear lucency through the epiphysis best seen on frog-leg lateral views (Fig. 73.2)
- Flattening and deformity of the epiphysis: necrotic bone weaker than normal bone
- Contrast-enhanced MRI and scintigraphy: reperfusion of the femoral head, either from recanalization of the existing vessels along the lateral column of the epiphysis or from neovascularization from vessels at the base of the epiphysis

Healing phase:

- Reossification of the epiphysis beginning at the periphery (Fig. 73.3)
- Remodeling until the patient reaches maturity: shape and sphericity of the femoral head is determined by containment within the acetabulum
- Coxa magna (broadening of the head)
- Broadening of the metaphysis
- Metaphyseal "cysts": focal deposition of cartilage within the metaphysis (Fig. 73.4)
- Coxa breva: shortening of the femoral neck from growth plate arrest
- MRI most sensitive to evaluate extent of osteonecrosis and femoral containment and physeal interruption

IMAGING PITFALLS: Although radiographs are usually abnormal at the time of presentation, radiographic findings can lag behind the initial insult by as much as 14 months. MRI and bone scintigraphy can detect early signs of osteonecrosis.

Imaging Strategy

Radiography should include frontal and frog-leg lateral views of both hips. MRI is recommended to detect early changes when radiographs are normal or in the later stages of disease to better assess severity and associated

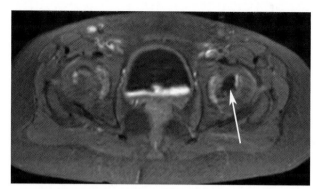

Figure 73.1. Axial contrast-enhanced T1 MR image in a boy with left hip pain shows decreased perfusion of the left femoral epiphysis (arrow).

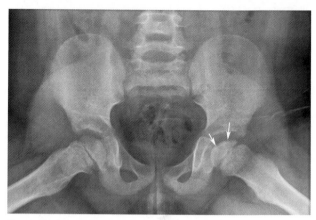

Figure 73.2. Frog-leg lateral view of the pelvis in a boy with left hip pain shows a subchondral fracture (arrows) with increased sclerosis, flattening and irregularity of the left femoral epiphysis.

complications. Sequences include: coronal T1, STIR; axial T1, T2 with fat suppression; sagittal: T1, T2 with fat suppression; dynamic pre- and postcontrast T1 gradient echo (GRE) with subtraction. Bone scintigraphy is utilized when MRI is unavailable or contraindicated.

Related Physics

Radionuclide scintigraphy is still commonly used in the workup of hip pain in children. Some data will be attenuated along its path to the detector by overlying structures such as soft tissue or bone. These seemingly photopenic regions can undergo a process known as "attenuation correction" to account for this. In modern single photon emission computed tomography (SPECT) systems this is done first by acquiring a CT image of the anatomy of interest prior to the injection of the radionuclide. Rays along the axial images of the CT

scan can be integrated and used as a proxy for attenuation along any specific path. Image reconstruction can be done by filtered back projection or iterative reconstruction. Filtered back projection is prone to streak artifacts where there is a highly discordant concentration of isotope such as in the urinary bladder. With an increase in computer speeds, iterative reconstruction is becoming the preferred algorithm as it is less prone to artifact and is mathematically capable of correcting for attenuation and blur related to depth. Artifacts on SPECT include center of rotation (COR), uniformity, stray magnetic field effects, and motion. COR artifacts are caused by a misalignment of the gantry's center of rotation relative to the center of rotation of the acquired data, which can cause streak artifacts and image blurring. Detector uniformity artifacts occur from nonuniform light across the sodium iodide

(A)

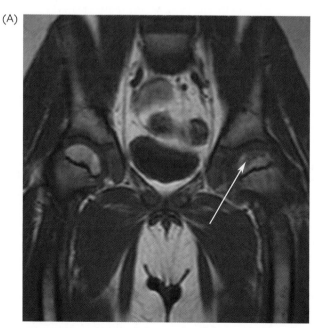

(B)

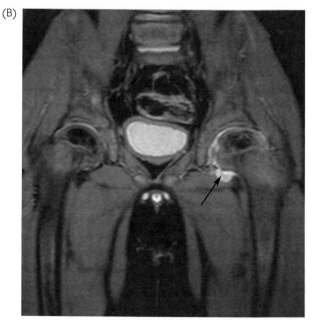

Figure 73.3. Coronal T1 (A) and STIR (B) MR images in a girl with advanced Perthes show flattening and irregularity of the femoral epiphysis (white arrow) with marrow edema along with a joint effusion (black arrow).

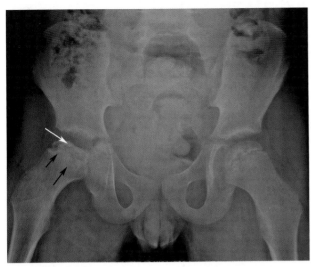

Figure 73.4. Frontal radiograph of the pelvis in advanced Perthes shows fragmentation of the right femoral epiphysis (white arrow) with metaphyseal cyst (black arrows) formation. There is widening of the joint space resulting from increased cartilage.

crystal, defective or uncalibrated photomultiplier tubes, or faulty electronics. This will create partial or complete circular arcs on the image, appearing brighter or darker than the true signal. When nuclear medicine cameras are located in close proximity to MRI or other magnetic fields, electrons generated within the photomultiplier tube may be misdirected resulting in inaccurate signal output from that tube. Patient or respiratory motion results in misregistration and image blurring.

Differential Diagnosis

- Toxic synovitis
- Septic hip
- Juvenile chronic arthritis
- Juvenile osteonecrosis
- Meyer dysplasia
- Slipped capital femoral epiphysis

Clinical Issues

The method of reperfusion forms the basis of the Modified Herring Classification that assesses prognosis based on the percentage of lateral pillar height that is maintained:

- Type A: full height of lateral pillar is preserved and no density change
- Type B: > 50 percent of lateral pillar height is preserved
- Type B/C border group: very narrow lateral pillar that is at least 50 percent of original height; lateral pillar with little ossification at least 50 percent of original height; lateral pillar that is 50 percent of original height and depressed relative to central pillar

- Type C: < 50 percent of lateral pillar is preserved

Treatment can be either conservative with immobilization or abduction bracing, or surgical with femoral and pelvic osteotomies to contain the hip. The lateral pillar classification and age at the time of onset of the disease strongly correlate with the outcome in patients with LCPD. Children 8 years of age or less who have type B hips at the time of onset have a favorable outcome regardless of treatment. Surgical treatment is favorable in those children who are more than 8 years of age and have B or B/C border group hips. Patients with type C hips at the time of diagnosis have a poor outcome regardless of treatment. Of those with LCPD, 60 to 70 percent of hips heal spontaneously without impairment at maturity, but a large number undergo premature degeneration (secondary osteoarthrosis), which is the most common long-term complication. Treatment does not influence the extent of necrosis or revascularization, however it can prevent deformity and possibly delay early osteoarthritis. Poorer prognosis has also been associated with > 20 percent epiphyseal extrusion from the acetabulum or > 50 percent epiphyseal involvement.

Key Points

- Legg-Calvé-Perthes disease is an idiopathic avascular necrosis of the proximal femoral epiphysis.
- LCPD most commonly affects 5- to 8-year-old Caucasian boys.
- Imaging findings include sclerosis, fragmentation and flattening of the capital epiphysis.
- MRI detects abnormalities up to 14 months earlier than plain radiography.
- Lateral pillar classification and age of onset of disease strongly correlate with prognosis.

Further Reading

Balasa W, Gruppo RA, Glueck CJ, Wang P, Roy DR, Wall EJ et al. Legg-Calve-Perthes disease and thrombophilia, *J Bone Joint Surg Am.* 2004;86:2642–2647.

Dillman RD, Hernandez RJ. MRI of Legg-Calve-Perthes disease. *AJR.* 2009;193:1394–1407.

Fabry, G. Clinical practice: the hip from birth to adolescence. *Eur. J Pediatr.* 2010;169:143–148.

Herring JA, Hui TK, Browne R. Legg-Calve-Perthes disease. Part 1: Classification of radiographs with use of the modified lateral pillar Stulberg classifications. *J Bone Joint Surg Am.* 2004;86(10):2103–2120.

Herring JA, Kim HT, Browne R. Legg- Calvé Perthes disease. Part II: Prospective multicenter study of the effect of treatment on outcome. *J Bone Joint Surg Am.* 2004;86(10):2121–2134.

Jaramillo D. What is the optimal imaging of osteonecrosis, Perthes and bone infarcts? *Pediatr Radiol.* 2009;39(Suppl 2):S216–S219.

CHAPTER 74

Slipped Capital Femoral Epiphysis

Paul Babyn, MD

Definition

Slipped capital femoral epiphysis (SCFE), also referred to as slipped upper femoral epiphysis, is defined as a type I Salter-Harris fracture through the proximal femoral physis. While the epiphysis remains intact within the acetabulum, loss of structural integrity along the physis results in displacement of the femoral neck and the appearance of a posteriorly and inferiorly displaced epiphysis.

Clinical Features

The most common hip disorder in adolescents, SCFE affects approximately 1 to 6 in 20,000 patients with a 2:1 male predominance. Metachronous bilateral involvement may occur in up to one-third of patients and synchronous involvement is not uncommon. The disorder is most common in patients 10 to 15 years of age shortly after the onset of puberty. Studies have reported greater prevalence in patients with obesity, African or Hispanic ancestry and endocrine disorders. Slipped capital femoral epiphysis may be classified by the chronicity of clinical symptoms and the stability of the joint. The presence of symptoms for less than 3 weeks distinguishes acute from chronic SCFE. Sudden exacerbation of chronic symptoms is known as acute-on-chronic SCFE. The ability to weight bear in the affected joint distinguishes stable from unstable conditions; in stable SCFE, the patient maintains the ability to weight bear, which is lost in unstable SCFE. In general, acute SCFE is associated with an unstable joint and intense pain unlike in chronic SCFE in which pain is mild and may subside with rest. An impending slip, or "pre-slip," of the capital femoral epiphysis may present as hip pain, but without clear radiographic evidence of slippage, although minor metaphyseal and physeal changes may be seen, including widening and irregularity of the physis and rarefaction of the proximal femoral metaphysis adjacent to the physis. If left untreated, pre-slips inevitably result in SCFE.

Anatomy and Physiology

Slipped capital femoral epiphysis results from shear forces along the proximal femoral physis, which leads to type I Salter-Harris fracture through the physis with subsequent displacement of the metaphysis relative to the epiphysis, usually inferiorly and superiorly. Risk factors for developing SCFE include biomechanical factors (obesity, trauma), which may increase the intensity of shear forces along the physis, as well as endocrinopathies (hypothyroidism, renal disease, and hypogonadism), which may decrease the structural integrity of physis. The combination of increased biomechanical stress and a weakened perichondrial ring during puberty, because of increased growth and hormonal changes, respectively, accounts for the high incidence of SCFE in patients between 10 and 15 years of age.

Imaging Findings

Radiography:
- Widening, lucency, and irregularity of the physis
- Sclerosis in the femoral neck caused by femoral head rotation
- Klein's line does not intersect with epiphysis on frontal view (Fig. 74.1)
- Bone remodeling
- Displacement of the epiphysis from the metaphysis anteriorly or posteriorly on lateral view
- Osteonecrosis, chondrolysis, and osteoarthritis in the hip joint

MRI:
- Abnormal morphology of head-neck junction
- High T2 SI indicative of stress and edema at the physis
- Synovitis
- Joint effusion

Based on radiographic findings, severity of SCFE may be classified as mild, moderate, or severe depending on extent of slippage of the metaphysis at the level of the epiphysis by less than one-third, one-third to two-thirds, and greater than two-thirds, respectively. Alternatively, severity of SCFE may be defined by the angle made by the capital epiphysis and the shaft of the femur, in which mild, moderate, and severe disease may be described by an angle of less than 30 degrees, between 30 and 50 degrees, and greater than 50 degrees, respectively.

Imaging Strategy

Imaging in patients with SCFE is typically conducted at initial diagnosis, as well as postoperatively. Radiography,

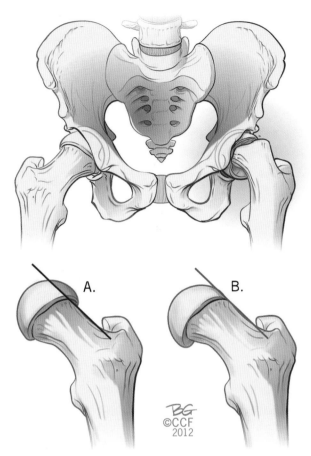

Figure 74.1. SCFE. Frontal illustration of the pelvis shows classic left SCFE with widening of the physis and superior migration of the metaphysis. Figure A shows a normal Klein's line (green) along the lateral border of the femoral metaphysis intersecting the femoral epiphysis. Figure B shows an abnormal Klein's line (red) that does not intersect the epiphysis consistent with SCFE.

are impeded by metal artifact, bone scintigraphy may be beneficial.

> **IMAGING PITFALLS:** Positioning patients with unstable joints in order to obtain frog-leg lateral views is not recommended because of patient discomfort and the possibility of exacerbating the slippage. True lateral views are recommended in these patients.

Related Physics

Body habitus typical for SCFE presents challenges in obtaining high-quality radiographic images. High spatial resolution is desired in order to detect subtle early changes of physeal widening and irregularity even before the "slip" has occurred. Imaging is performed in the Bucky with grid using large cassettes at high resolution despite the massive amounts of data generated. Body habitus poses challenges regarding exposure control and noise. A small focal spot cannot generate high enough exposure output so that a large focal spot is chosen. Automatic exposure control may be augmented with a density control adjuster of +1 to +2 that will increase the mA without increasing the exposure time. Noise is controlled by use of a grid and exposure augmentation. As there is risk for bilateral disease, bilateral imaging is required necessitating gonadal shielding.

Differential Diagnosis

- Hemarthrosis
- Fracture
- Septic arthritis
- Acute osteomyelitis
- Legg-Calvé-Perthes disease
- Juvenile rheumatoid arthritis
- Transient synovitis

Common Variants

Although the metaphysis is usually displaced anteriorly and superiorly, the orientation of slippage may differ depending on the mechanism of injury. In addition, radiologists should recognize bilateral SCFE, which is not uncommon in patients with previous unilateral SCFE.

Clinical Issues

When the patient experiences only mild symptoms, SCFE may go undiagnosed for lengthy periods. Surgery is the treatment of choice to prevent further slippage and promote physeal closure. Improved prognosis with fewer complications has been reported following urgent treatment within 24 hours of diagnosis. Therefore, SCFE should be treated as an emergency upon diagnosis and confirmation by imaging. In patients with previous SCFE, special attention should

with frontal and frog-leg lateral views, remains the primary modality, and CT and MRI may provide valuable additional information when radiography is inconclusive. Because of the lack of ionizing radiation and improved tissue contrast, MRI is preferred. For surgical planning, CT and MRI volume reconstructions may be of value. In patients with clinical symptoms, but negative radiographic findings, MRI or bone scintigraphy may assist in the identification of impending SCFE, or "pre-slips." Imaging at initial diagnosis should be used to rule in rather than rule out SCFE, especially in patients with clinical symptoms in whom one or more risk factors are identified.

MRI of the pelvis, including both hips, include the following sequences: coronal STIR, T1; axial T1, T2 with fat suppression; sagittal T1, T1 FLASH, T2. Postoperative radiographic imaging should be conducted to detect early signs of complications. In unilateral SCFE, postoperative imaging should also focus on identifying signs of slippage in the contralateral hip, especially if the patient experiences decreased range of motion or pain. In complicated cases, CT or MRI may be necessary. When both CT and MRI

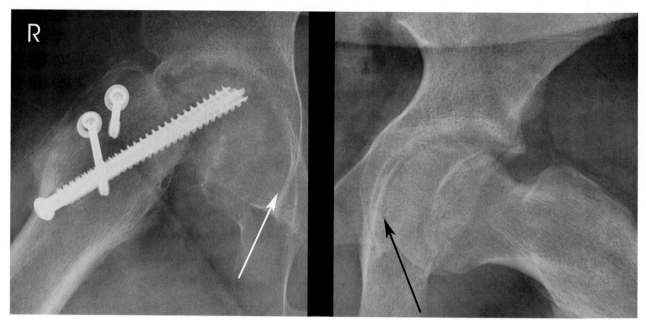

Figure 74.2. Frog-leg lateral radiograph of the right hip in a teen following SCFE fixation shows a noticeable decrease in thickness of the cartilage with joint space narrowing (white arrow) resulting from chondrolysis which may be seen prior to or following treatment. Left hip shows normal cartilage thickness (black arrow).

be focused to identifying early signs of slippage in the contralateral hip. Prophylactic screw or pin fixation may be indicated in these patients. Complications of SCFE may be either idiopathic or iatrogenic. Forceful fixation and more severe, unstable cases are associated with greater incidence and severity of complications, such as chondrolysis, osteonecrosis, and osteoarthritis. Chondrolysis is defined as > 2-millimeter decrease in cartilage thickness compared with

normal hip, or total cartilage thickness of < 3 millimeters in cases with bilateral involvement (normal cartilage thickness should be ~ 4 to 5 millimeters in patients 10 to 15 years of age Fig. 74.2). This may be seen initially, but is more frequently seen following treatment. Osteonecrosis presents as patchy radiolucency and sclerosis, usually in the femoral head (Fig. 74.3). If clinically suspected, bone scintigraphy or MRI should be requested. Osteoarthritis may result from

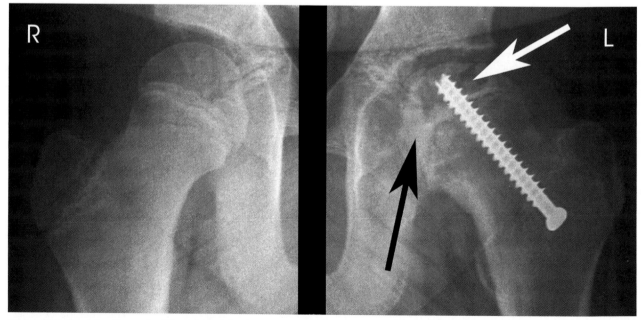

Figure 74.3. Frontal radiograph of the left hip following screw fixation for SCFE shows fragmentation, lucency (white arrow), and sclerosis (black arrow) consistent with avascular necrosis. Right hip is normal.

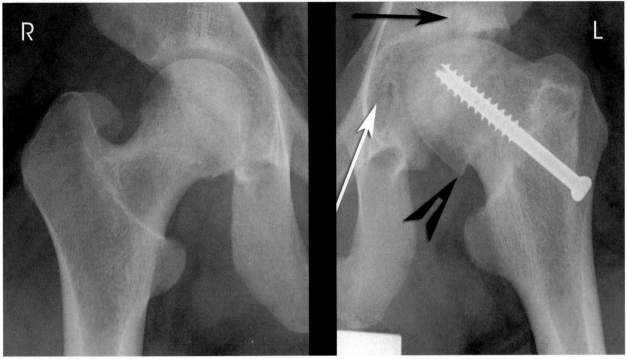

Figure 74.4. Frontal radiograph of the left hip after osteotomy and screw fixation for SCFE shows lucency (white arrow), sclerosis (black arrow), and spurring (arrowhead) in the femoral neck resulting from osteoarthritis. Right hip is normal.

metaphyseal impingement, even if only temporarily prior to treatment, or poor anatomic alignment after treatment. There is typically bony lucency in the femoral head and a hump in the femoral neck (Fig. 74.4). There may also be femoral head impingement. CT or MRI may be helpful.

Key Points

- Approximately 2:1 male predominance
- Type I Salter-Harris fracture through the physis
- Displacement of the metaphysis while the epiphysis remains within the acetabulum
- Risk factors include obesity, trauma, and endocrinopathies
- Common complications include avascular necrosis, chrondrolysis, and osteoarthritis

Further Reading

Dwek JR. The hip: MR imaging of uniquely pediatric disorders. *Magn Reson Imaging Clin N Am.* 2009;*17*(3):509–520, vi.

Fabry G. Clinical practice: the hip from birth to adolescence. *Eur J Pediatr.* 2010;*169*(2):143–148.

Hubbard AM. Imaging of pediatric hip disorders. *Radiol Clin North Am.* 2001;*39*(4):721–732.

Laine JC, Kaiser SP, Diab M. High-risk pediatric orthopedic pitfalls. *Emerg Med Clin North Am.* 2010;*28*(1):85–102, viii.

Tins B, Cassar-Pullicino V, McCall I. Slipped upper femoral epiphysis: imaging of complications after treatment. *Clin Radiol.* 2008;*63*(1):27–40.

CHAPTER 75

Achondroplasia

Shawn E. Parnell, MD

Definition

Achondroplasia is the most common nonlethal skeletal dysplasia. It is characterized by rhizomelic disproportionate short stature, enlarged head with prominent forehead, short hands, exaggerated lumbar lordosis, and normal cognitive development.

Clinical Features

Birth incidence is approximately 1 in 10,000 to 1 in 30,000. Achondroplasia is a disproportionate short-limbed dwarfism with proximal portions of the extremities being shorter than the middle and distal segments (rhizomelia). Affected individuals have a relatively enlarged head with prominent forehead (frontal bossing), midface hypoplasia, and depressed nasal bridge. In infancy, there is a prominent thoracolumbar kyphosis. In older children and adults there is accentuation of the lumbar lordosis. The fingers are short and nearly the same length. As a result of poor enchondral bone formation in achondroplasia, the skull base is small relative to the calvarium (as the latter is formed from membranous bone). Resultant foramen magnum stenosis can contribute to cervicomedullary compression and has been associated with sudden infant death, sleep apnea, respiratory disorders, hyperreflexia, and clonus.

Anatomy and Physiology

Achondroplasia is an autosomal dominant disorder caused by a mutation of the fibroblast growth factor receptor 3 (FGFR3) gene on chromosome 4. This mutation leads to unregulated signal transduction through the receptor and resultant inappropriate growth plate differentiation and deficient endochondral growth. Eighty percent of cases are caused by spontaneous mutation.

Imaging Findings

- Shortened femurs or humeri and increased biparietal diameter may be seen on third-trimester prenatal ultrasound (US)
- Frontal bossing and midface hypoplasia on lateral skull films (Fig. 75.1)
- Decreased size of skull base and foramen magnum, with keyhole-shaped appearance of the latter on cross-sectional imaging (Fig. 75.2)
- Small thorax with shortened ribs
- Short pedicles (lateral view of spine), decrease of interpediculate distance from the upper to lower lumbar spine (frontal view of spine) (Fig. 75.3A)
- Thoracolumbar gibbus deformity (kyphosis) in infancy (Fig. 75.3B)
- Congenital spinal stenosis related to shortened pedicles and narrow interpediculate distance: may be seen throughout the spine, but is often most prominent in the lumbar spine
- Flat acetabular roofs, narrow sciatic notches, short wide iliac wings (Fig. 75.4)
- Rhizomelic shortening of long bones (Fig. 75.5)
- Relatively long fibulae
- Trident-shaped hands

> **IMAGING PITFALLS:** Severe forms of hypochondroplasia may have similar clinical and radiographic findings to achondroplasia. Genetic testing may be needed to differentiate between the two entities.

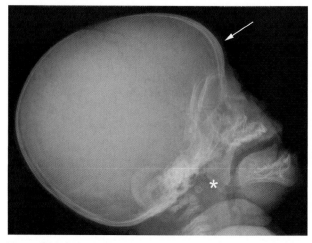

Figure 75.1. Lateral view of the skull demonstrates frontal bossing (arrow), midface hypoplasia, and small skull base typical of achondroplasia. Note the enlarged adenoids (*)

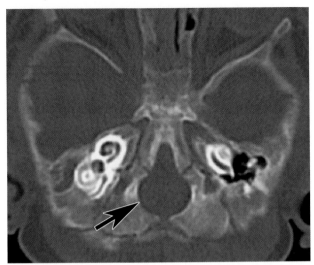

Figure 75.2. Axial noncontrast CT of skull base in a 2-month-old patient with achondroplasia demonstrates narrowing of the foramen magnum, with characteristic "keyhole" shape (arrow). Fluid in the right mastoid air cells may represent normal variation in this age group, although eustachian tube dysfunction is more common with achondroplasia.

(A) 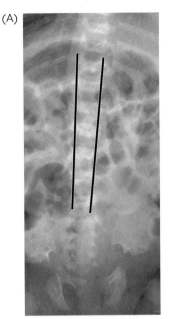 (B)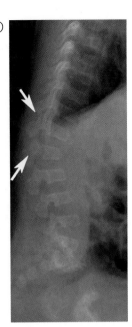

Figure 75.3. Frontal lumbar spine radiograph (A) in an infant with achondroplasia demonstrates narrowing of the inferior interpediculate distance (black lines); lateral view (B) demonstrates short pedicles and typical thoracolumbar gibbus deformity seen in infancy (arrows).

Imaging Strategy

In a child with suspected skeletal dysplasia, a skeletal survey should be obtained. This typically includes anteroposterior (AP) and lateral views of the skull, lateral view of the cervical spine, AP and lateral views of the thoracolumbar spine, AP view of the chest, AP view of the pelvis, and frontal views of all extremities, to include the posteroanterior (PA) view of hands and AP view of feet. In addition, noncontrast head CT can be obtained to evaluate for degree of foramen magnum narrowing. For evaluation of central sleep apnea, hyperreflexia, or clonus, MRI of the cervical spine can also be obtained. Later in life, symptomatic lumbar stenosis is also well-evaluated by lumbar spine MRI.

Related Physics

Achondroplastic patients may undergo many radiographic studies in their lifetime especially if surgical limb lengthening techniques are undertaken. As achondroplasia is predominantly rhizomelic, radiographs will more often involve proximal arms and legs as well as pelvis, posing risk to adjacent sensitive organs. With this comes an increase in the cumulative absorbed dose over a patient's lifetime. Epidemiologically, the factors that are more important than absorbed dose are organ-specific and effective dose as these are most critical in determining future cancer risk. Despite our best efforts at shielding the pediatric patient, internal scatter to lung, thyroid, gonads, breast, and the gastrointestinal tract is inevitable. Organ-specific dose is the amount of energy deposited per unit mass in that organ, whereas the effective dose is an equivalent full-body dose

(obtained by multiplying the organ dose by a tissue weighting factor) giving the overall sensitivity of the tissue to radiation-induced cancer. There are no known thresholds below which radiation is safe, therefore we continue with the current dogma of "as low as reasonably allowable." One suggestion that could be considered for patients who will require multiple serial radiographs would be to reduce the mAs and *increase* the kVp (reducing absorption) with postprocessing to win back the contrast, in a so-called "minimal dose fracture series."

Differential Diagnosis

- Hypochondroplasia: a member of the achondroplasia group of skeletal dysplasias, hypochondroplasia results from FGFR3 mutations. Findings for hypochondroplasia are less severe, but qualitatively similar to achondroplasia.
- Thanatophoric dysplasia: also part of the achondroplasia group, thanatophoric dysplasia is a more severe disorder with bowed appearance of long bones, more severe shortening of ribs, and increased platyspondyly, with characteristic U- and H-shaped vertebra on frontal spine radiographs. Perinatal lethality is typical with this condition, secondary to respiratory insufficiency or cord compression at the craniocervical junction.
- Homozygous achondroplasia: if both parents contribute mutations for achondroplasia, the bone findings are more similar to thanatophoric dysplasia, and

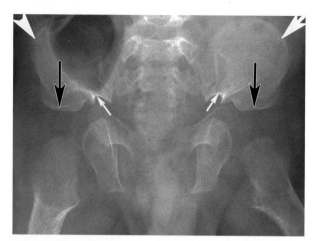

Figure 75.4. Frontal pelvis radiograph in an infant with achondroplasia shows flat acetabular roofs (black arrows), narrow sciatic notches (white arrows), and short wide iliac wings (arrowheads).

death from respiratory insufficiency in infancy is common.

- SADDAN dysplasia: defined as severe achondroplasia with developmental delay/acanthosis nigricans

Clinical Issues

A number of respiratory, otolaryngologic, neurologic, and orthopedic issues are associated with achondroplasia. Respiratory difficulties in infancy may result from the narrow thorax, small nasal passages, adenoidal hypertrophy, and transient muscular hypotonia. Severe obstructive sleep apnea can result in cardiorespiratory failure and death. Because of the multifactorial nature of obstructive sleep apnea in these patients, tonsillectomy and adenoidectomy may not be curative. Recurrent otitis media is also common secondary to midface hypoplasia and short eustachian tubes and may require myringotomy tube placement. Cervicomedullary compression can occur in infancy, with resultant neurologic impairment of the extremities manifesting as hyperreflexia, clonus, and eventual paresis. Later in life, lumbar lordosis develops, and lumbar stenosis is worsened by presence of intervertebral disc bulges and osteophyte formation. Treatment is reserved for symptomatic patients, with occipital decompression in infancy and lumbar laminectomies in older patients. Hydrocephalus can present in infancy secondary to foramen magnum stenosis, but typically stabilizes without intervention. It is recommended to monitor head growth every 6 months during the early years of life. In older patients, jugular foramen stenosis and resultant jugular hypertension may also result in hydrocephalus. Decompression is necessary in up to 17 percent of patients. Thoracolumbar gibbus deformity usually disappears as truncal hypotonia resolves, however it may become fixed in more than 10 percent. To help prevent this, caregivers should avoid putting these infants in an unsupported seated position during the first year of life. An orthosis may be used for support. Tibial bowing is also common, and when needed, corrective osteotomies are usually performed in the teenage years.

Key Points

- Most common nonlethal skeletal dysplasia
- Abnormal enchondral bone formation caused by mutation in FGFR3
- Rhizomelic disproportionate short stature
- Frontal bossing, midface hypoplasia
- Spinal stenosis, narrow foramen magnum
- Characteristic pelvis with flat acetabular roofs and narrow sciatic notches
- Differential diagnosis includes other members of the achondroplasia (FGFR3 mutation) group, including hypochondroplasia and thanatophoric dysplasia

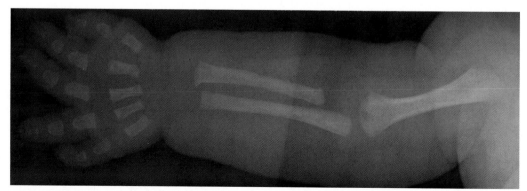

Figure 75.5. Right upper extremity radiograph in a patient with achondroplasia demonstrates relative shortening of the humerus characteristic of rhizomelia.

Further Reading

Baujat G, Legeai-Mallet L, Finidori G, Cormier-Daire V, Le Merrer M. Achondroplasia. *Best Practice & Research Clinical Rheumatology.* 2008;*22*(1):3–18.

Lachman RS. *Taybi and Lachman's Radiology of Syndromes, Metabolic Disorders and Skeletal Dysplasias.* Fifth Edition. Philadelphia, PA: Mosby Elsevier; 2007:865–870.

Richette P, Bardin T, Stheneur C. Achondroplasia: from genotype to phenotype. *Joint Bone Spine.* 2008;*75*:125–130.

Spranger JW, Brill PW, Poznanski AK. *Bone Dysplasias: An Atlas of Genetic Disorders of Skeletal Development.* Second edition. New York, NY, Oxford University Press and Urban & Fisher Verlag; 2002:83–89.

Superti-Furga A, Unger S, The Nosology Group of the International Skeletal Dysplasia Society. Nosology and classification of genetic skeletal disorders: 2006 revision. *Am J Med Genet A.* 2007;*143*(1):1–18.

CHAPTER 76

Osteogenesis Imperfecta

Unni Udayasankar, MD and Ihsan Mamoun, MD

Definition

Osteogenesis imperfecta (OI) is a heritable connective tissue disorder characterized by extremely fragile bones with or without secondary characteristics such as blue sclera, abnormal teeth (dentinogenesis imperfect), hearing loss, short stature, and scoliosis.

Clinical Features

The primary clinical manifestation of OI is frequent, multilevel fractures that result in deformed limbs. Osteogenesis imperfecta has a highly variable clinical presentation, ranging from a mild form with no deformity, normal stature, and few fractures to a form that is lethal during the perinatal period. To assess prognosis and to help assess the effects of therapeutic interventions, OI has been classified into various types. The most widely used classification (Sillence) distinguishes four clinical types. Type II has subtypes A, B, C based on imaging features. Type V is not fully characterized but is believed to be autosomal dominant as are types I to IV. Types VI to XI are autosomal recessive and are uncommon. It is the four Sillence subtypes that prevail clinically (Table 76.1).

Anatomy and Physiology

Most cases are caused by mutations in genes encoding type 1 collagen found in skin, ligaments, and bone. This leads to a qualitative or quantitative reduction in type 1 collagen, which is the basic defect resulting in the skeletal and extraskeletal manifestations. The gene mutations tend to be either inherited or new mutations. The inherited mutations show increased recurrence risk with subsequent pregnancies. The degree of histologic change in bone is well-correlated with the clinical severity of the disease.

Imaging Findings

Prenatal US:
- Difficult in milder forms of the disease, most useful in severe forms (types II and III)
- Decreased calvarial ossification: increased transparency resulting from hypomineralization of the skull permits clear delineation of fetal brain detail; skull may deform/compress with transducer pressure
- Femur length usually < 5th percentile*
- Angulated long bones*
- US gap along the length of a long bone*
- Narrow thorax with beaded appearance of the ribs*
- Platyspondyly*

* Results of in utero fractures

Radiography:
Head:
- Multiple wormian bones (Fig. 76.1)
- Basilar invagination (25 percent)
- Middle ear ossicle fractures or fixation anomalies
- Neural foraminal narrowing

Spine:
- Thoracic scoliosis or kyphosis
- Vertebral compression fractures
- Platyspondyly or biconcave appearance resulting from multiple microfractures

Chest:
- Multiple rib fractures (Fig. 76.2)
- Pectus excavatum or carinatum
- Valvular or aortic anomalies (rare)

Pelvis:
- Protrusio acetabulae
- Flat acetabular roof

Other:
- Diffuse osteopenia with multiple fractures (Fig. 76.3)
- Slender gracile long bones with more severe involvement of the lower extremities
- Cortical thinning
- Trumpet-shaped or cystic metaphysis
- Hyperplastic callus formation
- Popcorn calcification in the metaphyseal/epiphyseal regions resulting from endochondral ossification of displaced and fragmented physis (Fig. 76.4)
- Pseudoarthrosis formation at the site of fracture healing
- Joint laxity
- Zebra-stripe sign: cyclic bisphonate treatment results in parallel sclerotic growth recovery lines in long bones

Table 76.1 – Expanded Sillence Classification of Osteogenesis Imperfecta

TYPE	CLINICAL SEVERITY	MUTATED GENE	MODE OF INHERITANCE
I	Mild non-deforming	*COL1A1/2*	AD
II	Perinatal lethal	*COL1A1/2*	AD
III	Severe	*COL1A1/2*	AD
IV	Moderate	*COL1A1/2*	AD
V	Moderate	Unknown	AD
VI	Moderate to Severe	Unknown	AR
VII	Moderate	*CRTAP*	AR
VIII	Severe to perinatal death	*LEPRE1*	AR

Imaging Strategy

Osteogenesis imperfecta is one of the more common skeletal dysplasias detected with prenatal US.

Most imaging features of OI are readily demonstrated on plain radiographs. Therefore, radiography remains the initial investigation of choice in patients with OI and MRI and CT play adjunct roles. Basilar invagination may be better demonstrated on CT or MRI. Wormian bones, otosclerosis, and middle ear ossicular fractures, if present, are also better seen on CT. CT densitometric temporal bone scanning may be helpful in some cases of OI with conductive hearing loss. Dual X-ray absorptiometry (DEXA) may be used to assess low bone mineral density in children with milder forms of OI.

Related Physics

The radiographic challenge with OI lies in imaging a skeletal system that has absolutely less mineralization because of thinner bones, thus reducing the intrinsic bone to soft-tissue contrast. In addition, the bones may not mount a significant reparative response following fracture, making it very difficult to rule out subtle fractures unless there is angulation. In this case, elimination of scatter is paramount and this is best performed "in the Bucky" regardless of patient size/age. The technique chosen should augment tissue contrast and would include low kVp (50 to 60), use of grid and automatic exposure control (AEC). In addition to preset techniques at the console, body-part-specific and view-specific imaging algorithms are used for processing

(A)

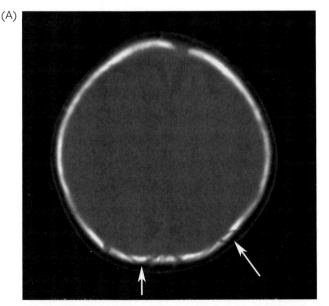

(B)

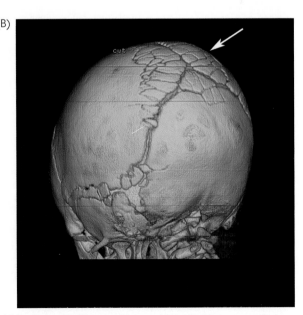

Figure 76.1. Axial brain CT (bone window; A) and volume-rendered 3-D reformatted image (B) in a child with OI shows multiple small wormian bones (arrows) in the posterior aspect of the sagittal and lambdoid sutures.

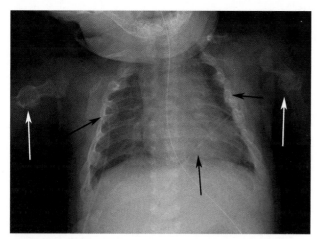

Figure 76.2. Frontal radiograph of the chest in a 6-month-old infant with OI demonstrates diffuse osteopenia with bilateral fractures of multiple ribs (black arrows), both humeri (white arrows) and bilateral radius and ulna. There is exuberant callus formation around the humeral fractures. This callus leads to the "beaded" appearance of the healing bones.

following image acquisition. These include image contrast, brightness, and degree of edge enhancement. Very short exposure times or maximal temporal resolution can be used in the younger patient, which will limit motion artifact and optimize spatial resolution.

Differential Diagnosis

Prenatal US:

- Lethal form of hypophosphatasia
- Thanatophoric dysplasia

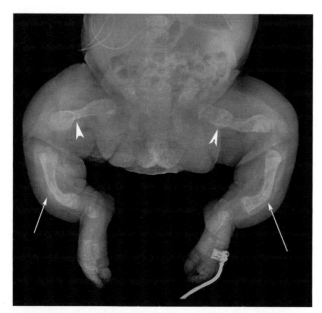

Figure 76.3. Frontal radiograph of the pelvis in an infant with OI demonstrates diffuse osteopenia with tibial bowing (arrows). There are fractures of both femora in various stages of healing (arrowheads).

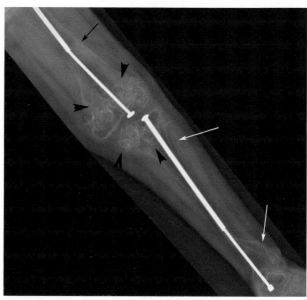

Figure 76.4. Frontal radiograph of the lower extremity in an 8-year-old girl with OI show telescoping rods in the femur and tibia with severe osteopenia. The distal fibula is severely gracile and bowed (white arrows). There is a remodeling fracture at the distal femoral diaphysis (black arrow). Classic "popcorn" calcifications are present in the distal femoral and proximal tibial epiphyses and metaphyses (arrowheads).

- Achondrogenesis type I
- Campomelic dysplasia

Radiography:

- Nonaccidental trauma
- Primary juvenile osteoporosis
- Secondary juvenile osteoporosis
- Malignant osteoporosis
- Hypophosphatasia
- Menkes (kinky-hair) syndrome

Common Variants

Type I is the most common variant. Few fractures result in mild deformity in this variant.

Clinical Issues

The presence of fractures of various ages in neonates and children could suggest nonaccidental trauma or child abuse. However, OI should be kept in mind in these cases. One should look for radiologic features or familial phenotypic findings that point to a diagnosis of OI. Skin biopsy or serum DNA analysis may be useful in these cases.

Hearing loss is a common secondary manifestation of OI that can occur in all subtypes. Although the hearing loss is mild and uncommon in childhood, the incidence and the decibel loss increase significantly in adulthood. Dentinogenesis imperfecta, malocclusion, tooth impaction, and or abnormal rates of tooth eruption are seen in some subtypes of OI.

Basilar invagination has been observed in approximately 25 percent of patients with OI, most often seen in type IV. Neurologic symptoms may result from compression of posterior fossa structures causing headache, trigeminal nerve dysfunction, horizontal nystagmus, sensory >motor dysfunction, intermittent vertigo, or compromised respiration. Headache occurring with sudden head movement (such as during a sneeze, laugh, or cough) is the most common symptom. Correction of long bone deformity in children with OI often requires multiple osteotomies with intramedullary nail fixation. Telescopic rods are often used, as these have the capacity to elongate as the child grows, thus decreasing the number of operative procedures in young children.

Key Points

- OI is one of the most common skeletal dysplasias.
- More severe forms can be detected on prenatal US.
- Diagnostic factors include: family history, genetic screening, clinical and histologic findings, and imaging findings.
- Multiple fractures on a background of thin and gracile bones raises nonaccidental trauma as a key differential consideration.

- Wormian bones are asymptomatic.
- Basilar invagination, middle ear ossicle abnormalities, and platyspondyly may be symptomatic and evident by head and neck imaging.

Further Reading

Forlino A, Cabral WA, Barnes AM, Marini JC. New perspectives on osteogenesis imperfecta. *Nat Rev Endocrinol.* 2011;7(9): 540–557.

Hayes M, Parker G, Ell J, Sillence D. Basilar impression complicating osteogenesis imperfecta type IV: the clinical and neuroradiological findings in four cases. *J Neurol Neurosurg Psychiatry.* 1999;66:357–364.

Schramm T, Gloning KP, Minderer S, Daumer-Haas C, Hörtnagel K, Nerlich A, Tutschek B. Prenatal sonographic diagnosis of skeletal dysplasias. *Ultrasound Obstet Gynecol.* 2009;34(2):160–170.

Taybi H, Lachman RS. *Radiology of Syndromes, Metabolic Disorders, and Skeletal Dysplasias.* Fourth Edition.: Mosby-Year Book;1996.

Van Dijk FS, Pals G, Van Rijn RR, Nikkels PG, Cobben JM. Classification of osteogenesis imperfecta revisited. *Eur J Med Genet.* 2010;53(1):1–5.

CHAPTER 77

Juvenile Idiopathic Arthritis

Mahesh Thapa, MD

Definition

The term "juvenile idiopathic arthritis" (JIA), which is defined as a chronic autoimmune inflammation of the joints in children, has replaced "juvenile chronic arthritis" and "juvenile rheumatoid arthritis." '

Clinical Features

Juvenile idiopathic arthritis is the most common chronic rheumatic disease of childhood. The International League of Associations for Rheumatology (ILAR) identifies seven subtypes: systemic arthritis; oligoarthritis; polyarthritis RF-negative (rheumatoid-factor-negative); polyarthritis RF-positive; psoriatic arthritis; enthesitis-related arthritis; and undifferentiated arthritis. Both seronegative and seropositive diseases are more common in girls, with the exception of Still's disease, which is seen equally in boys and girls. Pain, swelling, and morning stiffness are the hallmarks and JIA classically features chronic involvement of one or more joints, lasting at least 6 weeks in a patient under 16 years of age. The knee is the most commonly affected joint in the body. Other commonly involved joints include wrist, ankles, hands, elbow, hip, shoulder, sacroiliac joints, feet, cervical spine, and temporomandibular joint.

Anatomy and Physiology

Juvenile idiopathic arthritis begins with synovial inflammation and overproduction of joint fluid. Synovitis progresses to synovial hyperplasia and formation of a highly cellular inflammatory pannus. This pannus eventually erodes the adjacent cartilage and bone resulting in articular destruction and ankylosis.

Imaging Findings

Early or Active Disease

Radiography:
- Soft-tissue swelling (especially hands and wrists)
- Periosteal reaction (after a few weeks of disease, most common in metacarpals, metatarsals, and proximal phalanges)
- Osteitis

MRI:
- Marrow edema: low T1, high T2 and proton density (PD) signal intensity (SI) +/- enhancement and poorly defined margins
- Synovitis and synovial proliferation (usually with effusion): low to intermediate T1 and high T2 SI with hyper-enhancement
- Joint fluid: low T1, high T2 SI, brighter T2 SI than synovium
- Cartilage: subtle irregularities, alteration of the normal smooth contour of the cartilage, blurring and obscuring of the typically sharp margins

Ultrasound (US):
- Hypoechoic and irregular synovial thickening
- Hypervascular synovium on power Doppler
- Effusion usually anechoic

Response to Therapy
- Decrease in the thickness and vascularity of the synovium
- Decrease in joint fluid

Advanced Disease
- Bone erosions (late finding; Fig. 77.1)
- First subchondral signs of erosion: low PD or T1 SI; high T2 SI; marrow enhancement; may coexist with periosteal reaction in fingers (better seen on radiographs); cortical break in at least one plane; well-circumscribed, juxtacortical lesion; loss of normal low signal in cortical bone; marked contrast enhancement
- Subchondral cysts
- Joint space narrowing (Fig. 77.2)
- Ankylosis: most common in the cervical spine (Fig. 77.3) and second and third carpometacarpal joints
- Osteoporosis
- Growth disturbances resulting from hyperemia: advanced bone age relative to chronologic age (Fig. 77.4); epiphyseal enlargement (especially knee, elbow, and hip)

Other Changes
- Tenosynovitis
- Meniscal atrophy

(A)

(B)

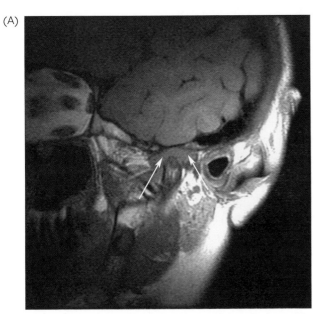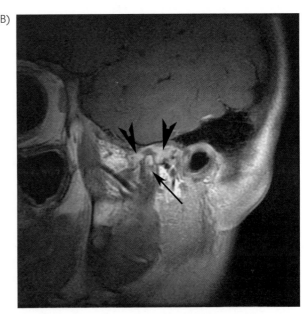

Figure 77.1. Sagittal oblique T1 MR image without contrast (A) in an 11-year-old boy with pauciarticular JIA shows grossly thickened synovium with pannus (arrows). Postcontrast image (B) shows multiple erosions of the mandibular condyle (arrows) with diffuse enhancement of the pannus (arrowhead). The disk is not identified and has likely been destroyed.

- Enthesitis
- Subclinical tendon rupture
- Bone infarct
- Ligament involvement
- Rheumatoid nodules

Imaging Strategy

Timely diagnosis can facilitate better clinical outcome. In the active phase articular synovitis can usually be adequately evaluated with clinical examination. Initial radiographs allow exclusion of other causes of pain and establish

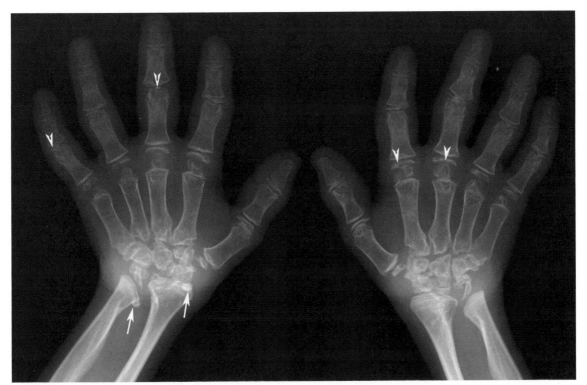

Figure 77.2. Frontal radiograph of both hands in an 8-year old-girl with severe systemic polyarticular JIA shows significant erosive disease throughout both hands and wrists with soft-tissue swelling, osteopenia, and joint space narrowing. There is some epiphyseal sclerosis (arrowheads), likely resulting from avascular necrosis. Soft-tissue calcifications (arrows) are likely dystrophic and can occur after joint injections.

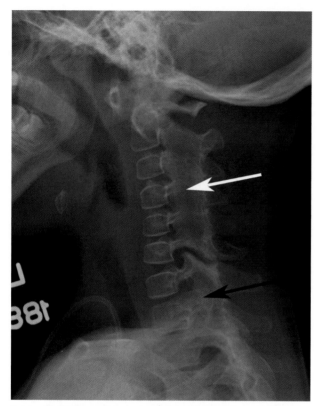

Figure 77.3. Lateral cervical spine radiograph in an 8-year-old girl with systemic polyarticular JIA shows fusion/ankylosis of the posterior elements at C2 to C6 (white arrow) as well as posterior fusion of C7 to T2 (black arrow).

Related Physics

Signal-to-noise in MRI is significantly affected by the choice of coil, and this becomes more important with smaller body parts such as the pediatric wrist and hand. Volume coils provide better radiofrequency (RF) homogeneity over a large volume with better depth imaging. These are often customized to the body part such as the birdcage coils used for head or knee imaging. Surface coils consist of a loop of conducting material placed on the region of interest using the body coil as the transmitter and the surface coil as the receiver. Surface coils can be closely draped over an area and are therefore more versatile in conforming to various body parts. Two coils in frequent use in pediatric imaging are the phased-array and quadrature coils. Phased-array coils offer a smaller sensitive volume where signals are additive in the coil resulting in lower detected noise and reduced aliasing. Quadrature coils are configured with two linearly polarized fields rotated 90 degrees to each other where signal is correlated and summed with significantly higher signal-to-noise. Coils can be combined when a larger field of view is required than could be imaged with a single coil.

a radiographic baseline. Unfortunately, radiographs cannot depict early synovial and cartilaginous involvement, and in general, will not be abnormal until the disease reaches an advanced stage. Ultrasound with high-frequency transducers and MRI have both been used for early assessment of the disease process. US can effectively depict the severity of the disease by allowing assessment of joint effusions, synovial thickening, cartilage destruction/thinning, and associated synovial cysts. Power Doppler can demonstrate the intense vascular nature of the pannus. Serial US is very useful in monitoring disease activity and for following response to therapy and may detect residual, new, or increased disease activity before it is clinically apparent. In addition, US can be used to accurately guide therapeutic intra-articular steroid injection. For depiction of early inflammatory change, synovitis, cartilage defects, and late manifestations of the disease, MRI is superior to US. Though not routinely used in standard clinical practice, studies have demonstrated that the rate of contrast-enhancement and dynamic contrast-enhancement measurements of the synovium can be used to assess the degree of inflammation. Quantitative MR assessment of the synovial volumes can also be obtained. Three-dimensional data can be further analyzed, with quantitative assessment of cartilage volume and thickness. Contour mapping may be of potential value in assessing response to treatment and establishing long-term prognosis.

Common Variants

- Seropositive JIA (5–15%): usually presents in adolescent females as polyarticular disease with soft-tissue swelling and advanced bone age in the hands; hand and foot erosions occur a few years after symptoms begin.
- Seronegative JIA (85%): pauciarticular (< four joints, usually large) is more common than polyarticular disease (often symmetric and very diffuse disease)
- Still's disease: seronegative form of JIA with systemic symptoms in children less than 5 years of age; polyarthritis, usually without bone changes, high fever, anemia, hepatosplenomegaly, lymphadenopathy, and leukocytosis
- Psoriatic arthritis: arthritis and two of the following: nail pitting, onycholysis, dactylitis, or a first degree relative with psoriasis
- Enthesitis-related arthritis (ERA): arthritis and/or enthesitis and at least two of the following: HLA-B27 antigen-positive; onset after age 6 years in a boy; sacroiliac joint tenderness and/or inflammatory lumbosacral pain; symptomatic acute anterior uveitis or a first-degree relative with ERA; ankylosing spondylitis; inflammatory bowel disease and sacroiliitis; acute anterior uveitis, or Reiter's syndrome.

IMAGING PITFALLS: Ultrasound is an operator-dependent modality, with only limited visualization of some joints. The acoustic window can be narrow, precluding complete assessment of the entire joint. The efficacy of US can be further

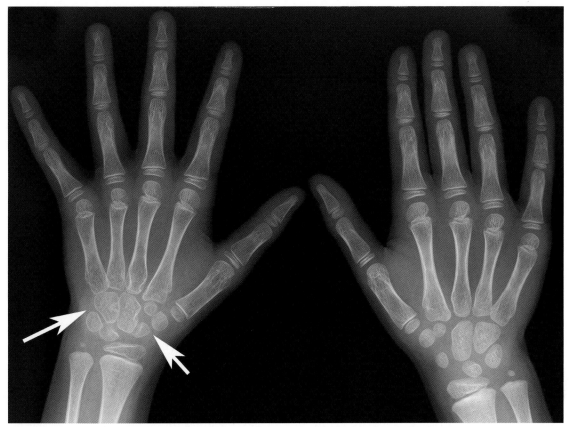

Figure 77.4. Frontal radiograph of the hands in a 5-year-old girl with polyarticular JIA, RF-negative, antinuclear antibody positive disease and decreased range of motion of her right wrist shows advanced bone age of the carpal bones (arrows) when compared to the normal left.

limited by the difficulty in positioning active children with swollen, painful joints.

Conventional spin echo MR sequences may limit distinction of thick synovium from synovial fluid given the similar signal intensity of the two.

Timing of MR imaging after contrast administration is important. Contrast passes quickly from the synovium to the joint fluid. One must image within 5 minutes of contrast injection to avoid mistaking contrast within the synovial fluid for enhancing synovium. This is particularly important when studying more than one joint or imaging in more than one plane post-contrast-administration.

Apparent bone marrow edema is a precursor of erosive disease in adults, however it is commonly seen in growing healthy children volunteers.

Clinical Issues

Growth disturbance is a significant complication in some children with JIA, generally resulting in premature fusion of the physis, growth stunting, and limb-length discrepancies. The mandible is affected in a significant number of patients resulting in malocclusion and facial asymmetry in childhood. Ten percent of children with arthritis have progressive disease that is disabling for them as adults.

Key Points
- MRI is the best modality for JIA.
- Important MR findings include joint effusion, synovial enhancement, bone edema, and erosions.
- JIA is indistinguishable from infection on imaging.

Differential Diagnosis
- Septic arthritis
- Post-traumatic synovitis
- Pigmented villonodular synovitis
- Infectious arthritis
- Hemophilia
- Leukemic arthritis

Further Reading

Avenarius DM, Ording Müller LS, Eldevik P, Owens CM, Rosendahl K. The paediatric wrist revisited-findings of bony depressions in healthy children on radiographs compared to MRI. *Pediatr Radiol.* 2012.

Buchmann RF, Jaramillo D. Imaging of articular disorders in children. *Rad Clin N Am.* 2004;*42*:151–168.

Hashkes PJ, Laxer RM. Medical treatment of juvenile idiopathic arthritis. *JAMA*. 2005;*294*(13):1671–1684.

Johnson K. Imaging of juvenile idiopathic arthritis. *Pediatr Radiol*. 2006;*36*:743–758.

Jordan A, McDonagh JE. Juvenile idiopathic arthritis: the paediatric perspective. *Pediatr Radiol*. 2006;*36*(8):734–742.

Magni-Manzoni S, Malattia C, Lanni S, Ravelli A. Advances and challenges in imaging in juvenile idiopathic arthritis. *Nat Rev Rheumatol*. 2012.

Petty, et al. ILAR classification of JIA. *The Journal of Rheumatology*. 2004;*31*:2.

Pruthi P, Thapa M. Infectious and inflammatory disorders. *Magn Reson Imaging Clin N Am*. 2009;*17*:423–438.

Tanturri de Horatio L, Damasio MB, Barbuti D, Bracaglia C, Lambot-Juhan K, et al. MRI assessment of bone marrow in children with juvenile idiopathic arthritis: intra- and interobserver variability. *Pediatr Radiol*. 2012.

Workie DW, Dardzinski B, Graham TB, et al. Quantification of dynamic contrast enhanced MR-imaging of the knee in children with juvenile rheumatoid arthritis based on pharmacokinetic modelling. *Magn Reson Imaging* 2004;*22*:1201–1210.

CHAPTER 78

VACTERL

Neil Mardis, MD

Definition

The acronym "VACTERL" refers to the association of multiple congenital anomalies including **V**ertebral, **A**norectal, **C**ardiac, **T**racheoesophageal fistula and/or **E**sophageal atresia, **R**enal, and **L**imb. This association was described in 1965 by the pediatric radiologist, John Kirkpatrick, however Quan and Smith in 1973 gave it the acronym VATER, which was later expanded to VACTERL.

Clinical Features

This condition is not a syndrome or a diagnosis but, rather, a nonrandom association of abnormalities of embryogenesis that occur in the first 4 weeks of gestation. It is rare for all of the anomalies to be present in one child, but the presence of one or more of these anomalies will prompt a search for the others. The incidence of VACTERL ranges between 1 in 6,250 and 1 in 3,333 births. Although there is not a single genetic defect that leads to VACTERL, various precipitating events have been suggested. The association is often encountered in children of diabetic mothers, although this is not a unifying feature.

Anatomy and Physiology

One compelling explanation for VACTERL lies in viewing the association as a primary developmental field defect. The concept of primary developmental fields was developed as "parts of the embryo in which the processes of development of complex structure appropriate to those parts are controlled and coordinated in a spatially ordered, temporally synchronized, and epimorphically hierarchal manner"(Opitz, 1982). It was Opitz's theory that during blastogenesis (the first 4 weeks of embryonic development) and organogenesis (gestational weeks 4 to 8), the fetus is of such small size that various developing fields (vertebral, anorectal, etc.) are in such close proximity spatially and temporally as to render the fetus a single developing field. Thus, a teratogenic insult of any etiology may affect what in later development may seem spatially disparate locations.

Imaging Findings

Vertebral:
- Vertebral segmentation anomalies: butterfly, hemivertebra, block, hypersegmented (Fig. 78.1)
- Sacral anomalies or agenesis
- Scoliosis
- Rib anomalies: supernumerary, fused, or bifid

Anorectal malformation (ARM):
- Any anorectal malformation, including anal stenosis, is included as a VACTERL association
- Anal atresia with or without fistula
- "Fistula" is simply the persistent communication of the hindgut to the genitourinary tract resulting from failure of separation during embryogenesis
- Hindgut may end blindly or terminate in the bladder, bladder neck, posterior urethra or on the perineum in boys, and in the vagina or on the perineum in girls

Cardiac:
- No specific cardiac disease is uniquely associated
- Septal defect most common
- Others: conotruncal abnormalities, tetralogy of Fallot, arch anomalies including coarctation, hypoplastic left heart, and total anomalous pulmonary venous connection

Esophageal Atresia:
- +/- one or two tracheoesophageal fistula(s) is a common feature of VACTERL
- Fistula from trachea to esophagus, best seen in lateral projection (Fig. 78.2)
- Fistula may be horizontal (H-type) or oblique (N-type)
- Distal fistula with EA: air within stomach and small bowel despite EA (prior to G-tube)
- Proximal fistula with EA: trachea to proximal esophageal pouch (uncommon) may occur as the only fistula or with a distal tracheoesophageal fistula (TEF); recurrent pneumonia/pneumonitis common prior to repair
- Enteric tube coiled in or ending in the proximal esophageal pouch
- Gas-filled large-caliber proximal esophageal pouch (frontal or lateral view)
- Gasless abdomen implies EA without distal TEF, may be longer-segment atresia than with TEF

Renal:
- Position (ptotic or pelvic kidneys)
- Fusion (horseshoe or cross-fused ectopia)
- Cystic dysplasia

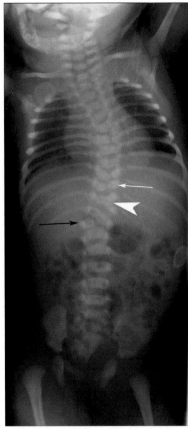

Figure 78.1. Frontal view of the entire spine in a newborn shows multiple vertebral segmentation anomalies including butterfly vertebra (white arrow), hemivertebra (black arrow), and fusion anomalies (arrowhead) in the thoracic, lumbar, and sacral regions.

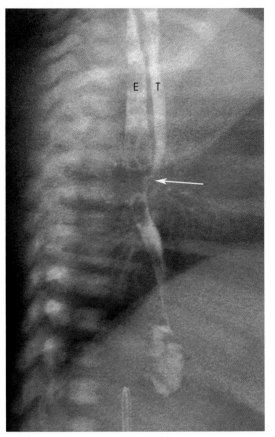

Figure 78.2. Lateral image from barium esophogram in child with recurrent pneumonias shows a tracheoesophageal fistula (arrow). Trachea (T), esophagus (E).

- Ureteropelvic junction obstruction
- Vesicoureteral reflux (with or without ectopic ureteral insertion)
- Agenesis

Limb anomalies:

- Radial ray anomalies: absence or hypoplasia of the radius, first metacarpal and thumb (Fig. 78.3)
- Other reported anomalies less common: triphalangeal thumb; transverse limb deficiencies; preaxial polydactyly; aplasia or hypoplasia of the humerus, tibia, fibula, and femur; radioulnar synostosis

Miscellaneous:

- Single umbilical artery
- Rib anomalies
- Sternal anomalies
- Sprengel deformity
- Klippel-Feil
- Hydrocephalus
- Encephalocele
- Agenesis of the corpus callosum
- Eye abnormalities

US:

- Distended distal rectal pouch can be seen with linear tranducer over perineum
- Presacral masses or anterior meningocele (part of Currarino triad)
- High incidence tethered cord

Radiography:

- Prone cross-table lateral image with skin marker at expected location of anus shows gas in distal rectal pouch
- Sacral segmentation anomalies common
- Urine mixed with meconium may calcify (boys with high or intermediate ARM)

Fluoroscopy:

- Colostogram: instill contrast into the distal limb of a colostomy to determine the point of communication of the hindgut with the GU tract in high or intermediate malformations
- Voiding cystourethrography (VCUG): contrast may reflux into the hindgut during bladder filling or voiding in boys with a high or intermediate ARM; hindgut does not connect to the urinary tract in girls unless they have a cloacal malformation

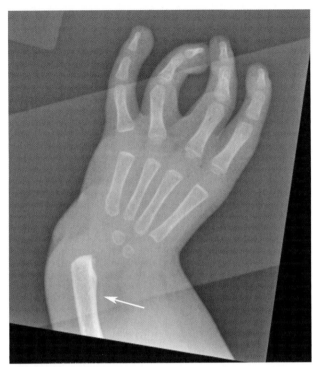

Figure 78.3. Frontal radiograph of the hand in a child with VACTERL reveals absence of the radius, first metacarpal, and thumb with a single forearm bone representing a dysmorphic ulna (arrow).

Imaging Strategy

Identification of one of the components of VACTERL association such as EA or TE fistula, anal atresia, or radial ray anomaly will often prompt a search for the other anomalies. Vertebral anomalies are a common feature of patients with the VACTERL association and may be detected on chest or abdominal radiographs that were obtained for another reason. The entire spine should be carefully scrutinized. Frontal and lateral radiographs are generally sufficient to evaluate for the presence and extent of vertebral defects. Patients with vertebral (particularly sacral) anomalies and/or anorectal malformations require US of the spine to rule out tethered cord. The presacral space can also be assessed for a presacral mass or meningocele that may be found in patients with Curarrino's triad of anorectal malformation, sacral anomaly, and presacral mass. If the spine US is abnormal, MRI is performed for presurgical planning. Transperineal US can be used to estimate the length of atresia. Distal colostogram is often performed to identify a communication between the hindgut and the GU tract, particularly in children with presumed high- or intermediate-level anorectal malformations prior to repair. MR imaging of the pelvic floor and anorectal region may be needed after repair if complications develop. Heart disease in patients with suspected VACTERL is typically first evaluated with echocardiography. Occasional use of cardiac MRI or conventional or CT angiography may be warranted for further evaluation of complex cardiac disease. If a TEF is suspected clinically, the radiologist may be asked to perform a barium swallow or esophogram. Small fistulas can be difficult to identify and separate from aspirated barium. Particular attention should be paid to patient positioning to optimize tangential depiction of the fistula. Renal US is recommended as a screening test. Further imaging with VCUG may be necessary to fully evaluate the urinary tract.

Radiography is usually sufficient to evaluate for limb abnormalities in patients with suspected VACTERL.

Related Physics

The diagnosis of VACTERL association often involves multiple imaging modalities. In order to create readable images for any cross-sectional modality, data must be reconstructed using a defined algorithm. Simple back-projection is the precursor to filtered back-projection, a method currently used for CT and PET imaging. The simple back-projection technique involves taking analog signal obtained at the detector and converting it to digital data and back-projecting it across image space. A map of the digital data as a function of angle of acquisition and recording detector number is referred to as a sinogram and functions as the raw data for back-projection. When rows of data from the sinogram are projected across image space, the resultant image will be blurry as a result of the mathematical process. For this reason digital filters are employed prior to back-projecting in an adaptation known as filtered back-projection. With faster computers, iterative reconstruction has been developed, holding a promise for more accurate images because of its ability to model the image chain more accurately. Iterative reconstruction first requires a baseline estimate of the object's shape which can be accomplished with a filtered back-projection image and then synthetic data are forward-projected through the image and compared to acquired data. Invariably the comparison is imperfect and there are multiple rapid iterative adjustments made to the image to bring the forward-projected data into greater concordance with the acquired data. Iterations are stopped when the level of concordance reaches a certain degree of accuracy.

Differential Diagnosis

- OEIS complex: omphalocele-extrophy-imperforate anus-spinal defects
- Cloacal malformation
- PHAVER syndrome: **P**terygia, congenital **H**eart **A**nomalies, **V**ertebral defects, **E**ar anomalies, and **R**adial defects
- Sirenomelia sequence
- Feingold syndrome
- TAR: thrombocytopenia and absent radius
- Holt Oram syndrome
- Casamassima-Morton-Nance syndrome
- Diabetic embryopathy

Clinical Issues

Classically, three of the features of VATER were required for inclusion in the association, however, currently no strict guidelines exist. More important than rendering the label of VACTERL is the understanding that when a particular defect such as esophageal or anal atresia is encountered, a thorough evaluation of the patient is required to search for less obvious but clinically significant anomalies.

Key Points

- VACTERL is an acronym for **V**ertebral, **A**norectal, **C**ardiac, **T**racheoesophageal fistula, **E**sophageal atresia, **R**enal, **L**imb.
- Any number of anomalies constitutes VACTERL.
- VACTERL is an association, <u>not</u> a syndrome.
- One anomaly should prompt thorough search for others through focused imaging.

Further Reading

Eltomey MA, Donnelly LF, Emery KH, Levitt MA, Peña A. Postoperative pelvic MRI of anorectal malformations. *AJR Am J Roentgenol*. 2008;*191*(5):1469–1476.

Kirkpatrick JA, Wagner ML, Pilling GP. A complex of anomalies associated with tracheoesophageal fistula and esophageal atresia. *Am J Roentgenol Radium Ther Nucl Med*. 1965;95:208–211.

Levin TL, Han B, Little BP. Congenital anomalies of the male urethra. *Pediatr Radiol*. 2007;*37*(9):851–862; quiz 945. Epub 2007 May 22.

Martinez-Frías ML, Frías JL. VACTERL as primary, polytopic developmental field defects. *Am J Med Genet*. 1999;83;13–16.

Opitz JM. The developmental field in clinical genetics. *J Pediatr*. 1982;*101*:805–809.

Quan L, Smith DW. The VATER Association. Vertebral defects, Anal atresia, T-E fistula with esophageal atresia, Radial and Renal dysplasia: a spectrum of associated defects. *J Pediatr*. 1973;*82*:104–107.

CHAPTER 79

Tarsal Coalition

L. Todd Dudley, MD

Definition
Tarsal coalition is the congenital fusion of two or more tarsal bones, frequently causing foot and ankle pain in children and adolescents.

Clinical Features
The pattern of inheritance is autosomal dominant with nearly full penetrance, but the same joint is not always affected between generations. The true prevalence is not known but is close to 1 percent in the United States, although cadaveric studies have reported incidence as high as 9 percent. The condition is bilateral in approximately 50 percent of cases, and there is a slight male predominance. The presenting symptom is usually pain or stiffness with activity, sometimes first noted after antecedent trauma, weight gain, or increased athletic activity. The incidence of pain increases with advancing ossification. Because calcaneonavicular coalition ossifies relatively early, it presents earlier (8 to 12 years of age); talocalcaneal coalition, however, is usually symptomatic in adolescence (12 to 16 years of age). Sometimes the diagnosis of tarsal coalition does not occur until adulthood, and many cases are asymptomatic. Some patients present with peroneal spastic flatfoot, a condition that includes pain, rigid valgus deformity of the hindfoot and forefoot, and peroneal muscle spasm. This condition does not reflect true peroneal muscle spasm, but rather peroneal muscle shortening to adjust for heel valgus and to maintain a less painful position for the subtalar joint.

Anatomy and Physiology
Tarsal coalition is caused by abnormal differentiation and segmentation of the primitive mesenchyme, resulting in lack of joint formation and is defined by anatomic location. Approximately 90 percent of cases are talocalcaneal (usually involving the middle facet) and calcaneonavicular (perhaps overrepresented because of its characteristic radiographic appearance). Although debatable, the two are probably equal in prevalence. "Talonavicular, calcaneocuboid, cubonavicular, and navicular-medial cuneiform types are much less common. There may be multiple coalitions in one foot. Coalition can occur in other joints, but this is frequently associated with other limb anomalies (such as fibular hemimelia). Tarsal coalition is also categorized by completeness of ossification. *Synostosis* refers to a complete osseous bar, *synchondrosis*, a cartilaginous bar, and *syndesmosis*, fibrous union.

Imaging Findings

Calcaneonavicular
Radiography:
- Best depicted on 45-degrees internal oblique radiographic view (Fig. 79.1)
- Proximity of articulating surfaces
- Synostosis: bony bar
- Fibrous or cartilaginous coalition: closely approximated surfaces often irregular
- Anteromedial calcaneus abnormally widened or flattened
- "Anteater's nose" sign: elongation and thickening of the anterior process (lateral radiograph) may indicate calcaneonavicular coalition
- Hypoplasia of the talus (uncommon)

CT:
- Broadening of the medial aspect of the anterior and dorsal calcaneus
- Close apposition of calcaneal process to navicular
- Joint-space narrowing and marginal reactive bone changes if fibrous or cartilaginous

MRI:
- Most pronounced in the sagittal plane
- Periarticular cortical changes
- Periarticular marrow edema on fluid-sensitive sequences

Talocalcaneal
Radiography:
- Most commonly involves the middle facet at the sustentaculum tali
- May be difficult to visualize on radiographs
- "C" sign: prominent inferior outline and C-shaped configuration of the medial talar dome and postero-inferior sustentaculum resulting from bone bridging between the talar dome and sustentaculum tali (low sensitivity, high specificity)

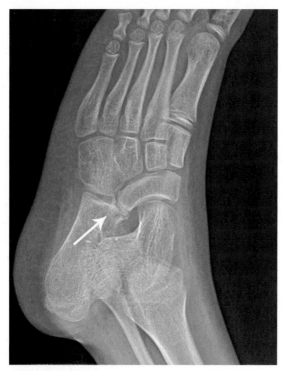

Figure 79.1. Oblique radiograph of the left foot in a 9-year-old boy with pain demonstrates nonosseous calcaneonavicular coalition characterized by joint-space narrowing (white arrow) and marginal reactive bone changes.

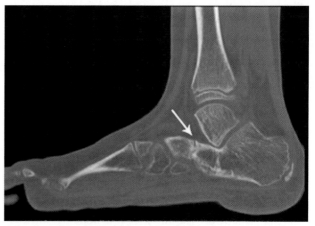

Figure 79.2. Sagittal CT image of the left foot in a 10-year-old boy with pain demonstrates the "anteater's nose" sign (arrow) from elongation and thickening of the anterior process of the calcaneus and osseous calcaneonavicular coalition.

- Low sensitivity noteworthy in young patients (under 12 years of age) and those with exclusive involvement of the posterior aspect of the middle facet
- Talar beak*: results from impaired subtalar joint motion causing the navicular to override the talus, periosteal elevation at insertion of the talonavicular ligament, and a cycle of osseous repair, which forms the beak (low sensitivity, specificity; Fig. 79.2)
- Narrowing of the posterior subtalar joint*
- Rounding of the lateral talar process*
- Lack of depiction of the middle facets on the lateral radiograph*
- "Ball in socket" tibiotalar joint on AP view (rare)*

CT:

- Best depicted in coronal plane
- Osseous coalition: bony bar bridging the middle talar facet of the subtalar joint
- Nonosseous coalition: joint-space narrowing and possibly reactive cystic and hypertrophic changes of the articulating surfaces
- Downsloping of the middle facet (normal sustentaculum slopes upward medially) (Fig 79.5)
- Involvement of posterior and anterior facets variable, and some are localized only to the posterior aspect of the middle facet

* Findings result from altered mechanics in weight bearing

MRI:

- Best seen in coronal plane
- Reactive changes and marrow edema on fluid-sensitive sequences (Fig. 79.3)
- Downsloping of sustentaculum tali and narrowing of the medial talocalcaneal joint space with cartilage, fibrous or bone signal intensity at the articulation (Fig. 79.4)

Imaging Strategy

Tarsal coalition is usually found incidentally on foot radiographs obtained for pain. In cases in which coalition is suspected clinically, the initial assessment should be with three routine radiographic views of the foot: anteroposterior, 45-degree internal oblique and lateral. Calcaneonavicular and talonavicular coalitions are usually readily seen on radiographs, whereas talocalcaneal coalition can only be suggested. The Harris-Beath radiographic view for talocalcaneal coalition has been replaced by cross-sectional imaging. If radiographs are equivocal or negative, but suspicion is still high, cross-sectional imaging is recommended. Scintigraphy is generally not used. If the index of suspicion for tarsal coalition is high, CT should be performed; not only is CT more cost-effective, but it is often requested for surgical planning where feasible. CT is not as sensitive as MR at finding other entities that cause pain; if the suspicion for coalition is low or moderate, MR should be considered. CT is performed in axial planes with coronal reformatted images, with both feet positioned symmetrically in the gantry. Acquired and reformatted images should be viewed with 3-millimeter intervals. Three-dimensional reconstruction images may be helpful, particularly for surgical planning. Routine MR ankle protocols suffice for tarsal coalition and include: sagittal and axial T1, proton density, and T2, as well as a fluid-sensitive sequence (STIR, proton density or T2 with fat suppression) to assess marrow signal.

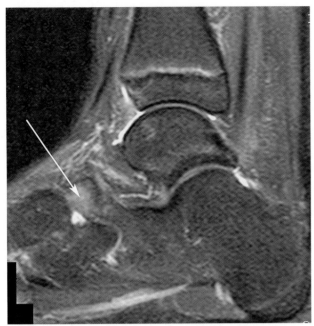

Figure 79.3. Sagittal STIR MR image of the hindfoot in a 14-year-old girl with pain shows high signal intensity (SI) in the elongated anterior calcaneal process and navicular (arrow) consistent with edema in osseous calcaneonavicular coalition.

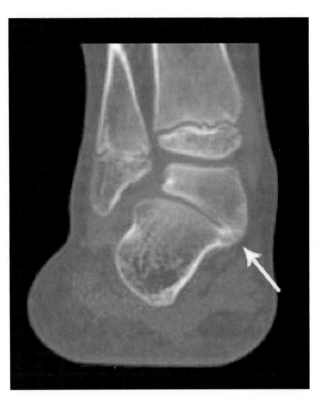

Figure 79.5. Coronal CT image of the right foot in a 12-year-old boy with pain demonstrates downward sloping of the medial aspect of the sustentaculum tali and middle facet (arrow) consistent with osseous middle facet talocalcaneal coalition.

Related Physics

Tarsal coalition can be imaged with CT or MRI and displayed using 3-D technologies. These include multiplanar reconstruction (MPR), maximum intensity projection (MIP), volume rendering (VR), and surface shaded display (SSD). Quantitative assessment can also be determined over areas of interest from the source data. Using MPR technology one can reconstruct and view images in three principle orthogonal planes as well as oblique planes of any angle. The reconstructed images are most often made from axial datasets, ideally where the voxels are cubic (i.e., isotropic voxel size). The imaging computer treats this as a volume of data permitting the user to slice through the volume in any orientation that is beneficial to diagnosis. The three principle faces on this volume are axial, coronal, and sagittal. For CT, MPR is best performed when the raw data are acquired at unity pitch, small detector width and reconstructed with thin contiguous images or greater thickness with 50 percent overlap. MIP images are produced by first defining a reference point of view for the volume of data. Next, the computer traces rays from behind the volume toward the viewing point. Only the voxel with the maximum Hounsfield unit or signal strength along each ray is displayed in a planar image, regardless of its position in the volume. This is particularly useful in bone imaging or CT arteriography. For VR, a threshold value is chosen and all voxels above this value are *retained* with those on the surface being displayed. This generates a true 3-D image. Surface shaded display is similar to VR in that voxels are chosen by a threshold with the refinement that voxels on the surface are *retained* and internal ones discarded resulting in a "hollow model" and a substantially reduced data size. Any true 3-D model can be used for quantitative assessment; in tarsal coalition one is capable of measuring the area/volume of the fibrous or cartilaginous articulation by tracing the areas on the MPR images and stacking them to produce a volume or tracing the volume directly from the VR.

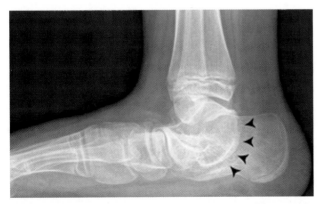

Figure 79.4. Lateral radiograph of the right foot in a 13-year-old girl with pain demonstrates pes planus and the "C" sign (arrowheads). Synostosis of the middle and posterior subtalar joints was confirmed by CT.

Differential Diagnosis

Talocalcaneal coalition:

- Inflammatory arthrofibrosis in middle subtalar facet
- Normal subtalar ligaments (medial talocalcaneal and interosseous talocalcaneal) which do not produce the osseous irregularity seen with coalition

Talar beak:

- Diffuse Idiopathic Skeletal Hyperostosis (DISH)
- Acromegaly
- Rheumatoid arthritis
- Athletes

Spastic flatfoot:

- Fracture
- Arthritis
- Tumor
- Inflammatory arthrofibrosis

Clinical Issues

Treatment of all patients with tarsal coalition begins conservatively and consists of orthotics, casting, NSAIDs, steroid injections, or physical therapy. If conservative management fails, surgery is usually performed. Calcaneonavicular and talocalcaneal coalitions may be treated with surgical resection. Recurrence may be prevented by interposition of the extensor digitorum brevis tendon (calcaneonavicular coalition) or fat (talocalcaneal coalition). Failure of resection is uncommon (between 10 and 23 percent of patients), usually attributed to arthritis, incomplete resection, or recurrent coalition. The final treatment attempt consists of joint fusion or arthrodesis.

Key Points

- Most common forms are calcaneonavicular and talocalcaneal

- Typical presentation is pain, which increases with advancing ossification
- Typical onset for calcaneonavicular is 8 to 12 years of age and for talocalcaneal is 12 to 16 years of age
- Classic radiographic findings for the two most common forms: "anteater's nose" sign (calcaneonavicular) and the "C"sign (talocalcaneal)
- Radiographs relatively insensitive for talocalcaneal coalition; CT recommended if suspicion high; MR preferred if suspicion low to identify other entities causing pain
- Classic cross-sectional imaging findings: joint-space narrowing, bony bar, abnormal articular orientation, reactive bone changes, marrow edema

Further Reading

Chapman VM. The Anteater nose sign. *Radiology*. 2007; *245*:604–605.

Emery KH, Bisset GS, Johnson ND, Nunan PJ. Tarsal coalition: a blinded comparison of MRI and CT. *Pediatr Radiol*. 1998;*28*:612–616.

Linklater J, Hayter CL, Vu D, Tse K. Anatomy of the subtalar joint and imaging of talo-calcaneal coalition. *Skeletal Radiol*. 2009;*38*:437–449.

Newman JS, Newburg AH. Congenital tarsal coalition: multimodality evaluation with emphasis on CT and MR imaging. *Radiographics*. 2000;*20*:321–332.

Rozansky A, Varley E, Moor M, Wenger DR, Mubarak SJ. A radiologic classification of talocalcaneal coalitions based on 3D reconstruction. *J Child Orthop*. 2010;*4*:129–135.

Taniguchi A, Tanaka Y, Kadono K, Takakura Y, Kurumatani N. C sign for diagnosis of talocalcaneal coalition. *Radiology*. 2003;*228*:501-5-5.

Upasani VV, Chambers RC, Mubarak SJ. Analysis of calcaneonavicular coalitions using multi-planar three-dimensional computed tomography. *J Child Orthop*. 2008;*2*:301–307.

CHAPTER 80

Rickets

Stephen L. Done, MD

Definition

Rickets is osteomalacia in growing bones resulting from inadequate calcium and phosphorus product, usually in the presence of sufficient cartilaginous and osteoid matrix.

Clinical Features

Rickets may be suspected clinically because of enlarged wrists, knees, and costochondral margins. The enlarged costochondral margins may be palpable. This is termed the "rachitic rosary." Genu vara is more common than genu valgum in weight-bearing children. Some children with rickets have poor linear growth, bone pain, late onset of walking, fractures, delayed suture closure, or delayed tooth eruption. Some infants or young children present with sudden onset of seizures or tetany resulting from severe hypocalcemia. Electrocardiographic findings may include long QT interval, U-waves and abnormal T-waves. Compromise of immune function may result in infections, most commonly pneumonia.

Anatomy and Physiology

Normal bone formation requires adequate and functional forms of vitamin D, calcium, and phosphate, as well as vitamin D receptors. Worldwide, most cases of rickets are nutritional in origin resulting from inadequate vitamin D intake or lack of sufficient sun exposure to provide endogenous production of this steroid hormone. Vitamin D is naturally acquired by eating oily fish and egg yolks. Lack of sufficient calcium in the diet is rare except in some regions of Turkey and Africa. Avoidance of sun exposure as a result of indoor living as well as avid use of sunscreens have led to decreased photosynthetic production of Vitamin D. Vitamin D is hydroxylated in the liver and kidneys to its most active form; it is essential for the adequate absorption of calcium from the gut and maintenance of proper calcium and phosphorous product necessary for normal mineralization of the skeleton. Rickets may develop secondary to renal or hepatic diseases that impair the hydroxylation pathway. Extreme phosphate wasting that occurs at the renal tubular level can cause rickets. This form of rickets is most often seen in hereditary x-linked hypophosphatemic rickets (XLHR), which was previously called vitamin-D-resistant rickets.

Understanding events that normally occur at the growth plate is useful when considering the radiographic findings in rickets (Fig. 80.1). Chondrocyte proliferation, enlargement, and apoptosis in the presence of a milieu of calcium and phosphorus result in calcification of the cartilage in the area of the growth plate known as the zone of provisional calcification (ZPC), the dense white line just beneath the growth plate. These cartilage struts are the primary trabeculae, which are also known as primary spongiosa. Blood vessels from the bone marrow invade this area, osteoclasts begin to resorb the primary trabeculae and subsequently produced trabeculae from the secondary spongiosa. This region of active bone formation also serves as a calcium reservoir that is used when a rapid source of calcium is needed to maintain serum calcium levels. The metaphyseal surface area is large and osteoclasts are abundantly present and are readily available for the work of dissolving bone.

Imaging Findings

- Earliest imaging finding is loss of ZPC resulting from lack of mineralization (Fig. 80.2)
- Fuzzy and indistinct trabeculae
- Metaphyseal fraying and flaring (Fig. 80.3)
- Cupped metaphysis: epiphysis driven into the soft proximal metaphyseal bone in older weight-bearing children
- Bowing: genu varum (bow-legged) or less often with genu valgum (knock-knees; Fig. 80.4)
- "Rachitic rosary": bulbous expansion at the metaphysis of anterior ribs (Fig. 80.5)
- Craniotabes: poor ossification of the skull with indistinct cortical margins and apparently widened sutures
- Secondary hyperparathyroidism: cortical tunneling and subperiosteal resorption of bone
- With treatment the zones of provisional calcification are reestablished and the bones begin to reossify with alternating lucent and dense bands (Fig. 80.6)
- Chambering: caused by occasional cartilage rests within the trabecular bone
- Pelvic, hip, and sacral deformity
- Insufficiency fractures in weight-bearing children

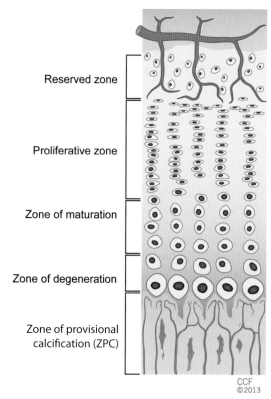

Reserved zone

Proliferative zone

Zone of maturation

Zone of degeneration

Zone of provisional calcification (ZPC)

CCF
©2013

Figure 80.1. Anatomy of the growing metaphysis.

- Premature closure of sagittal suture often with dolichocephaly (XLHR)
- Nephrocalcinosis (XLHR)

Imaging Strategy

Rickets, like any metabolic bone disease in children will be most easily detected in areas of rapid bone growth.

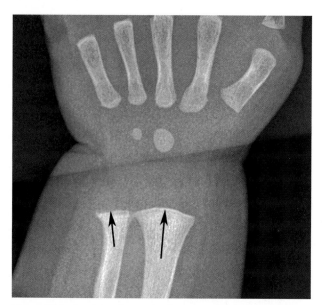

Figure 80.2. Frontal radiograph of a normal infant wrist. The ZPC is calcified cartilage and appears on the radiograph as a dense white line (arrows). Cartilage calcification is always more dense than the ossification of bone.

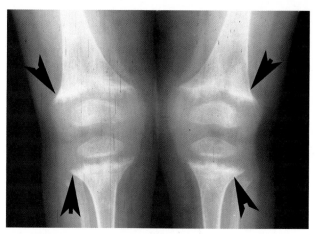

Figure 80.3. Frontal radiograph of the knees in a child with active rickets. Prior to therapy metaphyses are frayed, cupped, and flared (arrowheads). The ZPC is absent and growth plate is widened.

These include the wrists and knees where loss of ZPC is easily recognized. Screening radiographs include a frontal view of the knees in infants and an AP view of the wrist in children.

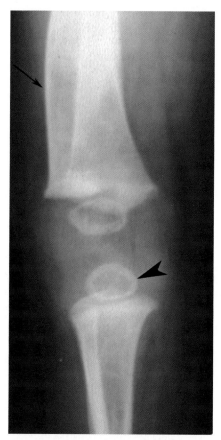

Figure 80.4. Frontal radiograph of the knee in a child with scurvy, which is a form of osteoporosis with adequate mineral (hydroxyapatite) but insufficient matrix. This image shows a ring epiphysis (arrowhead) and normal ZPC. Sheathing periosteal new bone (black arrow) is a result of subperiosteal hemorrhage.

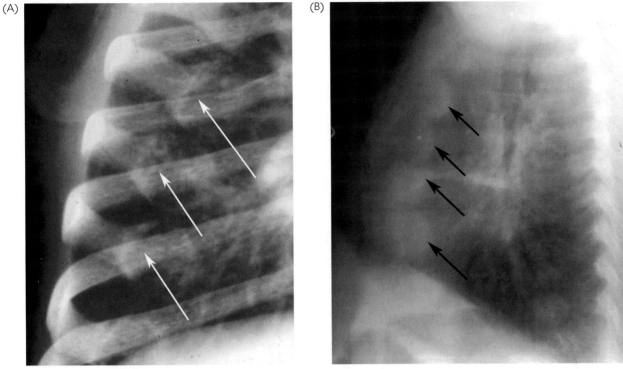

Figure 80.5. Frontal radiograph of the chest with rib detail (A) in an infant with rickets shows the "rachitic rosary" resulting from widening and flaring of the anterior metaphyses of the growing ribs (white arrows). Lateral radiograph (B) shows severe demineralization of all bones and wide cupped bulbous rib ends (black arrow).

Related Physics

In order to properly evaluate the trabecular pattern and ZPC in infants, all aspects of high-resolution imaging must be employed while ensuring lowest possible radiation dose to the patient. High-resolution parameters include small focal spot, high-resolution film, high-resolution computed radiography (CR) or direct radiography (DR) plates and monitors. A CR cassette can be processed in standard (200 micron) or high-resolution (100 micron) modes. Most DR systems are 160 microns without dual option. The smaller cassettes (8 x 10 and 10 x 12) are always read out in high-resolution mode whereas the 14 x 17 cassettes are generally read out in standard mode (high-resolution generates much more data which is time-intensive and this is further increased with larger cassettes). For infants with suspected rickets the smaller cassettes are used. High-resolution radiography requires the highest-resolution black-and-white monitor for optimal viewing.

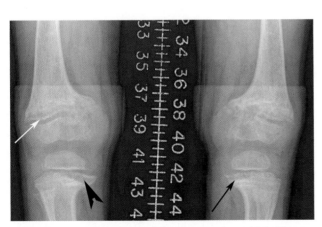

Figure 80.6. Frontal radiograph of the knees in a child with active rickets following treatment shows the new ZPC has become calcified and is dense (white arrow). The old ZPC is also calcified (black arrow). Intervening cartilage is slow to calcify or resorb and will take time to fully resolve (black arrowhead).

Differential Diagnosis

- Insufficiency fractures from osteoporosis (Fig. 80.7A)
- Scurvy (Fig. 80.7B)
- Metaphyseal chondrodysplasia
- Congenital syphilis
- Nonaccidental trauma (especially if less than 6 months of age)

Common Variants

- Hypophosphatemic rickets: a true form of congenital rickets that exists despite adequate intake of vitamin D; unique in that manifestation of rickets at the knees usually out of proportion to wrists
- Congenital rickets: rare and may be seen in infants born of mothers who are suffering from end-stage renal disease, have severe pre-eclampsia, are severely malnourished or severely vitamin-D-deficient

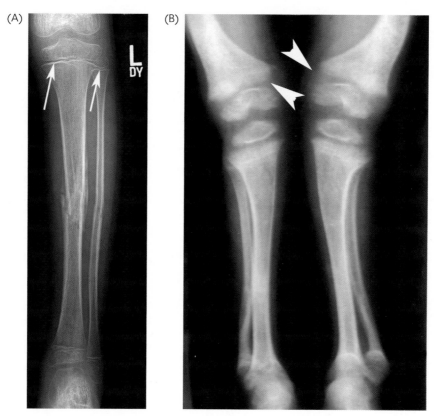

Figure 80.7. Frontal radiograph of the tibia fibula (A) in a child with disuse osteoporosis from fracture. Osteoporosis is a condition of insufficient bone, the matrix is lacking and trabeculae are resorbed by osteoclasts. Zones of provisional calcification (ZPC) (white arrows) are well-maintained. Frontal radiograph of the lower extremities (B) in a child with nutritional rickets (osteomalacia in growing bones) where matrix is adequate but mineralization is inadequate shows the trabeculae are present, but fuzzy and indistinct. ZPC is absent and metaphyses are brush-like and frayed, and the growth plate (white arrowhead) is axially widened. The bones are soft and bend with weight bearing. Genu valgum is present.

- Renal osteodystrophy (secondary hyperparathyroidism): may have the unusual finding of rickets in a skeleton that is overall more densely ossified than usual, and there may be coexisting soft-tissue calcification
- Oncogenic rickets: paraneoplastic process resulting from decreased renal tubular function secondary to a substance produced by some mesenchymal or connective tissue neoplasms; results in decreased renal production of 1.25 (OH)$_2$ D resulting in hypophospatemic rickets; resolves on removal of tumor
- Some medications used to treat solid tumors can also result in renal tubular dysfunction leading to acquired hypophosphatemic rickets

IMAGING PITFALL: Frequently the distal ulna may be misinterpreted as representing rickets when it is slightly cupped. This is a common normal variant.

Key Points

- Rickets is osteomalacia in growing bones.
- Insufficient Ca-P product most commonly from dietary insufficiency of vitamin D, insufficient sunlight, or ingested calcium.
- ZPC fails to calcify at the metaphysis.
- Metaphysis is frayed, splayed, and disarrayed with widening and decrease in normal density of the ZPC.
- Rickets appears as alternating bands of density with healing.
- Rickets must be differentiated from disuse or osteoporosis from scurvy.

Further Reading

Bloom E, Klein EJ, Shushan D, Feldman KW, Variable presentations of rickets in children in the emergency department. *Pediatric Emergency Care.* 2004;*20*:126–13.

Chapman T, Sugar N, Done S, Marasigan J, Wambold N, Feldman K. Fractures in infants and toddlers with rickets. *Pediatr Radiol.* 2010;*40*(7):1184–1189. Epub 2009 Dec 9.

Griscom NT, Jaramillo D. "Osteoporosis," "Osteomalacia," and "Osteopenia." *AJR*. 2000;*175*:267–268.

Holick MF. Resurrection of vitamin D deficiency and rickets, *Journal Clinical Investigation*. 2006;*116*:2062–2072.

Holick MF. Vitamin D deficiency, *New England Journal Medicine*. 2007;*357*:266–281.

Perez-Rossello JM, Feldman HA, Kleinman PK, Connolly SA, Fair RA, Myers RM, Gordon CM. Rachitic changes, demineralization, and fracture risk in healthy infants and toddlers with vitamin D deficiency. *Radiology*. 2012;*262*(1):234–241. Epub 2011 Nov 21.

Pezeshk P, Carrino JA. Rickets and osteomalacia. In: Weissman, BN, ed. *Imaging of arthritis and metabolic bone disease*. Philadelphia, PA: Elsevier; 2009:660–667.

Shore RM, Metabolic bone disease. In: Slovis, TL, ed. *Caffey's Pediatric Diagnostic Imaging*. Eleventh edition. Philadelphia, PA: Elsevier;: 2008;2728–2732.

Slovis TL, Chapman S, Evaluating the data concerning vitamin D insufficiency/deficiency and child abuse, *Pediatric Radiology*. 2008;*38*:1221–1224.

CHAPTER 81

Fibromatosis Colli

Victor J. Seghers, MD, PhD

Definition

Fibromatosis colli is benign fibroblastic soft-tissue proliferation within the sternocleidomastoid muscle (SCM) presenting in the newborn period. It is also known as sternocleidomastoid tumor of infancy, pseudotumor of infancy, and congenital muscular torticollis.

Clinical Features

Fibromatosis colli affects 0.4 percent of live births with slight male predominance. This condition often presents within the first few weeks of life as a firm nontender nodule or mass, usually in the distal two-thirds of the SCM, right side more than left, and it is rarely bilateral. Coexisting involvement of the trapezius muscle has been reported. The lesion achieves maximum size within 4 weeks after onset and typically resolves over the next 4 to 8 months. Up to 30 percent of infants with fibromatosis colli present with torticollis. The head tilts towrd the affected side and the chin turns away. A small number of patients develop ipsilateral hemifacial and hemicranial microsomia as a result of chronic torticollis. Bilateral involvement is rare, but results in apparent shortening of the neck and upturning of the chin. Other associated abnormalities include developmental dysplasia of the hip, rib anomalies, clubfoot, metatarsus adductus, scoliosis, mental retardation, and seizure disorders.

Anatomy and Physiology

The cause of fibromatosis colli is uncertain, but the favored pathophysiology is fibrous reaction to injury of the SCM from intrauterine crowding or during difficult birth. One theory suggests that injury results in venous outflow tract, local edema, degeneration of muscle fibers, and ultimately fibrosis of the muscle. The disorder is associated with breech presentation at birth, forceps delivery, and primiparous birth.

Imaging Findings

US:

- Fusiform thickening in the distal two-thirds of the sternocleidomastoid muscle (Fig. 81.1)

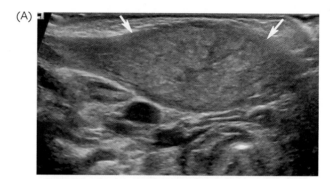

(A)

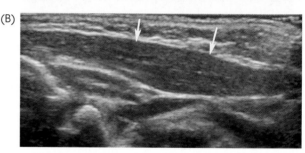

(B)

Figure 81.1. Sagittal US of the right neck (A) in a 20-day-old with enlarging right neck mass shows fusiform dilation of the distal SCM resulting from a poorly defined intramuscular mass with heterogenous but predominantly hyperechoic echotexture (arrows). Sagittal US of the left neck (B) shows the normal appearance of the SCM (arrows).

- Intramuscular mass with well-defined margins
- No invasion of adjacent soft tissues
- Lesion moves synchronously with SCM muscle on real-time imaging
- Lesion and muscle show variable echotexture and characteristics, often either homogeneously isoechoic or slightly hypoechoic

CT and MRI:

- Lesion is often isodense with the remainder of the muscle on CT (Fig. 81.2)
- Variable signal intensity and enhancement of the lesion on MRI
- Enlargement of the SCM
- Preservation of adjacent fascial planes
- Mass effect upon surrounding structures
- Uncommonly intralesional hemorrhage or calcification

(A)

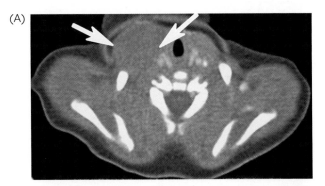

(B)

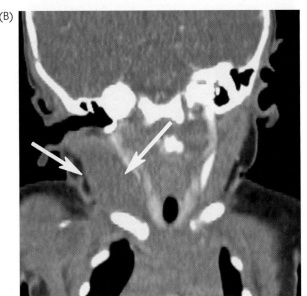

Figure 81.2. Axial (A) and coronal (B) contrast-enhanced CT in a 4-month-old with refractory torticollis shows swelling of the right SCM (arrows) with ipsilateral torticollis with head tilt.

Imaging Strategy

If the history is typical, no imaging is required. When non-muscular causes of torticollis are suspected or when there is a palpable neck mass without torticollis, imaging may be employed. Ultrasound is the preferred imaging modality because of lower cost, absence of ionizing radiation, and no need for sedation. CT and MRI are reserved for atypical cases where US is not diagnostic. If imaging exams demonstrate a lesion in the sternocleidomastoid with irregular margins that extends outside the muscle, is unusually hyperemic, or has significant regional lymphadenopathy, other etiologies should be considered.

Related Physics

Fibromatosis colli should be a straightforward US diagnosis but still presents problems for some radiologists largely as a result of improper US technique. This invariably renders images with poor signal-to-noise and/or contrast-to-noise ratios. The SCM has a characteristic echogenic raphe or septation that separates the medial and lateral bellies and it is identification of this raphe on US that will make the correct

diagnosis of fibromatosis colli. This septation will not be seen with poor signal-to-noise as it will have the same echogenicity as the surrounding muscle. Contrast-to-noise ratio speaks to the ability to see an object as different from its background when significant noise is present. In this case, the object of interest is the muscle boundary as it relates to the body behind it. The heterogeneity of the muscle body is caused by its high inherent noise. Contrast-to-noise equals the echogenicity of the boundary minus the echogenicity of the muscle divided by the standard deviation of the echo signal in the muscle.

Differential Diagnosis

- Classic hemangioma
- Sarcoma: rhabdomyosarcoma, infantile fibrosarcoma, granulocytic sarcoma
- Infantile fibromatosis or myofibromatosis
- Lipoblastoma or lipoblastomatosis

Clinical Issues

Treatment is usually limited to simple stretching exercises. Up to 90 percent of cases spontaneously resolve within 4 to 8 months. Surgery is reserved for the severe refractory cases after 1 year of age to prevent permanent contracture, facial asymmetry, or plagiocephaly.

Key Points

- Fibromatosis colli is a benign fibroblastic tumor of infancy, located within the SCM.
- Fibromatosis colli typically appears within a few days after birth as a palpable mass/torticollis.
- Spontaneous gradual resolution is typical after 4 to 8 months.
- US demonstrates variable echotexture fusiform dilation of the distal two-thirds of the SCM with no surrounding tissue invasion or adenopathy.
- Treatment is often conservative, consisting of observation and physiotherapy.
- Developmental facial and skull malformations in refractory cases may require surgical intervention.

Further Reading

Crawford SC, Harnsberger HR, Johnson L, Aoki JR, Giley J. Fibromatosis colli of infancy: CT and sonographic findings. *AJR*. 1988;*151*:1183–1184.

Lowry KL, Estroff JA, Rahbar R. The presentation and management of fibromatosis colli. *Ear Nose Throat J*. 2010;*89*(9):E4–E8.

Murphey MD, Ruble CM, Tyszko SM, Zbojniewicz AM, Potter BK, Miettinen M. Musculoskeletal fibromatoses: radiologic-pathologic correlation. *Radiographics*. 2009;*29*: 2143–2176.

Robbin MR, Murphey MD, Temple HT, Kransdorf MJ, Choi JJ. Imaging of musculoskeletal fibromatosis. *Radiographics*. 2001;*21*:585–600.

CHAPTER 82

Osteochondritis Dissecans

Robert C. Orth, MD, PhD

Definition

Osteochondritis dissecans (OCD) is an intra-articular condition characterized by injury and separation of a fragment of bone from the surrounding subchondral bone with or without disruption of the overlying articular cartilage. The resulting lesion is also referred to as an osteochondral fracture or defect.

Clinical Features

The overall incidence is unknown, but there is a male predominance and a peak in the teen years. Children with OCD typically present with vague and poorly localized pain. Symptoms tend to be chronic at presentation and worsen with activity. Locking and effusion are also common. Up to one-third have minimal or no symptoms with lesions discovered incidentally.

Anatomy and Physiology

Multiple causes have been implicated and include ischemia and genetic factors, but most lesions are likely initiated by chronic and repetitive trauma. The increased incidence of OCD in active athletes lends credence to chronic repetitive microtrauma as the most likely etiology. The result is microfractures through the subarticular bone that may also involve the epiphyseal and articular cartilage. This can lead to an unstable fragment if synovial fluid dissects through the fracture (Fig. 82.1).

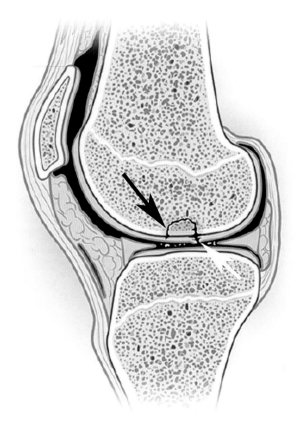

Figure 82.1. Osteochondritis dissecans. Fracture may be isolated to the subarticular bone (black arrow) or may involve overlying cartilage with a flap (white arrow) or circumferential fissure; dissection of synovial fluid through the fracture leads to an unstable fragment.

Imaging Findings

Radiography:

- Most common in lateral aspect of the medial femoral condyle but may occur at other locations including the lateral femoral condyle, trochlea, patella, tibia, elbow, talus, and hip
- Lucent, well-localized, subchondral epiphyseal lesion
- Loose bodies if the osteochondral fragment contains enough ossified subchondral bone

MRI:

- T1 hypointense and variably T2 hyperintense (Fig. 82.2)

- MR highly sensitive and specific in differentiating stable from unstable OCD lesions in adults
- Unstable lesions have the potential to detach and become loose bodies (Fig. 82.3)

Features of instability in adults (* indicates questionable significance in isolation in children):

- T2 hyperintense rim* surrounding the OCD lesion (Fig. 82.4)
- Cyst(s)* surrounding the OCD lesion (Fig. 82.5)
- T2 hyperintense fracture line extending through the articular cartilage overlying the OCD lesion
- Fluid-filled osteochondral defect

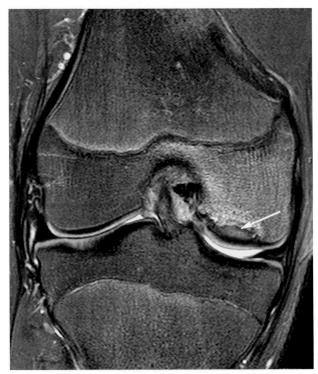

Figure 82.2. Coronal T2 MR image with fat suppression in a 14-year-old male with right medial knee pain for 7 months and no known injury shows an OCD lesion (arrow) at the lateral aspect of the medial femoral condyle with moderately increased signal intensity and surrounding bone marrow edema.

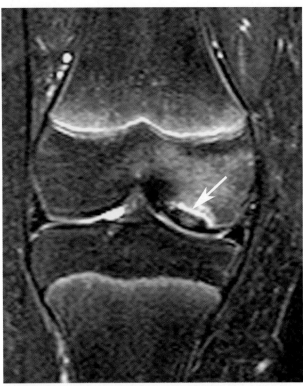

Figure 82.4. Coronal T2 MR image with fat suppression in a 12-year-old female with medial knee pain shows an OCD lesion (arrow) at the lateral aspect of the medial femoral condyle surrounded by a rim of high signal intensity. She continued to have pain following conservative treatment and subsequently underwent arthroscopic drilling of the lesion.

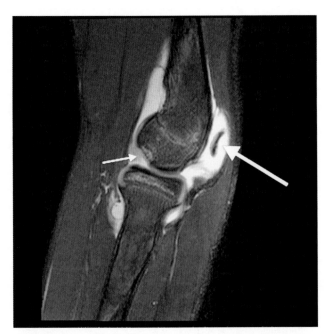

Figure 82.3. Sagittal T2 MR image with fat suppression following intra-articular injection of gadolinium in a 13-year-old active male baseball player with knee pain and swelling shows an OCD lesion of the right capatellum (small arrow) and associated loose body (large arrow).

Features of instability in juvenile OCD when present together (sensitivity/specificity 100%):

- Multiple cysts including one > 5 millimeters
- High T2 signal rim equal to fluid intensity
- Multiple breaks in the subchondral bone on T2
- Second outer rim of low T2 signal

Imaging Strategy

The modality of choice is MRI to fully characterize osteochondral lesions and direct treatment. The choice of pulse sequences depends on the location of pain and institutional preferences. A potential protocol to evaluate OCD of the knee could include: sagittal proton density (with or without fat supression); sagittal T2 with fat suppression; coronal T2 with fat suppression; coronal T1; and axial T2 with fat suppression; high-resolution heavily T2-weighted sequence for cartilage assessment (optional).

Related Physics

Presurgical planning with MRI can often include high-resolution imaging of cartilage, which creates a large dataset. This is one of many examples of why most modern radiology departments require high-speed, high-capacity picture archiving and communication systems (PACS). The

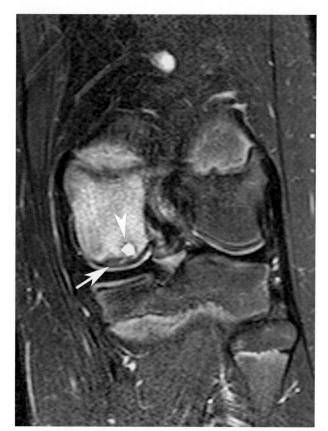

Figure 82.5. Coronal T2 MR image with fat suppression in an 11-year-old female with knee pain shows a 5-millimeter cyst (arrowhead) adjacent to an OCD lesion (arrow) at the lateral aspect of the medial femoral condyle.

Differential Diagnosis
- Normal variant ossification
- Cortical irregularity of the distal femoral metaphysis
- Acute osteochondral fracture
- Stress or insufficiency fracture
- Avascular necrosis

Common Variants
Normal variation in the ossification patterns of the femoral condyle can mimic stage 1 OCD and is distinguished by:

- Location: more toward inferior, posterior, and central portions of the femoral condyle
- Accessory ossification centers will be well-corticated
- Bony spiculations
- Normal overlying cartilage signal
- Lack of bone marrow edema

Clinical Issues
Juvenile OCD (prior to physeal closure) has a better prognosis than adult OCD with high rates of healing following rest and nonoperative conservative treatment. Operative treatment of unstable lesions may include arthroscopic microfracturing, surgical fixation of the OCD lesion at the donor site, and/or cartilage debridement.

Key Points
- Separation of intra-articular subchondral bone from surrounding bone
- Peak in teen years with male predominance
- Uncertain etiology
- Instability criteria by MR differ between pediatric and adult patients
- Juvenile OCD responds better to conservative treatment than adult OCD

components of PACS systems include hardware, software, communication protocols and infrastructure. The hardware includes image display, routers, and image archival systems (servers, tape, spinning disk, etc.). The software applications include the hospital information system (HIS) and electronic medical record (EMR), radiology information system (RIS), voice recognition dictation system and Digital Imaging and Communications in Medicine (DICOM) reader platform. The infrastructure is what connects the hardware and can include fiberoptic cable, coppernet or wireless networks. The speed of transmission of images is determined by bandwidth, which is given in bits per second. For example, one 256 x 256 x 16 bit MR image is approximately 1 megabit (M) so that an entire study of 400 images or 400 M bits would be optimally transmitted in 7 minutes at a bandwidth of 1 M/second or 40 seconds at a bandwidth of 10 M/second. These times are actually an overestimation as many factors will decrease network efficiency such as traffic, choke points in the network that run at slower rates, hardware failure, and routing queues. This is analogous to trying to drive home at rush hour versus later in the evening. Efficiency in imaging will ultimately be affected by the degree of systems integration between the HIS, RIS, PACS and the dictation system.

Further Reading
Gebarski K, Hernandez RJ. Stage-I osteochondritis dissecans versus normal variants of ossification in the knee in children. *Pediatric Radiology*. 2005;35(9):880–886.

Hughes JA, Cook JV, Churchill MA, Warren ME. Juvenile osteochondritis dissecans: a 5-year review of the natural history using clinical and MRI evaluation. *Pediatric Radiology*. 2003;33(6):410–417.

Kijowski R, Blankenbaker DG, Shinki K, Fine JP, Graf BK, De Smet AA. Juvenile versus adult osteochondritis dissecans of the knee: appropriate MR imaging criteria for instability. *Radiology*. 2008;248(2):571–578.

O'Connor MA, Palaniappan M, Khan N, Bruce CE. Osteochondritis dissecans of the knee in children. A comparison of MRI and arthroscopic findings. *The Journal of Bone and Joint Surgery*. 2002;84(2):258–262.

CHAPTER 83

Osteochondroma

Stuart Morrison, MB, Ch.B, FRCP

Definition

Osteochondroma is defined as an outgrowth of bone and cartilage from the surface of a bone. Continuity of the lesion with the underlying cortex and medullary canal is diagnostic. "Exostosis" literally means an outgrowth of bone and is no longer an acceptable synonym for an osteochondroma.

Clinical Features

Osteochondroma is the most common pediatric bone tumor. A solitary osteochondroma presents as a painless lump frequently close to a joint and radiographs are ordered for further characterization. The majority of osteochondromas are noted in childhood and adolescence. The true incidence is unknown, as many cases are discovered incidentally on radiographs obtained for other reasons. Multiple familial osteochondromas (MFO) is a separate autosomal dominant disease characterized by a large numbers of osteochondromas throughout the skeleton. Every bone, except the calvarium, can be involved. Being autosomal dominant, one parent has the disease unless there is a new mutation, which occurs in 10 percent of cases. A frequent complication of hereditary MFO is short stature.

Anatomy and Physiology

An osteochondroma is a developmental lesion rather than a true tumor, as it forms from a displaced growth plate. Experimentally, osteochondromas can be produced by removing a portion of the growth plate and transferring it to the metaphysis. The lesions grow until skeletal maturity; any growth beyond that time is unusual and worrisome. Most osteochondromas arise in the long bones including femur, humerus, tibia, and fibula in order of frequency. The spine is rarely involved with a predilection for the posterior neural arch. In most cases, MFO is caused by mutations in the genes exostocin 1 (EXT1) and exostocin 2 (EXT2).

Imaging Findings

Radiography:
- Broad-based/sessile type (Fig. 83.1)
- Pedunculated type has a slender stalk
- Medullary cavity is continuous with parent bone

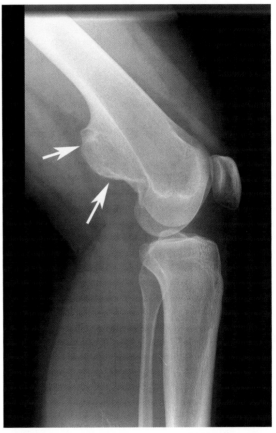

Figure 83.1. Lateral X-ray radiograph of the knee demonstrates a posterior sessile osteochondroma (arrows) from distal femoral metaphysis. Cartilage cap is not visible radiographically.

- Abnormal modeling of adjacent metaphysis (common; Fig. 83.2)
- Growth away from the adjacent joint or growth plate
- Variable calcification of the cartilage cap (Fig. 83.3)
- Cartilage cap is thickest during childhood and thins during adulthood and may eventually become absent

MRI/CT:
- Medullary cavity extends through base of lesion
- Cartilage cap follows physis in signal intensity
- Lesion may impinge on adjacent vital structures (nerves, vessels; Fig 83.4)

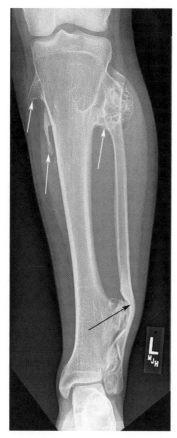

Figure 83.2. Hereditary multiple osteochondromas. Frontal radiograph of the left knee in a child with MFO shows multiple pedunculated and sessile osteochondromas (white arrows) arising from metaphyses and growing away from the adjacent joint. Distal tibial osteochondroma is deforming by pressure and scalloping the adjacent fibula cortex (black arrow).

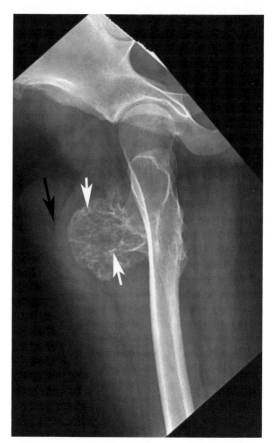

Figure 83.3. Frontal frog-leg lateral radiograph of the right hip in a teen with a palpable mass shows a large cauliflower-shaped solitary osteochondroma arising from femoral metaphysis with calcification (white arrows) in the cartilage cap. Note displacement of adjacent soft tissues (black arrow).

Imaging Strategy

Plain radiographs in two orthogonal planes are usually sufficient to diagnose an osteochondroma. Osteochondromas that occur in anatomically complex areas such as the bony pelvis, pectoral area, and spine may be further evaluated by either CT or MRI (Fig. 83.3); MRI is the preferred imaging modality to eliminate exposure to radiation.

> **IMAGING PITFALLS:** A cartilage cap thicker than 2 centimeters on MRI or CT in the skeletally mature patient strongly correlates with development of a secondary chondrosarcoma. However, increased thickness of the cartilage cap is normal in younger growing patients and should not be concerning.

Related Physics

Multiple familial osteochondroma is imaged with routine acquisitions including T1, spin density, T2 and T2*. At the

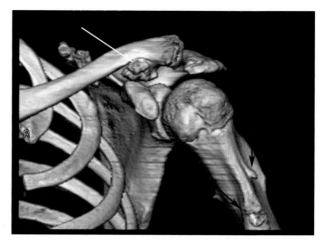

Figure 83.4. Coronal 3-D CT volume-rendered reconstruction of the left shoulder in a child with neuropraxia and pain shows the unusual position of an osteochondroma (white arrows) from inferior surface of lateral clavicle growing toward the coracoid process. Note osteochondromas (black arrows) around proximal humeral metaphysis.

molecular level the difference between these lies in the molecular environment of the hydrogen proton. The spin density (or proton density) image is made purely from the total density of hydrogen atoms (hydrogens/mm³). This sequence is highly sensitive to free water, which is the component of most disease processes, while maintaining excellent anatomic detail because of its high signal-to-noise ratio. Spin echo, also known as spin lattice, refers to the fact that protons are embedded in a lattice or local structure within a tissue, and this is unique to each tissue type and state of matter. The application of an RF pulse will cause randomly oriented spins to align themselves to the direction of the static magnetic field. The de-alignment of these spins toward their thermal distribution is characterized by the T1 relaxation time, which is unique for each tissue. The T1 actually represents the recovery of signal along the z-axis. T1 varies with the field strength such that an increase in B_0 will increase the precessional frequency of the protons in tissue rendering lesser differences between protons within fat, tissue, and water, leading to decrease in image contrast. The greatest benefit of higher field strength is to T2 and not to T1, as T2 is less susceptible to field strength. T2 is also known as spin-spin interaction and refers to the decay constant for signal on the y-axis. This occurs after the 90-degree followed by the 180-degree rephasing pulse. A higher field strength leads to a better T2 image, not because of improvements in T1 or T2, but because of increased signal-to-noise ratio. T2* is a "real-world" measurement of the ideal T2 constant. T2* is always less than T2 because of ever-present magnetic field homogeneities. When inhomogeneities in field strength are small, T2* approaches T2. In general, T2* differs from T2 by several milliseconds. Ferromagnetic or paramagnetic particles, such as contrast agents, will decrease T1 and T2. Typical T1/T2 relaxation values in milliseconds are seen in Table 83.1.

TISSUE	T1	T2
Muscle	1,130	35
Cartilage	1,060	42
Synovial fluid	2,850	1,210
Subcutaneous fat	288	165
Marrow fat	288	165

In brain, typical values are as follows: water = 3,000/3,000 milliseconds; gray matter = 810/100 milliseconds; white matter = 680/90 milliseconds; and fat = 240/85 milliseconds. Ferromagnetic or paramagnetic particles such as contrast agents will decrease T1 and T2.

Differential Diagnosis

- Parosteal osteosarcoma
- Metachondromatosis: very rare bony dysplasia of multiple osteochondromas and intraosseous enchondromas frequently involving fingers

- Langer-Giedion syndrome: contiguous gene syndrome of trichorhinophalangeal syndrome and multiple osteochondromas
- Potocki-Shaffer syndrome: contiguous gene syndrome of multiple osteochondromas and parietal foramina/skull ossification defects
- Supracondylar spur from the distal humerus: incidence of 3 percent; antero-medial bony outgrowth that points toward the elbow joint; ligament from the spur can attach to the medial epicondyle and compress the median nerve

Common Variants

- Subungual exostosis: osteochondroma arises under the nail bed most frequently from the great toe
- Epiphyseal osteochondroma or Trevor's dysplasia epiphysealis hemimelica: osteochondroma presents as a pedunculated mass arising from the epiphysis, most commonly in the lower extremity
- Bizarre parosteal osteochondromatous proliferation of bone: hands and feet simulating osteochondromas; arises from cortical surface with no alteration of the underlying bone or continuity with the medullary space

Clinical Issues

Longitudinal growth of a bone is most frequently adversely affected by the sessile type of osteochondroma. Lesions can cause pressure on adjacent neurovascular structures leading to neuropathy. Examples include peroneal nerve compression leading to foot drop from a proximal fibular osteochondroma and spinal cord compression from a posterior neural arch osteochondroma. Vascular injury occurs most commonly from an osteochondroma at the posterior knee causing popliteal artery pseudoaneurysm. A bursa can develop over the tip of a large osteochondroma and, with continued friction, can lead to inflammation. Pressure changes can develop at adjacent bones and joints such as impingement from a large femoral neck osteochondroma limiting movement of the hip joint. Compression of a distal tibial osteochondroma on the adjacent fibula can produce deformity around the ankle joint with a talar tilt. Similar deformity and growth disturbance in the forearm can produce a Madelung deformity at the wrist. Fracture of an osteochondroma is infrequent.

Malignant change almost never occurs in childhood. Pain and continued growth are the best predictors of malignant transformation. Lesions transform to a low-grade peripheral chondrosarcoma. Less than 1 percent of solitary osteochondromas and 3 to 5 percent of hereditary osteochondromas undergo malignant change. Radionuclide bone scan is no longer of value to assess for malignancy. There has been no cost/benefit analysis to support routine surveillance. Radiation is described both experimentally and following therapy as a cause of osteochondromas. The earlier the age when radiation is administered, the more likely the development of osteochondromas, emphasizing the increased sensitivity of the younger child to radiation. Osteochondromas were the commonest skeletal finding with an incidence of 24 percent in children receiving therapeutic radiation below 5 years of age and none in older children in one series of 58 children.

Key Points

- Most common bone tumor of childhood
- Continuity of the lesion with the underlying cortex and medullary canal is diagnostic
- Sensitivity of younger skeleton (<5 years) to radiation-induced osteochondroma
- Complications occur from local pressure effect on adjacent structures
- MFO is a separate autosomal dominant disease with a higher incidence of malignant change

Further Reading

Bernard SA, Murphy MD, Flemming DJ, Kransdorf MJ. Improved differentiation of benign osteochondromas from secondary chondrosarcomas with standardized measurement of cartilage cap at CT and MRI imaging. *Radiology.* 2010;*255*(3):857–865.

Fletcher BD, Crom DB, Krance RA, Kun LE. Radiation-induced bone abnormalities after bone marrow transplantation for childhood leukemia. *Radiology.* 1994;*191*:231–235.

Murphy MD, Choi JJ, Kransdorf MJ, Flemming DJ, Gannon FH. Imaging of osteochondromas: variants and complications with radiologic-pathologic correlation. *Radiographics.* 2000;*20*(5):1407–1434.

Schmale GA, Wuyts W, Chansky HA, Raskind W, Hereditary multiple osteochondromas gene reviews. NCBI Bookshelf. Available at: http://www.ncbi.nlm.nih.gov/books/NBK1235/. Accessed 2012

Taitz J, Cohn RJ, White L, Russell SJ, Vowels MR. Osteochondroma after total body irradiation: an age-related complication. *Pediatr Blood Cancer.* 2004;*42*(3):225–229.

CHAPTER 84

Jeune Syndrome

Neil Mardis, MD

Definition

Asphyxiating thoracic dysplasia (ATD), also known as Jeune syndrome or thoracopelviphalangeal dysplasia, is a short-limbed dysplasia characterized by short horizontal ribs, which compromise lung development and function often leading to lethal respiratory distress in the neonatal period.

Clinical Features

Overall, the degree of thoracic dysplasia is highly variable ranging from severely shortened ribs with associated thoracic insufficiency incompatible with postnatal life to very mild, clinically and radiographically occult rib dysplasia without respiratory symptoms. There is often multiorgan disease that primarily affects the kidneys and to a lesser extent the liver, pancreas, and retina. The syndrome has been estimated to occur in 1 per 100,000 to 130,000 live births. In addition to the variable thoracic dysplasia, patients are of short stature with short limbs and broad, short hands and fingers. The chest is typically narrow with a small internipple distance and small thoracic circumference. Pectus anomalies may coexist. Patients may have tachypnea, repeated respiratory infections, noisy breathing, exercise intolerance and fatigue related to restrictive lung disease with alveolar hypoventilation. Severe respiratory compromise may lead to death in the first 2 years, but respiratory status tends to improve after 2 years of age. Renal insufficiency secondary to glomerular fibrosis and sclerosis as well as tubular disorders can begin as early as 2 years of age in some patients. This leads to progressive nephropathy and chronic renal failure. Death in patients aged 3 to 10 years is usually secondary to renal disease. Proliferation of periportal biliary radicals is often seen at histopathologic examination and may lead to periportal fibrosis although clinical manifestations are uncommon. Retinal disease occurs in 15 percent of patients and usually first manifests as decreased night vision. Intelligence is usually normal.

Anatomy and Physiology

Affected persons have abnormal enchondral ossification related to chondrocyte columns that are poorly formed and insufficient in number. The lungs have normal architecture but are hypoplastic as a result of limited size of the rib cage, particularly during the first 2 years of life. Those with renal disease may have glomerular fibrosis or sclerosis, interstitial fibrosis. There may be renal tubular concentrating defects, with proteinuria and abnormal resorption of phosphate and uric acid. A gene locus for ATD has been mapped to 15q13 in some affected individuals. A chromosome 12 deletion has been described. Mutations have been found in the DYNC1H1 gene and the IFT80 gene (mapped at 3q24) in other patients.

Imaging Findings

Radiography:
- Small, bell-shaped thorax with short horizontal ribs (Fig. 84.1)
- Expansion of the costochondral junction
- High clavicles resemble bicycle handlebars
- Small pelvis with a trident appearance of the medial acetabular roof at the sacrosciatic notch (Fig. 84.2)
- Proximal femoral ossification centers abnormally present at birth in two-thirds of patients (normally not seen until 4 to 6 months)
- Metaphyseal cupping in the metacarpals and phalanges of the infant with ATD
- Cone-shaped epiphyses are noted in the hands later in childhood
- Polydactyly may be present however there is a lower frequency of involvement than that noted in other short-rib polydactyly syndromes (such as Ellis-van Creveld)
- Shortening of the long bones of the extremities varies in severity
- Skeletal features, including the rib-shortening, become progressively less radiographically apparent as the patient ages (Fig. 84.3); patients with milder degrees of thoracic dysplasia may have deceptively normal appearing chest radiographs by early or late childhood

US/CT:
- Renal disease: cystic dysplasia with macrocysts
- Hepatic fibrosis or mild bile duct dilation
- Pancreatic cysts are uncommon and may be seen with exocrine insufficiency

(A)

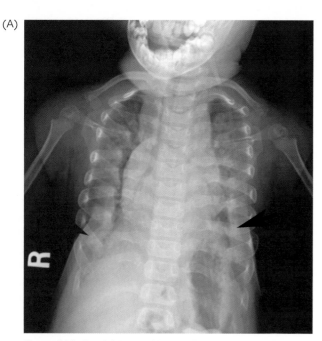

(B)

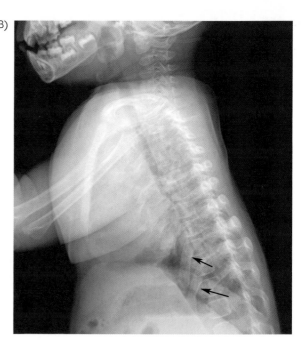

Figure 84.1. Frontal (A) and lateral (B) radiographs of the chest in a child with Jeune syndrome show severe rib shortening (arrows). This patient later underwent thoracic expansion with vertical expandable prosthetic titanium ribs (VEPTR) to improve pulmonary function.

Imaging Strategy

The initial workup includes a full skeletal survey. Frontal and lateral views of the skull and axial skeleton and individual frontal views of the chest, abdomen, pelvis, extremities, and hands should be obtained. Three-dimensional CT imaging with shaded surface display may help with surgical planning for primary or repeated efforts to repair clinically significant chest wall abnormalities. Screening US of the abdomen to evaluate for renal (or less commonly hepatic

and pancreatic) disease should also be performed. In older children, liver enzyme abnormalities will often indicate liver disease before it is appreciated on US.

Related Physics

Evaluation for syndromes in the newborn is a multidisciplinary process in which radiography plays an important role. The skeletal survey is performed at the table-top and includes multiple images of several body systems including the chest, abdomen, pelvis, and extremities. Each requires separate imaging parameters in the absence of automatic exposure control (AEC). All of these techniques are available as presets at the console in the fixed-base radiology setting. Portable requests should be discouraged as none of the presets are available and patient positioning can be challenging leading to potential decreased resolution and increased dose. The chest is evaluated for gross morphology, which does not require high-dose/resolution. Suggested technique would be 60 kVp and 1 mAs. The abdomen and pelvis are also evaluated for morphology/shape but here a higher mAs such as 2 to 2.5 is required in imaging through less air and greater bone and soft tissue. The extremities are evaluated in greater detail for normal development, shape, size, and abnormal soft-tissue calcification or deformity. Suggested technique would be 60 kVp and 1.6 mAs.

Figure 84.2. Frontal radiograph of the pelvis in a patient with Jeune syndrome shows short iliac bones and narrow sacrosciatic notches (arrows). The acetabular margin resembles a trident (arrowheads).

Differential Diagnosis

- Chondroectodermal dysplasia (Ellis-van Creveld syndrome): patients with Ellis-van Creveld (EvC) also demonstrate shortening of the ribs with a resultant

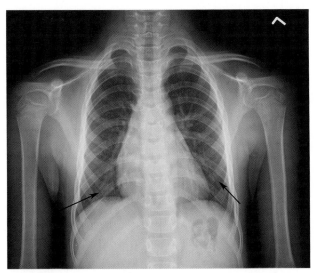

Figure 84.3. Frontal view of the chest in a 6-year-old patient with milder manifestations of Jeune syndrome shows subtle rib shortening (arrows) and chest wall narrowing that could easily be overlooked.

are proteins that produce directed movement along microtubules and the same gene is affected in patients with short-rib polydactyly type III (Verma-Naumoff syndrome), which is a severe condition with prenatal demise.

Clinical Issues

It can be difficult to differentiate Jeune syndrome from other short-rib polydactyly conditions. Clinicians often rely on radiologic features to help narrow the differential diagnosis and stratify genetic testing. In severe cases, the most pressing clinical issue is thoracic insufficiency. Patients surviving early infancy are subject to repeat pulmonary infections often resulting in significant morbidity. Chest reconstructive surgery has been performed to increase pulmonary function.

Key Points

- Narrow thorax with short ribs
- Varying degrees of restrictive lung disease ranging from prenatal or infant death to mild thoracic insufficiency
- Brachydactyly, polydactyly, and limb shortening (micromelia)
- Retina, kidneys, and liver often affected
- Renal disease often leads to death at 3 to 10 years

narrow thorax; degree of rib shortening is typically less severe in patients with EvC and rarely leads to life-threatening pulmonary insufficiency; pelvis in EvC has a similar trident appearance with mesomelic shortening of the long bones; frequency of polydactyly approaches 100 percent in EvC, which may help in discrimination; accessory oral frenula or fusion of the upper lip and gums, hypoplastic nails, and congenital heart disease (most commonly an atrial septal defect) seen only with EvC.

- Barnes syndrome (thoracolaryngopelvic dysplasia): autosomal dominant condition is also typified by a small thorax and pelvis; laryngeal stenosis provides a unique discriminating feature.
- Short rib-polydactyly (SRP) syndromes: Saldino-Noonan syndrome (type I SRP), Majewski (type II SRP), Verma-Naumoff (type III SRP), and Beemer-Langer (type IV SRP); all are autosomal recessive and can be difficult to differentiate from Jeune syndrome and EvC.

Variants

- ATD1: prototype as described above
- ATD2: results from a mutation in the IFT80 gene located on chromosome 3q24-q26; intraflagellar transport gene is necessary for the development and maintenance of cilia; shortening or bowing of the femurs and polydactyly or brachydactyly without renal or hepatic disease seen in ATD1
- ATD3: caused by a mutation in the DYNC2H1 gene located on chromosome 11q14.3-q23.1 located at gene locus 11q13.5; this gene encodes dyneins, which

Further Reading

Beales PL, Bland E, Tobin JL, Bacchelli C, Tuysuz B, Hill J, Rix S, Pearson CG, Kai M, Hartley J, Johnson C, Irving M, Elcioglu N, Winey M, Tada M, Scambler PJ. IFT80, which encodes a conserved intraflagellar transport protein, is mutated in Jeune asphyxiating thoracic dystrophy. *Nat Genet.* 39:727–729.

Brueton LA, Dillon MJ, Winter RM. Ellis-van Creveld syndrome, Jeune syndrome, and renal-hepatic-pancreatic dysplasia: separate entities or disease spectrum? *J Med Genet.* 1990;27:252–255.

Jeune M, Beraud C, Carron R. Asphyxiating thoracic dystrophy with famial characteristics. *Arch Fr Pediatr.* 1955;12(8):886–891.

Keppler-Noreuil KM, Adam MP, Welch J, Muilenburg A, Willing MC. Clinical insights gained from eight new cases and review of reported cases with Jeune syndrome (asphyxiating thoracic dystrophy). *Am J Med Genet A.* 2011;155A(5):1021–1032.

Morgan NV, Bacchelli C, Gissen P, Morton J, Ferrero GB, Silengo M, Labrune P, Casteels I, Hall C, Cox P, Kelly DA, Trembath RC, Scambler PJ, Maher ER, Goodman FR, Johnson CA. A locus for asphyxiating thoracic dystrophy, ATD, maps to chromosome 15q13. *J Med Genet.* 2003;40:431–435.

Yerian LM, Brady L, Hart J. Hepatic manifestations of Jeune Syndrome (asphyxiating thoracic dystrophy). *Semin Liver Dis.* 2003;23:195–200.

CHAPTER 85

Cleidocranial Dysplasia

Alan E. Schlesinger, MD

Definition

Cleidocranial dysplasia (CCD) is an autosomal dominant skeletal dysplasia characterized by abnormal hypoplastic clavicles and delayed (or absent) closure of the cranial sutures and fontanelles. It is also known as cleidocranial dysostosis (although this is technically incorrect as this disorder is now classified as a dysplasia rather than a dysostosis).

Clinical Features

The incidence of CCD is approximately 1 in 1,000,000 individuals, it involves all ethnic groups, and males and females are affected equally. Closure of the anterior fontanelle as well as fusion of the sagittal and metopic sutures is delayed (and they may remain open throughout life). There is delay in ossification of the skull leading to a soft skull in infancy. The nasal bridge may be depressed and the forehead is broad. Patients can present with failure to shed deciduous teeth, delayed eruption of teeth, and supernumerary teeth. Patients with CCD are more prone to sinus and middle ear infections. In the thorax, hypoplasia of the clavicles can lead to the ability to bring the shoulders together. There may be an associated skin dimple. If the scapulae are hypoplastic, the shoulders can be small and sloping. The ribs can be short with potential resultant respiratory distress. Mothers with CCD often require Caesarian delivery because of dysplastic changes in the pelvis. The second metacarpal is excessively long as a result of an accessory epiphysis; the remaining bones of the hands and feet are short. The nails can be hypoplastic, dysplastic, or absent. Overall height is diminished with disproportionate shortening of the limbs (especially the upper limbs) relative to the trunk. Intelligence is normal in patients with CCD.

Anatomy and Physiology

Cleidocranial dysplasia is the result of mutations of the CBFA1 gene on chromosome 6p21. This gene codes for a protein that is part of the bone morphogenetic protein signaling cascade and is involved in differentiation of osteoblasts and in chondrocyte differentiation.

Imaging Findings

US:

- Prenatal US: small or absent clavicles; pubic bone defect; skull abnormalities as below

Radiography:

- Wormian bones, delayed ossification of the skull, delayed closure of sutures and fontanelles, supernumerary teeth (Fig. 85.1)
- Poor pneumatization of the paranasal sinuses and mastoid air cells
- Brachycephaly
- Frontal bossing
- Absent parietal bone ossification and/or parietal foramina
- Partial or (rarely) complete absence of the clavicles (commonly the lateral or middle thirds; Fig. 85.2)
- Two separate clavicular segments that are not fused (variant)
- Small scapulae
- Short ribs
- Absent ossification of pubic bone in early infancy with subsequent wide symphysis pubis, hypoplastic iliac wings, large/tall femoral head ossification centers (Fig. 85.3)
- Pseudoepiphyses in metatarsals and metacarpals (Fig. 85.4)
- Dysplasia of fifth middle phalanx (and less commonly the second middle phalanx), cone-shaped epiphyses, shortening of the distal phalanges of the hand
- Delayed skeletal maturation

Imaging Strategy

A child with presumed CCD should have a complete skeletal survey. This examination should include separate AP views of the hands and feet. Occasionally, CT with 3-D reconstructions may be helpful in evaluating the cranial anomalies.

Related Physics

The workup of any skeletal dysplasia requires many radiographs, which may be repeated over time. Through

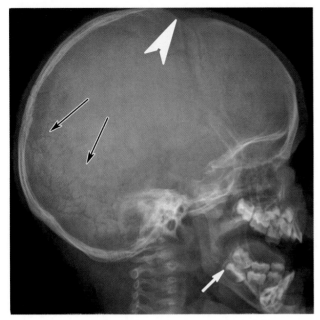

Figure 85.1. Lateral skull radiograph in a child with CCD demonstrates a wide anterior fontanelle (arrowhead), wormian bones (black arrows), and supernumerary teeth (white arrows).

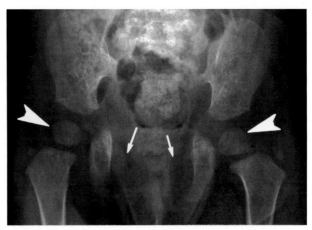

Figure 85.3. Frontal pelvic radiograph in a child with CCD demonstrates poorly ossified pubic bones (arrows) and large, tall femoral head ossification centers (arrowheads).

the study of many children imaged in this way, one is able to determine the radiobiologic effects of a population. Epidemiology is the study of outcome of this group matched to a control group of the same demographics who have not been imaged. Though cleidocranial dysplasia has not been specifically followed to determine incidence of excess cancers from imaging, information is available from other groups showing an increased incidence of solid organ and hematologic malignancies in children exposed in Chernobyl and Hiroshima. These disasters exposed people to one large dose whereas radiologic imaging exposes to smaller doses repeated over time. The field of radiobiology studies the malignancy rate from radiation exposure compared to that from

background radiation and this is referred to as the excess cancer risk. Not only is this important, it is also important to understand changes in the temporal nature of the onset of the cancer. This is referred to as the latency period. For hematologic malignancies the latency can be as short as

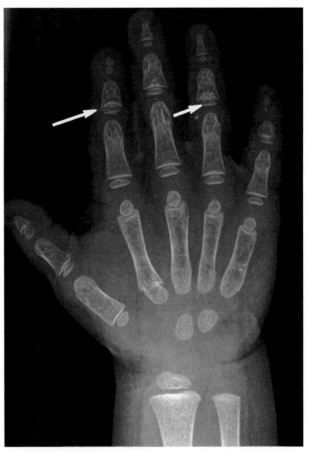

Figure 85.4. Frontal hand radiograph shows small distal phalanges, dysplastic second and fifth middle phalanges, and cone-shaped epiphyses in the middle phalanges of the second and fourth fingers (arrows).

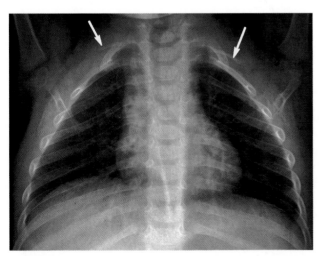

Figure 85.2. Frontal chest radiograph in a child with CCD reveals hypoplastic clavicles (arrows).

7 years; with solid-organ tumors the latency is closer to two to four decades. This becomes more of an issue in pediatrics where the remaining life expectancy is longer than in adults.

Differential Diagnosis

- Congenital pseudoarthrosis of the clavicle
- Pyknodysotosis: persistently open fontanelle and cranial sutures with osteolysis of the lateral clavicle
- Mandibuloacral dysplasia: delayed closure of cranial sutures, wormian bones, and clavicular hypoplasia
- Yunis-Varon syndrome: has many of the features of CCD but can be differentiated by the fact that these patients have hypoplasia or aplasia of the thumbs or great toes and have micrognathism

Common Variants

Parietal foramina-cleidocranial dysplasia has changes of CCD with accompanying parietal foramina, however, the dental anomalies are not present in this condition. The CDAGS syndrome (**c**raniosynostosis, **d**elayed closure of the fontanelles, cranial **d**efects, clavicular hypoplasia, **a**nal and **g**enitourinary malformations, and **s**kin eruption) is a related disorder that is genetically distinct from CCD but shares many imaging and clinical findings.

Clinical Issues

Dental procedures may be necessary to treat the delayed shedding of the deciduous teeth, delayed eruption of the permanent teeth, and the supernumerary teeth. Sinus and middle ear infections may require aggressive therapy. Although fontanelles eventually close in most patients, helmets may be warranted to prevent injury for high-risk activities, especially if the defects are large. The dysplastic changes in the pelvis lead to a higher Caesarean section rate in women with CCD.

Key Points

- Hypoplasia of the clavicles
- Dental anomalies including delayed shedding of deciduous teeth, delayed eruption of teeth, and supernumerary teeth
- Wide cranial sutures and delayed closure of the anterior fontanelle
- Pelvic anomalies including underdevelopment of the pubic bones

Further Reading

Lachman RS. Cleidocranial dysplasia. In: *Taybi and Lachman's Radiology of Syndromes, Metabolic Disorders and Skeletal Dysplasias.* Fifth edition. Philadelphia, PA: Mosby; 2007:913–915.

Mendoza-Londono R, Lammer E, Watson R, et al. Characterization of a new syndrome that associates craniosynostosis, delayed fontanel closure, parietal foramina, imperforate anus, and skin eruption: CDAGS. *Am J Hum Genet.* 2005;77:161–168.

Mundlos S. Cleidocranial dysplasia: clinical and molecular genetics. *J Med Genet.* 1999;36:177–182.

Spranger JW, Brill PW, Poznanski A. Cleidocranial dysplasia. In: *Bone Dysplasias.* Second edition. New York, NY: Oxford University Press;2002:393–398.

CHAPTER 86

Blount Disease

L. Todd Dudley, MD

Definition

Also known as tibia vara, Blount disease is a progressive deformity that theoretically results from abnormal stress or changes in the posteromedial proximal tibial physis, causing focal growth suppression, genu varum, and potentially mild limb-length discrepancy. Although there are various subtypes described in the literature, the two categories originally described by Blount remain useful: infantile-onset and adolescent- or late-onset. Although radiographic findings in both groups are similar, the clinical features vary depending on age of onset.

Clinical Features

Infantile Form

The infantile form of Blount disease usually becomes evident at 1 to 3 years of age. It essentially begins as normal bowing that progresses beyond infancy. The findings are typically symmetric and bilateral, though not always. This condition is more often seen in early walkers, African-Americans, obese children, and those with a positive family history. The children may demonstrate "in-toeing," if their feet are rotated medially as a result of internal rotation of the tibia. The lateral collateral ligament of the knee may become lax. There is a painless varus force during the stance phase of ambulation.

Adolescent Form

The adolescent form differs from the infantile form in that the age of onset is usually between 8 and 14 years. The tibial abnormality is more likely to be unilateral and painful. It often affects African-Americans and obese individuals, sometimes developing after a period of rapid weight gain.

Anatomy and Physiology

Normal development of the knee begins with mild infantile bowing, which is likely a result of in utero molding. Normal bowing gradually corrects and converts to mild valgus alignment by age 2 to 3 years as a result of normal weight-bearing with ambulation. Ultimately, in adulthood, there is a normal minimal varus alignment. In Blount disease, excessive stress at the proximal medial tibial physis alters endochondral bone formation, resulting in a degree of delayed ossification and subsequent medial tibial growth arrest. Additional changes are seen initially in the medial epiphyseal cartilage and the medial meniscus, both of which enlarge to help maintain a normal femoral tibial angle. Continued abnormal stress on the posterior and medial tibial physis results in decreased growth in this region. The asymmetric growth at the proximal tibial physis results in tibia vara.

Imaging Findings

Radiography:
- Depression, irregularity, and beaking or fragmentation of the posterior medial tibial metaphysis (Fig. 86.1A)
- Wide physis medially from growth arrest or laterally from traction
- Lateral subluxation of the tibia and medial tibial plateau in the intercondylar notch
- Metaphyseal-diaphyseal angle > 11 degrees (Fig. 86.1B)
- Adducted tibia (tibia vara) without significant diaphyseal bowing

MRI:
- Earliest change is high T2 signal intensity (SI) in medial tibial epiphyseal cartilage even before radiographic changes
- High T1 SI in medial meniscus
- Low T1 SI in medial tibial metaphysis
- Beaked appearance of the medial metaphysis
- Gradual development of vertical orientation of medial physis
- Bony bridging in the damaged physis

Imaging Strategy

Weight-bearing standing frontal radiographs are the mainstay of Blount imaging. CT or MR may be used for assessing the degree of proximal tibial growth plate fusion and to aid in treatment planning.

Related Physics

Multiplanar MR imaging for pre-surgical planning requires gradient coils in three planes (xy, xz, yz). The geometry of

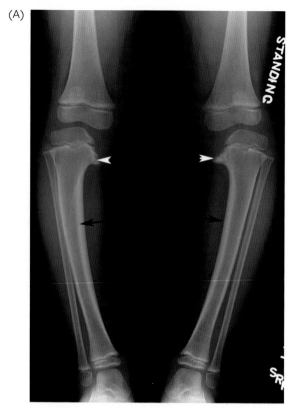
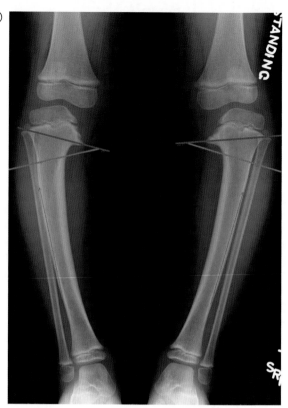

Figure 86.1. Weight-bearing frontal view of the distal femurs and tibias (A) in a 4-year-old female with bilateral tibia varus shows medial cortical thickening (arrows) of the tibiae without significant lateral tibial diaphyseal bowing; medial tibial metaphysis is depressed, beaked and irregular bilaterally (arrowheads). Figure (B) demonstrates the tibial metaphyseal-diaphyseal angle (right 26 degrees, left 20 degrees) determined by the intersection of a line perpendicular to the lateral tibial diaphyseal cortex (red) and a line connecting the two most inferior points of the tibial metaphysis (blue); angle of greater than 11 degrees is suggestive of Blount disease.

the coils is unique in that one must provide gradients along the three principle axes while maintaining an open bore at each end. Two pairs of saddle coils are embedded along the long axis of the bore to create gradients in the x and y directions (right-to-left and anterior-to-posterior, respectively) with one pair of Helmholtz for z-axis (cradiocaudad) gradient. These create a uniform variation in magnetic field strength such that for the z-gradient in a 1.5 Tesla magnet, the strength at the head may be 1.54 Tesla and at the feet 1.46 Tesla, for example. The gradients permit Fourier analysis of data to allow localization in the slice, frequency, and phase directions and are specified in milliTesla per meter (mT/m). Slew rate is used to characterize how quickly a gradient can change over time and is given in mT/m per second (mT/m/s). Higher slew rates allow for faster imaging and are found on higher-end systems. Eddy currents are undesirable currents that are generated by the changing magnetic fields in conductors (gradients). The currents set up "wave-like" artifacts in the image and can cause localized heating in leads and tissue. There are several electronic methods in use to compensate for eddy currents; these are beyond the scope of this discussion.

Differential Diagnosis

- Physiologic bowing
- Focal fibrocartilaginous dysplasia of the proximal tibia (lesion usually slightly more distal)
- Physis trauma
- Osteochondroma
- Enchondroma

Variants

Femoral involvement is not a defining feature of Blount disease and the relative significance of coexisting femoral abnormalities is debated but worth considering. Coexistent focal widening of the distal medial femoral physis on MRI has been described. Distal femoral varus has been reported in some cases of late-onset tibia vara and may be important when planning surgical correction.

Clinical Issues

The severity of the changes is described by the Langenskiöld classification, which ranges from I to VI (Fig. 86.2). Higher stages denote greater abnormality. Prior to characteristic

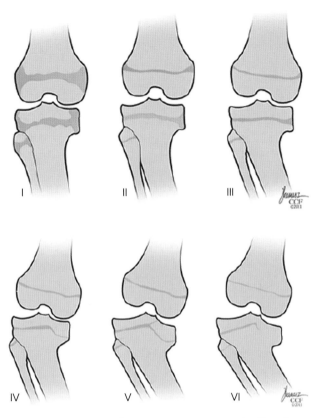

I   II   III

IV   V   VI

Figure 86.2. Langenskiöld classification system for Blount disease. The classifications are determined by the degree of medial ephiphyseal downsloping and medial epiphyseal overgrowth with higher grades showing greater degrees of genu vara deformity.

Treatment of the infantile form initially involves bracing during waking weight-bearing hours beginning at age 18 to 24 months, usually for 2 years. Realignment osteotomy is definitive treatment of both adolescent form and infantile form that fails conservative treatment. Surgery tends to be most effective before 5 years of age. Primary surgical repair after age 6 to 8 years often results in recurrence. Physeal bony bars complicate treatment.

Key Points

- There are two forms of Blount disease, infantile-onset and adolescent-onset.
- Radiographic features of both forms involve inferior depression, irregularity and beaking of the medial tibial metaphysis.
- Tibial metaphyseal-diaphyseal angle > 11 degrees is suggestive of Blount in a child with progressive tibia vara.
- Infantile Blount may be distinguished from physiologic bowing: physiologic bowing usually also involves the femur and progressively improves after 18 months, resolving by age 3 years.
- MRI can aid in differentiating physiologic bowing from Blount.

tibial changes, differentiation between physiologic bowing and infantile Blount disease may be impossible. Physiologic bowing usually also involves some bowing of the femurs and usually progressively improves after 18 months and resolves by age 3 years. Progressive genu vara is one of the most reliable features of infantile Blount. Levine and Drennan proposed a potential method for differentiating between normal bowing and infantile Blount disease. This method involves measuring the metaphyseal-diaphyseal angle, with normal physiologic bowing measuring ≤ 11 degrees and Blount disease > 11 degrees in most cases. MR may help differentiate physiologic bowing from infantile Blount disease with features listed under Imaging Findings.

Further Reading

Cheema JI, Grissom LE, Harcke HT. Radiographic characteristics of lower-extremity bowing in children. *Radiographics.* 2003:23:871–880.

Craig JG, van Holsbeeck M, et al. The utility of MR in assessing Blount disease. *Skeletal Radiol.* 2002(31):208–213.

Ecklund K, Jaramillo D. Patterns of premature physeal arrest: MR imaging of 111 children. *AJR Am J Roentgenol.* 2002;178(4):967–972.

Eggert P, Viemann M. Physiologic bowing or infantile Blount's disease. Some new aspects on an old problem. *Pediatr Radiol.* 1996;(26):349–352.

Feldman MD, Schoenecker PL. Use of the metaphyseal-diaphyseal angle in the evaluation of bowed legs. *J Bone Joint Surg Am.* 1993;75(11):1602–1609.

Gordon JE, King DJ, Luhmann SJ, Dobbs MB, Schoenecker PL. Femoral deformity in tibia vara. *J Bone Joint Surg Am.* 2006;88(2):380–386.

Neurological

CHAPTER 87

Dandy-Walker Malformation

Nadja Kadom, MD

Definition

Dandy-Walker malformation (DWM) was named in 1954 in honor of the neurosurgeons Walter E. Dandy and Arthur E. Walker who first described patients with this entity in 1914 and 1942, respectively. Dandy-Walker malformation is characterized on imaging by a combination of complete or partial agenesis of the vermis, large posterior fossa fluid collection communicating with the fourth ventricle, an enlarged posterior fossa, and elevation of the torcular herophili.

Clinical Features

The incidence of DWM is low, approximately 1 in 30,000 births. Although 40 percent of patients with DWM are intellectually normal, it may cause intellectual disabilities in 40 percent of patients and borderline disabilities in 20 percent. There is an association of approximately 70 percent between DWM and other central nervous system (CNS) malformations such as hydrocephalus (80 percent), agenesis or hypoplasia of the corpus callosum, interhemispheric cysts, abnormal gyration, heterotopias, occipital meningoceles, brainstem and dentate nucleus malformations, and hamartomas. Additional systemic abnormalities include cardiac, genitourinary, intestinal, facial, and limb malformations.

Anatomy and Physiology

It is generally accepted that DWM most likely results from abnormal development of the roof of the rhombencephalon. Specifically, in the membranous part of the rhombencephalon there is an intimate developmental relationship between neuroblastic proliferation forming the vermis, the cerebellar hemispheres (the vermis being formed prior to the cerebellum), the choroid plexus, Blake's pouch cyst, and the evolving CSF openings (foramen of Luschka and Magendie). Disturbance in development of one of these structures may cause subsequent abnormal development of a related structure, which may lead to DWM. Key features of DWM include partial or complete agenesis of the vermis and a large fluid-filled bony posterior fossa with occipital bone thinning and bulging. Both of these features contribute to large appearance of the fourth ventricle and

its communication with the posterior fossa fluid (Fig. 87.1). Other features are elevation of the transverse venous sinuses and the torcular herophili, sometimes above the level of junction of the lambdoid sutures (so-called "lambdoid-torcular inversion"), and cerebellar hypoplasia. When assessing the vermis and cerebellum, one must understand what establishes a diagnosis of agenesis versus hypoplasia or atrophy. In agenesis or partial agenesis the organ or parts of the organ are absent. In contrast, hypoplasia refers to underdevelopment and atrophy refers to deterioration of the organ.

Imaging Findings

CT and MRI:

- Axial MRI: vermian agenesis when no vermis at all seen throughout the posterior fossa
- Various degrees rotation of partial vermis (Fig. 87.2)
- Partial vermian agenesis similar to prominent mega cisterna magna (Fig. 87.3) and posterior fossa arachnoid cyst
- Sagittal MRI: elevation of transverse venous sinuses and torcular herophili
- "Lambdoid-torcular inversion": lambdoid suture lies below the level of the torcular herophili
- +/– Hydrocephalus resulting from aqueductal stenosis
- +/– Callosal dysgenesis

> **IMAGING PITFALLS:** A small vermis can be seen in many disorders. Use multiplanar imaging before making a diagnosis of DWM or variant.

Common Variants

Currently, DWM, Dandy-Walker variant (DWV), and mega cisterna magna (MCM) are considered a "complex" or "continuum" of DW. Some authors also include Blake's pouch cyst in this spectrum. Dandy-Walker variant lacks enlargement of the bony posterior fossa (but has abnormalities of vermis/cerebellum) and MCM lacks abnormalities of vermis and cerebellum (but can have an enlarged posterior fossa). Blakes pouch cyst is similar to MCM but with displacement of the choroid plexus posteriorly underneath the vermis.

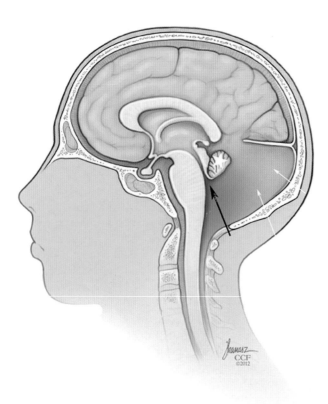

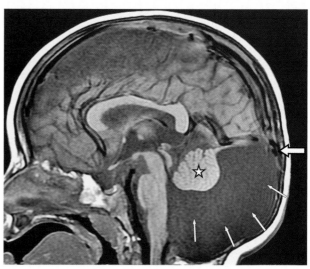

Figure 87.2. Sagittal midline T1 MR image of the brain in a child with DWM shows hypoplastic and abnormally rotated vermis (star), large fourth ventricle that communicates with the posterior fossa fluid (thin arrows), elevation of the torcular herophili (thick arrow), and an overall enlarged bony posterior fossa with calvarial thinning.

Figure 87.1. Dandy-Walker spectrum. The triad includes enlarged posterior fossa with elevation of the straight sinus and torcular herophili (white arrows), small uplifted or absent vermis (star) and communication of the fourth ventricle with CSF-filled posterior fossa (black arrow).

Imaging Strategy

MRI is the best imaging modality for evaluation of DWM. Recommended sequences include sagittal T1, axial T2, axial FLAIR, coronal T2 or FLAIR, and contrast enhancement if Blake's pouch cyst is a diagnostic consideration. Patients with DWM and hydrocephalus may undergo multiple CT scans and radiographs over a lifetime for evaluation of shunt function. In these cases, a low-mA CT technique is recommended for routine follow-up imaging.

Related Physics

The digital repository for the storage of image information is k-space. If we use the analogy of an "orchestra," each point in k-space represents every signal of the same spatial frequency in the image; all instruments in each of the string sections represent *all* points in the image of the same "pitch." This information is organized according to magnitude such that the signals representing larger objects (low spatial frequency) are stored nearest the center and those representing the smallest objects and sharpness of edges (high spatial frequency) are placed on the periphery. The signal placed in k-space is also oriented orthogonal to its location; signals oriented along the x-axis in k-space correspond to objects along the y-axis in the image and

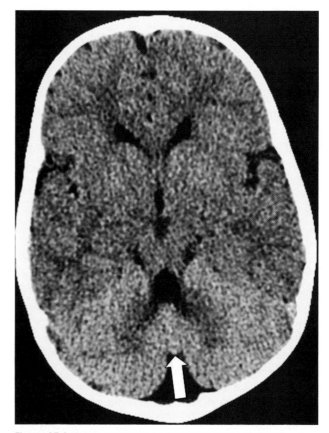

Figure 87.3. Axial unenhanced CT image of the vermis in suspected DWM shows a small vermis (arrow) suggesting hypoplasia, however subsequent MR imaging showed a normal vermis with a prominent posterior fluid space resulting from an arachnoid cyst.

vice versa. As an example, when imaging the head, the silhouette is the largest recognizable symbol in the image and therefore its signal in k-space would be near the center. The sulci and gyri (intermediate-sized structures) would be located at intermediate distance between center and periphery of k-space. Finally, fine nuances in structure as well as noise would be located at the periphery and corners; this portion contains very little diagnostic information especially given the inferior spatial resolution of MRI to CT. The importance of this is that k-space need not be filled in its entirety in order to obtain diagnostic images. The order of k-space filling can be manipulated to minimize the effects of patient motion, minimize reconstruction time, and limit distracting noise in the image.

Differential Diagnosis

- Dandy-Walker variant (DWV)
- Other posterior fossa cysts/prominent fluid spaces (mega cisterna magna, arachnoid cyst, Blake's pouch cysts) (Fig. 87.4)
- Small cerebellum (various cerebellar hypoplasias, cerebellar atrophies—hereditary and acquired) (Fig. 87.5)

Clinical Issues

The majority of patients with DWM have hydrocephalus (approximately 80 percent). The severity of clinical deficits that are related to hydrocephalus depend on the time of diagnosis and success of shunt placement. Therefore, patients would greatly benefit from early diagnosis and genetic counseling, preferably prenatally. Studies have

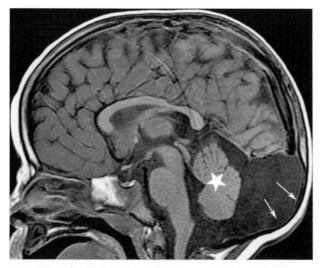

Figure 87.4. Sagittal midline T1 MR image of the brain in a patient with arachnoid cyst or mega cisterna magna (MCM) shows enlarged posterior fossa with bone thinning (arrow), and some elevation of the torcular herophili, however the vermis (star) is completely normal, allowing the radiologist to rule out DWM or DWV with confidence.

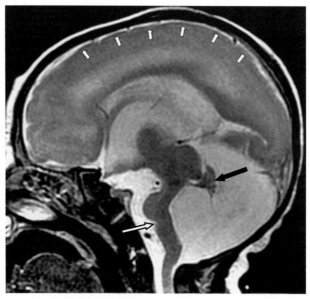

Figure 87.5. Sagittal midline T2 MR image of the brain in a patient with Walker-Warburg syndrome (WWS), a congenital muscular dystrophy, shows some features that overlap with DWM, such as cerebellar hypoplasia (black arrow) and large posterior fossa with elevation of the torcular herophili. However, there are additional abnormalities in WWS, including abnormal white matter, lissencephaly (short white arrows), pontine clefts, (large white arrow) and brainstem deformity.

shown that fetal MRI and ultrasound (US) are both valuable in identifying the "classic" DWM, but fetal US is inferior to fetal MRI when some of the classic signs are absent and differentiation of DWV from MCM or other cerebellar abnormalities is necessary. In general, a diagnosis of DWM should be made with caution, as it implies additional genetic defects and an approximately 60 percent chance of abnormal mental development. With partial absence of the vermis, one must assess multiple planes in order to confidently diagnose DWM.

Key Points

- Rare
- Posterior fossa disorder with "classic features" including complete or partial agenesis of the vermis, enlarged posterior fossa, enlarged fourth ventricle that communicates with posterior fossa fluid and elevation of the torcular herophili
- Spectrum: DWM, DWV, MCM, Blake's pouch cyst
- Differentiate from other entities with vermis hypoplasia or atrophy
- Fetal MRI superior to US for diagnosis
- Early diagnosis, genetic counseling, intervention important

Further Reading

Congenital malformations of the brain and skull. In: Barkovich AJ, ed. *Pediatric Neuroimaging*. Fifth Edition. Philadelphia, PA: Lippincott, Williams and Wilkins; 2012:477–480.

Klein O, Pierre-Kahn A, Boddaert N, Parisot D, Brunelle F. Dandy-Walker malformation: prenatal diagnosis and prognosis. *Childs Nerv Syst*. 2003;*19*(7–8):484–489. Epub 2003 Jul 16.

Kollias SS, Ball WS Jr, Prenger EC. Cystic malformations of the posterior fossa: differential diagnosis clarified through embry-ologic analysis. *Radiographics*. 1993;*13*(6):1211–1231. Review. PubMed PMID: 8031352.

Patel S, Barkovich AJ. Analysis and classification of cerebellar malformations. *AJNR Am J Neuroradiol*. 2002;*23*(7):1074–1087.

Ten Donkelaar HJ, Lammens M. Development of the human cerebellum and its disorders. *Clin Perinatol*. 2009;*36*(3):513–530. Review.

Wg Cdr A Alam, Gp Capt BN Chander, Sqn Ldr M Bhatia. Dandy-Walker variant: prenatal diagnosis by ultrasonography. *MJAFI*. 2004;*60*(3).

CHAPTER 88

Chiari Malformations

Korgün Koral, MD

Definitions

Chiari I malformation refers to descent of pointed cerebellar tonsils below the level of foramen magnum (opisthion-basion line) greater than 6 millimeters in the first decade and greater than 5 millimeters in the second decade with or without syrinx (syringohydromyelia). Chiari II malformation refers to lumbar myelomeningocele associated with a small posterior fossa and multiple brain abnormalities.

Clinical Features

Patients with Chiari I malformation generally present with headaches, characteristically in the occipital region. When a syrinx is present, signs and symptoms related to myelopathy may be present. Patients with Chiari II malformation have the skin defect repaired at the site of the lumbar myelomeningocele in the first days of life. Approximately 80 percent of these patients subsequently develop obstructive hydrocephalus.

Anatomy and Physiology

In Chiari I malformation (Fig. 88.1), the cerebellar tonsils lie below the level of the foramen magnum, altering the cerebrospinal fluid flow dynamics in the region of the cervicomedullary junction. Continued abnormal increased movement of the neural tissues against the walls of the posterior fossa and foramen magnum result in cerebellar tonsillar gliosis and syrinx formation, generally in the cervical spinal cord. Chiari II malformation (Fig. 88.2) is hypothesized to result from incorrect expression of the cell adhesion molecule resulting in failure of closure of the posterior neuropore of the developing neural tube. In Chiari II malformation, the distal spinal cord terminates as a neural placode at the level of the lumbar myelomeningocele, which results in tethering. The posterior fossa is small, forcing the cerebellar vermis—and not the tonsils (chracteristic of Chiari I)—to herniate into the dorsal cervical spinal canal. The cerebral aqueduct is generally compromised, resulting in obstructive hydrocephalus.

Imaging Findings

The presence of Chiari I may be suspected from CT, but definitive diagnosis is made on brain MR. The diagnosis is made if the tips of the cerebellar tonsils extend 6 millimeters or more

below the level of the foramen magnum. On MR imaging, sagittal midline images show a shortened clivus and retroflexed odontoid process (Fig. 88.3). The cerebrospinal fluid spaces around the cervicomedullary junction are effaced and the cerebellar tonsils "wrap" around the cervicomedullary junction. The posterior fossa is small. The fourth ventricle is either normal or near normal in shape. Associated developmental abnormalities of the cervical spine such as assimilation of C1 to the clivus and Klippel-Feil syndrome are common. A syrinx is present in 20 to 65 percent of patients with Chiari I malformation. The sine qua non of the Chiari II malformation is a lumbar myelomeningocele (Fig. 88.4). Other imaging findings that may be found in patients with Chiari II include:

- Inferior cerebellar vermis herniation into the cervical spinal canal
- Small, compressed fourth ventricle (if "normal," suspect entrapment)

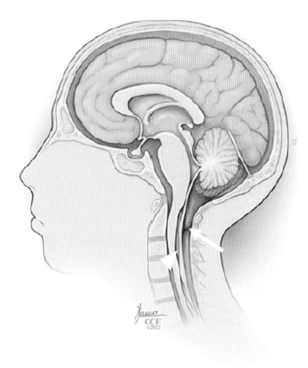

Figure 88.1. Chiari I: inferior descent of pointed cerebellar tonsils below the foramen magnum (arrow) and cervical cord syrinx (arrowhead).

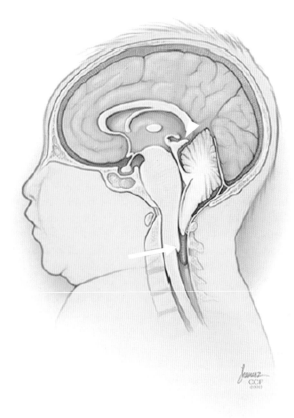

Figure 88.2. Chiari II: Small posterior fossa and cerebellar herniation superiorly and inferiorly, medullary kinking (arrow), and tectal beaking (arrowhead). There is often scalloping of the clivus and large massa intermedia with callosal dysgenesis.

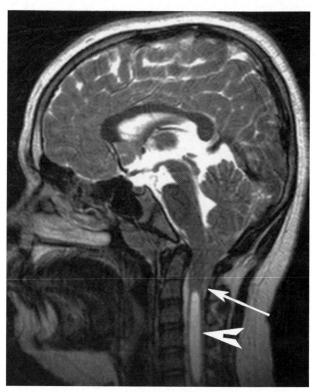

Figure 88.3. Sagittal T2 MR image of a 9-year-old female with Chiari I malformation shows pointed cerebellar tonsils (arrow) and the tips of the cerebellar tonsils lie more than 2 centimeters below the level of foramen magnum. An expansile cervical spinal cord syrinx is present (arrowhead).

- Scalloping of petrous apices and dorsal clivus
- Tectal beaking (Fig 88.5)
- Cervicomedullary kink (caused by compression by the dentate ligament on the inferiorly displaced spinal cord)
- Cerebellar "towering" through the heart-shaped, widened tentorial incisura
- Thickened massa intermedia
- Hypogenesis of corpus callosum (generally of the splenium and rostrum)
- Interdigitation of medial gyri (resulting from a fenestrated falx cerebri)
- Heterotopic gray matter (Fig 88.6)
- Lacunar skull/stenogyria
- Obstructive hydrocephalus
- Syringomyelia is much less common than in Chiari I, but may be present in Chiari II

Imaging Strategy

In Chiari I malformation, sagittal T1- and T2-weighted and axial FLAIR (or T1-weighted) images of the brain are generally sufficient. A phase-contrast cerebrospinal fluid flow study allows for dynamic evaluation of the cerebrospinal fluid pathway. The study is generally performed at the midline sagittal plane using a velocity encoding gradient of 5 to 10 centimeters per second. Spine imaging is performed using sagittal T2-weighted (or STIR), T1-weighted, and axial T2-weighted images of the spinal cord. Axial T1-weighted images of the lumbosacral spine may be obtained to exclude low-lying cord or thickening of filum terminale.

In Chiari II malformation, imaging is performed to assess concomitant abnormalities of the supratentorial brain and for assessment of hydrocephalus. It is important to use head CT sparingly for evaluation of the ventricular size, as patients with shunted hydrocephalus undergo neuroimaging for ventricular size surveillance throughout their entire life. Rapid brain MR (HASTE, TS FFE) allows for evaluation of the ventricular size in less than 30 seconds without exposing the patient to ionizing radiation. If a patient with Chiari II malformation has epilepsy, an epilepsy imaging protocol is employed to identify subtle cortical dysplasia or gray matter heterotopia. Spine imaging is performed when a syrinx is suspected or for assessment of complication of detethering surgery (i.e., development of an epidermoid at the site of attempted release).

Related Physics

K-space is the digital "orchestra" for the storage of image information where each point in k-space represents every

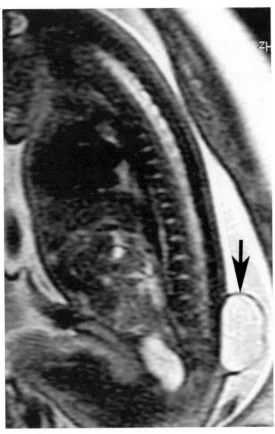

Figure 88.4. Sagittal ultrafast fluid-sensitive MR image in a term fetus with Chiari II malformation shows a membrane-covered lumbar myelomeningocele (arrow).

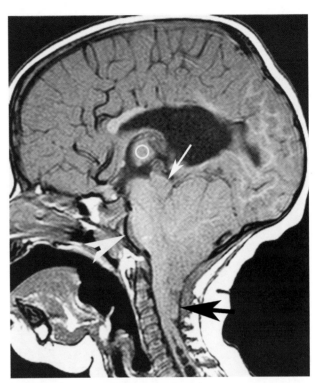

Figure 88.5. Sagittal T1 image in a 23-month-old female shows the classic changes of Chiari II malformation including small posterior fosssa, inferior herniation of cerebellum (black arrow), tectal beaking (white arrow), prominent massa intermedia (circle), scalloping of basiocciput (arrowhead), and hypogenetic corpus callosum. There is an expansile cervical syrinx.

signal of the same spatial frequency in the image; each "instrument" represents *all* points in the image of the same "pitch." High-spatial-frequency information is stored at the periphery and low-frequency information near the center of k-space; it is the low- and mid-frequency information that is most valuable in MRI, especially given its lower spatial resolution than CT. The original MR signal from each volume is a complex waveform, which contains multiple frequencies. This is akin to music from the entire string section from the orchestra. Once the signal is acquired, it undergoes a process known as Fourier transformation, which deconstructs the signal into component parts based on its frequency; this is akin to separating into each type of instrument in the string section (bass, cello, viola, violin, etc.). The information from Fourier transformation is then sent to fill k-space akin to filling the chairs in the orchestra.

Differential Diagnosis

■ Chiari I malformation may be "acquired" in certain syndromes (e.g., Crouzon, Pfeiffer), which are characterized by premature closure of the sutures resulting in a small skull base and posterior fossa.

■ In severe chronically shunted hydrocephalus, the cerebellum may herniate cranially through the tentorial incisura because of the collapsed brain; but there is no myelomeningocele.

Common Variants

Chiari III malformation is very rare. It consists of intracranial stigmata of Chiari II malformation in addition to an occipital and upper cervical encephalocele where there is herniation of the cerebellum, brain stem, and cervical spinal cord (Fig. 88.7). Isolated vermis hypoplasia (Fig. 88.8) is unrelated to the Chiari malformations and may be syndromic.

Clinical Issues

In Chiari I malformation, surgical decompression is achieved by suboccipital craniectomy with or without resection of posterior arch of C1. Depending on the degree of tonsillar herniation, the cerebellar tonsils may have to be resected. Tonsillar resection requires opening of the dura, which in turn increases the risk of infection and pseudomeningocele formation. The size of the concomitant syrinx usually diminishes following suboccipital craniectomy. If the syrinx persists and the patient remains symptomatic,

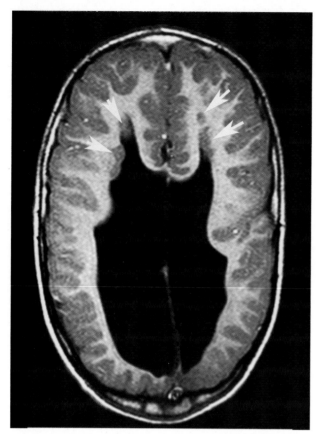

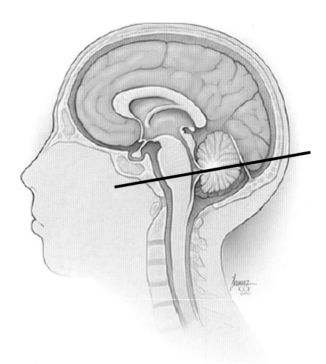

Figure 88.8. **Vermian hypoplasia:** Defined as less than 50 percent of the vermis lying below the horizontal line drawn through the widest point of the fourth ventricle, the fastigial point (line).

Figure 88.6. Axial T1 image in a 7-year-old child with Chiari II malformation shows subependymal gray matter heterotopia (arrows) along the frontolateral ventricle walls.

a stent may be placed connecting the syrinx cavity to the subarachnoid space.

The incidence of Chiari II malformation has decreased more than 50 percent following widespread use of maternal folic acid supplementation. Prenatal surgery for myelomeningocele repair has decreased the need for shunting and improved motor outcomes at 30-month follow-up. The degree of disability in Chiari II malformation is related to the level of the open neural tube defect. Patients with defects higher than L2 are generally nonambulatory. Urinary and gastrointestinal dysfunction is common.

Key Points

- Chiari I is much more common than Chiari II.
- The cerebellar tonsils herniate in Chiari I; the cerebellar vermis herniates in Chiari II.
- Coexisting brain abnormalities are common in Chiari II.
- Syrinx is more common in Chiari I than Chiari II.
- Lumbar myelomeningocele is sine qua non of Chiari II.
- Prenatal myelomeningocele repair is beneficial in Chiari II.

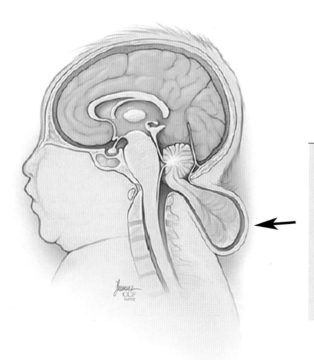

Figure 88.7. Chiari III: Findings of Chiari II plus an occipital cephalocele (arrow).

Further Reading

Adzick NS, Thom EA, Spong CY, Brock JW, Burrows PK, Johnson MP, et al. A randomized trial of prenatal versus postnatal repair of myelomeningocele. *N Engl J Med.* 2011, Feb 9.

Congenital malformations of the brain and skull. In: Barkovich AJ, ed. *Pediatric Neuroimaging.* Fifth edition. Philadelphia, PA: Lippincott, Williams and Wilkins; 2012:491–501.

Naidich TP, Blaser SI, Delman BN, McLone DG, Dias MS, Zimmerman RA, et al. In: Atlas, SW, ed. *Magnetic Resonance Imaging of Brain and Spine.* Fourth edition. Philadelphia, PA: Lippincott, Williams and Wilkins; 2009:1364–1447.

Disorders of neural tube closure. In: Osborne AG, ed. *Diagnostic Neuroradiology.* St. Louis, MO: Mosby-Year Book, Inc; 1994:15–23.

CHAPTER 89

Encephaloceles

Julie H. Harreld, MD

Definition

An encephalocele is the herniation of neural tissue through an osseous defect of the skull. Encephaloceles may be considered as *anterior* (in front of the coronal suture or involving the orbit or nasal cavity) or involving the *convexity*.

Clinical Features:

Overall incidence ranges from 1:300 to 1:10,000 live births. Occipital (convexity) encephaloceles comprise approximately 75 percent of encephaloceles in Western nations and are more common in females and multiple gestations, whereas frontoethmoid (anterior) encephaloceles are more common in Asia and have no gender predominance. Occipital or other convexity encephaloceles are generally diagnosed prenatally. Overall mortality is approximately 33.3 percent. Microcephaly, hydrocephalus, large size (>50mm), and presence of significant neural tissue within the encephalocele carry a poor prognosis. Clinical features include developmental delay and features of hydrocephalus. Associated congenital anomalies that are poor prognostic indicators include agenesis of the corpus callosum, cerebellar dysgenesis, and cortical dysplasia. Parietal encephaloceles have a higher incidence of associated anomalies and a poorer prognosis. Although "form fruste" *atretic* occipital or parietal cephaloceles may escape prenatal diagnosis, they may be associated with other brain abnormalities, ranging from anomalous draining veins to Walker-Warburg (cerebro-oculomuscular) syndrome.

Whereas encephaloceles may be occult, they may present with CSF leak or recurrent meningitis. Sincipital (frontoethmoidal, nasoethmoidal or nasoorbital) encephaloceles may be diagnosed earlier because of dysmorphia (midline facial swelling, hypertelorism, or proptosis), or may present later in life with persistent nasal obstruction or CSF rhinorrhea. Lateral transsphenoidal encephaloceles may occur as a result of sphenoid dysplasia in neurofibromatosis. Median/midline transsphenoidal encephaloceles may be associated with pituitary/hypothalamic abnormalities, midline facial and brain anomalies, optic disc anomalies ("Morning Glory" anomaly or coloboma), and/or Moyamoya syndrome.

Anatomy and Physiology

Unlike open neural tube defects, encephaloceles most likely arise from a postclosure defect in the overlying neural-crest derived mesenchyme forming the skull. Defects in any of the numerous enchondral ossification centers of the skull base may also occur, with subsequent herniation of intracranial contents. Ingestion of folic acid has been proven to decrease the occurrence of this defect.

Imaging Findings

Occipital/occipitocervical and other convexity lesions:

- Herniation of CSF and brain tissue through skull defect (Fig 89.1) (Fig 89.2)
- Hydrocephalus (60 percent)
- Associated CNS abnormalities including agenesis of the corpus callosum, cerebellar dysgenesis, cortical dysplasia, or microcephaly
- MR venography: herniation of dural sinuses

Anterior (Sincipital/Basal) lesions:

- Herniation of CSF and brain tissue through anterior skull defect into the sinuses, nasopharynx, or other anterior skull base defect (Fig 89.3) (Fig 89.4),
- Midline craniofacial and brain abnormalities
- Ocular/orbital anomalies
- Pituitary gland, hypothalamus, anterior cerebral arteries may be contained in transsphenoidal encephaloceles
- Basal encephaloceles associated with Moyamoya syndrome

IMAGING PITFALLS:
- Incomplete ossification of the skull base is normal in infants, and anterior encephalocele should not be assumed (MRI should be performed if there is suspicion for encephalocele).
- Vascular imaging is key to surgical planning.
- Associated CNS anomalies are negative prognostic indicators and should be carefully ruled out.

Imaging Strategy

Neuroimaging is performed for prognosis and surgical planning. To best delineate the neural tissue component,

(A)

(B)

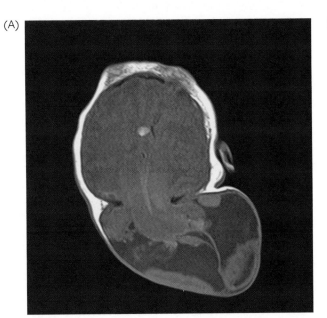

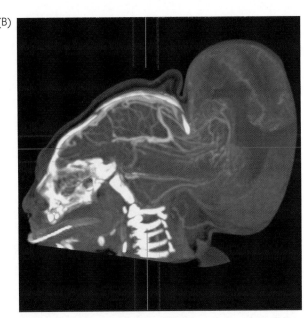

Figure 89.1. Axial T1 MR image (A) and sagittal reconstruction of CT venogram (B) in a baby with occipital encephalocele show microcephaly, herniation of vascular structures and large size, which carry a poor prognosis. An encephalocele that is larger than the head size is termed a "giant encephalocele"; other CNS anomalies are often present.

MRI should be performed in multiple planes in all patients. For surgical planning, CT imaging with multiplanar and 3-D reconstructions can help define the osseous defect. MR venography (MRV) should be performed to evaluate the venous sinuses, as their presence in the defect complicates surgery. MR angiography (MRA) should also be performed if the occipital enchephalocele is large. For basal encephaloceles, MRA should also be performed, as these have been associated with Moyamoya, increasing the risk of operative complications.

Related Physics

Using an "orchestra" analogy, the signal acquired from the image is initially complex akin to the orchestra members sitting randomly in the music hall tuning up. Fourier

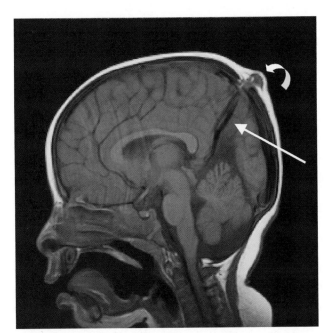

Figure 89.2. Sagittal T1 MR image in a child with atretic parietal encephalocele (curved arrow) shows the persistent falcine sinus (straight arrow), a frequent accompanying vascular anomaly. (Image courtesy of Dr. Zoltan Patay, St. Jude Children's Research Hospital, Memphis, TN)

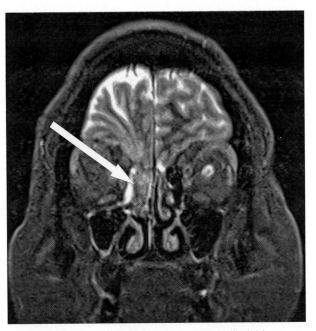

Figure 89.3. Coronal STIR MR image in a child with right nasoethmoidal (sincipital) encephalocele demonstrates CSF and brain tissue within the encephalocele (arrow).

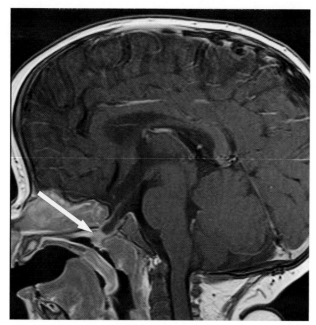

Figure 89.4. Sagittal midline contrast-enhanced T1 image in a child with transsphenoidal encephalocele shows ectopic enhancing pituitary tissue (arrow). Endocrine, ocular, and/or vascular anomalies may be present.

transformation organizes the "sounds" by pitch (frequency); the lowest frequencies (basses) are identified and placed on the right side of the stage entering from stage left—center of k-space—followed by low-mid frequencies (cellos), high-mid (violas) and finally high frequencies (violin). Image efficiency is optimized by filling the center of k-space first and this can be done in a variety of ways. The corollary to this is that the least efficient method of k-space filling would be in raster fashion—having *individual* section members enter the stage in order of frequency (violin, viola, cello, bass) rather than by *section* based on stage location forcing the basses to move through seated violins, etc.

Differential Diagnosis

- Gliocele—protrusion of a glial-lined cyst through an osseous defect
- Meningocele—protrusion of meninges and CSF only
- Pseudomeningocele—postoperative collection not bordered by dura
- Spontaneous temporal lobe encephalocele—may present with middle ear effusions/infections or progressive hearing loss, or with medically refractory temporal lobe epilepsy

Variants

Chiari III malformation is a rare herniation of posterior fossa contents through a low occipital or high cervical

defect, in combination with the brain findings of Chiari II. Hydrocephalus, hydromyelia, and tethered cord are usually present. Occipital encephalocele is a feature of Meckel-Gruber syndrome and has been associated with Dandy-Walker malformation.

Clinical Issues

A greater amount of neural tissue within the sac and the presence of associated CNS or non-CNS abnormalities are associated with a poorer prognosis. Nonfunctional neural tissue is generally excised and the dura closed in watertight fashion; cranioplasty is not generally performed. Postoperative complications include hydrocephalus and infection.

Key Points

- Occipital encephaloceles are the most common in the Western population and are more common in females and multiple gestations.
- Nasoethmoidal encephaloceles are most common in the southeast Asian population, with no gender predominance.
- Size of sac, neural component, and accompanying CNS abnormalities such as microcephaly or hydrocephalus are prognostic.
- Basal encephaloceles may be occult and present with repeated subclinical meningitis, nasal obstruction, and/or CSF rhinorrhea.
- Vascular evaluation with MRA/MRV provides essential preoperative information.

Further Reading

Baradaran N, Nejat F, El Khashab M. Cephalocele: report of 55 cases over 8 years. *Pediatr Neurosurg.* 2009;*45*(6):461–466.

Kiymaz N, Yilmaz N, Demir I, Keskin S. Prognostic factors in patients with occipital encephalocele. *Pediatr Neurosurg.* 2010;*46*(1):6–11.

Mahapatra AK, Suri A. Anterior encephaloceles: a study of 92 cases. *Pediatr Neurosurg.* 2002;*36*(3):113–118.

Martinez-Lage JF, Poza M, Sola J, et al. The child with a cephalocele: etiology, neuroimaging, and outcome. *Childs Nerv Syst.* 1996;*12*(9):540–550.

Naidich TP, Altman NR, Braffman BH, McLone DG, Zimmerman RA. Cephaloceles and related malformations. *AJNR Am J Neuroradiol.* 1992;*13*(2):655–690.

Padmanabhan R. Etiology, pathogenesis and prevention of neural tube defects. *Congenit Anom (Kyoto).* 2006;*46*(2):55–67.

Teng E, Heller J, Lazareff J, et al. Caution in treating transsphenoidal encephalocele with concomitant moyamoya disease. *J Craniofac Surg.* 2006;*17*(5):1004–1009.

Wind JJ, Caputy AJ, Roberti F. Spontaneous encephaloceles of the temporal lobe. *Neurosurg Focus.* 2008;*25*(6):E11.

CHAPTER 90

Holoprosencephaly

Gisele Ishak, MD

Definition

Holoprosencephaly (HPE) is a spectrum of congenital structural forebrain anomalies, defined by lack of formation of midline structures and variable degree of interhemispheric cerebral fusion. It is divided into alobar (the most severe), semilobar (intermediate) and lobar (the least severe) forms.

Clinical Features

With an incidence of 1 per 10,000 live births, HPE is uncommon. Clinical severity relates to degree of hemispheric and deep gray nuclei fusion. Patients may have seizures, dystonia, hypotonia, mental retardation, pituitary/hypothalamic dysfunction (present in 70 percent of alobar HPE resulting from hypothalamic nonseparation). The severity of symptoms correlates with basal ganglia fusion. Craniofacial malformations are often associated with HPE and correlate with the severity of brain malformations. These include cyclopia, proboscis, midline facial clefting, single central incisor, and metopic suture synostosis.

Anatomy and Physiology

Maternal diabetes is a well-established teratogen in HPE. In some there is an inherited or de novo chromosome abnormality, disrupting the dorsoventral patterning of the rostral neural tube during early embryogenesis. This results from impaired cleavage of the prosencephalon with a gradient seen in which the separation of the hemispheres and development of the falx cerebri progress from the occipital pole to the frontal pole of the cerebrum.

Imaging Findings

Absence of the septum pellucidum is seen in all types of HPE. Olfactory nerves may be absent and myelination may be delayed, predominantly in more severe cases of fusion. Absent or azygous anterior cerebral artery may also occur.

Alobar HPE

- No falx cerebri or corpus callosum.
- Cerebrum is a pancake-like mass anteriorly.
- Monoventricle is continuous with a dorsal cyst (Fig. 90.1)
- Basal ganglia, hypothalami, and thalmi are fused.

Semilobar and lobar HPE

- Falx cerebri is variably absent, predominantly present posteriorly (Fig 90.2).
- Anterior corpus callosum is absent at the site of cerebral fusion.
- Basal ganglia, thalami, hypothalami may be partly fused (Fig 90.3).
- May be challenging to distinguish lobar from semilobar HPE, however, if the posterior half of the body of the corpus callosum (in addition to the splenium) is formed, it can be classified as lobar HPE.

Imaging Strategy

The diagnosis of the more severe forms of HPE (alobar and semilobar) is often suspected on prenatal ultrasound, and fetal MRI can better classify the anomaly and associated findings. Postnatal CT scan or (preferably) MRI confirms the diagnosis, the anatomic subtype, and associated central nervous system anomalies. MR sequences should include sagittal T1, axial T1 or inversion recovery, axial FLAIR, axial T2, coronal T2 (best to look for olfactory nerves), and axial diffusion.

Related Physics

There is no one-size-fits-all approach to k-space filling but instead one should base this decision on each indication and sequence. The choice of method involves a balance between speed of imaging and content of the image. Infant brain imaging is able to record and display fine detail (high spatial-frequency) necessary to make eloquent diagnoses. It is important, therefore, to use techniques that more completely fill k-space, which is done at the expense of temporal efficiency. Techniques that optimize spatial resolution in infant brain MR include spin echo with sequential k-space filling or fast spin echo with fast or turbo filling of k-space. Diffusion weighted imaging can use echo planar k-space filling as the signal generated by the restricted motion of water molecules is more important than spatial resolution. The goal with fetal brain imaging, on the other hand, is to detect structural deformities that are not necessarily in the high-spatial-frequency domain. Images of sufficient quality can be generated using single-shot fast spin echo

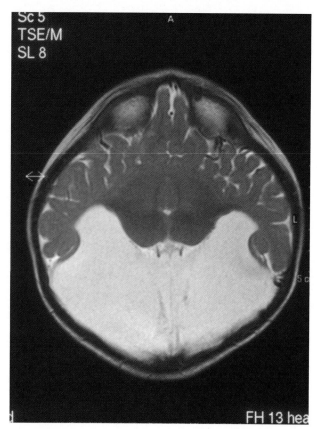

Figure 90.1. Axial T2 MR image in a newborn with seizures shows a monoventricle and a pancake-like cerebral tissue anteriorly, fusion of the deep gray matter nuclei, and absence of the third ventricle. No interhemispheric fissure or falx seen and the corpus callosum (not shown) is absent. Findings are consistent with alobar holoprosencephaly.

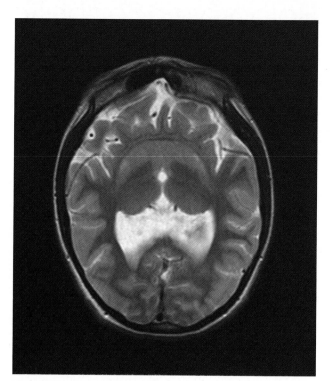

Figure 90.2. Axial T2 MR image in an adolescent with developmental delay shows presence of the posterior falx with anterior fusion involving the frontal lobes and basal ganglia. Frontal horns and septum pellucidum are absent, thalami are separate, and the third ventricle is present. Findings are consistent with semilobar holoprosencephaly.

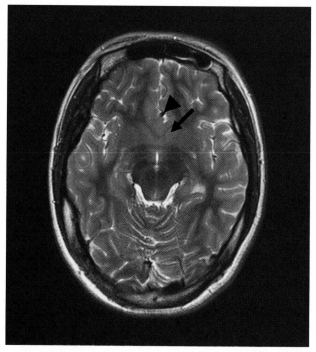

Figure 90.3. Axial T2 MR image in an adolescent with developmental delay shows a focal region of interhemispheric inferior frontal lobe fusion adjacent to the anterior commissure (arrow). There is an azygous anterior cerebral artery (arrowhead). The most anterior aspect of the corpus callosum (not shown) is absent at the site of the fusion. Findings are consistent with lobar holoprosencephaly.

with half Fourier transformation. This technique ignores high-frequency in favor of mid- and low-frequency information to create diagnostic images.

Differential Diagnosis

- Agenesis of the corpus callosum with interhemispheric cyst (much better prognosis than HPE)
- Hydranencephaly: the falx is present and the residual cerebral tissue is seen along the tentorium and the thalami and basal ganglia may be spared

Common Variants

Middle interhemispheric variant of holoprosencephaly (MIV), or syntelencephaly (Fig. 90.4), is the main variant characterized by interhemispheric fusion of the posterior frontal and parietal lobes. This is associated with callosal dysgenesis at the level of the interhemispheric fusion. The anterior frontal, occipital lobes and basal ganglia are separated. Thalami may be fused in 33 percent. Myelination is typically normal and patients are less affected clinically. Another variant is the solitary medial maxillary central

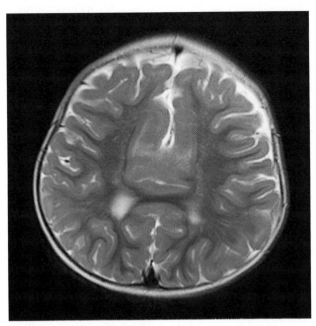

Figure 90.4. Axial T2 MR image in a child with seizures shows fusion of the posterior frontal and parietal lobes, presence of anterior and posterior interhemispheric fissures, and absence of the septum pellucidum (not shown). This is consistent with middle interhemispheric variant of HPE.

incisor, one of several microforms of autosomal dominant holoprosencephaly. Septooptic dysplasia is considered a mild holoprosencephaly variant.

Clinical Issues

Severely affected children typically do not survive beyond early infancy, although a significant number of more mildly affected children survive past 12 months. Management includes hormone replacement therapy for pituitary dysfunction, antiepileptic drugs for seizures, and ventriculoperitoneal shunt placement for hydrocephalus, which necessitates follow-up imaging with CT or MRI. Genetic counseling and risk assessment depend on determination of the specific cause of HPE in each individual.

Key Points

- HPE is a congenital malformation with abnormal development of midline structures.
- Maternal diabetes is a known teratogen.
- In some cases, there is an inherited or de novo chromosome abnormality, disrupting the dorsoventral patterning of the rostral neural tube during early embryogenesis.
- HPE is a spectrum of disorders (alobar, semilobar and lobar) respecting a gradient of development in which separation of the cerebral hemispheres progresses form posterior to anterior.
- Craniofacial malformations follow the severity of the intracranial malformation and include cyclopia, proboscis, midline facial clefting, single central incisor and metopic suture synostosis.
- Middle interhemispheric variant is a distinct clinical and radiologic type.

Further Reading

Congenital malformations of the brain and skull. In: Barkovich AJ, ed. *Pediatric Neuroimaging*. Fifth edition. Philadelphia, PA: Lippincott, Williams and Wilkins; 2012:446–454.

Hahn JS, Barnes PD. Neuroimaging advances in holoprosencephaly: refining the spectrum of the midline malformation. *Am J Med Genet C Semin Med Genet*. 2010;154C(1):120–132.

Levey EB, Stashinko E, Clegg NJ, Delgado MR. Management of children with holoprosencephaly. *Am J Med Genet C Semin Med Genet*. 2010;154C(1):183–190.

CHAPTER 91

Hemimegalencephaly

Janet R. Reid, MD, FRCPC

Definition

Hemimegalencephaly (HME) is a rare sporadic congenital condition characterized by overgrowth of one hemisphere of the brain secondary to malformation of cortical development; it is also known as unilateral megencephaly or macrencephaly.

Clinical Features

The incidence is unknown but there is a male predominance. The head is large and asymmetric. Patients have seizures that are difficult to control associated with significant developmental delay and mental retardation. Hemiparesis and severe developmental delay are invariably present. Functional or anatomic hemispherectomy may be the treatment of choice for intractable seizures. There are no defining laboratory tests.

Anatomy and Physiology

Hemimegalencephaly is caused by an early (first-trimester) disruption of the pathway of neuron development and organization in the brain. Abnormalities along entire pathway from germinal matrix proliferation, migration along the radial glial fibers, and cortical organization result in overgrowth and disorganization of the hemisphere with polymicrogyria, pachygyria, and subependymal heterotopia. This implies lack of normal neural regulation although specific biochemical causes have not been found (Fig. 91.1).

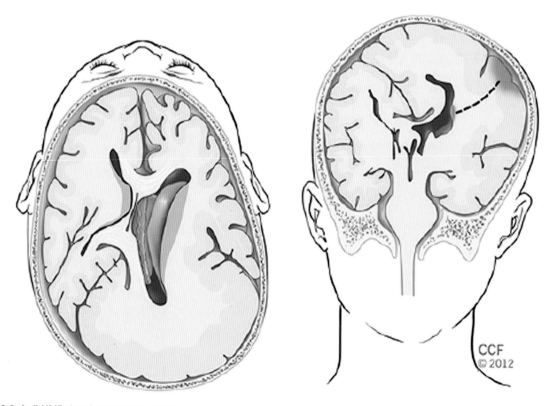

Figure 91.1. Left HME showing possible points of disordered embryologic development. Disorders may occur at any or all points along the pathway including germinal matrix proliferation (small red disk), migration along the radial glial fibers (dotted line), and cortical organization (red patch in periphery).

Imaging Findings

Hemimegalencephaly may be suspected on prenatal US with large head circumference and biparietal diameter with asymmetry. The involved hemisphere may be diffusely increased in echogenicity. Postnatal US will show the same. In addition, dystrophic calcification may be found in the dysplastic brain tissue. Because of its superior contrast resolution, MR provides the most detail and will show:

- Enlarged hemisphere
- Ipsilateral enlargement of the lateral ventricle (Fig. 91.2)
- Overgrowth of the occipital lobe with infolding (Fig. 91.3)
- Accelerated or undermyelination (Fig. 91.4)
- Polymicrogyria
- Pachygyria: thickened cortex with blurring of the gray white junction on T2 (Fig. 91.5)
- Dystrophic calcification
- Subependymal and hemispheric heterotopia
- Small/dysmorphic ipsilateral basal ganglia and thalami

IMAGING PITFALLS: It is important not to miss malformations involving the contralateral hemisphere that might preclude surgical hemispherectomy for intractable seizures.

Imaging Strategy

A child with intractable seizures and suspicion for underlying malformation of cortical development should have MRI. This should include the following sequences:

- Sagittal and axial T1 or inversion recovery
- Axial fast T2; coronal T2
- Axial proton density or FLAIR
- Axial diffusion
- Coronal T1-weighted volume such as MPRAGE
- Axial multiplanar gradient echo

In addition PET and SPECT with fusion imaging may be helpful in localizing a seizure focus to assist in surgical planning. Most commonly PET and SPECT will show global decreased metabolic activity in the involved hemisphere.

Related Physics

As white matter myelinates, it becomes "brighter" on T1. This has been simplistically linked to the lipid component in myelin. Although the reasons have not been entirely worked out, it is more likely that the increase in brightness (or T1 shortening) relates to binding of water and lipids (cholesterol and galactocerebrosides) on the surface of the myelin. Increased signal in unmyelinated white matter on

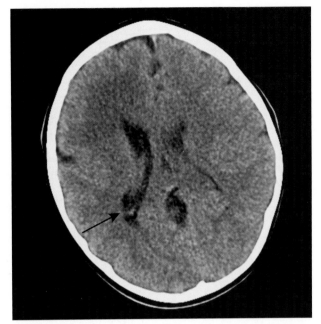

Figure 91.2. Axial unenhanced CT in an 8-month-old boy with intractable seizures shows right hemisphere malformation of cortical development and enlargement of the right hemisphere and atrium (arrow) of lateral ventricle consistent with HME.

T2 is reflective of axonal and extracellular free water. With myelination, signal drops (T2 shortening) and this is most likely related to tighter packing and organization as well as saturation of the polyunsaturated fatty acids in the myelin. A mature myelination pattern is expected by 6 months of

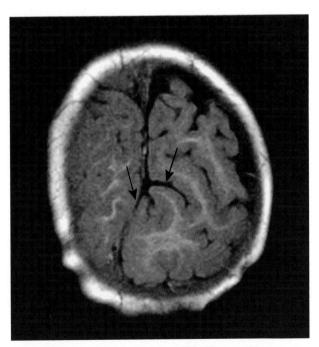

Figure 91.3. Coronal T1 multiplanar GRE MR image in a 6-month-old girl with intractable seizures and hemiplegia shows left hemisphere overgrowth and occipital infolding (arrows) consistent with HME.

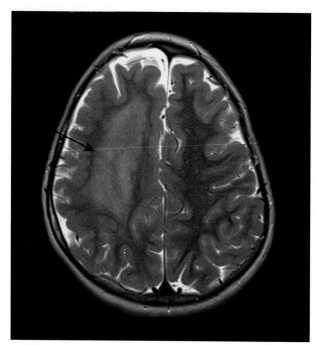

Figure 91.4. Axial T2 MR image in a 2-year-old boy with developmental delay and hemiplegia shows high signal in white matter of the right hemisphere consistent with delayed myelination (arrow) in HME.

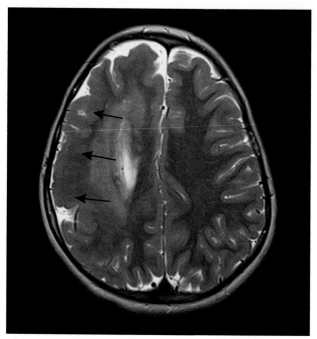

Figure 91.5. Axial T2 MR image in a 2-year-old boy with developmental delay and hemiplegia show s thickened right cortex (arrows), blurred gray/white interface, and shallow sulci consistent with pachygyria in HME.

age on T1-weighted sequences and by 22 to 36 months of age on T2-weighted sequences.

Differential Diagnosis

- Hemispheric malformation of cortical development
- Contralateral atrophy from a prior remote ischemic event during prenatal development
- Contralateral Rasmussen encephalitis
- Neurocutaneous syndrome (see below)

Common Variants

Hemimegalencephaly may be isolated or occur in conjunction with:

- Hemihypertrophy +/- Klippel Trenaunay syndrome
- Neurofibromatosis type I
- Epidermal Nevus Syndrome
- Proteus syndrome
- Hypomelanosis of Ito
- Tuberous sclerosis
- A rare variant of HME involves the entire ipsilateral brainstem and cerebellum as well as the supratentorial brain

Clinical Issues

A child with HME may undergo functional or anatomic hemispherectomy for intractable seizures that necessitates

follow-up imaging with CT or MRI. Findings may include postoperative subdural hemorrhage, hydrocephalus, fluid collections in the immediate period followed by gradual shift of the normal hemisphere into the surgical bed resulting in distortion of the intracranial contents. There is a relatively high morbidity and mortality associated with hemispherectomy.

Key Points

- Sporadic congenital anomaly
- Macrocephaly with large ventricle *on the side of the large hemisphere*
- Disorder of proliferation, migration, *and* organization
- May also be malformations of cortical development involving the opposite hemisphere
- Isolated or part of a neurocutaneous syndrome
- Rare involvement of the ipsilateral brainstem and cerebellum in addition to supratentorial brain

Further Reading

Congenital malformations of the brain and skull. In: Barkovich AJ, ed. *Pediatric Neuroimaging*. Fifth edition. Philadelphia, PA: Lippincott, Williams and Wilkins; 2012:407–411.

Broumandi DD, Hayward UM, et al. Best cases from the AFIP: hemimegalencephaly. *RadioGraphics*. 2004;24:843–848.

Crino PB. Molecular pathogenesis of focal cortical dysplasia and hemimegalencephaly. *Journal of Child Neurology*. 2005;20:330–336.

Hung P-C, Wang H-S. Hemimegalencephaly: cranial sono-graphic findings in neonates. *Journal of Clinical Ultrasound.* 2005;33(5):243–247.

Salamon N, Andres M, et al. Contralateral hemimicrencephaly and clinical-pathological correlations in children with hemi-megalencephaly. *Brain.* 2006;*129*:352–365.

Sasaki M, Hashimoto T, et al. Clinical aspects of hemimegalen-cephaly by means of a nationwide survey. *Journal of Child Neurology.* 2005;*20*:337–341.

Sato, Yagashita A, et al. Hemimegalencephaly: a study of abnor-malities occurring outside the involved hemisphere. *American Journal of Neuroradiology.* 2007;*28*:678–682.

Tinkle BT, Schorry EK, et al. Epidemiology of hemimegalen-cephaly case series and review. *American Journal of Medical Genetics.* 2005;*139A*:204–211.

CHAPTER 92

Closed Spinal Dysraphism

Nadja Kadom, MD

Definition

Spinal dysraphism that is associated with direct exposure of neuronal tissue through lack of skin covering is called "open spinal dysraphism" (OSD), and spinal dysraphism protected by overlying skin is termed "closed spinal dysraphism" (CSD). Some authors still use the term "occult spinal dysraphism" or "spina bifida (occulta)" synonymously with CSD. These terms were traditionally used for patients with nonfused vertebral posterior elements in the absence of any symptoms or other abnormalities; they are confusing and should be abandoned altogether.

Clinical Features

The spectrum of clinical presentation in CSD is broad. Some patients are asymptomatic and up to 80 percent of patients have skin lesions (pigmentation, dimples, hair patches, hemangiomas, sinus tracts). Tethered cord syndrome (TCS) describes clinical symptoms that may occur in patients with CSD. Patients with TCS present with progressive neurological deterioration affecting bowel and bladder function (incontinence), as well as difficulty walking, weakness, and foot deformities. The pathophysiology of TCS is traction on the conus medullaris and its adjacent nerve roots during postnatal growth of the spine and spinal cord resulting from immobilization of the conus. The treatment is usually surgical.

Occasionally spinal dysraphism associated with cord tethering may mimic adolescent idiopathic scoliosis and MRI spine imaging is therefore recommended in the presurgical (orthopedic) workup for these patients. Additional clinical indications for imaging of the spine for CSD include: spinal subcutaneous mass, clinical symptoms of TCS, anorectal malformations, children of diabetic mothers, spinal skin lesions, and abnormal fetal imaging studies.

Anatomy and Physiology

Neurulation is the process by which the central nervous system forms in vertebrate embryos. In primary neurulation the initial neural plate creases inwardly until the edges come in contact and fuse to form a tube. To complete the process of primary neurulation the tube must also separate from the ectoderm (with subsequent fusion of the skin overlying the tube) and separate from the neural crest cells (the latter then further differentiate into paraspinal neural structures). In secondary neurulation part of the tube (the caudal spine) forms by hollowing of a solid precursor, called the caudal cell mass. Abnormal primary or secondary neurulation can result in spinal dysraphism, a failure of complete formation of the spinal elements.

Entities of CSD are divided into those with a subcutaneous mass and those without. Closed spinal dysraphism with subcutaneous mass comprises meningocele, lipomyelocele and lipomyelomeningocele, as well as terminal myelocystocele and nonterminal myelocystocele. The embryologic mechanism in the formation of meningocele is unknown. Terminal myelocystocele is the result of abnormal secondary neurulation and all others are caused by abnormal primary neurulation, specifically nondysjunction (cervical myelocystocele) and premature dysjunction (lipomyelocele and lipomyelomeningocele).

Varieties of CSD without associated subcutaneous mass are further classified into simple and complex entities. Simple lesions include dermal sinus (resulting from abnormal primary neurulation with nondysjunction), intradural lipoma dermoid/epidermoid, filum lipoma (resulting from abnormal primary neurulation with premature dysjunction), and tight filum (resulting from abnormal secondary neurulation). The filum terminale short "filum," is thought to be a remnant of the caudal cell mass after formation of the distal conus and junction of the conus with the upper spinal cord. Its MRI appearance is equal to that of the cauda equina nerve roots, and it is easily identified as the midline structure that arises from the tip of the conus. It should always be measured at the L5/S1 level and its normal diameter is usually no more than approximately 1 millimeter. A persistent terminal ventricle is an ependyma-lined fluid cavity of the conus and essentially considered a normal variant related to secondary neurulation.

Complex lesions include dorsal enteric fistula, neurenteric cyst, diastematomyelia, caudal regression syndrome, and segmental spinal dysgenesis. Dorsal enteric fistula, neurenteric cyst, and diastematomyelia are all related to abnormalities of the notochord. The notochord is an embryologic structure that lies between the neural tube dorsally and the endoderm ventrally. Dorsal enteric fistula is the result of a split notochord, allowing communication of bowel with the dorsal skin. Neurenteric cysts are a result of incomplete separation of the notochord from the endoderm resulting in cysts that usually become symptomatic in the second and third decades of life through compression of neuronal structures. Diastematomyelia is characterized by a split of the spinal cord, usually in association with a focal bony or cartilaginous bar that separates the spinal canal into separate dural compartments. Below the bony bar the two spinal cords may or may not join again. Diastematomyelia may be asymptomatic or associated with scoliosis and/or TCS. Caudal regression syndrome is a result of abnormal secondary neurulation and represents a spectrum of disorders that range from total or partial unilateral sacral agenesis to sirenomyelia ("mermaid syndrome") with complete fusion of the lower limbs. Segmental spinal dysgenesis is of unknown origin and includes several entities: segmental agenesis/dysgenesis of thoracic or lumbar spine and segmental pathology of spinal cord/nerve roots. Patients usually present with congenital paraparesis/paraplegia and deformed limbs.

Imaging Findings

Each entity within the group of CSD is named according to its constituents: the suffix "-cele" refers to a lesion that goes beyond the margins of the spinal canal; the syllable "meningo" stands for meninges and CSF and usually indicates that the lesion is raised above the skin level; "myelo" stands for neuronal tissue and "lipo" for fat. It becomes a bit complicated when the "cyst" is added to the name, meaning a cyst has formed inside the spinal cord and extends beyond the spinal canal. (Fig 92.1) (92.2)

A tight filum may be thicker than usual or normal in appearance and may be a diagnosis of exclusion in patients with clinical TCS. A filar lipoma refers to varying degrees of fat in the filum with associated thickening, bright on T1 and T2 and dark on fat-suppressed sequences. Fat/lipoma within the filum must be differentiated from an intradural lipoma (Fig. 92.3), which is separate from the filum but in most cases also attached to the conus and thus the cause of cord tethering. A dermal sinus is a small skin defect that courses deep and is usually best seen clinically. It may communicate with the intrathecal space and cause infections. A persistent terminal ventricle is a fluid-filled cavity in the conus, lined by ependyma, and should be differentiated from syrinx and cystic masses of the conus. Dorsal enteric fistula may contain bowel, which makes the diagnosis easy. Neurenteric cysts have mostly cystic appearance, but certain types may contain various tissue types, such as bone, cartilage, and fat. The diagnosis of diastematomyelia (Fig. 92.4) is made by identifying the split halves of the spinal cord with or without a bony or cartilaginous bar that separates the spinal canal.

The task for the radiologist is to find the cause of TCS so it can be treated early for a better chance of maximal

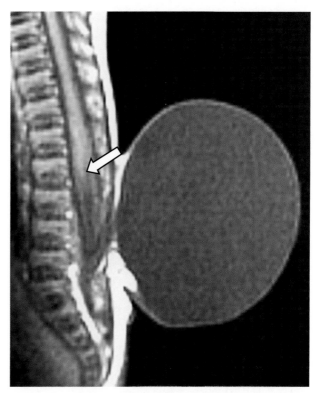

Figure 92.1. Sagittal midline unenhanced T1 MR image of the lumbosacral spine in a newborn with a back lesion shows a large lesion under the dorsal lumbosacral skin with fluid-isointense T1 signal consistent with meningocele. There is a dorsal defect in the spine but otherwise normal conus at L2 (arrow) and cauda equina.

reversal of symptoms. The normal position of the tip of the conus varies considerably in adults, from T11 to the upper third of L3. The likelihood of cord tethering is much higher for a conus tip positioned below the L2/3 disc level than above. The diagnosis of tethered cord may more confidently be made in the presence of additional findings, such as any form of a "-cele" or fatty tissue to which the conus may be attached.

Imaging Strategy

A newborn with a deep or high sacral dimple or other suspicious cutaneous lesion should undergo spine ultrasound screening to rule out tethered cord. Any positive case will require MRI for further characterization prior to surgical correction. Any older infant or child with clinical suspicion for CSD should undergo a spine MRI. The goal of the imaging evaluation is to accurately evaluate the level of the conus, the integrity of the spinal elements, to identify fatty lesions, to assess the craniocervical junction, and to screen the kidneys and dorsal skin. In scoliosis patients, one should add sequences to assess vertebral body shape and paraspinal soft tissues for masses (coronal T2-weighted images). The following sequences are recommended: sagittal T1 (entire spine) to assess the craniocervical junction, intrathecal fatty lesions, integrity of the

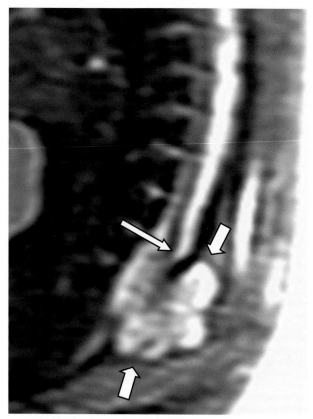

Figure 92.2. Sagittal single-shot FSE T2 MR image of the lumbosacral spine in a fetus shows a lobulated T2 bright lesion (thick arrows) and an associated defect in the posterior spinal elements. The conus is abnormally low, at the midportion of L3, and appears attached to the intrathecal portion of the lesion (thin arrow). In order to differentiate this lesion from OSD, it is necessary to assess the brain for features of Chiari II malformation. It may be difficult to see skin covering a lesion when the spine is positioned closely against the placenta, as in this patient. The lobulated shape of this lesion was not typical for a meningocele, and ultrasound in this patient showed fatty echotexture. Imaging diagnosis after birth was lipomyelomeningocele.

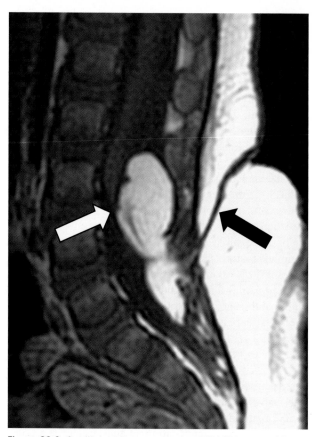

Figure 92.3. Sagittal midline unenhanced T1 MR image of the lumbosacral spine in a child with recurrent meningitis shows a large T1 bright mass in the dorsal intrathecal space to which the low lying conus is attached at upper L4 (white arrow). This patient also has lower lumbar subcutaneous fatty mass with a curvilinear track extending from the dorsal skin surface to the L5/S1 level with apparent termination dorsally at the fatty mass. Note the deficiency of the dorsal spinal elements. The findings represent an intradural lipoma with tethered cord and a subcutaneous lipoma with sinus tract (black arrow).

spinal elements and sinus tracts; sagittal T2 (entire spine) to define the vertebral bodies through bright T2 signal of the disc spaces; axial T1 (LS spine) to assess integrity of the spinal elements, fatty intrathecal lesions; axial T2 (entire spine) to assess kidneys and screen for terminal ventricle or syrinx; fat-suppressed T1 or T2 will confirm the fatty nature of lesions; diffusion-weighted images to differentiate epidermoids and dermoids from other cysts; and sagittal fat-suppressed T2 images and contrast-enhanced sequences to rule out intrathecal connection and infectious/inflammatory complications.

Related Physics

Ultrasound (US) is the best imaging modality to screen babies with sacral dimple for possible tethered cord (occult spinal dysraphism) as it offers superior spatial resolution over MRI without the need for sedation or contrast agents.

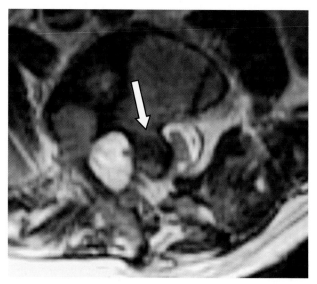

Figure 92.4. Axial T2 MR image at L5 in a child with scoliosis shows diastematomyelia with a bony bar (arrow) dividing the spinal canal into separate dural compartments.

Ultrasound imaging is cross-sectional and is characterized by three base resolution measures including axial, lateral, and elevational or slice thickness resolution. Axial resolution is predominantly determined by the transducer wavelength and the number of oscillations per pulse (spatial pulse length). For example, a 10-megahertz transducer will have 5 times better near field resolution than a 2-megahertz transducer; however with depth the resolution will decrease more quickly with higher-frequency transducers. The axial resolution is typically 2 to 3 times the size of a single wavelength because of multiple cycles in the spatial pulse length. Lateral resolution is defined by the length and not the width of the transducer footprint and number of elements used to create the beam. Lateral resolution can vary with depth in transducers with multiple focal zones where the resolution will be optimal at the level of the focal zone. Slice thickness is the third dimension, which is often overlooked in ultrasound. Elevational or "slice thickness" resolution is entirely a function of the width of the transducer. As the neural elements are relatively superficial in the newborn, the highest-frequency transducer can be used and the midline posterior cartilaginous elements of the spine serve as an excellent acoustic window. Nerve root movement can also be imaged given the real-time properties of US. The cauda equina lies in a CSF bath within the thecal sac, which enhances nerve conspicuity and identification of the level of the conus medullaris.

Differential Diagnosis

The diagnostic considerations in patients with TCS include all entities of OSD:

- Myelocele
- Myelomeningocele
- Hemimyelocele
- Hemimyelomeningocele

> **IMAGING PITFALLS:** Conus level may be inaccurate in patients with lumbosacral transitional vertebrae when counting vertebral bodies from the sacrum to the cervical spine.

Common Variants

Determination of the level of the conus may be difficult in the presence of transitional lumbosacral vertebrae, which has a prevalence of up to 21 percent in the general population. It is therefore recommended to acquire images that enable counting from the cervical spine to the sacrum.

Although the risk of TCS is higher for a conus position below the L2/3 disc level, it should be noted that TCS can also occur in patients with a normal conus position on imaging. Conversely, patients with an abnormally low conus position may not have TCS.

Clinical Issues

In fetal life it may be more difficult to differentiate the various forms of spinal dysraphism. Typically, CSD without a subcutaneous mass is missed by fetal imaging methods whereas CSD with a subcutaneous mass could be mistaken for a form of OSD (Fig. 92.2). Evaluation of the brain for features of Chiari II malformation helps to separate open from closed defects in most cases.

Key Points

- Disorders of embryonal spine development
- Numerous entities
- May present with tethered cord syndrome
- Determine conus level correctly by counting from top (cervical) to bottom (sacral)
- US for screening in newborns
- MRI for positive US and presurgical planning

Given the wide variety of entities that can be associated with TCS and the vast differences in treatment and prognosis, the radiologist's input is invaluable. It has been postulated that clinical deficits in TCS may be related to hypoxic damage to the conus and it has been shown that surgical detethering results in improved blood flow. Clinical outcomes after surgery vary widely and may in part be related to timing of intervention.

Further Reading

Congenital anomalies of the spine. In: Barkovich AJ, ed. *Pediatric Neuroimaging*. Fifth edition. Philadelphia, PA: Lippincott, Williams and Wilkins; 2012:857–917.

Bulas D. Fetal evaluation of spine dysraphism. *Pediatr Radiol*. 2010;*40*(6):1029–1037. Epub 2010 Apr 30. Review.

Medina LS. Spinal dysraphism: categorizing risk to optimize imaging. *Pediatr Radiol*. 2009;*39*(Suppl 2):S242–S246. Review.

Rossi A, Cama A, Piatelli G, Ravegnani M, Biancheri R, Tortori-Donati P. Spinal dysraphism: MR imaging rationale. *J Neuroradiol*. 2004;*31*(1):3–24. Review.

Rufener SL, Ibrahim M, Raybaud CA, Parmar HA. Congenital spine and spinal cord malformations—pictorial review. *AJR Am J Roentgenol*. 2010;*194*(Suppl 3):S26–S37. Review.

CHAPTER 93

Neurofibromatoses

Nadja Kadom, MD

Definition

Neurofibromatoses, comprised of neurofibromatosis type 1 (NF1), neurofibromatosis type 2 (NF2), and schwannomatosis, belong to the family of neurocutaneous syndromes. They are characterized by genetic defects of tumor suppressor genes causing tumor growth in various parts of the body, many affecting the central nervous system (CNS). Although they share a similar name, NF1 and NF2 are genetically very different with few overlapping characteristics. Both are autosomal dominant disorders with full penetrance. The nerve sheath tumors are the common feature for all of the neurofibromatoses.

Clinical Features

The most common of the neurofibromatoses is NF1, with a birth frequency of approximately one in 3,000. The genetic defect has been localized to chromosome 17, where the protein neurofibromin is encoded, which acts as a tumor suppressor. Neurofibromatoses type 1 is defined by the presence of at least two major disease symptoms :

- First-degree relative with NF1
- Six or more café au lait patches which are present at birth or appear in first few years of life
- Axillary or groin freckling
- Two or more neurofibromas or one plexiform neurofibroma
- Lisch nodules in the iris
- Optic pathway glioma
- Osseous dysplasia of the sphenoid wing
- Pseudoarthrosis of the long bones

Benign neurofibromas are the cardinal disease manifestation, but NF1 patients may also develop malignant peripheral nerve sheath tumors (MPNST), de novo or by malignant transformation of existing neurofibromas. Optic pathway gliomas are seen in 15 percent of NF1 patients and may be asymptomatic or present with loss of visual acuity. Gliomas can also occur in any other part of the brain, commonly in the cerebellum and brainstem. Most gliomas are pilocytic astrocytomas, but higher-grade gliomas can develop.

NF2 is less common than NF1 with a birth incidence of 1 in 25,000 and has been localized to chromosome 22, which encodes the protein merlin, another tumor suppressor. The National Institutes of Health Criteria for NF2 is bilateral vestibular schwannoma *OR* first-degree relative with NF2 and either unilateral vestibular schwannoma or two of the following: meningioma, schwannoma, glioma, neurofibroma, juvenile lens opacity. Vestibular schwannomas typically do not occur until the second or third decade of life. Therefore, the classic adult presentation of progressive sensorineural hearing loss, tinnitus, and imbalance is not seen in children. Instead, pediatric patients often present with symptoms related to the other tumors characteristic of the disease, including seizures, peripheral nerve dysfunction, myelopathy, and visual loss.

Schwannomatosis is very rare and the pathogenesis has not been defined. There is only a 15 percent familial incidence. Clinical symptoms typically do not occur until the second or third decade. The most common clinical presentation is pain. The Children's Tumor Foundation Criteria for the diagnosis of schwannomatosis is age > 30 years *AND* two or more nonintradermal schwannomas and no vestibular tumor on MRI and no constitutional NF2 mutation.

Anatomy and Physiology

Neurofibromatosis type 1 neurofibromas are benign peripheral nerve tumors containing a mixture of schwann cells, fibroblasts, perineural cells, mast cells, and nerve axons. This is in contrast to schwannomas, which consist entirely of schwann cells. Four different types of neurofibromas have been described: cutaneous (in 99 percent of patients, itching and stinging), subcutaneous (may cause pain), spinal nerve (may compress adjacent structures), plexiform (in 60 percent of patients, involving multiple fascicles of large nerves, neurological deficits and disfigurement).

Imaging Findings

CT and MRI:

Neurofibromatosis type 1

Central nervous system:
- Plexiform neurofibroma: characteristic "target" appearance on T2 with a muscle isointense center and a bright rim (Fig. 93.1), however, this pattern can also be seen with extraaxial schwannomas
- Malignant transformation of neurofibromas (Fig. 93.2): enlargement, peripheral contrast enhancement, perilesional edema, internal cyst formation

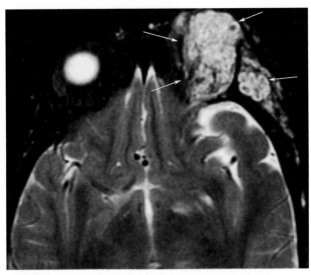

Figure 93.1. Axial T2 fat-saturated MR image in a 14-year-old girl with NF1 shows a mass (arrows) in the left orbit and left infratemporal fossa with "target" appearance: dark T2 signal centrally and bright T2 signal peripherally, typical of neurofibroma. There is also widening of the left middle cranial fossa subarachnoid space resulting from left sphenoid wing dysplasia.

- Optic gliomas (Fig. 93.3): can be diagnosed when there is abnormal enlargement of the optic nerve pathways, with or without contrast enhancement
- Sphenoid wing dysplasia: usually occurs in conjunction with plexiform neurofibroma in distribution of the ophthalmic nerve (V1)

Additional CNS features with unknown pathophysiology and clinical importance:

- Benign nonenhancing T2 bright lesions of infratentorial brain, as well as midbrain and basal ganglia
- Thickening of the corpus callosum
- T2-weighted signal increase and swelling of the hippocampi

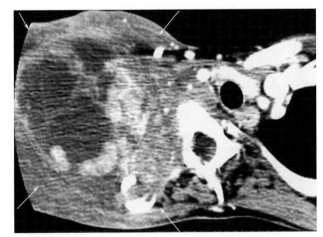

Figure 93.2. Axial contrast-enhanced CT image of the lower neck/shoulder region in a 14-year-old boy with NF1 shows a large right-sided mass (arrows) with peripheral contrast enhancement, cyst formation, and perilesional edema consistent with MPNST.

Bone :

- Widened neural foramen from spinal nerve neurofibromas or dural ectasia
- Pseudoarthrosis of a long bone
- Scoliosis: typically high thoracic in location
- Anterolateral tibia bowing: in contrast to the idiopathic tibial bowing that is typically posteromedial

Vascular:

- Vasculopathy: may develop in NF1 patients and affect the circle of Willis ranging from varying degrees of stenoses to Moyamoya disease
- Renal artery stenosis

Neurofibromatosis Type 2

- Vestibular schwannomas (Fig. 93.4): typically iso- to hypointense to gray matter on T1, mostly brighter than brain tissue on T2, and generally show contrast enhancement
- Meningiomas: dural based masses with T2 signal isointense to gray matter and contrast enhancement
- Ependymomas: posterior fossa or spinal intramedullary masses with bright T2 signal and contrast enhancement

IMAGING PEARLS: Fifty % of patients who present with MRI findings including the typical T2 brain lesions and optic glioma have NF1.

Imaging Strategy

Neurofibromatosis Type 1:

Patients with NF1 may undergo MRI to assist in making the diagnosis (usually young children and/or sporadic

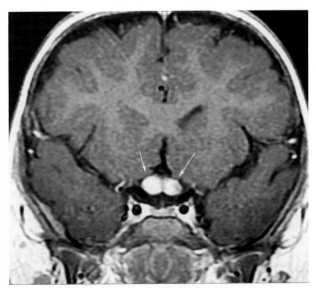

Figure 93.3. Coronal contrast-enhanced T1 MR image of a 17-month-old boy with a family history of NF1 shows bilateral enhancing lesions and expansion of the optic chiasm (arrows) consistent with optic glioma.

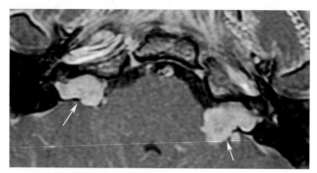

Figure 93.4. Axial contrast-enhanced T1 fat-saturated MR image of the internal auditory canals (IACs) in a 15-year-old boy with NF2 shows bilaterally enhancing schwannomas extending from the IACs into the cerebellopontine angles (arrows).

forms of NF1), screen for optic pathway glioma, monitor optic pathway glioma with or without treatment, or monitor for development of MPNST.

MRI should include:

- Coronal and axial T2 and postcontrast fat-saturated T1 orbits and chiasm: to evaluate optic chiasm lesions
- Axial or coronal T2/PD/FLAIR brain: to evaluate T2 lesions of the brain parenchyma
- Coronal postcontrast T1 fat-saturated brain: to evaluate cranial nerve neurofibromas frequently involving the trigeminal nerve
- Coronal postcontrast fat-saturated T1 or coronal T2 fat-saturated spine: to evaluate for spinal nerve neurofibromas
- Axial and sagittal postcontrast T1 spine: to evaluate for possible cord compression from spinal lesions
- Coronal T2 fat-saturated, postcontrast brain with T1 fat suppression: to evaluate for plexiform neurofibroma and features of malignant transformation
- MR arteriogram including Circle of Willis: to evaluate for vasculopathy

Neurofibromatosis Type 2:
MRI should include:

- High-resolution axial and coronal T2 and postcontrast T1 images of the brain in the same plane (usually does not require fat saturation) to evaluate vestibular schwannomas
- T2 and isovolumetric T1-weighted images of the brain postcontrast for meningiomas

Related Physics

Spin echo has long been the workhorse for basic MR imaging especially for T1-weighted imaging. All other sequences are built from this basic model of application of a 90-degree slice selective pulse followed by a 180-degree rephasing pulse and readout at time "TE." The main drawback is the long scan time required. Dual echo spin echo applies two 180-degree pulses that in turn generate proton density images (at a short TE) and

T2-weighted images (at a longer TE). Fast spin echo applies a 90-degree pulse followed by multiple 180-degree pulses, each of which is accompanied by a TE (readout). The number of 180-degree rephasing pulses is given by the echo train length (ETL) or "turbo factor" whereby the scan time is reduced by the same factor. A fast spin echo (FSE) sequence with an ETL of 9 will reduce the scan time by a factor of 9 over SE technique. Unfortunately a greater ETL does not mix well with shorter TE and results in image blur. For this reason FSE technique is best applied to T2 (with longer TE) rather than T1.

Differential Diagnosis

- Optic glioma: also occurs in patients without NF1, has slightly different morphology and imaging features and may have a different clinical course
- Optic nerve meningioma: evaluate if the mass is located peripheral (meningioma) versus intrinsic (glioma) to the nerve
- Pediatric suprasellar masses: craniopharyngioma, hypothalamic glioma, germ cell tumor or histiocytosis of the pituitary region
- T2 lesions in NF1: demyelinating disease, inflammatory disease, metabolic syndromes, or acute disseminated encephalomyelitis (ADEM)
- Meningioma: internal auditory canal (IAC) and spinal meningioma can appear identical to schwannoma
- Cranial and spinal nerve sheath tumors: neurofibromas and schwannomas are difficult to differentiate by imaging
- Metastatic disease to the internal auditory canal: hematogenous or extension from other posterior fossa tumors, such as atypical teratoid rhabdoid tumor

Common Variants

Several genetic variants of NF1 exist. Mosaicism can occur by mutation in early or late embryonic life, the latter causing a segmental NF1 which involves only one body segment. There is also an NF1 mutation that causes isolated symmetric multiple spinal nerve fibromas and café au lait lesions in the absence of other signs of NF1.

Clinical Issues

In NF1 patients, optic gliomas can cause visual loss; other brain gliomas can occur and some may have higher malignancy grade. In addition, approximately 50 percent of pediatric NF1 patients have cognitive deficits, including symptoms of attention deficit hyperactivity disorder (ADHD). Significant disfigurement from neurofibromas can represent a major source of psychological distress; some neurofibromas cause pain, and there is a lifetime 10 percent risk of MPNST. Patients with NF1 may develop cardiovascular complications, such as congenital heart defects, arteriovenous fistulae and malformations, vessel stenosis or occlusion, and hypertension related to renal artery stenosis (Fig. 93.5).

For pediatric NF2 patients the main clinical issues are seizures resulting from meningiomas and facial nerve palsy

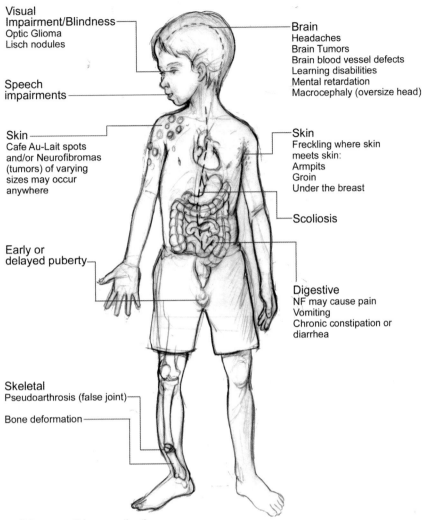

Visual
Impairment/Blindness
Optic Glioma
Lisch nodules

Speech
impairments

Skin
Cafe Au-Lait spots
and/or Neurofibromas
(tumors) of varying
sizes may occur
anywhere

Early or
delayed puberty

Skeletal
Pseudoarthrosis (false joint)

Bone deformation

Brain
Headaches
Brain Tumors
Brain blood vessel defects
Learning disabilities
Mental retardation
Macrocephaly (oversize head)

Skin
Freckling where skin
meets skin:
Armpits
Groin
Under the breast

Scoliosis

Digestive
NF may cause pain
Vomiting
Chronic constipation or
diarrhea

Other possible complications:
Delayed in learning to walk or talk. Short stature. Poor school performance. Increase in
size and number of tumors during pregnancy. Severe itching, psychosocial burdens
and cancer.

Figure 93.5. Neurofibromatosis Type 1. The complete clinical spectrum.

related to vestibular schwannoma; hearing loss usually develops later in life.

Key Points

- NF1 and NF2: Autosomal dominant disorders with full penetrance
- NF1: Neurofibromas and optic pathway glioma
- NF2: Bilateral vestibular schwannoma, neurofibromas, ependymomas, meningiomas
- Schwannomatosis: Multiple schwannomas excluding intradermal and vestibular types

Further Reading

Congenital malformations of the brain and skull. In: Barkovich AJ, ed. *Pediatric Neuroimaging*. Fifth edition. Philadelphia, PA: Lippincott, Williams and Wilkins; 2012:570–593.

Lu-Emerson C, PS. The neurofibromatoses. Part 2: NF2 and schwannomatosis. *Rev Neurol Dis*. 2009;6(3):E81–E86.

Mentzel HJ, Seidel J, Fitzek C, Eichhorn A, Vogt S, Reichenbach JR, et al. Pediatric brain MRI in neurofibromatosis type I. *Eur Radiol*. 2005;15(4):814–822.

Wasa J, Nishida Y, Tsukushi S, Shido Y, Sugiura H, Nakashima H, et al. MRI features in the differentiation of malignant peripheral nerve sheath tumors and neurofibromas. *AJR Am J Roentgenol*.; 194(6):1568–1574.

CHAPTER 94

Tuberous Sclerosis

Sumit Pruthi, MD

Definition

Tuberous sclerosis (TS) is an autosomal dominant genetic disease characterized by the development of multiple benign hamartomatous lesions in multiple organs and tissues throughout the body.

Clinical Features

The diagnosis of TS is made clinically from predefined major and minor criteria that include the presence of one or more of the following lesions: skin (angiofibromas, shagreen patch); retina (hamartomas);nails (periungual fibromas); heart (rhabdomyomas); kidneys (angiomyofibromas); brain ("tubers," nodules, malformations of cortical development); lungs (lymphangioleiomyomatosis in females after puberty); bone (cysts and sclerotic bone lesions); aorta (coarctation, aneurysm); and bowel (polyps). The classic triad of mental retardation, epilepsy, and adenoma sebaceum is uncommon.

Although commonly associated with cognitive impairment, only 50 percent of affected patients have below average intelligence and about 75 percent have epilepsy. Evidence suggests that early onset of seizures (before 5 years of age) and tuber burden are risk factors governing the onset and degree of cognitive impairment. Neuroimaging plays an important role not only in making the presumptive diagnosis but also in defining the full extent of central nervous system involvement. Characteristic abnormalities are present on neuroimaging studies in more than 95 percent of affected patients, with some detected prenatally, and may predate clinical manifestations by years.

Anatomy and Physiology

Most cases of TS result from spontaneous mutations, with an autosomal dominant heritance pattern in subsequent generations. The genetic disorder is encoded at the TSC1 locus on chromosome 9q34 and TSC2 locus on chromosome 16p13. The TSC1 and 2 loci are important regulators of the size of organs and cells, and they work in concert to control the mTOR pathway which is critical in the development of certain benign tumors such as renal angiomyolipomas. Proteins tuberin and hamartin are TSC gene products and important regulators in this pathway.

Imaging Findings

Cerebral Hamartomas ("Tubers")

These are the most characteristic lesions of tuberous sclerosis pathologically. Rarely solitary, numbers can vary from as few as two to as many as 20 to 30 tubers. They are most often supratentorial, frequently seen in the frontal lobe. Ten to fifteen percent of affected patients have infratentorial tubers. On CT, tubers are low in attenuation and usually do not enhance. About half calcify, seen best on CT. On MRI they are easily detected in 95 percent of patients, in 80 percent solely by their abnormal signal and in 20 percent because of expansion of the involved gyri. In neonates, they appear hyperintense compared to the surrounding unmyelinated white matter on T1-weighted images and hypointense to white matter on T2 images (Fig. 94.1). The lesions eventually become iso- to hypointense on T1-weighted images and hyperintense to white and gray matter on T2/FLAIR images (Fig. 94.2). Contrast enhancement occurs in 5 percent of the cases and does not indicate malignant degeneration, as neoplastic degeneration of cortical tubers is extremely rare.

Subependymal Hamartomas/Nodules (SENs)

Subependymal hamartomas/nodules appear as discrete or confluent nodular foci lining the lateral ventricles. The caudothalamic groove near the foramen of Monro is the most common location. Calcification, best detected by CT, is rare in the first year of life with an increase with the age of the patient (Fig. 94.3). Nodules are hyperintense on T1-weighted images and hypointense on T2-weighted images in the infant and as the myelin matures, they gradually become isointense with the white matter on T1 and iso- to hyperintense on T2-weighted images (Fig. 94.4) secondary to either increased cellularity or the presence of hydrated calcium.

Giant Cell Tumors (GCT)

A GCT is an enlarging subependymal nodule that is usually located near the foramen of Monro (Fig. 94.5). Seen in approximately 5 percent to 10 percent of cases, GCTs differ from SENs in size, tendency to enlarge, and characteristic location. Given the precarious location, enlargement may

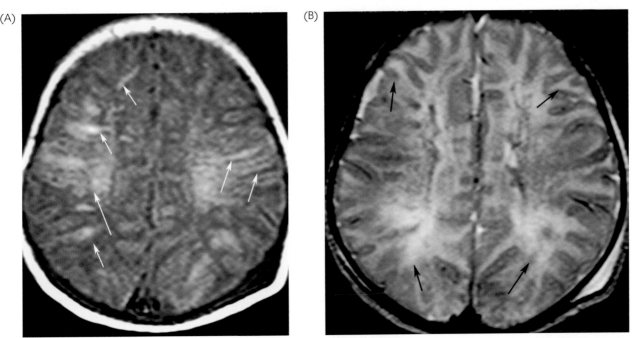

Figure 94.1. Axial noncontrast T1 GRE MR image (A) in an infant shows multiple linear hyperintensities (white arrows) most consistent with subependymal hamartomas. They are easily identifiable along the background of immature white matter. Axial T2 MR image (B) at the same level reveals linear hypointensities (black arrows), far less than seen on T1-weighted images, highlighting that many more tubers can be seen on T1 than T2-weighted imaging before complete myelin maturation.

result in hydrocephalus. Neither signal intensity nor the presence or absence of enhancement is useful in making the distinction between benign SEN and GCT. Size greater than 12 millimeters has been suggested as a defining criterion for GCT, however progressive enlargement of SEN rather than absolute size is a more reliable sign. At some centers, GCT is resected if there has been interval growth; whereas at others, ventricular obstruction is the only indication for

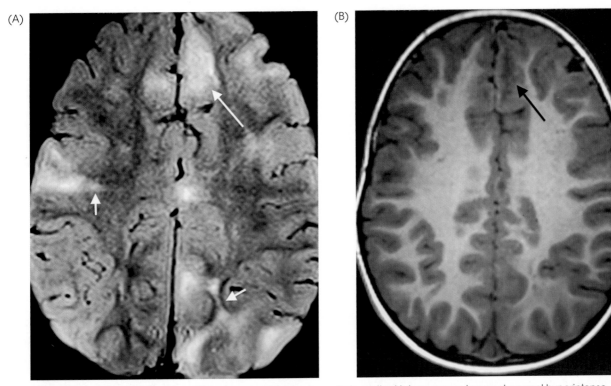

Figure 94.2. Axial FLAIR MR image (A) in a young child shows multiple cortical tubers appearing as abnormal hyperintense signal along the cortex and subcortical region with some areas showing gyral expansion (large white arrow). Linear hyperintense white matter lesions are seen extending centrally from the tuber (small arrows). Axial noncontrast T1 GRE MR image (B) shows a corresponding hypointense cortical tuber (black arrow). Many more cortical tubers are seen on FLAIR than on T1.

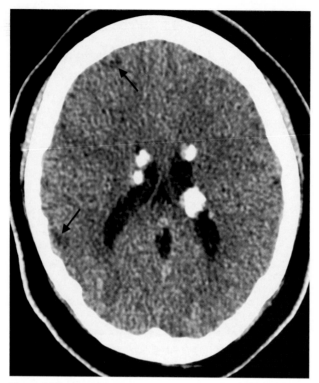

Figure 94.3. Axial noncontrast CT image in a child with seizures shows multiple easily identifiable calcified subependymal nodules. Cortical tubers (black arrows) appear as hypodense areas involving the cortex and subcortical region.

resection. Lesions may occasionally stabilize spontaneously. Oral rapamycin therapy (an mTOR inhibitor) has shown promise in inducing regression of GCT and may be an alternative to surgical resection.

White Matter Changes

Four distinct patterns of white matter lesions on MR imaging have reported: straight or curvilinear bands that extend from ventricles through the cerebrum; wedge-shaped lesions; nonspecific tumefactive or conglomerate foci; and cerebellar radial bands. These lesions are benign and are believed to represent disorganized, dysplastic or gliotic white matter or malformations of cortical development including balloon cell hyperplasia.

Imaging Strategy

The findings can be suspected on multiple modalities including fetal MRI, postnatal US and CT. The modality of choice is MRI for diagnosis and characterization of lesions in a child with seizures and suspicion for underlying TS, including: sagittal T1 volume gradient imaging such as MPRAGE with axial and coronal reconstructions; contrast-enhanced axial and coronal T1; axial fast T2; coronal T2; axial FLAIR; and axial diffusion.

> **IMAGING PITFALLS:** The imaging appearance of cortical tubers and SENs on CT and MRI depends upon the age of the patient and degree of white matter myelination.
>
> For successful imaging of cerebral lesions in neonates and young infants with tuberous sclerosis, T1-weighted sequences (preferably volumetric) are necessary.

Related Physics

Whereas spin echo (SE) and fast spin echo (FSE) sequences make use of a 90-degree pulse followed by one or a series

(A)

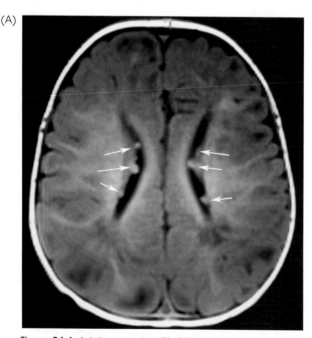

(B)

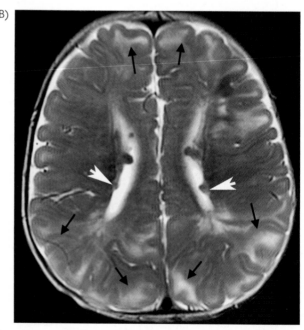

Figure 94.4. Axial noncontrast T1 GRE MR image (A) in a child with mature myelination pattern shows multiple subependymal nodules (white arrows) that appear isointense to surrounding white matter. Axial T2 MR image (B) at the same level shows several subependymal nodules (white arrowheads) that appear hyperintense to surrounding matter, secondary to either cellular lesions or the presence of hydrated calcium. Cortical tubers (black arrows) are numerous.

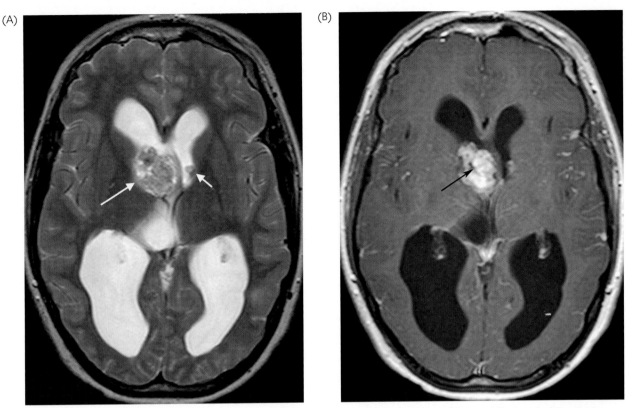

Figure 94.5. Axial T2 MR image (A) in a child with known TS shows a large hypointense mass (large white arrow) at the right foramen of Monroe extending into the frontal horn causing mild associated hydrocephalus, most consistent with GCT. There is also a smaller mass at the left foramen of Monroe (small white arrow). Axial contrast-enhanced T1 MR image (B) shows intense lesion enhancement (black arrow).

of 180-degree pulses, gradient echo technique applies a flip angle of less than 90 degrees and instead of a 180-degree pulse, applies a bipolar gradient pulse that reverses precessional direction within plane without flipping protons by 180 degrees. This reversal of precessional direction causes rephasing and signal reformation at each echo time (TE). The flip angle used in gradient echo is between 10 and 80 degrees whereby a larger angle renders greater T1 weighting and lower angle renders greater T2 weighting. In gradient echo imaging, "T2" is more appropriately referred to as "T2*", as the signal generated is a true representation of the free induction decay, whereas in spin echo imaging, "T2" reflects free induction *plus* the effects of the 180-degree rephasing pulse. Advantages include low SAR (specific absorption rate), absence of cross talk, and shorter scan time because of decreased flip angle. The disadvantages of gradient echo are inferior spatial resolution, susceptibility to field inhomogeneities, and increased artifacts at tissue interfaces. The artifact created at interfaces between tissues of differing properties can be used to one's advantage, and this is true in TS. Gradient echo is very sensitive to mineral such as iron in hemoglobin and methemoglobin or calcium, both of which will appear as dark signal with "blooming" on brain imaging. Calcifications in TS may be so subtle that they are only seen on GRE.

Differential Diagnosis

- Subependymal hemorrhage: premature infants
- Subependymal nodular heterotopia: absence of associated calcifications or contrast enhancement helps easily differentiate the heterotopia from SEN
- Focal neoplasm: solitary tubers (proton MR spectroscopy studies and perfusion imaging may be helpful in such cases by showing increased myo-inositol and normal perfusion in tubers)

Clinical Issues

Neurologic involvement in tuberous sclerosis complex is the most frequent cause of disease-related disability. Patients usually have multiple tubers, and identifying the one responsible for the onset of epileptogenic activity is often the most difficult and unfortunately the most important task both for the radiologist and clinician. The prognosis and cognitive outcome of the disease are critically influenced by timely surgical resection of the epileptogenic tuber. Neuroimaging is vital for presurgical evaluation in localizing the presumed epileptogenic focus. Diffusion tensor imaging (DTI), positron emission tomography (PET), and magnetoencephalography (MEG) have shown promise in improving the sensitivity for lesion detection. Diffusion tensor imaging provides information regarding both the magnitude (apparent diffusion coefficient) and the direction of water diffusion (fractional anisotropy) within a voxel. Tubers with significantly higher ADCs and lower FA are thought to have increased epileptogenic potential. Similarly, large areas of FDG-PET hypometabolism within tubers correlate with increased epileptogenic potential more so than tumor size alone. Tubers with increased [11C] methyl-L-tryptophan (AMT) PET are thought to be more epileptogenic than those without. Also, MEG shows promise in improving precise localization of epileptic foci for surgical resection in TS patients, especially if used in conjunction with PET/MRI fusion imaging.

Key Points

- Tubers, SENs and white matter abnormalities are best visualized on T1-weighted sequences before myelin maturation and can be easily missed or underestimated on fluid-sensitive sequences.
- Fluid inversion-recovery (FLAIR) sequence and magnetization transfer sequences depict more tubers and white matter anomalies than conventional SE images in older children and adults.
- Cortical tubers and SENs show variable contrast enhancement and the presence or absence of enhancement has no clinical significance.
- Progressive growth is the most reliable distinction between a benign SEN and a GCT.

Further Reading

The phakomatoses. In: Barkovich AJ, ed. *Pediatric Neuroimaging*. Fifth edition. Philadelphia, PA: Lippincott, Williams and Wilkins; 2012:593–604.

Baskin HJ Jr. The pathogenesis and imaging of the tuberous sclerosis complex. *Pediatr Radiol*. 2008; *38*:936–952.

Kalantari BN, Salamon N. Neuroimaging of tuberous sclerosis: spectrum of pathologic findings and frontiers in imaging. *AJR*. 2008;*190*:W304–W309.

Osborn AG. Disorders of histogenesis: neurocutaneous syndromes. In: *Diagnostic Neuroradiology*. First edition.:Mosby Elsevier ; 1994:93–98.

CHAPTER 95

Congenital Central Nervous System Infections

Nadja Kadom, MD

Definition

The acronym "TORCH" (**T**oxoplasmosis gondii), **O**ther (AIDS, lymphocytic choriomeningitis), **R**ubella, **C**ytomegalovirus (CMV), **H**erpesvirusis a widely used term that refers to congenital infections that can affect the central nervous system (CNS) and other parts of the body.

Clinical Features

It is important to know that in the United States some of the TORCH infections are becoming less prevalent and that some new infections have gained more attention in pregnant women. Congenital toxoplasmosis is declining in the United States as a result of high preexisting immunity in pregnant women (approximately 38 percent) and successful counseling for precautions regarding domestic cats. Congenital rubella syndrome (CRS) has significantly decreased in the United States as a result of successful immunization programs. The most commonly recognized congenital infection in the United States is now CMV, with an incidence of <100 per 10,000 live births (90 percent of these being asymptomatic). An increasing number of congenital syphilis (Treponema pallidum) is noted in the United States. Lymphocytic choriomeningitis (LCM), HIV, and Chagas disease (Trypanosoma cruzi) are of rising concern. Both systemic and neurological complications can result from intrauterine infections. Features in infants that raise suspicion for intrauterine infection include jaundice, hepatomegaly or splenomegaly, rash, intrauterine growth retardation, and chorioretinitis. Neurologic manifestations of congenital infection in neonates include microcephaly, hydrocephalus, seizures, meningoencephalitis, abnormal muscle tone, sensorineural hearing loss, and a variety of ophthalmologic anomalies.

Anatomy and Physiology

The effects of infections on the developing brain depend both on the time at which the infection occurs as well as the type of infectious agent. For example, rubella infection prior to 16 weeks gestation more likely causes ophthalmologic abnormalities, congenital heart disease, and sensorineural hearing loss, although rubella infection after gestational week 20 is more likely to be "silent" (without neurological deficits). Some infectious agents have very specific effects: rubella is the only infection to cause congenital heart lesions; varicella zoster causes unusual skin scarring ("cicatrix"); osteopathy is more common with syphilis and rubella; and chorioretinitis more likely relates to either toxoplasmosis or LCM infections. Because CMV affects the brain during the critical period of germinal matrix proliferation, migration, and cortical organization, it therefore shows characteristic dystrophic lesions (with calcifications) along this pathway (Fig. 95.1).

Imaging Findings

The key imaging findings in congenital infections are patchy white matter lesions, calcifications, possible cortical malformations, and ventriculomegaly. Ventriculomegaly can be caused by both volume loss and hydrocephalus. Sensorineural hearing loss may not show structural abnormalities on CT and MR of the temporal bones. It can be very challenging to differentiate various infectious causative agents based on imaging findings. However, certain infectious agents are more common and/or are more likely to show a certain pattern of imaging abnormalities:

- Toxoplasma: scattered calcifications, ventriculomegaly from volume loss or hydrocephalus
- Rubella: periventricular or parenchymal calcifications, microcephaly, microophthalmia
- CMV: 50 percent with periventricular calcifications; also periventricular leukomalacia, polymicrogyria, pachygyria, lissencephaly (Fig. 95.2)
- Herpes simplex: dense calcifications of basal ganglia and thalami, hemispheric cysts, lissencephaly

IMAGING PITFALLS: Brain calcifications are not specific for congenital infections.

Imaging Strategy

In most cases ultrasound (US), CT, and MRI will all be useful in the evaluation of congenital infections with CNS involvement. The benefits of US are use at the bedside of clinically unstable infants and identification of periventricular echogenic lesions, ventriculomegaly, and periventricular

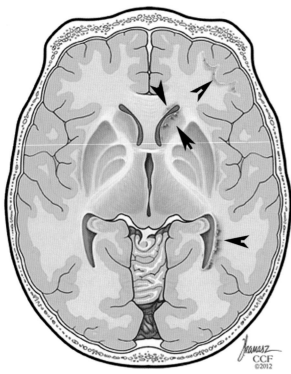

Figure 95.1. Medical Illustration: CMV. Typical distribution of calcifications in CMV infection (arrows) are along paths of proliferation, migration, and cortical organization.

cysts. CT is most useful in detection of calcifications, extent and pattern of ventriculomegaly, and it may also show signs of cortical malformations. For visualization of white matter lesions, cortical malformations, and various causes of ventriculomegaly, MR is the best modality. MR sequences should be geared toward visualization of the cortex (best achieved with 3-D T1 images, such as sagittal SPGR), evaluation of white matter lesions to differentiate from hereditary congenital diseases (best achieved with axial and/or coronal T2/FLAIR, DWI), and differentiation of types of ventriculomegaly/hydrocephalus (3-D T2 images of the midline are helpful, such as CISS or FIESTA). Susceptibility-weighted sequences may help in detection of calcifications. Fetal MR (Fig. 95.3) can be helpful in patients with abnormal US findings and for further evaluation of brain abnormalities, such as white matter volume loss, cortical malformations, delayed cortical maturation, and hemorrhages that can be seen in congenital infections.

Related Physics

TORCH infection may be imaged by MRI in the fetus or the newborn. The uncorrected magnetic field in MRI is not completely homogeneous because of imperfections in superconductors, the local environment, and external magnetic fields. It is therefore necessary to compensate for inhomogeneities in order to produce high-quality images. Inhomogeneities can exist in all three principle planes as well as any combination of these. Historically, compensations were accomplished through inserting small iron shimstock at strategic locations within the magnetic bore (passive shimming). These physical methods have been replaced by electronic shim coils (active shimming) on modern systems.

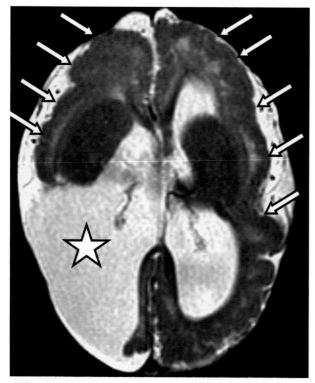

Figure 95.2. Axial T2-weighted MR image in a patient with congenital CMV shows bilateral cortical malformations with loss of deep cortical sulci, causing a lissencephalic appearance (small arrows). There is also a large right cerebral schizencephaly (star).

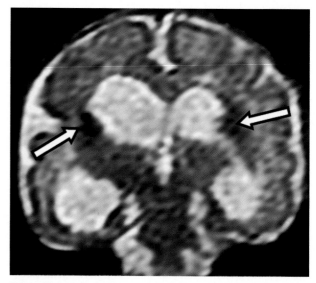

Figure 95.3. Coronal single-shot fast-spin-echo T2 fetal MR image through the thalami in a 32-week gestational fetus shows bilateral T2 dark areas of the ventricular walls (arrows), compatible with small germinal matrix hemorrhages. There is associated ventriculomegaly. There were positive maternal CMV titers.

These act in a similar manner to gradient coils but without change over time. Geometrically, shim coils are distributed in a modern MR system in a fashion similar to gradient coils with a pair for each of xy, xz, yz directions.

Differential Diagnosis

- Aicardi-Goutieres syndrome (AGS, also called "pseudo-TORCH" (Fig 95.4)) can present with any calcification pattern, therefore mimicking any congenital infection (Fig. 95.4). In contrast to the static encephalopathy seen in congenital infections, AGS is a progressive disease with onset usually in the first year of life.
- Cockayne syndrome: calcifications in the basal ganglia, cerebrum and cerebellum, short stature, characteristic facial features with marked enophthalmos and a beaked nose, deafness, and mental decline
- Fahr's disease: calcifications in the basal ganglia, cerebrum and cerebellum, movement disorders and behavioral anomalies
- Metabolic disease from diminished parathyroid function (hypo- and pseudohypoparathyroidism)
- Other genetic disorders with microcephaly, ventriculomegaly, and white matter abnormalities on imaging that can be mistaken for congenital infectious disease include congenital muscular dystrophies (such as Walker-Warburg syndrome; Fig. 95.5) and incontinentia pigmenti

Clinical Issues

Testing and treatment protocols for pregnant women have changed over the years through advances in laboratory medicine, immunization programs, counseling, and new treatment options. For toxoplasmosis, given high prevalence of antibodies in pregnant women (38 percent) and known transmission path from domestic cats, preventive counseling alone is now considered most cost-effective. Chances of rubella infection are very low in the United States given high immunization levels of the general population. CMV remains a diagnostic challenge: high IgG titers do not exclude reinfection and IgM titers stay high for several months, making it difficult to determine exact time of infection. Syphilis testing is now recommended for the initial prenatal exam. The HIV mother-to-child-transmission (MTCT) rates before, during, and after birth is estimated to be 40 percent. In some developed nations MTCT-prevention programs consisting of antiretroviral drugs to HIV-seropositive mothers and infants in combination with avoidance of breastfeeding have reduced the infection rates to less than 2 percent. In nations with limited health-care resources, the number of HIV-seropositive pregnant women receiving treatment increased to 33 percent in 2007 but further improvements remain on the agenda of the World Health Organization (WHO). Issues

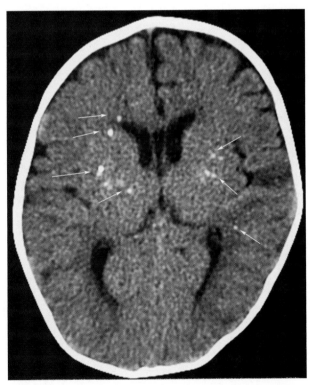

Figure 95.4. Axial noncontrast CT image in a newborn with Aicardi-Goutieres syndrome (AGS, "pseudo-TORCH") shows multiple punctate calcifications throughout the basal ganglia and around the right frontal horn and left trigone (arrows).

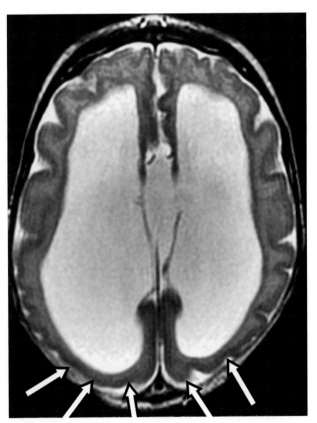

Figure 95.5. Axial T2-weighted MR image in a patient with Walker-Warburg syndrome shows ventriculomegaly and abnormal posterior cortex with thickened gray matter with pachygyria/lissencephaly (arrows), as can also be seen in congenital infections.

that threaten MTCT-prevention success rates in developed nations are racial/ethnic factors and young maternal age (teens), resulting in a delay in treatment initiation. In addition, some providers do not offer routine HIV testing to all pregnant women, and in those women that undergo testing and test seronegative initially, a seroconversion may occur later during their pregnancy and may be missed.

Key Points
- TORCH infection is a congenital condition.
- CMV is the most common etiology.
- Early gestational injury is worse.
- Calcifications are sensitive but not specific.

Further Reading
Bale JF Jr. Fetal infections and brain development. *Clin Perinatol.* 2009;36(3):639–653. Review.

Infections of the developing and mature nervous system. In: Barkovich AJ, ed. *Pediatric Neuroimaging.* Fifth edition. Philadelphia, PA: Lippincott, Williams and Wilkins; 2012:954–1050.

Kriebs JM. Breaking the cycle of infection: TORCH and other infections in women's health. *J Midwifery Womens Health.* 2008;53(3):173–174.

Kulkarni AM, Baskar S, Kulkarni ML, Kulkarni AJ, Mahuli AV, Vittalrao S, et al. Fetal intracranial calcification: pseudo-TORCH phenotype and discussion of related phenotypes. *Am J Med Genet A.* 2010;152A(4):930–937.

Malinger G, Lev D, Zahalka N, Ben Aroia Z, Watemberg N, Kidron D, et al. Fetal cytomegalovirus infection of the brain: the spectrum of sonographic findings. *AJNR Am J Neuroradiol.* 2003;24(1):28–32.

Sun MT, Yang SS, Juan CJ, Lin SH. Symmetrical brain calcifications. *Am J Med.* 2010;123(2):131–133.

Tong KA, Ashwal S, Obenaus A, Nickerson JP, Kido D, Haacke EM. Susceptibility-weighted MR imaging: a review of clinical applications in children. *AJNR Am J Neuroradiol.* 2008;29(1):9–17. Epub Oct. 9, 2007. Review.

CHAPTER 96

Acute Disseminated Encephalomyelitis

Sumit Pruthi, MD

Definition

Acute disseminated encephalomyelitis (ADEM) is generally a monophasic, nonvasculitic, inflammatory, acute demyelinating disease affecting the central nervous system (CNS), often preceded by an antecedent febrile infection or immunization and less commonly drug ingestion.

Clinical Features

Although ADEM often occurs 7 to 14 days after a viral infection or immunization, in some cases no definite history of prior infection or immunization is elicited. It usually presents with a wide range of multifocal neurologic abnormalities. The most common presenting signs/symptoms relate to motor deficits (including ataxia, paraparesis, etc.), brainstem dysfunction, and varying levels of altered consciousness. Males and females are equally affected. Though it can present at any age, ADEM is more common in children and young adults, with a mean age of 7.1 years and a peak range of 3 to 10 years of age. There is a seasonal risk with a peak in the winter and spring, the lowest incidence occurring in July and August. A single clinical event of ADEM can evolve over a period of 3 months, with fluctuations in clinical symptoms and severity and new lesions that can appear while the patient is on treatment. The clinical presentation or paraclinical tests do not allow a specific and unequivocal diagnosis of ADEM. The diagnosis is generally made after excluding other pathologies that can mimic ADEM. Cerebrospinal fluid (CSF) findings in ADEM often show evidence of inflammation and include either pleocytosis or elevated protein. Unfortunately, in many cases the CSF is normal or nonspecific with serological testing for infecting pathogens rarely being positive. The most important diagnostic tool for ADEM is brain magnetic resonance imaging (MRI). Some consider the diagnosis of ADEM only if the MRI is consistent with disseminated CNS demyelination, highlighting the importance of imaging in this patient population. High-dose corticosteroids is the treatment of choice followed by IV immunoglobulin (IVIG) and/or plasmapheresis. Prognosis is excellent for most patients.

Anatomy and Physiology

Numerous viral and bacterial pathogens and many vaccinations have been associated with ADEM. Based on pathologic similarities to experimental allergic encephalomyelitis (the animal model of inflammatory demyelination), ADEM is thought to be an autoimmune disorder where the host-cell-mediated response to an infecting pathogen cross-reacts with the myelin autoantigens in the CNS. Pathologically, this results in a diffuse perivenular inflammatory process with resultant confluent areas of demyelination with characteristic sparing of the axons.

Imaging Findings

- Moderate to large areas of demyelination (low-density on CT, prolonged T1 and T2 on MRI)
- Ill-defined, confluent bilateral lesions with asymmetric involvement (Fig. 96.1)
- Centrifugal lesions at the junction of the deep cortical gray and subcortical white matter

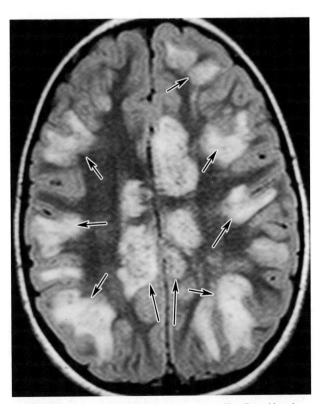

Figure 96.1. Axial FLAIR MR image in a teen with altered level of consciousness and paraparesis shows multiple foci of T2 prolongation located bilaterally and asymmetrically at the gray-white matter junction (arrows).

- Deep cerebral nuclei involvement in approximately 50 percent
- Brainstem, spinal cord, and cerebellar white matter involvement in 30 to 50 percent (Fig. 96.2)
- Variable lesion enhancement, mainly during subacute phase
- Long segment confluent lesions in the spinal cord (Fig. 96.3)
- Complete or partial resolution of lesions on followup MR confirming the monophasic nature of the disease (Fig. 96.4)
- T2 changes evolve over time with worsening of imaging findings despite clinical improvement
- Often delay in appearance of lesions on MR; normal MR does not exclude ADEM

Imaging Strategy

A CT scan of the brain may be normal and is often not helpful in establishing a diagnosis. Brain MRI with addition of spine MRI in certain appropriate clinical situations is the modality of choice for imaging these patients. The MRI is abnormal in the majority of cases and may even show early subtle features of the disseminated CNS demyelination associated with ADEM.

Related Physics

One can maximize the value of MRI by creating a protocol that has considered volume of the desired region of interest (ROI), both T1- and T2-weighted images, three orthogonal planes, and several specialized sequences. The ideal study images the smallest area to include the ROI and limited surrounding tissue. Studies that use a large field of view (FOV) will generate high signal to noise ratio (SNR) but very little detail and will often be nondiagnostic. The combination of T1 and T2 provides the anatomic detail as well as information about tissue properties such as increased free water (most commonly associated with pathology). By including all three image planes one can triangulate pathology within tissues. This can also be achieved through volumetric imaging with multiplanar reconstruction. Several special sequences are often included such as diffusion-weighted imaging in brain studies and angiographic sequences in cardiac studies.

Differential Diagnosis

- Multiple Sclerosis (see Table 96.1)
- Infectious meningoencephalitis (pial enhancement does not occur in ADEM and suggests meningoencephalitis; moreover response to corticosteroid therapy

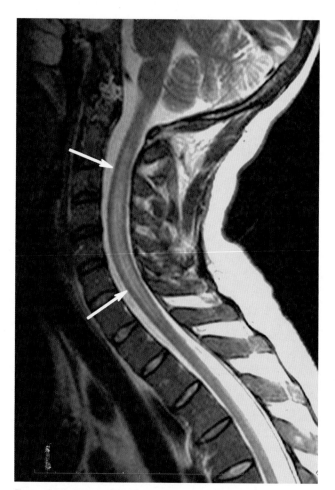

Figure 96.3. Sagittal T2 MR image of the cervical cord in a teen with dysesthesia shows a swollen cord with widespread confluent high-signal areas extending from C2 to C7 (arrows). This patient also had multiple intracranial bilateral and asymmetrical lesions at the gray-white matter junction.

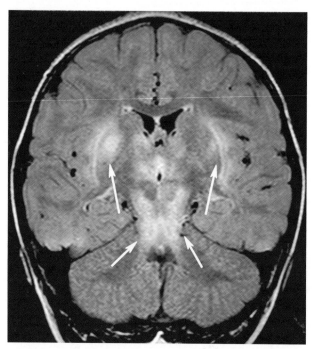

Figure 96.2. Coronal FLAIR MR image in a child with paraparesis shows abnormal hyperintensity involving bilateral basal ganglia and thalami with extension into the brainstem (arrows).

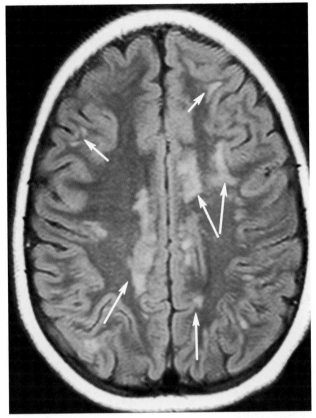

Figure 96.4. Axial FLAIR MR image in a teen with altered level of consciousness and paraparesis following 1 month of treatment with steroids shows near complete resolutions of the lesions with few residual foci of abnormal T2 prolongation (arrows).

is poor in infectious encephalitis and follow-up scans may show severe encephaloclasia)
- Collagen vascular diseases
- Vasculitis from Whipple disease, Bechets disease, primary CNS vasculitis; lesions of vasulitis often show restricted diffusion in the acute phase in contrast to increased water diffusivity of ADEM lesions
- Mitochondrial cytopathies: history & presentation are very different
- Tumor

Clinical Issues

The most important differential diagnostic consideration is multiple sclerosis (MS) with significant differences in therapeutic options and prognosis. It is difficult to make that distinction at presentation with confidence, although some of the clinical and radiologic features may point toward one or the other. Several distinguishing features are listed in Table 96.1.

In a child with a first attack, the presence of two of the following criteria favors MS over ADEM with a sensitivity of 81 percent and specificity of 95 percent:

- Absence of a diffuse bilateral lesion pattern
- Black holes (T1 hypointense lesions)
- Two or more periventricular lesions

Table 96.1 – Comparison of ADEM to Multiple Sclerosis

	ADEM	MS
Prevalence/demographics	■ Uncommon ■ Young age group ■ No sex predilection	■ Relatively common ■ Adolescents ■ Female predominance
Clinical aspects	■ Monophasic disease ■ Preceding history of infection/vaccination ■ Polysymptomatic ■ Alerted mental status & fever frequent ■ Bilateral optic neuritis ■ Excellent response to treatment with favorable prognosis	■ Multiphasic disease ■ Variable ■ Monosymptomatic ■ Rare ■ Mononuclear optic neuritis ■ Variable with relapses common
Labs	■ Elevations of the WBC of > 50 cells/millimeter can be seen ■ Oligoclonal bands variable	■ Highly atypical ■ Frequent
Imaging	a. No prior evidence of demyelination b. Extensive lesion load c. Confluent & ill-defined lesions d. Mainly along gray-white matter junction with rare involvement of corpus callosum e. Deep gray matter & posterior fossa f. Lesions can rarely be hemorrhagic g. No new lesions on follow-up MRI (after 6 months)	a. Recurrent b. Few lesions at onset c. Well-defined lesions d. Dawson's finger lesions e. Uncommon to involve deep gray or posterior fossa f. Virtually never hemorrhagic g. By definition the lesions are disseminated in space & time

Rare Variants:

- Multiphasic disseminated encephalomyelitis
- Relapsing disseminated encephalomyelitis
- Weston-Hurst syndrome: a rare hemorrhagic variant of ADEM

Key Points

- Criteria to facilitate diagnosis of ADEM include history of recent infection, a monophasic disease course, disseminated CNS disease with neurologic findings, and absence of metabolic or infectious disorders.
- CT may yield false-negative results in the presence of ADEM, despite widespread changes seen on MRI.
- Imaging may lag behind clinical progress.
- Imaging often shows widespread, bilateral multifocal, or extensive white matter lesions at the gray-white junction.
- Deep gray nuclei are frequently involved.

Further Reading

Callen DJ, Shroff MM, Branson HM, et al. Role of MRI in the differentiation of ADEM from MS in children. *Neurology.* 2009;*72*(11):968–973.

Krupp LB, Banwell B, Tenembaum S. Consensus definitions proposed for pediatric multiple sclerosis and related disorders. *Neurology.* 2007;*68*(16, Suppl 2):S7–S12.

Menge T, Hemmer B, Nessler S, et al. Acute disseminated encephalomyelitis: an update. *Arch Neurol.* 2005;*62*(11):1673–1680.

Murthy SN, Faden HS, Cohen ME, Bakshi R. Acute disseminated encephalomyelitis in children. *Pediatrics.* 2002;*110*(2 Pt 1):e21.

CHAPTER 97

Leukodystrophies

Paritosh C. Khanna, MD and Russell P. Saneto, DO, PhD

Definition

Leukodystrophies are a heterogeneous group of neurological disorders that comprise metabolic defects in the production and/or maintenance of myelin (dysmyelination), permanently delayed or deficient myelination (hypomyelination), or a frank destruction of myelin (demyelination). The most common conditions are described here.

Clinical Features

Clinical features are variable and depend on the disorder. Variability in MRI appearance within a disease entity is influenced by different ages of onset. Lifespan depends on extent of involvement with more severe forms often demonstrating more numerous and significant neurologic manifestations and early death.

Anatomy and Physiology

Diseases Initially Affecting the Periventricular White Matter

- Metachromatic leukodystrophy (MLD): lysosomal enzyme arylsulfatase-A deficiency with accumulation of sulfatide
- Krabbe disease or globoid cell leukodystrophy (GLD): lysosomal enzyme galactosylceramidase I deficiency with accumulation of cerebroside and psychosine
- X-linked adrenoleukodystrophy (ALD): peroxisomal enzyme acyl-CoA synthase deficiency with accumulation of very long chain fatty acids

Diseases Initially Affecting Subcortical White Matter

- Megalencephalic leukodystrophy (MLC): MLC1 gene mutation with large coalescent vacuoles in myelinated brain resulting in subcortical cysts and macrocephaly
- Pelizaeus-Merzbacher disease (PMD): X-linked recessive primary proteolipid protein defects result in breakdown of noncompacted myelin (T2 bright, because of bound water) resulting in patchy myelin deficiency with involvement of subcortical U-fibers and microcephaly

Metabolic Disorders Affecting Gray and White Matter

- Canavan disease: enzyme aspartoacylase deficiency with accumulation of N-Acetyl Aspartate (NAA) with macrocephaly
- Alexander disease: glial fibrillary acidic protein (GFAP) gene *de novo* mutation with increased destruction of white matter and formation of fibrous, eosinophilic deposits—Rosenthal fibers and macrocephaly

Imaging Findings

In general all conditions will have delayed myelination and abnormal white matter resulting in decreased attenuation on CT and increased T2/FLAIR signal on MRI in distributions as described below. On MR spectroscopy all will demonstrate increased choline, myoinositol; MLD may have normal and the remainder can have a decreased NAA peak. Only Canavan has an increased NAA peak.

Metachromatic Leukodystrophy

- Symmetric confluent T2-hyperintensity
- "Tigroid" and "leopard-skin" patterns of demyelination (from sparing of the perivascular spaces)
- Periventricular white matter
- Spares the subcortical U-fibers
- May have reduced or restricted diffusion in early stages
- No contrast enhancement
- Corpus callosum, internal capsule, corticospinal tracts frequently involved
- Sometimes T2-hyperintensity of cerebellar white matter
- Later, volume loss from white matter paucity

Krabbe

- Increased signal on T2/FLAIR weighted MRI involving thalamus, caudate, corona radiata and posterior limbs internal capsule signal
- Same areas show increased density on CT early in course of disease
- Optic nerves may be enlarged
- Increased diffusion noted in affected white matter
- Enhancement of lumbar nerve roots on spine MRI

(A)

(B)

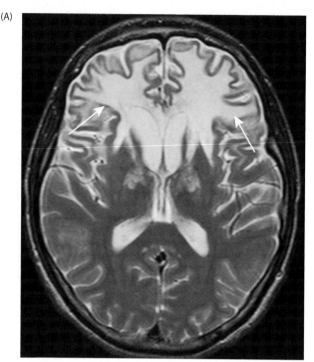

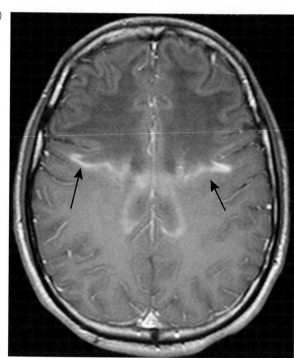

Figure 97.1. Axial T2 (A) and contrast-enhanced T1 (B) MR images in a 16-year-old male with anisocoria and changing pupil exam shows *predominantly frontal* lobe involvement with hyperintense frontal subcortical, deep and periventricular white matter signal with enhancement of the actively inflamed zone of the leading edge (small arrows) in this patient with variant x-linked adrenal leukodystrophy. Note bifrontal lateral ventriculomegaly from volume loss.

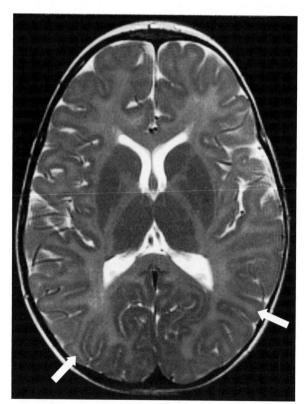

Figure 97.2. Axial T2 (A) and parasagittal T1 (B) MR images in a 4-year-old girl with macrocephaly and seizures demonstrate diffuse T2 white matter signal abnormality with sparing of internal capsules and subcortical CSF-equivalent cysts (white arrows) consistent with megalencephalic leukodystrophy with subcortical cysts.

X-Linked Adrenoleukodystrophy

- Posterior periventricular white matter involvement but may be frontal in children presenting at older age (Fig 97.1a and b).
- Three-zone pattern:
  - Innermost: T1-hypointense, T2-hyperintense (gliosis and scarring).
  - Intermediate: active inflammation and breakdown in the blood-brain barrier. T2-isointense/hypointense, enhances (actively inflamed).
  - Outer: T2-hyperintense, nonenhancing (leading edge of active demyelination). Symmetric T2-hyperintensity along descending pyramidal tracts is common. Increased diffusion noted in affected white matter.

Megalencephalic Leukodystrophy

- Subcortical CSF-equivalent cysts on all sequences and on CT
- Diffuse T2/FLAIR white matter signal abnormality with sparing of internal capsules (Fig 97.2)

Pelizaeus-Merzbacher Disease

- Near-complete lack of myelination
- Diffuse homogeneous T2-hyperintensity involving subcortical U-fibers
- Early involvement of internal capsule
- Rarely, heterogeneous or "tigroid" pattern of myelination caused by preserved myelin islands in perivascular areas

(A)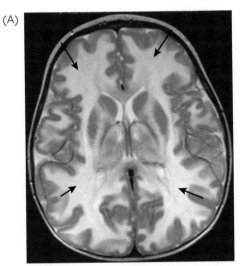

(B)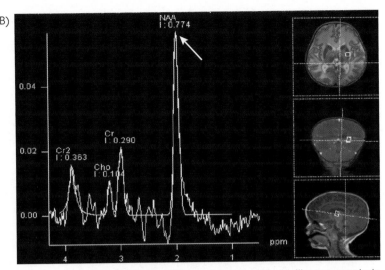

Figure 97.3. Axial T2 MRI (A) and MRI spectroscopy image at TE of 135 milliseconds (B) in an 8-month-old boy with macrocephaly and developmental delay show diffuse T2-hyperintensity (black arrows) involving white matter, including the subcortical U-fibers, internal and external capsules, and a prominent NAA peak (white arrow) consistent with Canavan disease.

Canavan

- Increased globus pallidus and thalamic signal noted on T2/FLAIR-weighted MRI early in course of disease
- May have reduced or restricted diffusion
- Diffuse T1-hypointensity and T2-hyperintensity involving white matter, with preferential involvement of subcortical U-fibers early in the disease (Fig 97.3a)
- Rapidly progressive disease has associated internal and external capsules and cerebellar white matter involvement
- Conspicuous volume loss in later stages
- Markedly elevated NAA on MR spectroscopy (Fig 97.3b)

Alexander

- Frontal lobe periventricular, deep and subcortical white matter typically affected
- Hypoattenuating on CT with periventricular T1-hyperintense/T2-hypointense band that may enhance (Fig 97.4a and b)
- Increased diffusion with loss of fractional anisotropy sometimes seen
- Subcortical white matter affected early
- Hyperintensity progresses posteriorly and to the internal and external capsules
- Cysts may develop in affected areas
- Other potentially enhancing areas: near tips of frontal horns, basal ganglia and thalami, optic chiasm, dentate nuclei and brainstem

IMAGING PITFALLS: Failure to include contrast-enhanced MRI and MRS in the protocol may result in diagnostic errors.

Imaging Strategy

Imaging should include the following sequences: Sagittal and axial T1 or T1-inversion recovery (inversion recovery) in children less than 1 year of age accentuates gray-white differentiation); axial T2; coronal T2; axial FLAIR; axial diffusion with ADC mapping; postcontrast three-plane T1; MR spectroscopy with evaluation of affected and normal-appearing white matter.

Related Physics

A method to interrogate brain chemistry noninvasively is MR spectroscopy (MRS). In MRS, each metabolite has a characteristic resonant frequency that can be encoded and identified. The metabolic elements that are most commonly evaluated are 1H (proton), 23Na (sodium), and 31P (phosphorus). There are two techniques for performing MRS: STEAM and PRESS. The acronym "STEAM" stands for stimulated echo acquisition mode, in which three 90-degree pulses are applied with short echo time (TE) and signals are averaged to generate a spectrum. This short-TE mode generates spectra for some metabolites that are particular to the developing infant brain such as myoinositol. The acronym "PRESS" stands for point resolved spectroscopy in which a 90–180–180 train of pulses is applied generating signal at an intermediate to long TE with greater signal-to-noise ratio (SNR). There are three common modes: single voxel, "slice" (2-D), and "volume" (3-D). It follows that with this progression there is an associated increase in SNR at the expense of time. Typical voxel dimension is 8 cm^3 which is extremely large by MR-imaging standards but is necessary to include enough nuclei to generate adequate SNR. In general the imaging time is equal to the product of the number of voxels in each dimension given by $t = TR \cdot Nx \cdot Ny \cdot Nz$, (where t = time, TR = repetition time,

(A)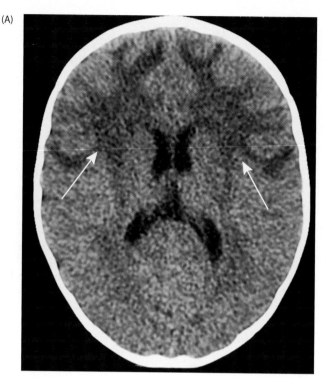

(B)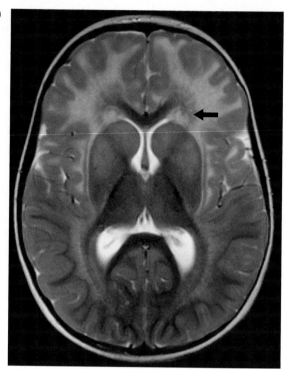

Figure 97.4. Axial unenhanced CT (A) and axial T2 MRI (B) images in a 13-month-old female with new onset seizure, residual paralysis, and posturing show decreased density on CT (white arrows) in the frontal lobe periventricular, deep and subcortical white matter and periventricular T2-hypointense band (black arrow) with T2 hyperintensity involving the deep and subcortical white matter consistent with Alexander disease.

N = number of voxels, and x, y, and z are each dimension). MR spectroscopy is more sensitive than specific to the presence of disease, however there are several conditions where MRS can be quite specific such as Canavan's Disease (markedly elevated NAA), peroxisomal disorders (abnormal peak at 3.35 ppm), maple syrup urine disease (abnormal peak at 0.9 to 1.0 ppm) and Leigh's disease spectrum (abnormal lactate peak).

Differential Diagnosis

- Acute disseminated encephalomyelitis (ADEM)
- Meningoencephalitis
- Hypoxic-ischemic encephalopathy
- Multiple Sclerosis
- Radiation and chemotherapy-induced leukoencephalopathy

Common Variants

X-linked adrenoleukodystrophy: atypical cases with unilateral or predominantly frontal lobe involvement may occur.

Clinical Issues

Long-term management is mainly supportive in most of the children that survive and with milder disease.

Key Points

- Anterior: Alexander
- Posterior: ALD
- Contrast-enhancing: both Alexander and ALD
- Macrocephaly: Alexander, Canavan
- Diffuse: Canavan (starts at U-fibers), MLD (spares U-fibers), Krabbe's (dense thalamus on CT), Pelizaeus-Merzbacher (homogeneous T2 signal)

Further Reading

Metabolic, toxic and inflammatory brain disorders. In: Barkovich AJ, ed. *Pediatric Neuroimaging*. Fifth edition. Philadelphia, PA: Lippincott, Williams and Wilkins; 2012:81–216.

Hypomyelination and leukodystrophies. In: Barkovich AJ, Moore KR, Jones, BV, et al., eds. *Diagnostic Imaging. Pediatric Neuroradiology*. First edition. Salt Lake City, UT: Amirsys; 2007:I1/44–1/51.

Cheon JE, Kim IO, Hwang YS, et al. Leukodystrophy in children: a pictorial review of MR imaging features. *Radiographics*. 2002;22(3):461–476.

Phelan JA, Lowe LH, Glasier CM. Pediatric neurodegenerative white matter processes: leukodystrophies and beyond. *Pediatr Radiol.* 2008; *38*(7):729–749. Epub Apr 30, 2008.

Schiffmann R, van der Knaap MS. Invited Article: An MRI-based approach to the diagnosis of white matter disorders. *Neurology.* 2009;*72*(8):750–759.

Steenweg ME, Vanderver A, Blaser S, et al. Magnetic resonance imaging pattern recognition in hypomyelinating disorders. *Brain.* 2010;*133*(10):2971–2982.

van der Knaap MS, Valk J. *Magnetic Resonance of Myelination and Myelin Disorders.* Third edition. Springer-Verlag Berlin Heidelberg 2005.

CHAPTER 98

Mitochondrial Cytopathies

Paritosh C. Khanna, MD and Russell P. Saneto, DO, PhD

Definition

Mitochondrial cytopathies (MCs) are a heterogeneous group of neurological disorders that demonstrate varied biochemical, neuroimaging, and clinical features, all of which have their origins in genetically determined mitochondrial dysfunction. Most disorders are related to abnormal activity of the five electron transport chain (ETC) subunits involved in oxidative phosphorylation or, less commonly, calcium homeostasis, innate immunity, and apoptosis.

Clinical Features

Incidence is 1:4,000. Although most patients demonstrate neurologic symptoms, some may have nonspecific symptoms and can demonstrate a fluctuating course that may result in variable presentations. Common neurologic symptoms include ataxia, external ophthalmoplegia, ptosis, gastrointestinal dysmotility and vomiting, peripheral neuropathy, swallowing and respiratory problems, dystonia, and seizures. Other patients present with episodic paresis, stroke-like episodes, hypotonia and psychomotor delay, and regression.

Characteristic clinical presentations for the more common mitochondrial cytopathies are described below:

Mitochondrial Encephalomyopathy, Lactic Acidosis, and Stroke-like episodes (MELAS): this is a progressive neurodegenerative disease that often presents with migraines preceding stroke-like events resulting in refractory partial seizures, muscle weakness, deafness, and slow progressive dementia.

Leigh's Syndrome: Leigh's is a progressive neurodegenerative disease that typically presents with delay in reaching developmental milestones, spasticity, brainstem dysfunction, dystonia, and abnormal eye movements. Many other organs are also affected.

Kearns-Sayre syndrome (KSS): this is a neurodegenerative disorder characterized by intellectual disabilities, progressive ophthalmoplegia, and ptosis. Other organ involvement manifests with complete heart block, cardiomyopathy, sensorineural hearing loss, and endocrine abnormalities.

Alpers syndrome: also known as hepatocerebral disease, Alpers is characterized by treatment-resistant seizures, psychomotor regression, and liver impairment.

Glutaric Aciduria (GA) type 1: GA type 1 is a neurodegenerative disease that commonly presents with neonatal macrocephaly and progresses to cerebral palsy-like signs including spasticity, muscle weakness and decreased tone. GA type 2 often appears in infancy with sudden metabolic crisis, acidosis, and low blood sugar.

Anatomy and Physiology

The heterogeneity of disease results from the involvement of two genomes, at the nuclear and mitochondrial level. This dual control results in a variety of clinical presentations and organ involvement caused by disordered ATP metabolism. There are a few defined syndromes as noted below, but many disorders do not have a well-defined phenotype because of genome interactions and other yet unknown modifying mechanisms.

MELAS: about 80% of patients have a mutation, adenine to guanine transition at the tRNA for leucine at position 3243 in the maternal origin mitochondrial DNA (mtDNA).

Leigh's Syndrome: this group of disorders results from multiple nuclear and mtDNA mutations including defects/deficiency of pyruvate dehydrogenase, cytochrome oxidase (ETC: complex IV), ATPase complex (ETC: complex V) mutations and other subunits and assembly factors of ETC enzyme complexes.

KSS: this results from an mtDNA deletion ranging from several bases up to seven kilobases resulting histopathologically in spongiform changes involving both gray and white matter of the tegmentum, basal ganglia, and white matter of the cerebrum and cerebellum.

Alpers Syndrome: Alpers results from an mtDNA depletion that presents at various ages depending on the type of mutation within the nuclear gene, polymerase gamma 1 gene (POLG).

Glutaric Aciduria: type 1 is caused by deficiency of glutaryl CoA dehydrogenase; GA type 2 results from deficiency in either electron-transfer flavoprotein or electron-transfer flavoprotein dehydrogenase. Both disorders are nuclear gene mutations.

Others: mitochondrial neuro-gastrointestinal encephalomyopathy (MNGIE), Myoclonus, Epilepsy with Ragged Red Fibers (MERRF), autosomal recessive/dominant progressive external ophthalmoplegia, Pearson syndrome, Leber hereditary optic neuropathy, retinitis pigmentosa, Friedrich's ataxia, etc.

Imaging Findings

MRI is one of the many diagnostic tools used in conjunction with biochemical testing and biopsy to arrive at the diagnosis of a ME. An MRI may be normal, may have nonspecific findings or may demonstrate strong pointers to underlying disease. MR spectroscopy demonstrates elevated lactate in most cases, however absence of this finding does not exclude an ME.

General features: these are variable with regions of brain destruction, volume loss, and mineralization. Disease typically affects both gray and white matter. There is bilateral, symmetric involvement of basal ganglia in many disorders: edema with/without restricted diffusion in the acute phase and atrophy in the chronic phase. The thalami, brainstem and deep cerebellar gray nuclei may also be involved. Subdural hemorrhages are noted in some cases.

MELAS (Fig. 98.1): stroke-like lesions, not conforming to known arterial territories and without venous etiology, with restricted diffusion and T2/FLAIR abnormalities involving the cortex. Multiple, temporally separated, transient and fluctuating episodes are characteristic.

Leigh's syndrome (Fig. 98.2): prototype mitochondrial disease, with hallmark neuroimaging findings. Progressive signal abnormalities, most frequency in the lentiform nuclei and caudate nuclei, but abnormalities involving the thalamus, periaquiductal gray, tegmentum, red nuclei, and dentate nuclei can be seen.

KSS (Fig. 98.3): increased CT attenuation of basal ganglia from mineralization. Cerebral and cerebellar atrophy often with T2/FLAIR hyperintense bilateral lesions observed in subcortical white matter, thalamus, basal ganglia (substantia nigra and globus pallidus), and brainstem.

Alpers syndrome: T2/FLAIR hyperintensities in the majority of patients within the occipital regions, deep cerebellar nuclei, thalamus, and basal ganglia. However, MRI can be normal.

Glutaric Aciduria types 1 and 2(Fig. 98.4). Enlarged extra-axial spaces and Sylvian fissures (secondary to prominent volume loss) in GA types 1 and 2. Subdural hematomas in GA type 1 secondary to stretched bridging veins. GA type 1 shows symmetrically decreased FDG-PET uptake in the basal ganglia, thalami, insular cortex.

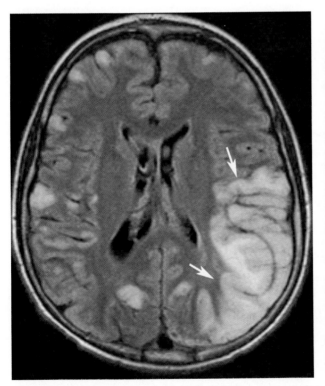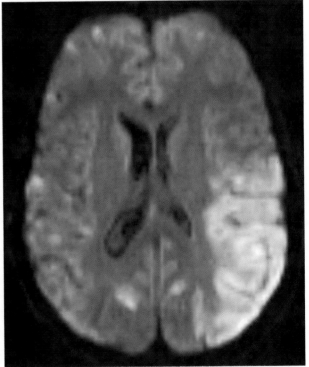

Figure 98.1. Axial FLAIR (A) and axial DWI (B) MR images in an 8-year-old male, normal until age 4 years, with right-sided paresis show a large area of FLAIR signal abnormality involving the left posterior temporal and parieto-occipital regions (arrows) with scattered cortical foci of abnormality in the right and left cerebral cortex. These areas show diffusion restriction on axial trace diffusion images suggesting a stroke-like episode consistent with MELAS.

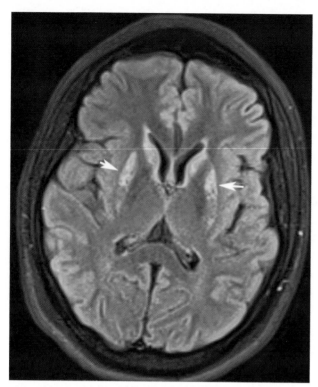
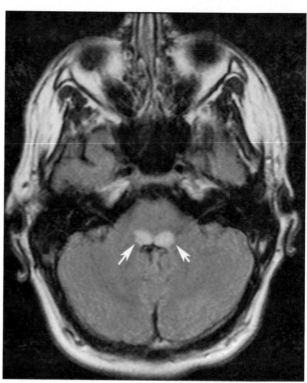

Figure 98.2. Axial FLAIR (A) MR image in an 18-year-old male with progressive dysphagia, dyspnea, and diplopia demonstrates abnormal increased FLAIR signal within the entirety of the bilateral caudate heads and putamina (arrows) with cystic foci within the anterior aspect of the putamen and cerebellar volume loss (not shown). Axial FLAIR (B) MR image in another patient demonstrates symmetric foci of FLAIR signal abnormality in the dorsal pons (arrows). Patients had cytochrome oxidase deficiency (Leigh's).

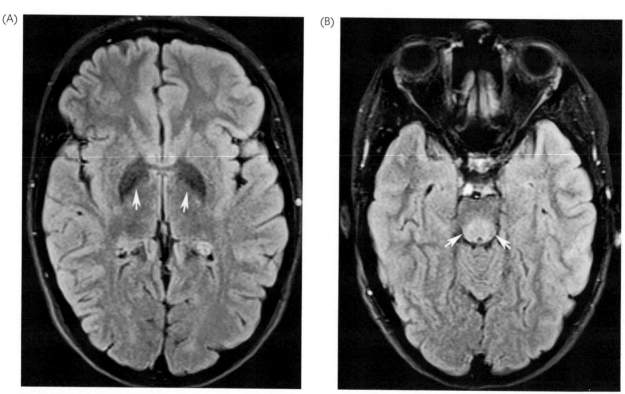

Figure 98.3. Axial FLAIR(A) MR image in a 15-year-old female, normal until age 10 years, with ophthalmoplegia, ptosis, and cardiac pacemaker shows greater than expected hypointense signal involving the globus pallidi (arrows). Axial FLAIR (B) MR image shows increased signal in periaqueductal gray matter extending into the brainstem (arrows) consistent with Kearns-Sayre syndrome (7 kb mtDNA deletion).

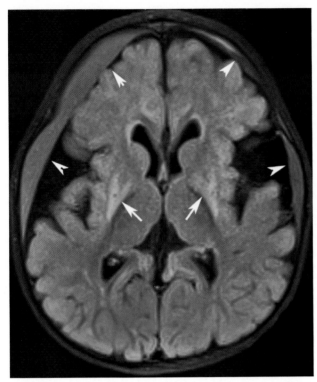 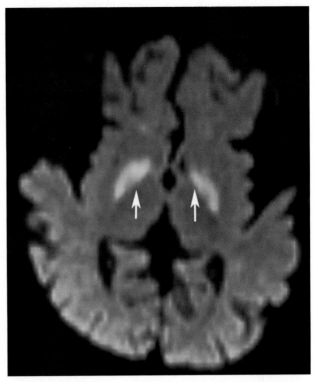

Figure 98.4. Axial FLAIR (A) MR image of a 1-month-old male with developmental delay demonstrates bilateral subacute subdural hemorrhages (arrowheads) with symmetric putaminal signal abnormality (arrows) consistent with GA type 1. Axial trace diffusion (B) MR image of another patient demonstrates restricted diffusion in bilateral putamina and globus pallidi (arrows); this acute exacerbation was precipitated by systemic infection and was consistent with GA type 2. In both patients there is significant bifrontal and peri-Sylvian volume loss with symmetric prominence of extraaxial spaces.

> **IMAGING PITFALLS:** Normal MRI and MRS do not exclude MC.

Imaging Strategy

Imaging should include the following sequences: Sagittal and axial T1; axial T2; coronal T2; axial FLAIR; axial diffusion with ADC mapping; postcontrast three-plane T1; MR spectroscopy with evaluation of affected and normal-appearing white matter and deep gray structures (highest concentration of mitochondria).

Related Physics

Brain chemistry can be interrogated noninvasively with MR spectroscopy (MRS). The nuclei most commonly evaluated are 1H (proton), 23Na (sodium), 31P (phosphorus). Proton spectroscopy provides the highest signal-to-noise because of the large amount of water. In pediatric neuroimaging, MRS has been used to further characterize tumors, stroke, seizure foci, metabolic disorders, infections, and leukodystrophies. MR spectroscopy produces a spectrum and not an image. The spectrum represents all metabolites in a voxel that has been manually placed in pathologic tissue by the radiologist. The metabolites generate spectral peaks that are at frequencies determined by their chemical structure and are distributed in a frequency range between 63 and 64 megahertz. Spectral information is converted to parts per million concentrations by integration of area under the peaks, and values are qualitatively reported as ratios of the major metabolites or relative heights of the peaks. It is important to place the voxel in brain and away from bone and scalp where there is a high fat content. A water-suppression technique is applied using either chemical shift selective (CHESS) or inversion recovery technique. The two main MRS techniques are stimulated echo acquisition mode (STEAM) and point resolved spectroscopy (PRESS). The STEAM mode is similar to GRE in applying a 90-degree refocusing pulse to collect signal; TE can be much shorter at the expense of signal to noise ratio (SNR). The spin echo technique of PRESS uses a 180-degree refocusing pulse generating higher SNR.

Differential Diagnosis

- Hypoxic ischemic encephalopathy in the neonate with symmetric restricted diffusion involving the basal ganglia
- Encephalitis
- Neurofibromatosis type 1
- Wilson disease
- Kernicterus
- Molybdenum cofactor deficiency

Common Variants

MELAS: diffuse white matter lesions are occasionally noted, involving periventricular white matter, centrum semiovale and corpus callosum.

Leigh's syndrome: the cytochrome-oxidase-deficient subtype demonstrates symmetric brainstem and cerebellar T2/FLAIR signal abnormalities.

Clinical Issues

Diagnosis may not be apparent until later in patients with milder forms of enzyme deficiency or in the face of stressful events such as infection or other metabolic stressors. Treatment for these disorders is challenging. In general, therapy includes the use of antioxidants, vitamins, replacement of respiratory chain cofactors, changes in diet, and medications treating specific symptoms (i.e., cardiac dysfunction and seizures).

Key Points

- Symmetric deep gray signal abnormality in earlier stages
- Volume loss, mineralization in later stages
- Punctate signal abnormality in basal ganglia, brainstem, and cerebellum in Leigh's

- Transient, recurrent, nonvascular strokes in MELAS
- Subdural collection in GA type 1
- Age of abnormal imaging presentation variable, may be brought out by stressors and heteroplasmy

Further Reading

Toxic and metabolic brain disorders. In: Barkovich AJ, ed. *Pediatric Neuroimaging*. Fifth edition. Philadelphia, PA: Lippincott, Williams and Wilkins;2012:81–226.

Hypomyelination and leukodystrophies. In: *Diagnostic Imaging. In:* Barkovich AJ, Moore KR, Jones, BV, et al., eds. *Pediatric Neuroradiology*. First edition. Salt Lake City, UT: Amirsys; 2007:I1/52–1/55.

Saneto RP, Friedman SD, Shaw DW. Neuroimaging of mitochondrial disease. *Mitochondrion*. 2008;8(5–6):396–413.

Schiffmann R, van der Knaap MS. Invited Article: An MRI-based approach to the diagnosis of white matter disorders. *Neurology*. 2009;72(8):750–759.

Strauss KA, Lazovic J, Wintermark M, Morton DH. Multimodal imaging of striatal degeneration in Amish patients with glutaryl-CoA dehydrogenase deficiency. *Brain*. 2007;130(Pt 7):1905–1920.

van der Knaap MS, Valk J. *Magnetic Resonance of Myelination and Myelin Disorders*. Third edition. Springer-Verlag Berlin Heidelberg 2005.

CHAPTER 99

Atlantoaxial Instability and Injuries

Crystal Sachdeva, MD and Jeffrey C. Hellinger, MD

Definition

Atlantoaxial instability (AAI) and injuries refers to underlying laxity of ligaments, abnormal osseous development, and/or acquired osseous or ligamentous abnormalities which impact the integrity of the articulation between the first (C1, atlas) and second (C2, axis) cervical vertebrae, leading to secondary osseous injury, spinal cord compression, or a combination thereof.

Clinical Features

In absence of predisposing factors, AAI is rare. Among those with underlying risk factors, most are asymptomatic. Diagnosis is typically made during screening radiography performed for baseline surveillance or medical clearance in patients with risk factors for AAI. Symptoms may be acute, subacute, or chronic. Nonspecific symptoms include headaches, neck pain, limited range of neck motion (in particular with flexion), and torticollis. Depending upon the degree of cord and cervical nerve compression, neurologic symptoms may include occipital neuropathy, postauricular pain and tenderness, upper-extremity paresthesia, distal muscle weakness, spasticity, gait disturbance, bowel/bladder dysfunction, and quadriplegia. Vertebral-basilar artery insufficiency may result if there is vascular compression. On physical exam, abnormal range of neck motion may be present, abnormally aligned cervical vertebrae may be palpated, and upper-extremity radiating parethesias may be elicited using a Spurling maneuver (axial load on the head with neck extension and lateral rotation toward each shoulder). Instability is confirmed by performing upper-extremity sensory, motor, and reflex neurologic exams with the neck in neutral position and in flexion.

Anatomy and Physiology

The atlantoaxial articulation is comprised of three synovial joints functioning as one unit. These joints include a median and two lateral articulations. The median atlantoaxial joint is located between the posterior surface of the anterior arch of C1 and the anterior surface of the dens of C2. Joint integrity is supported by the transverse, apical, and alar ligaments. The lateral articulations are between the inferior articular facets of the C1 lateral mass and the superior articular facets of the C2 lateral mass; joints are supported by capsular ligaments to the articular surfaces. The atlantoaxial articulation maintains cervical spine alignment, spinal canal morphology, and spinal cord function during cervical spine motion. Normal motion for the atlantoaxial unit consists of a combination of pivotal and translational rotary rotation. The median articulation is important for cervical spine lateral rotation, whereas the lateral joints are important for anterior-posterior rotation and transmitting the weight of the skull. During flexion and extension, the transverse and alar ligaments limit the posterior motion of the odontoid process in relation to the anterior arch of C1. Increased laxity and instability between the body of the atlas and the odontoid process of the axis will result in increased mobility at the C1-C2 articulation. Mobility may occur in anterior, posterior, or lateral directions during normal or abnormal flexion, extension, distraction, and/or rotational strain and related mechanical forces, resulting in variable subluxation to complete dislocation of C1 and C2 with secondary fractures; all injuries should be considered unstable. Posterior subluxation (e.g., cervical spine hyperflexion or hyperextension) may result in spinal cord impingement with the potential for neurologic compromise and occasionally death. Children younger than 8 years are prone to injury to the C1-C3 vertebrae as the fulcrum of motion is at the C2-C3 level and children have increased spinal mobility because of weak cervical musculature, increased head to body size, ligament laxity, immature vertebral joints, and angled articular facets. These factors contribute to high torque and shearing factors at the atlantoaxial joint, with rotatory subluxation being the more common mechanism of injury in this age group. Additional predisposing conditions include:

Congenital
- C1 anterior arch hypoplasia
- C1 occipitalization
- Odontoid aplasia
- Odontoid hypoplasia
- Os terminale
- Os odontoideum (Fig. 99.1)
- C1 anterior arch hypoplasia

Inflammatory
- Ankylosing spondylitis
- Psoriatic arthritis

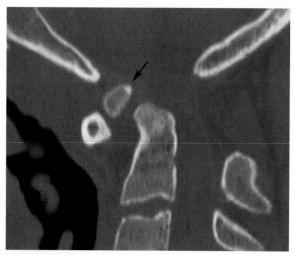

Figure 99.1. Cervical spine CT confirms the antlantoaxial subluxation and demonstrates an os terminale (arrow), which is separate from, unfused, and angulated in its relationship to the dens.

- Reiter syndrome
- Rheumatoid arthritis (25%)
- Systemic lupus erythema

Syndromic
- Trisomy 21 (15 to 25%)
- Marfan syndrome

Infectious
- Alveolar abscess
- Cervical adenitis
- Mastoiditis
- Otitis media
- Retropharyngeal abscess (Fig. 99.2)
- Osteomyelitis
- Discitis

Traumatic
- Chronic (e.g., repetitive)
- Remote (e.g., nonunion)

Among individuals with Trisomy 21, the frequency of asymptomatic AAI is 10 to 20 percent (Fig. 99.3). Symptomatic AAI occurs in 1 to 2 percent of patients with Trisomy 21. In patients with rheumatoid arthritis, cervical involvement occurs in 25 to 80 percent.

Imaging Findings

Suspected fractures, subluxations, and soft-tissue injuries should be distinguished from normal variant anatomy. The relationship between the anterior arch of C1 and the odontoid process (dens) of C2 is used to evaluate for instability such that AAI in children is defined by an atlantodental interval (ADI) of greater than 5 millimeters between the

(A)

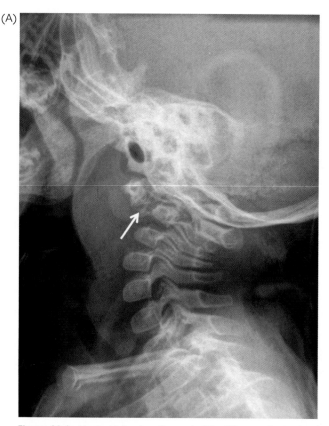

(B)

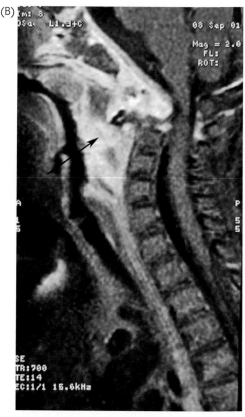

Figure 99.2. Neutral lateral radiograph (A) of the cervical spine in a 6-year-old girl with fever, neck pain, neck swelling, and limited range of motion, who was found to have a retropharengeal abscess with C1-C2 osteomyelitis and instability demonstrates moderately extensive prevertebral soft-tissue swelling with widening of the AAI (white arrow). Sagittal T2 MR image of the cervical spine (B) demonstrates extensive inflammation anterior to the cervical spine (black arrow), infiltrating the C1-C2 articulation.

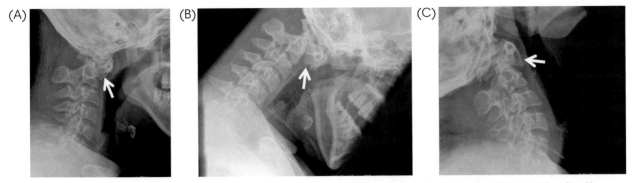

Figure 99.3. Neutral (A), flexion (B), and extension (C) lateral radiographs of the cervical spine in a 17-year-old male with Trisomy 21 and C1-C2 instability demonstrate fixed C1-C2 subluxation with significant widening (arrows) of the AAI (9 mm) (white arrows).

C1 arch and the dens (Fig. 99.4). Of critical importance is recognition of discontinuous anterior cervical, posterior cervical, or spinolaminar lines on a lateral projection, malalignment of the C1 and C2 lateral masses on a frontal projection, malalignment of the C1 arch and the dens on a frontal projection and an abnormal ADI on a lateral projection (Fig. 99.5).

Altantoaxial instability is classified as follows:

Type I: <3-millimeter anterior rotatory displacement of C1 on C2 (intact transverse ligament).
Type II: 3- to 5-millimeter anterior displacement of C1 on C2 with one of the lateral masses serving as a pivot point (probable transverse ligament injury). The distance narrows between the posterior C1 arch and the dens, typically <1.8 millimeters.
Type III: > 5-millimeter anterior displacement of C1 on C2 (transverse and/or alar ligament injury).
Type IV: posterior displacement of C1 on C2.

Soft-tissue edema or hemorrhage causes widening of the retropharyngeal or retrotracheal space, widening of the prevertebral space with displacement of the fat stripe, and deviation of the larynx or trachea. Signs of abnormal vertebral body alignment include a loss of normal lordosis, acute kyphotic angulation, torticollis, widening of the interspinous distance, and rotation of the vertebral bodies. Widening of joint articulations and fractures may be directly visualized using frontal, lateral, or oblique projections. The odontoid radiograph is most useful for identifying congenital anomalies and fractures of the dens as well as rotational displacement of the dens relative to the C1 arch and malalignment of the lateral masses. Key findings may include a decrease in the ADI with widening of the lateral masses, ipsilateral to rotation and increase in the ADI with narrowing of the lateral masses, contralateral to rotation. Both CT and MRI will depict the degree of spinal canal narrowing and cord compression. Spinal cord compression will result in increased signal intensity on T2.

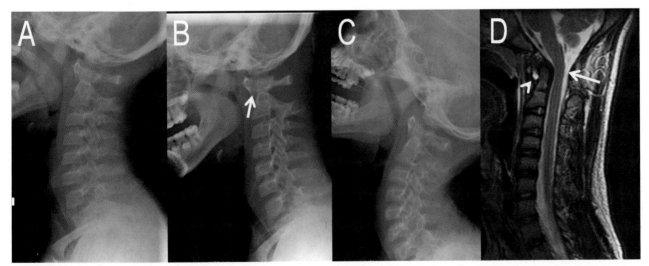

Figure 99.4. Neutral (A), flexion (B), and extension (C) lateral radiographs of the cervical spine in an 18-year-old female with Trisomy 21 and C1-C2 instability demonstrate a normal AAI on neutral and extension positioning, with moderate widening (7.5 mm) of the AAI during flexion (arrow). Sagittal T2 MR image (D) confirms anterior subluxation of C1 on C2. In addition, there is fluid in the C1-C2 articulation (arrowhead). Subluxation results in mild anterior thecal sac effacement (arrow) without cord atrophy or signal abnormality.

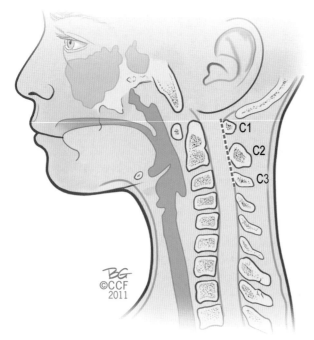

Figure 99.5. Both this lines in the pediatric cervical spine. Spinolaminar line is a smooth continuous line at C1-C3 (red dotted line).

Imaging Strategy

A child with a history of head, neck, or spine trauma, and/or symptoms suggestive of spinal cord impingement should have cervical spine radiography with a minimum of anteroposterior (AP), lateral, and odontoid (open-mouth) radiographs. If these studies are negative and there remains a high index of suspicion, real-time flexion and extension radiographs should be obtained. Alternatively, if instability is detected or known, flexion and extension views may be obtained to evaluate the degree of mobility. A CT scan should be obtained when the radiographs are suboptimal and have not answered the clinical questions and for more detailed assessment of fractures, subluxations, or dislocations identified on radiographs (Fig. 99.6). An MRI should be performed for evaluation of soft tissues, spinal cord, discs, ligaments, edema, and hemorrhage.

Related Physics

For cross-sectional imaging, spatial resolution is determined by the size of the voxels which have coordinates in the x, y and z directions. In MRI these are referred to as phase, frequency (readout), and slice-select directions. Spatial resolution and noise are competing properties. Reducing voxel size will increase spatial resolution at the expense of increased noise resulting from decrease in signal. At the MRI console one can manipulate all three dimensions of the voxel independently. The x-y direction in axial imaging refers to the phase and frequency directions and their product is referred

to as the "matrix size." A larger matrix size will give higher resolution. Increasing the number of phase encoding steps will incur a time penalty, whereas increasing the number of frequency encoding steps will not. By decreasing the slice thickness in the z direction (effectively increasing the number of slices in the same volume) one would require several stepped acquisitions through the entire volume at the expense of time. One strategy for more complete anatomic coverage in the slice-select direction without increased time from additional acquisitions is to increase the interslice gap while maintaining the slice thickness and resolution. In general the gap does not exceed 30 percent of the slice thickness. In summary, the voxel is usually square in the x-y plane with customarily a larger z dimension.

Differential Diagnosis

- Brachial plexus injury
- Cervical spine disease
- Concussion
- Repetitive head injury
- Thoracic outlet syndrome
- Torticollis
- Vertebral and disc injury
- Sprain/strain injuries
- Discogenic pain syndrome
- Facet syndrome
- Radiculopathy

Common Variants

Normal anatomic variants that may simulate AAI or injury include the following:

- Pseudosubluxation: physiologic anteroposterior offset of cervical spine vertebral bodies secondary to ligamentous laxity; occurs frequently at C2-C3. The posterior cervical line difference is < 2millimeters.
- Overriding anterior atlas arch onto the odontoid process: occurs in 20% of children up to 4 years of age.
- Cervical spine straightening with absence of lordosis: seen up to the age of 16 years and is demonstrated by a widened C1-C2 space upon flexion.
- Prominent prevertebral soft tissues during respiration: this will occur during expiration and may be a normal finding in infants.

Clinical Issues

When symptomatic, AAI warrants treatment. Unstable injuries are treated surgically with fusion of C1-C2 vertebrae. Postoperative complications may include hemorrhage into the spinal canal and paralysis from cord compression. Postoperative imaging includes radiographs, CT, and MRI. Given the potential for serious neurologic sequelae from AAI, it is recommended that patients with risk factors

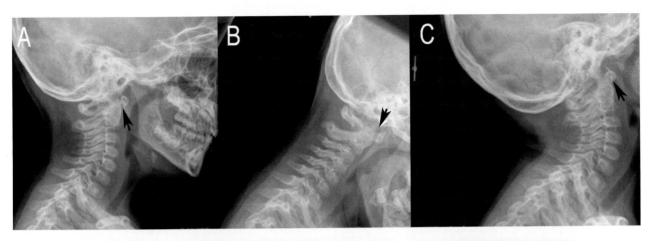

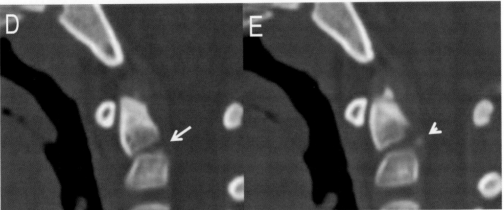

Figure 99.6. Neutral (A), flexion (B), and extension (C) lateral radiographs of the cervical spine in a 4-year-old girl in a restrained motor vehicle crash who sustained a dens fracture with C1-C2 instability demonstrate a normal AAI in neutral and at extension, with mild widening of the AAI during flexion (3.5 mm) (black arrows). Cervical spine sagittal CT images (D, E) demonstrate an angulated, oblique transverse fracture through the base of the dens (white arrow), associated with a small posterior fracture fragment (arrowhead).

undergo screening neurologic consultation with cervical spine radiography. If AAI is identified, patients are typically restricted from activities that require moderate to extensive flexion and extension motion.

Key Points

- AAI results in increased mobility between the first two cervical vertebrae and can cause severe neurological symptoms if there is associated spinal cord compression.
- Common risks for AAI include Trisomy 21 and rheumatoid arthritis.
- Children < 8 years of age may sustain injury to C1C3 spine.
- An ADI > 3 mm may be suggestive for AAI, with definite AAI when ADI >5 mm.
- Common physiological variants of the pediatric spine can simulate AAI.

Further Reading

Hockberger RS, Kirshenbaum KJ, Doris PE. Spinal injuries. In: Rosen P, et al., eds. *Emergency Medicine: Concepts and Clinical Practice.* Fourth edition. St. Louis, MO: Mosby-Year Book; 1998.

Leshin L. Down syndrome and craniovertebral instability: topic review and treatment recommendations. *Pediatric Neurosurgery.* 1999; *31*(2):71–77.

Lustrin SB, Karakas SP, Ortiz AO, et al. Pediatric cervical spine: normal anatomy, variants, and trauma. *RadioGraphics.* 2003;23:539–560.

Nontraumatic subluxation. In: Beers MH, et al., eds. *The Merck Manual.* Eighteenth edition. West Point: Merck & Co; 2006:328–329.

CHAPTER 100

Dermoids and Epidermoids

Christopher Daub, MD, Zachary Bailey, MD, and Lisa H. Lowe, MD

Definition

Dermoids and epidermoids are unilocular, ectoderm-lined cysts that can present at numerous locations throughout the body. Unlike teratomas, they are not neoplasms. The clinical features and characteristics of these masses are dependent on their location and contents. Epidermoids consist of squamous epithelium lining and internal debris mostly consisting of desquamated keratin and cholesterol. Dermoids contain dermal appendages (sebaceous glands, hair, etc.) in addition to squamous epithelial lining. The varied contents of dermoids accounts for their complex imaging features.

Clinical Features

Dermoids tend to present in midline locations, and epidermoids are typically located off midline. Periorbital/facial and glabellar (nasal bridge) dermoids tend to present at birth with palpable, firm, visibly apparent superficial masses. They are commonly located adjacent to sutures and may have an associated sinus track with or without skin stigmata (i.e., dimple, sinus track, skin tag, or tuft of hair). Intracranial dermoids (also called teratomas) commonly present in the second to fourth decade with headaches and/or seizures resulting from mass effect or chemical meningitis from leakage of internal contents. Posterior fossa dermoids, which are associated with Klippel-Feil syndrome, often present with an occipital dimple, palpable mass, and/or sinus track with or without superimposed infection.

Abdominal and pelvic dermoids/epidermoids tend to present in older children when large in size because of their deep location. They may be asymptomatic and detected incidentally, or cause symptoms secondary to local mass effect such as abdominal pain or constipation, as can occur with retroperitoneal dermoids. Ovarian dermoids are bilateral in 15 to 20 percent of cases and often present with abdominal pain, caused by torsion or rupture, that may mimic appendicitis.

Anatomy, Physiology, and Embryology

Most periorbital/cranial dermoids and epidermoids likely arise between 3 and 5 weeks gestation resulting from failure of surface ectoderm to separate from the underlying neural tube or abnormal sequestration of surface ectoderm elements. Intracranial dermoids are thought to arise earlier in embryologic development than epidermoids. They tend to be midline in location and are most commonly found in the suprasellar cistern and frontonasal regions. Less commonly, they are found in the posterior fossa within the fourth ventricle or midline vermis. Glabellar dermoids occur when skin elements are pulled into the prenasal space by the regressing dural diverticulum that retreats after extending through the foramen cecum to contact the tip of the nose during embryogenesis. Epidermoids are thought to arise later in embryologic development, are more laterally located (off midline), and are most commonly found in the cerebellopontine angle, around the fourth ventricle and parasellar region. Slow growth of dermoids/epidermoids is related to intraluminal accumulation of debris from desquamation and/or glandular secretions.

Ovarian dermoids, otherwise known as mature cystic teratomas of the ovary, are congenital neoplasms usually derived from at least two of the three germ cell layers. Hypothetically they occur as a result of failure of cell division (meiosis II or meiosis I) in a premeiotic cell. Thus, they are formed of pluripotential cells and can contain multiple structures including hair, teeth, fat, skin, muscle, and endocrine tissue.

Imaging Findings

Dermoids have a variety of appearances because of their heterogenous contents including soft tissue, fat, and calcifications. Echogenicity on ultrasound, attenuation on CT and signal characteristics on MRI depend on the contents of the mass. Periorbital/facial and cranial dermoids tend to be located in the midline or adjacent to sutures (Fig. 100.1). They are most often well-defined and do not enhance. Glabellar dermoids/epidermoids may have a sinus tract extending toward the tip of the nose or a tract extending intracranially (Fig. 100.2). Specific signs of intracranial extension include an enlarged foramen cecum and/or a bifid crista galli. Epidermoids tend to be off midline in location and, on MRI, have signal characteristics that follow water as well as restricted diffusion (Fig. 100.3).

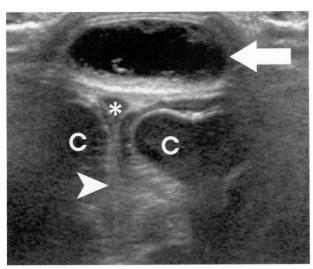

Figure 100.1. Coronal ultrasound in an 8-week-old female with a scalp lump proven to be a dermoid demonstrates a well-defined midline cystic scalp mass (arrow). Also noted are the sagittal sinus (asterisks), falx cerebri (arrowhead), and cerebral hemispheres (C).

Abdominal and ovarian dermoids appear as mixed solid and cystic masses that are heterogeneous in echotexture, attenuation, and signal intensity. Abdominal radiographs may show mass effect or calcifications including teeth. Hyperechoic foci with posterior acoustic shadowing (teeth) and an echogenic dot-dash pattern (hair) are seen on ultrasound (Fig. 100.4). Dermoids with large calcifications may cause so much acoustic shadowing on ultrasound

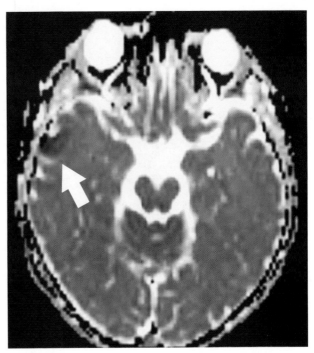

Figure 100.3. Axial ADC map in a 7-year-old male with an incidental mass seen on a CT performed for trauma shows a well-defined mass with restricted diffusion in the right temporal lobe (arrow). The lesion was bright on T2- and diffusion-weighted images (not shown) consistent with epidermoid.

that much of the mass is obscured, a finding known as the "tip of the iceberg" sign. On CT and MRI, abdominal and ovarian dermoids may contain mass-like mobile clumps of internal hair and debris, a finding known as a Rokitansky nodule (Fig. 100.5). Ovarian enlargement and/or free fluid caused by associated torsion may be seen as well.

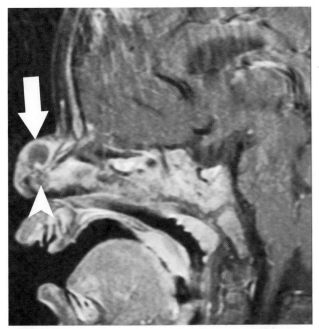

Figure 100.2. Sagittal contrast-enhanced T1 fat-suppressed MR image in an 8-month-old male with an intra- and extranasal mass since birth reveals a well-defined, peripherally enhancing bilobed mass with components located superficial, extranasal (arrow) and deep, intranasal (arrowhead) to the nasal bones consistent with dermoid.

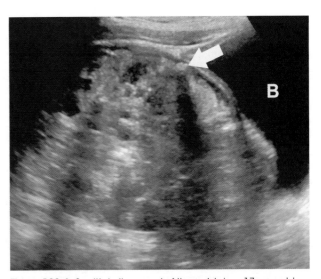

Figure 100.4. Sagittal ultrasound of the pelvis in a 17-year-old female with abdominal pain shows a large solid adnexal mass above the bladder (B) with small internal cysts and calcifications (arrow) showing posterior acoustic shadowing consistent with dermoid.

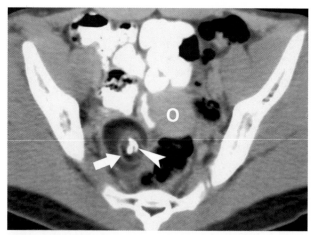

Figure 100.5. Axial contrast-enhanced CT image in a 15-year-old female with right lower quadrant pain shows a well-defined, right adnexal mass containing fat, soft tissue, and calcification. Within the mass is a nodule of debris or Rokitansky nodule (arrow), with a centrally located tooth-shaped calcification (arrowhead) consistent with dermoid/epidermoid. Note the normal left ovary (O).

Imaging Strategy

The imaging strategy of dermoids and epidermoids depends on lesion location. Although superficial lesions may be screened with ultrasound, head and neck dermoids often require CT or MRI for complete characterization. Glabellar dermoids, in particular, require both CT and MRI to evaluate for possible sinus tracts and intracranial extension. Ultrasound and CT are typically utilized to evaluate ovarian and abdominal dermoids.

> **IMAGING PITFALLS:** CT and MRI are both required in order to fully evaluate glabellar dermoids for intracranial extent, sinus tracts, and other intracranial anomalies.

Differential Diagnosis

Cranial dermoids adjacent to sutures have such a typical appearance that they require no further differential diagnosis. Similarly, ovarian dermoids contain tissues from all three germ cell layers (fat, fluid, and soft tissue) giving a pathognomonic appearance. The fact that epidermoids tend to follow fluid signal and have restricted diffusion are helpful features to narrow the differential diagnosis. One caveat is that restricted diffusion may be seen with abscesses.

Several specific differential diagnoses deserve mention:

Glabellar dermoid:
- Cerebral heterotopia (or nasal gliomas)
- Encephalocele (which can occur intra- and/or extranasally)

Cerebellopontine angle tumor:
- Arachnoid cyst
- Acoustic schwannoma
- Meningioma

Related Physics

Dermoids and epidermoids require MRI for definitive imaging and this can be performed on systems with magnetic field strengths from 0.3 to 7 Tesla. A practicing radiologist should understand the difference between field strengths as these impact safety and clinical value. In general, higher static field strength allows for more proton recruitment and therefore renders images with greater signal-to-noise. Field strengths for clinical magnets are specified in units of Tesla (T). For weaker magnets and in reference to the area outside the MR room, the unit gauss is used where 1 T = 10,000 gauss. Controlled access is maintained within five gauss of the magnet, delineated by a safety line referred to as the "5 gauss line." Alternatively, a series of doors and barriers will serve the same purpose in an MRI department. MR uses the properties of the magnetic dipole, which is a simple bar magnet having a north and south direction. The body's protons can be thought of as having a magnetic north and south and when a proton spins on its principle axis it has a magnetic dipole moment. Like a spinning top, this is associated with angular momentum. Again like the spinning top, when a 90-degree RF pulse is imposed on the proton it not only tips but begins to precess. This dipole moment forms the vector that is measured as signal in MRI. Several biologically relevant nuclei can be considered for MRI, all of which have an unpaired proton in the nucleus. These include hydrogen, C-13, O-17, N-23, and P-31, and all of these occur in physiologically important molecules such as ATP, ADP, etc.

Clinical Issues

Definitive treatment for dermoids and epidermoids is surgical resection, as the lesions tend to enlarge slowly over time with resultant mass effect on adjacent structures. Care must be taken to ensure complete resection of the lesion's capsule and any associated sinus tract in order to prevent recurrence.

Key Points

- Dermoids tend to be midline in location, more often contain fat, and have a variable appearance depending on their composition.
- Epidermoids tend to be off midline, follow fluid signal and show restricted diffusion on MRI.
- Both CT and MRI are required to fully evaluate glabellar dermoids/epidermoids.
- Ovarian dermoids may present with symptoms that mimic appendicitis resulting from mass effect, rupture, or associated torsion.

Further Reading

Caldarelli M, Massimi L, Kondageski C, Di Rocco C. Intracranial midline dermoid and epidermoid cysts in children. *J Neurosurg.* 2004;*100*(Pediatrics 5):473–480.

Lowe LH, Booth TN, Joglar JM, Rollins NK. Midface anomalies in Children. *RadioGraphics*. 2000;*20*:907–922.

Patel MD, Feldstein VA, Lipson SD, Chen DC, Filly RA. Cystic teratomas of the ovary: diagnostic value of sonography. *Am J Roentgenol AJR*. 1998;*171*(4):1061–1065.

Smirniotopoulous JG, Chiechi MV. Teratomas, dermoids, and epidermoids of the head and neck. *Radiographics*. 1995;*15*:1437–1455.

Yang DM, Jung DH, Kim H, Kang JH, Kim SH, Kim JH, Hwang HY. Retroperitoneal cystic masses: CT, clinical, and pathologic findings and literature review. *RadioGraphics*. 2004;*24*(5):1353–1365.

Brainstem Tumors

Ronald Rauch, MD

Definition

The three most common types of brainstem tumor encountered in a pediatric practice are diffuse pontine glioma, dorsally exophytic glioma, and tectal plate glioma, each with distinct histologic properties leading to wide variability in natural history and prognosis.

Clinical Features

Diffuse Pontine Glioma

This is the most common form of brainstem neoplasm seen in a pediatric practice, accounting for 55 to 80 percent of brainstem neoplasms. The tumors usually present in the second half of the first decade of life with cranial neuropathies and headache. Unfortunately, diffuse pontine gliomas have a very poor prognosis, with reported 3-year survival rates of less than 10 percent.

Dorsally Exophytic Glioma

Patients present with headache, vomiting and ataxia secondary to aqueductal occlusion and hydrocephalus; approximately 50 percent of patients present with cranial nerve deficits. Tumors may grow from the dorsal aspect of the pons, pontomedullary junction, or medulla and extend into the cisterns behind the brainstem and beneath the cerebellum and at times can extend up through the foramen of Magendie. These tumors have a much more favorable prognosis than the diffuse pontine gliomas with a 2-year survival of 100 percent with event-free survival of 67 percent.

Tectal plate glioma

The tumors originate in the quadrigeminal (tectal) plate along the posterior margin of the aqueduct of Sylvius, are slow-growing and only come to clinical attention when they cause hydrocephalus through obstruction at the cerebral aqueduct. Owing to their slow growth, these tumors have a favorable prognosis.

Anatomy and Physiology

Diffuse Pontine Glioma

The histology of pontine glioma is most often a fibrillary astrocytoma, a World Health Organization (WHO) grade II tumor. However, some of these tumors are anaplastic astrocytoma (WHO grade III) or rarely glioblastoma (WHO grade IV) neoplasms. It should be noted that the true histology at time of diagnosis is usually not obtained because the diagnosis is usually made radiographically and biopsy is avoided because there would be a great risk of neurosurgical complication if biopsy were done. Based on limited histologic/genetic material, it has been found that there is a higher frequency of P53 gene mutations in these tumors than in other posterior fossa tumors.

Dorsally Exophytic Glioma

These are most commonly pilocytic astrocytomas, similar in histology to juvenile pilocytic astrocytomas of the cerebellum.

Tectal Plate Glioma

The tumors are primarily low-grade fibrillary astrocytomas or less often pilocytic astrocytomas.

Imaging Findings

Diffuse Pontine Glioma

Diffuse pontine gliomas typically show expansion of the pons on CT and MR. The enlarged pons may appear to nearly encase the basilar artery and leave little cerebrospinal fluid space ventrally. The fourth ventricle is usually narrowed but patent and hydrocephalus at presentation is uncommon (Fig. 101.1). Tumors are generally hypodense on CT scan (Fig. 101.2).

On MRI, they are hypointense on T1 and hyperintense on T2 and FLAIR involving more than 50 percent of the cross-sectional area of the pons (Fig. 101.3). Tumors may spread into the midbrain or into the medulla. There is variable enhancement but little to no enhancement is more common. Diffusion restriction is unusual except in rare cases of grade IV astrocytomas. Leptomeningeal spread of disease is rare at presentation.

Dorsally Exophytic Glioma

These pilocytic astrocytomas appear as elsewhere in the brain. The tumor is most often dorsal to the medulla and may displace the fourth ventricle upward. On noncontrast

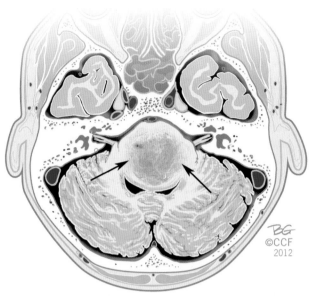

Figure 101.1. Diffuse pontine glioma. This tumor (arrows) infiltrates the entire pons surrounding cranial nerve nuclei and vital pathways with ill-defined borders making it impossible to remove surgically.

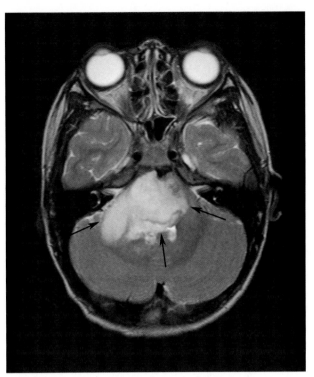

Figure 101.3. Axial T2 MR image in a 2-year-old child with headaches shows T2 hyperintensity and expansion of pons (arrows).

CT scan, they are hypoattenuating and on MRI they are hypointense on T1 and hyperintense on fluid-sensitive sequences with intense enhancement following intravenous contrast, often with a cyst or nonenhancing component

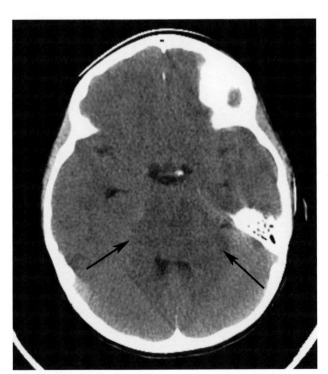

Figure 101.2. Axial noncontrast CT image in a child with headaches shows an expanded, low-density pons (arrows) consistent with diffuse pontine glioma.

(Fig. 101.4). Diffusion restriction and leptomeningeal spread of this benign tumor are rare.

Tectal Plate Glioma

The best way to detect these tumors is by their distortion of normal anatomy of the quadrigeminal plate. These tumors are often isodense compared to brain and difficult to detect on CT scan (or may be missed entirely). For this reason one should obtain MRI in all cases of apparent aqueductal stenosis to exclude a tectal plate glioma. On MRI tumors are iso- to hypointense on T1 (Fig. 101.5A) and iso- to hyperintense on T2. Enhancement is rare unless the tumors are pilocytic astrocytomas where they will often show intense enhancement (Fig. 101.5B).

Imaging Strategy

A child with cranial neuropathy and suspicion for a brainstem tumor should have MRI with: sagittal and axial T1 or inversion recovery; axial and sagittal T2; axial and sagittal FLAIR; axial diffusion; postcontrast images in all three planes.

Related Physics

All brainstem tumors should undergo definitive MR imaging, and it is important to understand some of the basic aspects of MR imaging in order to develop a knowledge base for more complex MR physics. MR imaging is produced by

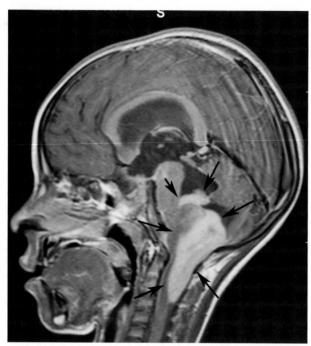

Figure 101.4. Sagittal contrast-enhanced T1 MR image in a 5-year-old female with vomiting and ataxia shows an enhancing lesion dorsal to the medulla (arrows) extending behind the brainstem and spinal cord, compressing the upper spinal cord, and also displacing the fourth ventricle upward consistent with dorsally exophytic glioma.

of a radiofrequency pulse forces the alignment 90 degrees off the magnetic field's axis. Because the proton has spin, this action results in precession of the proton's magnetic moment or vector, akin to a spinning top, as it makes its way back to align with the magnetic field. The rate at which the precession occurs in revolutions per second is directly proportional to the external magnetic field strength B_0; this is known as the Larmor frequency and is given in megahertz. The Larmor frequency (ω_0) can be calculated using the Larmor equation: $\omega_0 = \gamma\,\beta_0$ where γ is the unique gyromagnetic moment of each nucleus with an unpaired proton and defines the precessional frequency; for H this is 42.6 megahertz per Tesla.

Differential Diagnosis

Diffuse Pontine Glioma
- Dysmyelination associated with neurofibromatosis type 1
- Encephalitis
- Langerhan's cell histiocytosis
- Vascular malformation

Dorsal Exophytic Glioma
- Posterior fossa tumors: medulloblastoma, ependymoma, and cerebellar astrocytoma

Tectal Plate Glioma
- Pineal cell tumors
- Lymphoma

eliciting a signal from a nucleus with an unpaired proton, the most common of which is H. When H atoms are placed in an external magnetic field, the unpaired proton will align itself in either a high- or low-energy state. The introduction

(A)

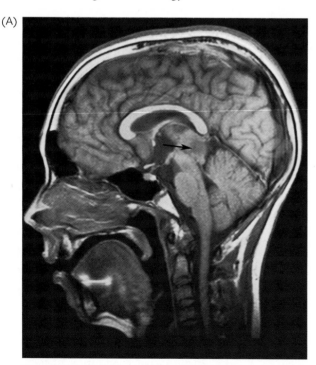

(B)

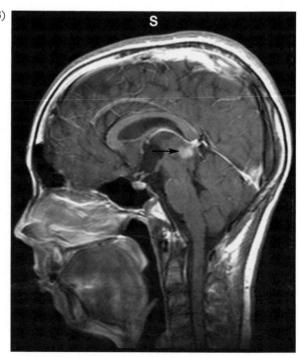

Figure 101.5. Sagittal noncontrast T1 MR image (A) in a 10-year-old male with headaches shows enlargement and slight hypointensity in the large bulky mass (arrow) in the quadrigeminal plate region. Sagittal contrast-enhanced T1 MR image (B) shows enhancement (arrow), as is typical of pilocytic astrocytomas, the most common type of tectal plate glioma.

(A)
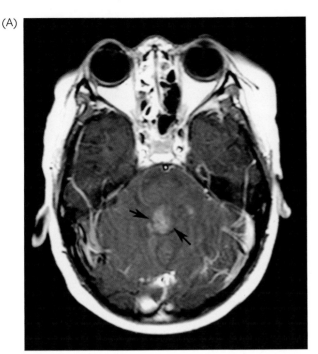

(B)
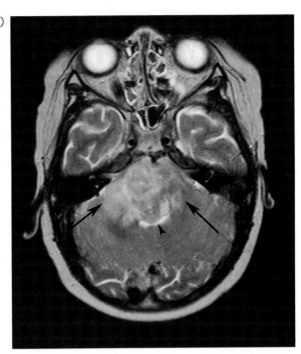

Figure 101.6. Axial contrast-enhanced T1 MR image (A) in a 2-year-old 9 months after chemotherapy shows new enhancement (arrows), suggesting the tumor has become more malignant with breakdown of the blood-brain barrier or there has been tumor necrosis caused by therapy. Pathology was diffuse pontine glioma. Axial T2 MR image (B) after chemotherapy shows growth of the tumor (arrows) with more mass effect on the fourth ventricle (arrowhead).

Clinical Issues

Diffuse Pontine Glioma

Because of the precarious location of these tumors, surgery generally has little if any role in treatment; the primary treatment is with radiation therapy. Chemotherapy provides only marginal improvement in the dismal prognosis of this tumor although clinical trials are ongoing. Enhancement often develops within the tumor after radiation (Fig. 101.6A). It can be challenging to determine if these changes are merely a result of radiation and associated tumor cell death or if the new enhancement and/or cystic or necrotic changes are a result of tumor growth. Continued follow-up imaging will often sort this out, but because the tumor is seldom truly cured, there may be a component of both radiation change and tumor growth producing the imaging changes. Transient marked improvement of diffuse pontine glioma is common after initial therapy followed by worsening with time (Fig. 101.6B).

Dorsally Exophytic Glioma

Complete surgical resection is the treatment of choice for exophytic glioma. Because complete excision is not always possible, there is a potential for tumor growth rendering a poorer prognosis than for cerebellar pilocytic astrocytomas in which complete resection is more often possible. Chemotherapy (or occasionally radiation) may be used at the outset or with tumor growth. Repeat surgery for residual tumor can improve prognosis.

Tectal Plate Glioma

Because of their precarious location and because most tectal gliomas are very slow-growing, treatment is restricted to shunting for hydrocephalus. Chemotherapy and/or radiation are employed for tumors that show growth over time.

Key Points

- Diffuse pontine gliomas are low-grade fibrillary astrocytomas that diffusely enlarge the pons without enhancement or hydrocephalus and are inoperable.
- Diffuse pontine gliomas may enhance on follow-up imaging, resulting from effects of treatment (within the tumor or in adjacent normal brain tissue) or from the tumor becoming a higher-grade astrocytoma.
- Dorsally exophytic gliomas are typical pilocytic astrocytomas dorsal to the brainstem, should NOT invade nor involve the entire brainstem, and have a fairly good prognosis with gross or subtotal resection.
- Tectal plate gliomas are low-grade fibrillary (or less often pilocytic) astrocytomas, remaining confined to the tectum and have a good prognosis.
- Tectal plate gliomas are treated by shunting the hydrocephalus.

Further Reading

Fischbein NJ, Prados MD, Wara W, Russo C, Edwards MS, Barkovich AJ. Radiologic classification of brainstem tumors:

correlation of magnetic resonance imaging appearance with clinical outcome. *Pediatr Neurosurg*. 1996;*242*:9–23.

Fuller C, Narendra S. Pilocytic astrocytomas and pilomyxoid astrocytomas and infiltrative astrocytoms. In: Adesina AM, Tihan T, Fuller C, Pouissaint TY, eds. *Atlas of Pediatric Brain Tumors*. New York: Springer; 2010.

Karajannis M, Allen JA, Newcomb EW. Treatment of pediatric brain tumors. *J Cell Physio*. 2008;*217*:584–589.

Koeller KK, Rushing EJ. From the archives of the AFIP pilocytic astrocytoma: radiologic-pathologic correlation. *Radiographics*. 2004;*24*:1693–1708.

Tortori-Donati P, Rossi A, Biancheri R, Garre, ML, Cama A. Brain tumors. In: Tortori-Donati A, Rossi A, Biancheri R, eds. *Pediatric Neuroradiology.*Berlin: Springer; 2005.

CHAPTER 102

Cerebellar Region Tumors

Ronald Rauch, MD

Definition

The three most common pediatric intracranial neoplasms below the tentorium but outside the brainstem are pilocytic astrocytoma, medulloblastoma, and ependymoma, each with unique histology and natural history.

Clinical Features

Pilocytic Astrocytoma

Pilocytic astrocytoma (previously called juvenile pilocytic astrocytoma because of its tendency to occur in children and young adults) can be found in many locations within the central nervous system, including in the optic nerve, hypothalamic-chiasmatic region, thalamus, cerebral hemispheres, brainstem, spinal cord, and cerebellum. Pilocytic astrocytomas are the second most frequent childhood cerebellar tumor. The peak age of pilocytic astrocytomas of the cerebellum is in the first decade. Pilocytic astrocytoma is a benign WHO (World Health Organization) grade I tumor. Children with this tumor typically demonstrate a good prognosis, with greater than 90 percent 10-year survival. Treatment is usually limited to surgical resection, and even children who have only a partial resection have a very good prognosis. Chemotherapy is usually reserved for patients who demonstrate growth of residual tumor or recurrence. Despite its low-grade and benign characteristics, up to 50 percent of these tumors demonstrate at least microscopic local invasion of the surrounding tissue. Although pilocytic astrocytomas are usually limited to the tumor site, spread along the cerebrospinal fluid pathways can be seen (with fairly good prognosis).

Medulloblastoma

Medulloblastoma is the most common cerebellar tumor of childhood. The typical patient is a male (approximately 3 males: 2 females) often under age 10 years (and almost always prior to age 20 years) with rapidly progressing symptoms of cerebellar dysfunction or nausea and vomiting typically for less than 3 months. The tumor is highly malignant, a grade IV WHO tumor, is locally invasive and often produces distant leptomeningeal metastasis. Surgery is the first line of treatment for medulloblastoma, with resection of as much of the tumor as possible, although if small amounts of tumor remain, there is usually a good response to radiation and chemotherapy. Tumors are designated as average risk unless the patient has a residual tumor burden of more than 1.5 cc of tumor or if there are known metastatic lesions or if the patient is under age 3 years at presentation (patients under age 3 years have a much higher risk of severe neurologic sequela from radiation, so radiation therapy is usually delayed until the patient reaches 3 years of age). Average-risk patients usually receive radiation to the entire nervous system with a boost to the tumor site and adjuvant chemotherapy. High-risk patients receive multidrug chemotherapy, and when those patients are over 3 years of age, they also receive radiation. After gross total tumor resection, 5-year survival rates are reported at above 70 percent.

Ependymoma

Ependymomas are not as common as pilocytic astrocytomas or medulloblastomas. Ependymomas are generally slow-growing and have a peak incidence in the first decade of life. The overall survival is affected by patient age and location of tumor, the latter affecting respectability. Overall 5-year survival is 45 percent.

Anatomy and Physiology

Pilocytic Astrocytoma

Tumors are composed of astroglial cells and with an abundance of cysts and characteristic "Rosenthal fibers" on special stains. Macroscopically the lesions are well-encapsulated and there is a tendency for macrocyst formation with a mural soft-tissue nodule (Fig. 102.1).

Medulloblastoma

Medulloblastomas are thought to arise from primitive cells. Earlier in life these undifferentiated cells are located in the midline and later migrate laterally and superiorly. This explains the midline location of tumors in younger children and the more lateral location in older children and adults (Fig. 102.2). In the past, medulloblastomas were lumped into the broad category of primitive neuroectodermal tumors (PNETs), but medulloblastoma is now known to be histologically and genetically separate from PNET.

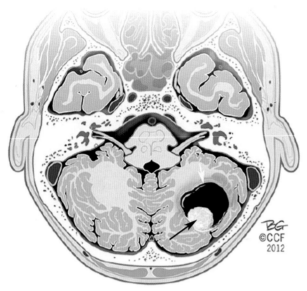

Figure 102.1. Pilocytic astrocytoma. Cyst (white arrow). with enhancing mural nodule (black arrow).

The tumor was named for the medulloblast, a cell that was at one time proposed to be the precursor for many cells of the cerebellum, but a medulloblast cell has never been identified. Medulloblastomas now are thought to either arise from primitive external granular layer cells or possibly from several different cell types.

Ependymoma

The histology of ependymoma of posterior fossa in children is either typical ependymoma (WHO grade II) or anaplastic ependymoma (WHO grade III). The tumor typically grows in the fourth ventricle and extrudes through the foramina of Lushka and Magendie (Fig. 102.3). Anaplastic

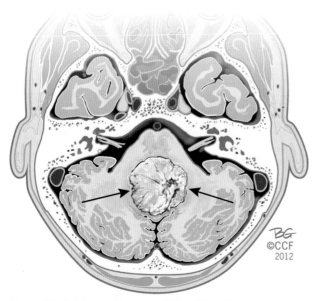

Figure 102.2. Medulloblastoma. Solid midline tumor (arrows).

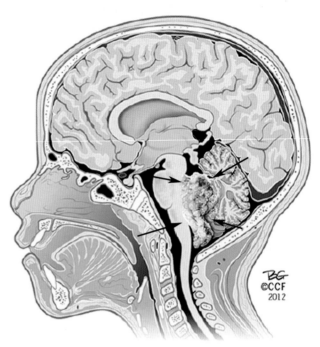

Figure 102.3. Ependymoma. Fourth ventricular mass that extrudes through the fourth ventricular formina (arrows).

ependymoma has a worse prognosis, grows more rapidly, and has a higher chance of CSF dissemination at time of diagnosis, but leptomeningeal spread with anaplastic ependymoma is still less common than in patients with medulloblastoma.

Imaging Findings

Pilocytic Astrocytoma

The classic appearance of pilocytic astrocytoma of the cerebellum, on both CT and MR, is a cyst with an enhancing nodule, found in 50 to 65 percent of pilocytic astrocytomas of the cerebellum. These tumors with a high cytoplasmic-to-nuclear ratio are usually hypodense on CT with occasional calcification. On MR, these neoplasms are T1 iso- or hypointense and T2/FLAIR hyperintense to cerebellar cortex.

There is no diffusion restriction. Surrounding edema is rare and minimal if present.

Tumor-related hemorrhage is also uncommon. Nearly all of these tumors show some enhancement and most show avid enhancement. As noted, the classic appearance is cyst with an enhancing nodule but with no enhancement of the cyst wall. Other patterns of enhancement are also seen including: enhancing nodule with enhancing cyst wall (Fig. 102.4) or a solid enhancing mass with no cyst, or even an enhancing mass with apparent central necrotic region. An enhancing wall is more often associated with tumor within the cyst wall and a nonenhancing wall usually indicates there is no tumor in the cyst wall, but this is not universally true.

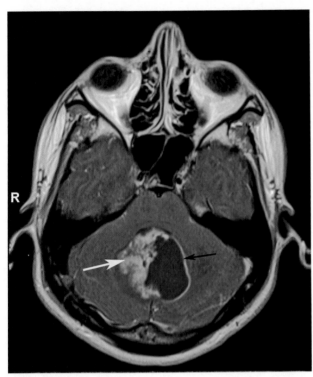

Figure 102.4. Axial contrast-enhanced T1 MR image shows a common appearance of a pilocytic astrocytoma, with enhancement of the tumor(white arrow) and enhancement of the cyst wall(black arrow).

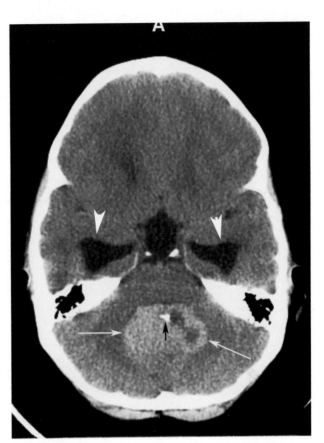

Figure 102.5. Axial noncontrast CT image in a child with headache shows a dense tumor(white arrows) with small calcification (black arrow) and necrotic regions arising from the vermis and filling the fourth ventricle. There is hydrocephalus with enlargement of the temporal horns of the lateral ventricles (arrowheads). Findings are consistent with medulloblastoma.

Medulloblastoma

These tumors are dense on CT because of the high nuclear-to-cytoplasm ratio (Fig. 102.5). Calcification is present in 10 to 40 percent. On MR these cellular tumors are usually hypo- or isointense to cerebellum on T1 and heterogeneous on T2 with surrounding vasogenic edema. The tumor often enhances on CT or MRI but the enhancement is variable and heterogeneous with regions lacking enhancement (Fig. 102.6). Enhancement may be totally absent in up to 20 percent. Diffusion restriction is common. Obliteration of the fourth ventricle with hydrocephalus is frequent at time of presentation. The tumor may extend through the foramen of Luschka or Magendie and may spread locally around the brainstem or spinal cord. Medulloblastomas have a moderately high frequency of distant CSF spread, present in up to one-third of cases at the time of diagnosis (Fig. 102.7). Leptomeningeal spread of tumor dramatically influences treatment and prognosis making it important to interrogate for distant spread early in the diagnostic evaluation. Because postoperative changes (such as hemorrhage or infection) can simulate or obscure leptomeningeal spread of disease, it is important to obtain an MR scan of the spine PRIOR to surgery if medulloblastoma is suspected. Metastatic lesions often show enhancement but some will not enhance. Although CSF cytology can detect some cases of leptomeningeal spread of medulloblastoma, MR is more sensitive than cytology, and a combination of MR plus cytology has the highest yield.

Ependymoma

Anatomy of the tumor is the most reliable way to make the diagnosis of ependymoma. The tumor lies in the fourth ventricle and often extends into foramen of Luschka (15 to 20 percent) and/or foramen of Magendie (up to 60 percent) and there is typically hydrocephalus at time of presentation. Other imaging characteristics are less definitive. The tumors are generally isodense or minimally hyperdense on CT. CT can also identify small calcifications that are present in up to 50 percent of these tumors (Fig. 102.8). Hemorrhage is uncommon (10 percent). On MRI, lesions are hypointense on T1 and heterogeneous with iso- to hyperintense signal on T2/FLAIR. Enhancement is often heterogeneous and a small number show no enhancement (Fig. 102.9). Diffusion weighted imaging usually shows values between the unrestricted diffusion of pilocytic astrocytoma and the diffusion restriction of medulloblastoma, but diffusion values for ependymoma can overlap with either pilocytic astrocytoma or medulloblastoma.

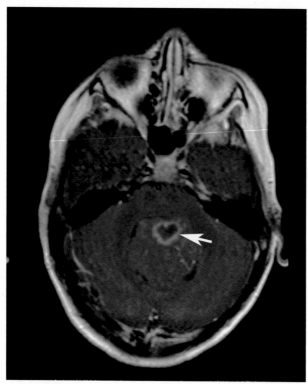

Figure 102.6. Axial contrast-enhanced T1 MR image in the same patient as Figure 102.5 shows some enhancement within the tumor (arrow).

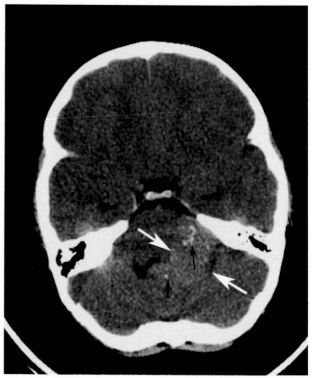

Figure 102.8. Axial noncontrast CT image in a patient with headache shows tumor(white arrows) in the fourth ventricle extending out through the foramen of Luschka. The tumor is slightly hyperdense and there are small calcifications(black arrows) present consistent with ependymoma.

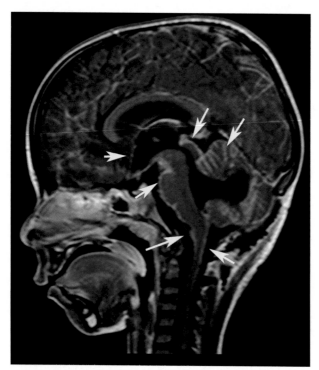

Figure 102.7. Sagittal contrast-enhanced T1 MR image in a patient with medulloblastoma shows extensive leptomeningeal enhancement(arrows) consistent with metastatic spread of disease.

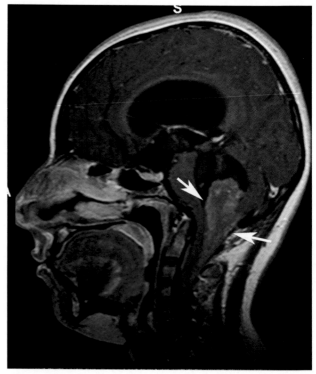

Figure 102.9. Sagittal contrast-enhanced T1 MR image shows an enhancing mass(arrows) in the mid-fourth ventricle extending down through foramen of Magendie.

Clinical Issues

Pilocytic Astrocytoma

If total excision can be achieved, no additional therapy is needed although many clinicians obtain follow-up MRI to assure the patient does not demonstrate tumor regrowth. If total excision of the pilocytic astrocytoma is not possible because of location of tumor with involvement of adjacent eloquent intracranial structures, chemotherapy may be given to help achieve local control and long-term survival. These patients are typically followed with frequent MR scans and may require repeat surgery to improve patient quality of life and longevity. Because there is a risk of tumor de-differentiation and of development of additional radiation-related problems including second tumors (especially in patients with pilocytic astrocytoma and neurofibromatosis type 1), radiation therapy is usually only used if other methods have failed and the tumor continues to grow.

Medulloblastoma

Total surgical resection produces best the outcome. If there is residual tumor seen after surgery, repeat surgery to attempt to achieve gross total resection is warranted if it is feasible. Radiation therapy induces changes of the brain parenchyma on MRI, seen as high signal intensity on T2 with variable enhancement. When such findings are discovered, short-term follow-up is warranted. Perfusion imaging may help differentiate tumor from radiation changes. However, differentiation between small tumor deposits and small foci of radiation change is frequently challenging (Figs. 102.10 and 102.11). Medulloblastoma may recur even after optimal therapy, either at the original tumor site or along leptomeningeal surface of the brain or spinal cord. Most recurrences are in the first few years after initial therapy. For this reason, most patients who are treated for medulloblastoma are followed on a regular basis with MRI every 2 to 4 months initially and then with longer periods between imaging after 3 to 5 years. The combination of high-quality neuroimaging with neurosurgery, radiation, and chemotherapy have significantly improved patient outcomes.

Ependymoma

If total resection is not possible, chemotherapy and radiation are used together, but survival chances are more guarded. Because ependymomas that arise more laterally within the fourth ventricle have a higher rate of spread through the foramen of Luschka and into the cerebellopontine angle where there are cranial nerves and essential arteries, these ependymomas are therefore often more difficult to fully resect. Thus ependymomas located laterally have a worse prognosis than those that arise in the midline.

Related Physics

Tumors of the posterior fossa may undergo PET imaging to determine activity and provide improved specificity for diagnosis. PET imaging requires isotopes with an inherent

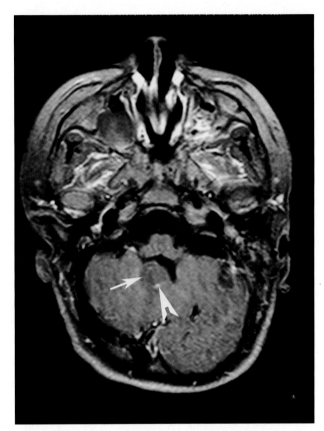

Figure 102.10. Axial contrast-enhanced T1 MR image with fat suppression in a child with vomiting shows tumor (arrow) located at right side of fourth ventricle with minimal enhancement (arrowhead), consistent with medulloblastoma.

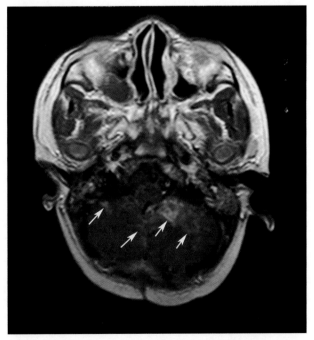

Figure 102.11. Axial contrast-enhanced T1 MR image in the same patient as Figure 102.10 11 months after gross total resection and radiation therapy shows new extensive enhancement (arrows) within cerebellum distant to the original tumor site. This represents effects of treatment and is not tumor as it resolved 9 months later.

energy instability. These elements are lightweight and lie in the second row of the periodic table. Examples are F18, O15, N, and C. None of these isotopes occur naturally and require a cyclotron for production. The radioisotope produced has unstable energy and charge. Because of this, decay occurs rapidly toward a stable state. The energy-to-mass decay occurs following the classic equation $e = mc^2$. This then balances the energy deficit. Each unstable nucleus decays via B+ emission where the nuclear force is overcome, allowing the B+ to be ejected from the nucleus and secondary anihilation of an orbital electron. The B+ must have energy equal to or greater than the binding energy to be released. This results in the production of two 511 KeV photons traveling in opposite directions thereby giving the basis for PET imaging. By attaching these light isotopes to metabolically important molecules such as FDG, metabolic processes can be imaged. The family of "light z" isotopes share the characteristic that they are designed to give up a B+ during decay.

Differential Diagnosis

Helpful differentiating points between the most common posterior fossa tumors:

- Most common tumors found in the cerebellar hemispheres: medulloblastoma and pilocytic astrocytoma
- Most common tumor to be found exclusively in the fourth ventricle: ependymoma
- Most common tumor to be hyperdense on CT: medulloblastoma
- Most common tumor to have restricted diffusion: medulloblastoma
- Most common tumor to have avid contrast enhancement: pilocytic astrocytoma
- Most common tumor to calcify: ependymoma
- Most common tumor to have surrounding vasogenic edema: medulloblastoma
- Tumor that shows no or little surrounding vasogenic edema: pilocytic astrocytoma

Other Tumors of the Cerebellum

- Atypical Teratoid/Rhabdoid Tumors (ATRT): rare, malignant tumors of young patients (<3 years of age) that can look like medulloblastomas or PNETs and often occur in the cerebellar hemisphere or near the foramen of Luschka; tumors are heterogeneous, slightly dense on CT, generally bright on T2 and dark on T1, with small cysts and calcifications and heterogeneous enhancement; local invasion is common.
- Gangliogliomas: low-grade tumors that can occur in the brainstem or cerebellum and in many other locations in the neuraxis; most frequently above the tentorium, especially in the temporal lobe; can look like pilocytic astrocytomas with a nodule and cyst; hypodense or less often, isodense to brain on CT; 10 to 30 percent have small calcifications; hypointense

on T1 and hyperintense on T2; usually appearing well-circumscribed and approximately half will show contrast enhancement
- Dysplastic gangliocytoma (also known by the eponym Lhermitte Duclos): very rare condition of the cerebellum most commonly seen in young adults but can be seen in pediatric patients; may be found incidentally when the patient is imaged for other reasons; termed a neoplasm by some and a dysplastic hamartoma with growth potential by others; may be part of Cowden disease with associated hamartomas of the breast and thyroid tissue and with increased risk for development of carcinoma; hypointense on T1, hyperintense on T2 with mass effect and striations of preserved but compressed cerebellar folia architecture (giving rise to the term "tiger-striped" lesion); almost never enhance and seldom calcify and are usually limited to one cerebellar hemisphere.

Key Points

- CT can help separate medulloblastoma (a fairly dense tumor) from other cerebellar region tumors, but all tumors in this region need MRI with contrast.
- Leptomeningeal spread of disease changes prognosis and treatment (not all leptomeningeal metastases enhance).
- MR scan of the spine should be done before surgery to evaluate for drop metastasis in medulloblastoma.
- Ependymoma is favored if there is a clear cleavage plane separating tumor in the fourth ventricle from the cerebellum.
- Best chance for cure in ependymoma is repeat surgery to achieve gross total tumor removal.

Further Reading

Fuller C, Narendra S, Tolicica I 1. Pilocytic astrocytomas and pilomyxoid astrocytomas, 2. Infiltrative astrocytoma, 3. Ependymal tumors, and Adesina AM and Hunter J. medulloblastomas. In: Adesina AM, Tihan T, Fuller C, Pouissaint TY, eds. *Atlas of Pediatric Brain Tumors*. New York: Springer; 2010.

Karajannis M, Allen JC, Newcomb EW. Treatment of pediatric brain tumors. *J Cell Physiol*. 2008;*21*:584–589.

Koeller KK, Rushing EJ. From the archives of the AFIP medulloblastoma: a comprehensive review with radiologic-pathologic correlation. *Radiographics*. 2003;*23*:1613–1637.

Koeller KK, Rushing EJ. From the archives of the AFIP pilocytic astrocytoma: radiologic-pathologic correlation. *Radiographics*. 2004;*24*:1693–1708.

Tortori-Donati P, Rossi A, Biancheri R, Garre ML, Cama A. Brain tumors In: Tortori-Donati A, Rossi A, Biancheri R, eds. *Pediatric Neuroradiology*. Berlin: Springer; 2005.

U-King-Im JM, Taylor MD, Raybaud C. Posteror fossa ependymomas: new radiological classification with surgical correlation. *Childs Nervous System*. 2010;*26*:1765–1772.

Yuh EL, Barkovich AJ, Gupta N. Imaging of ependymomas: MRI and CT. *Childs Nerv System*.2009;*25*:1203–1213.

CHAPTER 103

Other Brain Tumors

Korgün Koral, MD

Definitions

Craniopharyngioma: a benign, partly cystic epithelial tumor of the sellar region presumably derived from Rathke pouch epithelium.

Germinoma: central nervous system germ cell tumors are morphological and immunophenotypic homologues of gonadal and other extraneuraxial germ cell tumors. Germinoma is the most common central nervous system germ cell tumor.

Choroid plexus papilloma: intraventricular, papillary neoplasms derived from choroid plexus epithelium.

Clinical Features

Craniopharyngioma is a rare, biologically nonaggressive tumor of the sella and suprasellar region. The incidence of craniopharyngioma peaks between 10 and 14 years of age. The majority of the pediatric craniopharyngiomas are adamantinomatous, which tend to present with cysts and calcifications compared to the papillary form seen more commonly in adults. These tumors typically present with headaches and visual field defects related to compression of the optic chiasm and tracts. Pituitary and hypothalamic dysfunction can also occur.

Germinomas are germ cell tumors (others include teratoma, endodermal sinus tumor, and choriocarcinoma) that most commonly present before the end of the second decade. The majority are found in the pineal region, suprasellar region being the second most common site. Pineal germinomas generally present with hydrocephalus and Parinaud syndrome (upward gaze palsy) whereas the suprasellar germinomas usually present with diabetes insipidus. In 10 to 15 percent of pineal germinomas there is synchronous tumor in the suprasellar region. Pineal germinomas are 10 times more common in males, in contrast to suprasellar germinomas where there is no sex predilection.

Choroid plexus papillomas are low-grade (World Health Organization [WHO] grade I) neoplasms that may result in communicating hydrocephalus caused by overproduction of cerebrospinal fluid (CSF). Choroid plexus carcinoma (WHO grade III) is characterized by parenchymal invasion and metastases. Although these tumors can occur at any age, most present in the first 5 years of life with severe hydrocephalus.

Anatomy and Physiology

Craniopharyngiomas may be difficult to treat because of their critical location near the pituitary gland/stalk, optic nerves/chiasm, and hypothalamus. It is not uncommon for neurosurgeons to leave the cystic and calcified component of the tumors intact because of risk of injury to adjacent optic apparatus and hypothalamus. Occasionally craniopharyngiomas develop extracranially in the nasopharynx or paranasal sinuses.

Pure germinomas contain two cell lines, small round blue cells (lymphocytes), and primitive germ cells. They are histologically similar to testicular seminomas. A subtype of germinoma contains syncytiotrophoblastic cells. These tumors have a poorer prognosis and an increased recurrence rate with elevated levels of human chorionic gonadotropin in the CSF.

For pediatric choroid plexus papillomas, the lateral ventricles (usually left) are the most common sites, although the fourth ventricle is the most common location in adults. Some choroid plexus papillomas arise from extraventricular choroid plexus tissue. These are commonly seen in the cerebellopontine angle cisterns and in the region of the foramen magnum.

Imaging Findings

Craniopharyngioma: on CT, coarse calcifications can be seen at the cyst walls or in the solid component of the tumors (Fig. 103.1). The cysts are generally in the suprasellar cistern, but they may extend into the prepontine and interpeduncular cisterns in 25 percent. The cysts may be hyperintense on T1-weighted images because of increased protein content. The solid components show intense enhancement with intravenous contrast both on CT and MR imaging (Fig. 103.2).

Germinoma: on CT, the lesions may be hyperdense, composed of high-cellularity small round blue cell tumors. On MR imaging, the pineal germinomas are iso- to hyperintense to gray matter on T1- and T2-weighted sequences and enhance intensely (Fig. 103.3). Restricted diffusion can also be observed, reflecting high cellularity. Larger lesions may have

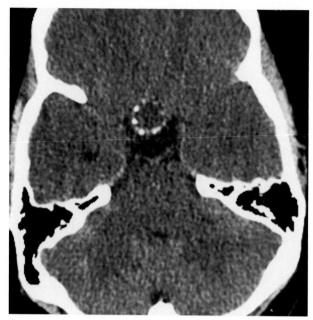

Figure 103.1. Axial noncontrast head CT in a 15-year-old female shows coarse calcifications in the walls of a suprasellar cyst consistent with craniopharyngioma.

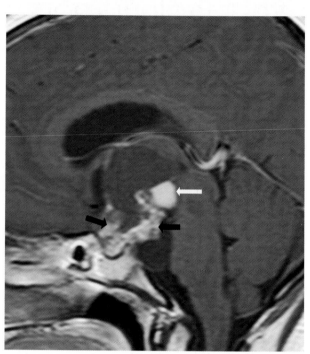

Figure 103.2. Sagittal contrast-enhanced T1 MR image in a 13-year-old female shows a complex mass with an enhancing solid component (black arrows) and a cyst with high protein content or hemorrhage (white arrow). Two other cysts are present: one displacing the third ventricle cranially and the other extending into the prepontine cistern consistent with craniopharyngioma.

regions of necrosis and cysts. The suprasellar germinomas involve the pituitary stalk and tuber cinereum and may extend to the floor of the third ventricle. Characteristically, absence of T1 shortening of neurohypophysis is noticed. A small germinoma may be not be readily apparent on imaging, therefore a child with diabetes insipidus and absent T1 shortening of neurohypophysis should be followed with MR imaging in 3 to 6 months to identify a presumed germinoma.

Choroid plexus papilloma: on CT, the tumors are usually iso- to hyperdense to brain and enhance intensely with contrast. The nodular, papillary surface contours of the choroid plexus papilloma are better appreciated on MR imaging aided by intense enhancement following intravenous gadolinium. When very large and arising from the lateral ventricles, choroid plexus papillomas may generate multiple CSF-filled cysts, which resolve following tumor resection (Fig. 103.4).

Imaging Strategy

Craniopharyngioma
- CT is important in distinguishing craniopharyngiomas from Rathke's cleft cyst, by demonstrating calcifications.
- Coronal reformations are particularly useful.
- Suggested sequences include: coronal T2 for assessment of optic apparatus; sagittal T1; axial diffusion; axial FLAIR; contrast-enhanced T1-weighted images in three orthogonal planes.

Germinoma
- Suggested sequences: sagittal T1; axial diffusion-weighted; axial T2; axial FLAIR; contrast-enhanced sagittal, coronal and axial T1; contrast-enhanced

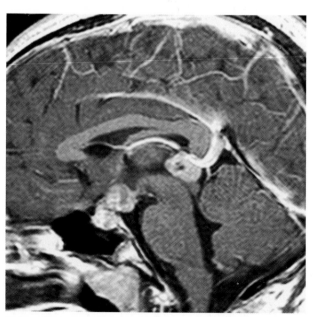

Figure 103.3. Sagittal contrast-enhanced T1 MR image in a 12-year-old male with germinoma demonstrates enhancing masses in the pineal gland and suprasellar cistern.

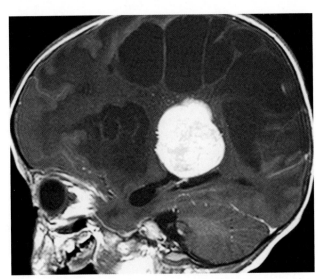

Figure 103.4. Parasagittal contrast-enhanced T1 MR image in a 19-month-old male with choroid plexus papilloma shows a large, enhancing mass in the right lateral ventricle intimately related to the choroid plexus in the temporal horn. Multiple fluid-filled extraaxial spaces are present in the cerebral hemisphere.

FLAIR is useful for identification of leptomeningeal tumor spread.

- Spine screening is mandatory with axial and sagittal contrast-enhanced T1-weighted images to evaluate for drop metastases.

Choroid Plexus Papilloma

- Suggested sequences: sagittal T1; axial diffusion; axial T2; axial FLAIR; contrast-enhanced sagittal, coronal and axial T1.
- MR spectroscopy is a useful tool for distinguishing choroid plexus papillomas (WHO grade I) from choroid plexus carcinomas (WHO grade III).

Related Physics

In a totally homogeneous medium, diffusion of a substance in water would occur randomly because of Brownian motion. An example would be adding a drop of red dye to water and returning an hour later to find that the water is uniformly pink. When a structure is present within a volume, diffusion becomes anisotropic because of high- and low-resistance paths present within the medium. An example of this would be placing a sheet of porous plexiglass in the water and repeating the experiment. In this case, one-half of the box would be darker in color than the other. Diffusion-weighted imaging (DWI) measures the rate of diffusion in each Cartesian direction. Diffusion will be restricted in certain conditions where architecture is distorted such as in stroke (edema), abscess (necrosis), and some tumors (high cellularity). There are also subtle differences in diffusion rate between normal tissues, so that DWI can demonstrate tissue interfaces. Diffusion weighted

imaging is performed using a fast single-shot echo planar sequence whereby two diffusion gradients are applied before and after the 180-degree pulse, in each of three Cartesian planes. This generates a "six-dimensional" image, where three of the dimensions are directional (x,y, and z) and the other three represent the diffusion rates (bx, by, bz). Two sets of images are rendered for interpretation: the "diffusion" images where diffusion restriction appears as high signal intensity and the apparent diffusion coefficient (ADC) map, where the converse is true. Diffusion tensor imaging is a method for depicting diffusional anisotropies as an interpretable image. In this image diffusion along the principle axes (x,y,z) are color-coded red, green, and blue with the intensity of the hue proportional to the magnitude of the diffusion in that direction. The eigenvalue is the magnitude and direction of diffusion within each voxel.

Differential Diagnosis

Craniopharyngioma

- Optic/hypothalamic pilocytic astrocytoma (does not calcify and generally can be identified as arising from the optic apparatus or hypothalamus)
- Rathke's cleft cyst (noncalcified primarily intrasellar lesion, which may occasionally extend into the suprasellar cistern and become symptomatic)

Germinoma

- Pineal: includes other germ cell tumors and pineal tumors (pineoblastoma, pineal cysts).
- Suprasellar region: includes Langerhans cell histiocytosis and, rarely, lymphocytic hypophysitis.
- Although presence of foci of T2 shortening has been suggested as an indicator in favor of germinoma over Langerhans cell histiocytosis, generally they are indistinguishable on imaging.

Choroid Plexus Papilloma

- Choroid plexus carcinoma (parenchymal infiltration is lacking in papillomas and is present in carcinomas; carcinomas may be multifocal and may disseminate into leptomeninges)
- Atypical choroid plexus carcinoma, a recently recognized subtype of intermediate aggressiveness
- Ependymoma and meningioma (characteristic nodular surface of choroid plexus papilloma helps to differentiate)

Clinical Issues

Patients with craniopharyngiomas may have decreased vision resulting from compromise of the optic apparatus. Following resection of sellar craniopharyngiomas, almost all patients develop hypothalamic obesity. Germinomas commonly present with CSF dissemination and invasion into the adjacent brain parenchyma. However, 5-year survival is approximately 90 percent related to their radiosensitivity. If elevated tumor markers, such as alphafetoprotein or beta hCG, can be demonstrated in the spinal fluid or blood, in the setting of a sellar or pineal mass, biopsy may be foregone. A new entity called atypical choroid plexus papillomas (WHO grade II) has been codified in the latest version of the WHO Classification of Tumors of the Central Nervous System.

Key Points

- Craniopharyngiomas: 90% will be cystic, 90 percent will have calcifications, 90% will enhance after contrast
- Germinomas: typically hyperdense on CT and hyperintense on T2-weighted images; highly radiosensitive
- Choroid plexus papilloma: papillomas are differentiated from carcinomas based on histologic, not radiologic or gross pathologic criteria

Further Reading

Intracranial, orbital, and neck masses of childhood. In: Barkovich AJ, ed. *Pediatric Neuroimaging*. Fifth edition. Philadelphia, PA: Lippincott, Williams and Wilkins;2012:637–807.

Souweidane MM. Brain tumors in the first two years of life. In: Albright AL, Pollack IF, Adelson PD, eds. Principle and Practice of Pediatric Neurosurgery. Second edition. New York, NY: Thieme Medical Publishers, Inc.; 2008:489–510.

Tomita T. Pineal region tumors. Craniopharyngiomas. In: Albright AL, Pollack IF, Adelson PD, eds. *Principle and Practice of Pediatric Neurosurgery*. Second edition. New York, NY: Thieme Medical Publishers, Inc.; 2008:585–605.

Wisoff JH, Donahue BR. Craniopharyngiomas. In: Albright AL, Pollack IF, Adelson PD, eds. *Principle and Practice of Pediatric Neurosurgery*. Second edition. New York, NY: Thieme Medical Publishers, Inc.; 2008:560–578.

CHAPTER 104

Spinal Cord Astrocytoma

Noah D. Sabin, MD

Definition

Spinal cord astrocytoma (SCA) is a primary intramedullary neoplasm of the spinal cord that arises from astrocytes.

Clinical Features

Spinal cord astrocytoma is the most common intramedullary spinal cord tumor in children accounting for approximately 60 percent of cases. There is no clear gender predominance in children although a predilection for males is seen in adults. The clinical characteristics of SCA are slowly progressive, usually over a period of months to years. Children most often present with neck and back pain, gait disturbance, torticollis, and scoliosis.

Anatomy and Physiology

Most frequently, SCAs are found in the cervicothoracic spinal cord. Fusiform enlargement of the cord is seen with the tumor often extending over several vertebral levels. Complete resection very difficult, if not impossible,because SCAs are typically situated eccentrically within the spinal cord and are usually infiltrative and extensive.

Imaging Findings

Magnetic resonance imaging (MRI), with its superior intrinsic contrast, provides the best imaging evaluation of SCA. The typical appearance of SCA is eccentric fusiform enlargement of the cervicothoracic spinal cord (often leading to enlargement of the bony spinal canal) spanning several vertebral levels with heterogeneous enhancement (Fig. 104.1). The tumor may lie centrally within the cord or may involve the entire cross-section of the cord. Some SCAs may not enhance although other tumors may demonstrate areas of intense enhancement (Fig. 104.2). The tumors are most often isointense to hypointense to the spinal cord on T1-weighted MRI images and hyperintense on T2-weighted images. Edema may extend superiorly and inferiorly from the tumor. Associated intratumoral, as well as rostral and caudal, "polar" cysts are sometimes seen (Fig. 104.3). The latter may not represent true tumor cysts but, rather, secondary hydromyelia. Hemorrhage is rare. Leptomeningeal spread of tumor most commonly occurs with higher-grade tumors (e.g., anaplastic astrocytoma).

Imaging Strategy

A child with a history of neck or back pain and symptoms and signs of myelopathy should undergo MR imaging of the entire spine with the following pulse sequences: sagittal and axial T1, sagittal and axial T2, postcontrast sagittal and axial T1 (without fat suppression).

> **IMAGING PITFALLS:** In rare cases, a spinal cord tumor can be missed because a limited MRI examination of the spine is requested when the clinical symptoms suggest a specific site (i.e., thoracic spine). However, a tumor can be located significantly higher than the symptoms suggest. Therefore, a MRI of the entire spine should be imaged.

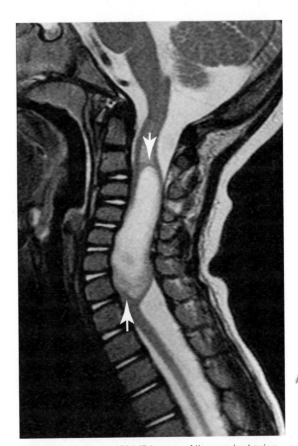

Figure 104.1. Sagittal T2 MR image of the cervical spine in a child with arm weakness demonstrates a high signal intensity mass (arrows) causing irregular fusiform enlargement of the cervical spinal cord consistent with SCA.

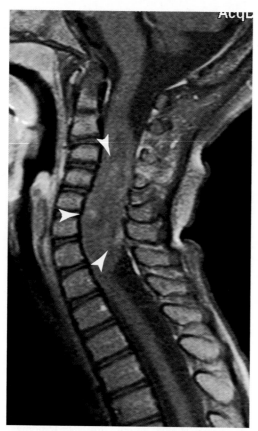

Figure 104.2. Sagittal contrast-enhanced T1 MR image of the cervical spine in a child with arm weakness demonstrates mild heterogeneous enhancement (arrowheads) of the SCA.

Related Physics

There are many artifacts associated with spinal cord imaging and knowledge of these is imperative for proper interpretation. These include metal or susceptibility, field inhomogeneity, radiofrequency, k-space, motion, chemical shift, Gibb's, aliasing, partial voluming, high-speed and high-field strength imaging. Only the last five will be discussed in this chapter, with the others found in the Choanal Atresia and Child Abuse (Cerebral) chapters. Gibb's artifact is seen as parallel ripples adjacent to structures with marked variation in signal intensity such as spine cord and cerebrospinal fluid. If imaged perfectly in frequency space, there would be a perfectly sharp transition from bright cord to dark CSF on T1 as an infinite number of frequencies would be needed to reconstruct the sharp edge in image space. However, in reality the number of frequencies used is truncated related to contraints in time and data resulting in "truncation" of data and sinusoidal ringing near the transition. Gibb's artifact can be minimized by increasing the matrix size in the phase direction (number of phase-encoding steps) without increasing the field of view (FOV). This comes at the expense of lower signal-to-noise and longer acquisition time. Aliasing occurs when the chosen FOV is smaller than the anatomy of interest resulting in information outside the FOV being subject to the radiofrequency (RF) energy. Signals within the FOV are arranged in k-space along a circular arc from 0 to 2π radians; signals outside the FOV occur from 0 to 4 pi radians, which are superimposed on the desired signals, therein leading to artifactual data. An

(A)

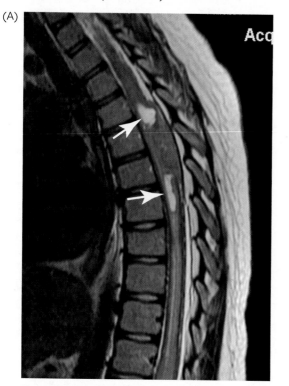

(B)

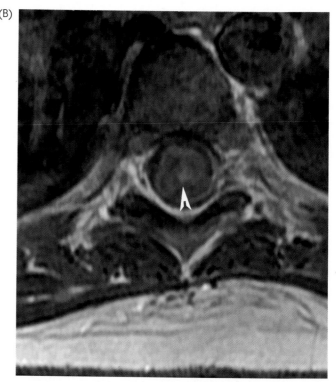

Figure 104.3. Sagittal T2 (A) and axial contrast-enhanced T1 (B) MR images of the thoracic spine in a child with leg weakness demonstrate an irregularly shaped mass with cystic degeneration (arrows) and heterogeneous enhancement (arrowheads) in the thoracic spinal cord consistent with SCA.

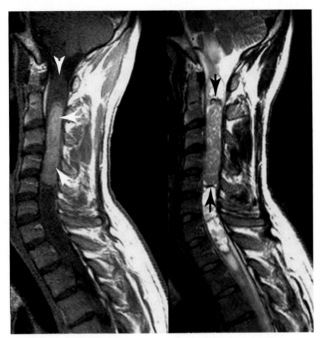

Figure 104.4. Contrast-enhanced sagittal T1 (A) and T2 (B) MR images of the cervical spine in a patient with spinal cord ependymoma reveal a mass with a prominent homogeneously enhancing component (white arrows). There are cystic areas at the superior and inferior poles (black arrowheads), and low signal intensity at the superior and inferior aspects of the enhancing mass on the T2-weighted image (black arrows) represents hemosiderin and is often referred to as the "cap sign." This finding is characteristic of spinal cord ependymomas although it is only seen in a subset of cases. (Images courtesy of Dr. Danielle Balériaux, Brussels, Belgium.)

example is the arms of a patient superimposed on the spine on a coronal image (with right to left phase encoding direction). This artifact is related to undersampling in the phase direction and corrected by increasing the FOV in the phase direction (at the expense of resolution) or increasing the number of phase encoding steps (at the expense of time). This latter technique is known as "phase oversampling." Another technique is to swap the phase and frequency direction, which in spine imaging is quite time-expensive. Tissues at the periphery of the bore where field lines are no longer parallel (as occurs with obese patients at the limits of bore size) will lead to spatial undersampling and zebra-like appearance or "moire" pattern. Partial volume artifact occurs when the thickness of the lesion is less than the slice thickness. This causes signals from adjacent tissues to superimpose on the lesion with resultant degradation in contrast-to-noise in the lesion. One can minimize this by decreasing image slice thickness. The most common single-shot artifact is known as N/2 ghosting which is the result of a multistep process. During signal acquisition, lines are written in k-space in a rastered fashion where alternating lines are written in opposite directions. Prior to image reconstruction the lines must be reversed, and during this process small errors in signal strength or position may occur. The mismatches create an additional faint image spaced at one-half the field of view in the phase direction because

every other line in k-space has been redirected. Likewise multishot suffers from the same vulnerability but the spacing is much less, with errors mostly caused by minor timing issues. Here, one will see multiple superimposed images that are offset much less than one-half the FOV in the phase direction. There are several electronic ways to minimize this. With greater field strength, most artifacts are accentuated as is the signal-to-noise.

Differential Diagnosis

- Spinal cord ependymoma: accounts for approximately 30 percent of intramedullary spinal cord tumors in children (as opposed to 60 percent in adults). In contrast to spinal cord astrocytomas, they are usually located centrally within the spinal cord, are sharply marginated and usually displace the surrounding spinal cord parenchyma rather than infiltrate it. This creates a good surgical cleavage plane that facilitates resection. Ependymoma is more vascular than astrocytoma with hemosiderin sometimes seen within and along the margins of the tumor. When a hemosiderin rim is present at one of the poles of the tumor it is called the "cap sign." This is seen only in a subset of tumors, but when present, is a very useful differential diagnostic clue. Spinal cord ependymomas often demonstrate intense, well-defined enhancement although heterogeneous enhancement may also occur (Fig. 104.4). The majority of spinal cord ependymomas are seen in the cervical spine with the remainder about equally distributed in the thoracic and lumbar regions. Despite the above, spinal cord ependymomas may be indistinguishable from cord astrocytomas.
- Spinal cord ganglioglioma: rare (approximately 1 percent of all spinal cord tumors) and grow very slowly so may see scalloping of adjacent bone. Composed of mixed ganglion and glial cells. Often indistinguishable from SCA.
- Hemangioblastoma: avidly enhancing nodule contacting a pial surface, often associated with extensive secondary intramedullary signal abnormalities (edema) or hydromyelia.
- Syringohydromyelia: cyst-like collection of CSF signal intensity within the spinal cord. Syringomyelia is secondary to a prior destructive intramedullary lesion (infarction, myelitis, contusion, etc.) In contrast, hydromyelia is the expansion of the central canal of the spinal cord and typically associated with an active causative lesion (e.g., Chiari I malformation, dysraphism).
- Myelitis: etiologies include autoimmune/inflammatory (multiple sclerosis, transverse myelitis, acute disseminated encephalomyelitis, Sjogren syndrome, etc.) as well as infection. Findings include cord enlargement and edema with variable enhancement.
- Spinal cord infarction: abrupt onset of symptoms.

Common Variants

Most SCA are low-grade (WHO grade I [pilocytic] or II diffuse fibrillary). The pilocytic type is common in children. Higher-grade astrocytomas, anaplastic astrocytomas (WHO grade III) and glioblastoma multiforme (WHO grade IV) of the spinal cord constitute approximately 10 to 15 percent of cases.

Clinical Issues

Lower-grade SCAs (WHO grades I and II) are associated with a better prognosis than higher-grade tumors (WHO grades III and IV). Patients with milder preoperative deficits have better outcomes. Spinal cord astrocytomas can be associated with neurofibromatosis type 1.

Key Points

- Intramedullary spinal cord neoplasm arising from astrocytes
- Most common intramedullary spinal cord tumor in children
- Usually eccentric fusiform enlargement of cervicothoracic spinal cord with heterogeneous enhancement
- Margins of tumor usually not well defined

Further Reading

Neoplasms of the spine. In: Barkovich AJ, ed. *Pediatric Neuroimaging*. Fifth edition. Philadelphia, PA: Lippincott Williams & Wilkins; 2012:924–952.

Huisman TAGM. Pediatric tumors of the spine. *Cancer Imaging*. 2009;9(special issue A):S45–S48.

Quinones-Hinojosa A, Gulati M, Schmidt MH. Intramedullary spinal cord tumors. In: Gupta N, Banerjee A, Haas-Kogan D, eds. *Pediatric CNS Tumors*. Berlin Heidelberg, Germany: Springer-Verlag; 2004:167–182.

Seo HS, Kim J-H, Lee DH, et al. Nonenhancing intramedullary astrocytomas and other MR imaging features: a restrospective study and systematic review. *AJNR Am J Neuroradiol*. 2010;31(3):498–503.

Smith JK, Lury K, Castillo M. Imaging of spinal and spinal cord tumors. *Semin Roentgenol*. 2006;41(4):274–293.

CHAPTER 105

Hypoxic Ischemic Injury

Gisele Ishak, MD

Definition

Hypoxic Ischemic Injury (HII) of the brain in neonates refers to irreversible brain damage that results from cerebral hypoperfusion and may be seen in preterm (<37 weeks gestational age) or term neonates. The manifestations vary according to the degree of hypoperfusion and gestational age of the patient at the time of insult.

Clinical Features

Hypoxic-ischemic injury is more common in preterm infants, involving up to 19 percent of infants born before 28 weeks. The prevalence of term HII ranges between 2 and 4 per 1,000 live term births.

Clinical signs of HII can be nonspecific at birth and should be suspected in case of intrapartum distress, low 5-minute Apgar score, fetal acidemia, depressed consciousness, bradycardia, hypotonia, and seizure. Infants who survive a severe insult typically develop quadriparesis, choreoathetosis, intractable seizure, and mental retardation. Patients with moderate injuries develop spastic diplegia or quadriplegic "cerebral palsy." In cases of mild HII, patients may recover completely or be mildly developmentally delayed.

Anatomy and Physiology

Hypoxic-ischemic injury is caused by diminished cerebral blood flow and hypoxemia. Because of differences in severity and duration of insult, brain maturity at time of insult, type and timing of imaging studies, there are variable patterns of brain injury. In general, mild to moderate ischemia in term infants manifests as damage to the less metabolically active watershed zones with shunting of blood to vital brain structures. Germinal matrix hemorrhage (GMH) (Fig. 105.1) and periventricular leukomalacia (PVL) occur in preterm infants with mild to moderate HII (Table 105.1). The germinal matrix, which is the precursor of neurons and glial cells, is most susceptible to ischemia and hemorrhage. It lines the walls of the lateral ventricles in fetal life and involutes by 34 weeks. The last portion to involute is located in the caudothalamic groove, where most of the germinal matrix hemorrhage originates. Previously thought to be related to ischemia in hypovascular watershed zones in the

preterm brain, PVL is now believed to be related to vulnerability of oligodendrocyte precursors, which disappear after 32 weeks gestational age, in concordance with the declining prevalence of PVL after 32 to 34 weeks gestational age. Profound ischemia in preterm and term infants manifests as damage to the areas of greatest metabolic activity that correspond to regions of advanced myelination, including the deep gray matter and brainstem.

Imaging Findings

Within the first 24 hours, diffusion-weighted MR imaging (DWI) is the most sensitive technique to show regions of injury. These regions will appear bright on T1- and T2-weighted MR imaging. Late imaging findings include atrophy of the injured structures with ex vacuo dilatation of the ventricles. Findings described herein are subdivided related to duration and severity of hypoxemia as well as gestational age.

Term Infant with Profound HII

- Deep gray matter (posterior putamina, ventrolateral thalami, hippocampi, dorsal brainstem) (Fig. 105.2)
- Cerebellar vermis
- Perirolandic cortex
- Corticospinal tracts

Term Infant with Mild to Moderate HII

- Watershed zones, predominantly parasagittal cortex and subcortical white matter and occasionally more diffuse involvement of the white matter (Fig. 105.3)

Preterm Infant with Profound HII

- Similar to term-infant profound pattern except that the basal ganglia and the perirolandic cortex are less involved because these areas do not myelinate until late (around 35 to 36 weeks gestational age).
- GMH and PVL may also occur.

Preterm Infant with Mild to Moderate HII

- Germinal matrix-intraventricular hemorrhage GMH-IVH

Initially PVL presents as increased periventricular echogenicity on ultrasound (US) and increased T2 signal on MRI

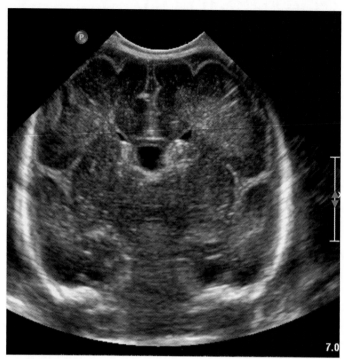

Figure 105.1. Coronal cranial ultrasound in a 2-day-old neonate born at 24 weeks gestation shows grade I germinal matrix hemorrhage in the caudothalamic groove bilaterally, more so on the left, with normal ventricular size and no intraventricuar extension. This is consistent with moderate HII. Periventricular hyperechogenecity is seen and is suspicious for PVL. Follow-up US showed cyst formation, confirming the diagnosis of PVL.

with subsequent cavitation and periventricular cyst formation at 3 to 6 weeks of age. Finally by 6 months of age, end-stage PVL (Fig. 105.4) results with resolution of cysts, progressive volume loss, ventriculomegaly, and thinning of the corpus callosum.

Imaging Strategy

Developmental immaturity makes it difficult to identify some of the clinical features of HII in preterm infants, and imaging plays an important role in early detection of HII. Intracranial US is an excellent screening modality for GMH and hydrocephalus, and can show increased echogenicity in involved deep gray matter or PVL. Where possible MRI should be considered the modality of choice for HII

and should include sagittal T1, axial T1 or inversion recovery, axial FLAIR, axial T2, coronal T2, axial diffusion (key sequence), and axial gradient echo (to check for hemorrhage). In addition, MRS may be helpful in demonstrating a lactate peak indicating anaerobic metabolism in damaged regions before conventional imaging becomes abnormal.

Related Physics

Several advanced acquisition techniques can be useful in MR imaging of infants with HII. These include flow compensation, angiography, diffusion, perfusion, and magnetization transfer. Flow compensation is employed to correct for spatial misregistration from flowing fluids. The magnitude of the correction depends on the velocity of the flowing fluid.

	Table 105.1 – Ultrasound grading system (originally described for CT but now widely used for US) for hypoxic ischemic brain hemorrhage in preterm infants with hypoxemia
GRADE	**IMAGING FINDINGS**
I	Subependymal hemorrhage with no intraventricular extension (Fig. 105.1)
II	Subependymal hemorrhage extending to the ventricles without ventricular enlargement
III	Subependymal hemorrhage extending to the ventricles with ventricular enlargement
IV	Periventricular parenchymal hemorrhagic infarction (thought to be caused by hemorrhage within a venous infarction and not extension of IVH, although almost always present together)

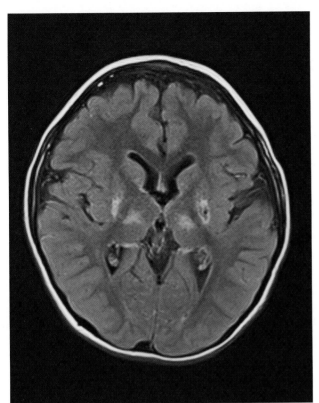

Figure 105.2. Axial FLAIR MR image in an 8-year-old child with spastic quadriplegia and seizure who suffered profound neonatal HII as a term infant shows abnormal signal in the ventrolateral thalami and posterior putamina.

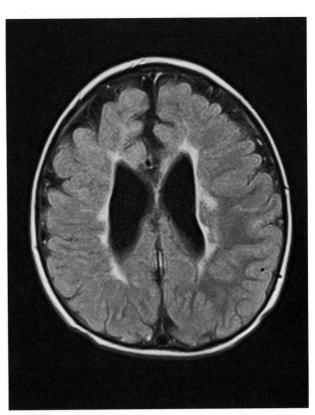

Figure 105.4. Axial FLAIR MR image in a 3-year-old with developmental delay and seizures shows increased signal in the periventricular white matter, with wavy contour of the lateral ventricles. Note that the deep sulci nearly abut the ventricular surface as a result of volume loss in the central white matter.

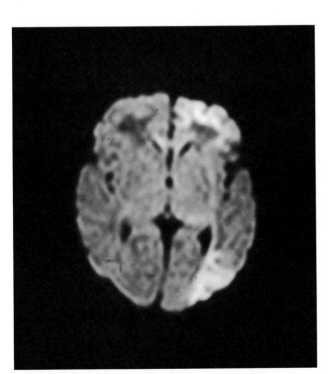

Figure 105.3. Axial DWI MR image in a 1-day-old term infant shows regions of diffusion restriction in the cortical and subcortical white matter of the left frontal and temporooccipital lobes in a watershed pattern consistent with mild HII.

One method involves mathematical correction (Taylor series expansion) and is best used for steady laminar flow with predictable direction and magnitude. The second method for flow compensation uses rephasing pulses in the flow direction to spatially rephase the protons and correct for misregistration. MR angiography uses three methods to image blood vessels: contrast-enhanced, time-of-flight and phase-contrast. Contrast-enhanced is performed after the intravenous injection of contrast that produces multiple planar images that can be rendered as maximum-intensity projections. This method is independent of flow direction. Time-of-flight is directionally dependent and uses a short-echo time (TE) sequence and flow compensation to rephase blood flowing into the slice to maximize its intensity and homogeneity. The rephasing is directly proportional to the velocity. Phase-contrast creates three phase images in the three orthogonal planes, which when added create a phase-contrast image with both flow direction and magnitude (velocity). When that image is subtracted from the preflow static image, the static protons are subtracted leaving just the flowing blood. Diffusion-weighted imaging uses the principle that cell membranes are destroyed in infarction and some tumors, so that there is no net diffusion across membranes. Perfusion is performed to evaluate areas of blood-brain barrier disruption or decreased cerebral perfusion in tumor or stroke. The method includes the injection of gadolinium followed by repeating multiple gradient echo sequences through the region of interest, observing for T2* effects (magnetic susceptibility) in areas that accumulate gadolinium chelate. From this, one obtains a qualitative value of mean transit time, time to peak, cerebral blood flow and blood volume. Perfusion images can be compared with diffusion to determine mismatches; areas that show diffusion restriction but no perfusion abnormality represent the penumbra of potentially viable tissue. Contrast-enhanced MR perfusion is technically challenging in infants as it requires the placement of a larger-caliber intravenous line and a large bolus of contrast. Magnetization transfer is a method employed to take advantage of the differences between the two environments in which protons exist. In a simple way, protons in normal tissue are bound to macromolecules (proteins) and those in diseased tissue are unbound and referred to as "free-water" protons. The bound protons exist in an inhomogeneous environment resulting in lower precessional frequency and shorter T2. By employing a saturation pulse at this lower frequency, the signal from free protons is enhanced, making disease more conspicuous.

Differential Diagnosis

Deep Gray Matter Lesions
- Metabolic disorders such as mitochondrial disease
- Kernicterus (abnormal signal in globus pallidus, not putamen or thalamus)

Periventricular White Matter Lesions
- Congenital infection (Cytomegalovirus).
- Inherited leukodystophy (Pelizaeus Merzbacher disease).
- Normal periventriuclar halo, which is seen as a normal hyperechoic blush. Suspect PVL if echogenicity is asymmetric, coarse, globular, or more hyperechoic than the choroid plexus.

Common Variants

The typical PVL pattern may occur in full-term neonates who are suffering from ischemia and sepsis. In addition, a mixed HII pattern involving the deep gray matter and the cerebral cortex/subcortical white matter may occur following a prolonged and profound episode of ischemia. If imaging and history are disconcordant, or if there is more than one child with HII per family involved, one should raise the possibility of inborn error of metabolism.

Clinical Issues

Hypoxic-ischemic injury is a significant cause of mortality and severe neurologic disability. There is a short therapeutic window of 2 to 6 hours during which interventions may be efficacious in reducing the severity of brain damage, thus it is essential to be familiar with the many patterns of injury for early diagnosis and management. Treatment consists largely of supportive care, seizure control, occupational, physical, and educational therapy, and rehabilitation.

Key Points
- DWI is the most sensitive modality in the acute period.
- Mild to moderate ischemia in preterm brain manifests as PVL or GMH-IVH.
- Mild to moderate ischemia in term brain involves cortex and subcortical white matter of watershed areas.
- Profound ischemia in preterm and term infants involves metabolically active central brain structures including deep grey matter structures
- Most common injury to the premature brain is PVL.
- PVL and GMH-IVH are uncommon after 34 weeks gestational age.

Further Reading

Argyropoulou MI. Brain lesions in preterm infants: initial diagnosis and follow-up. *Pediatr Radiol.* 2010;*40*(6):811–818. Epub 2010 Apr 30.

Brain and spine injuries in infancy and childhood. In: Barkovich AJ, ed. *Pediatric Neuroimaging.* Fifth edition. Philadelphia, PA: Lippincott, Williams and Wilkins; 2012:243–310.

Chao CP, Zaleski CG, Patton AC. Neonatal hypoxic-ischemic encephalopathy: multimodality imaging findings. *Radiographics.* 2006;*26*(Suppl 1):S159–S172.

Huang BY, Castillo M. Hypoxic-ischemic brain injury: imaging findings from birth to adulthood. *Radiographics.* 2008;*28*(2):417–439.

Twomey E, Twomey A, Ryan S, Murphy J, Donoghue VB. MR imaging of term infants with hypoxic-ischaemic encephalopathy as a predictor of neurodevelopmental outcome and late MRI appearances. *Pediatr Radiol.* 2010;*40*(9):1526–1535.

CHAPTER 106

Vein of Galen Malformation

Kay L. North, DO, Julianne Dean, DO, and Lisa H. Lowe, MD

Definition

Vein of Galen malformations (VOGMs) are congenital lesions composed of multiple arteriovenous shunts draining into a persistant median prosencephalic vein of Markowski (the precursor of the vein of Galen).

Clinical Features

The clinical manifestations of VOGM are dependent on the type and severity of the malformation. The most common type of VOGM (choroid form) presents in neonates with an intracranial bruit and severe high-output cardiac failure secondary to pulmonary hypertension. Flow reversal in the aorta can lead to myocardial ischemia and renal hypoperfusion followed by cardiorespiratory and renal failure, respectively. The second most common type of VOGM (mural form) presents later in the first year of life and has smaller shunts producing milder cardiac manifestations. The mural form of VOGM and smaller choroid malformations may present with an enlarged head circumference (macrocephaly) secondary to hydrocephalus. Other signs may include developmental delay, seizures, dilated scalp veins, proptosis, and epistaxis. Older children, adolescents, and adults with small malformations may also present with headaches, seizures, and intracranial hemorrhages resulting from the presence of microaneurysms within the lesion.

Anatomy and Physiology

In the developing brain, the choroid plexus provides arterial circulation and the large median prosencephalic vein of Markowski serves as venous drainage. Later, as the cortical arterial network and internal cerebral veins develop and mature, the primitive system is replaced and gradually involutes whereby the vein of Markowski becomes the great cerebral vein, or the vein of Galen. In some patients, however, the anterior segment of the median prosencephalic vein of Markowski progressively enlarges to form the dilated venous component of VOGM. Vein of Galen malformations are divided into two types based on the characteristics of the fistula including the choroidal (90 percent) and mural types, however, mixed forms may also occur. The choroidal type has an arteriovenous connection with multiple arteries, including the choroidal arteries forming an arterial nidus that drains via the anterior wall of the prosencephalic vein. The mural type is a direct arteriovenous fistula involving a few larger-caliber connections to the wall of the median vein of prosencephalon. Pathophysiologically, VOGM causes increased venous return to the right atrium, leading to increased pulmonary blood flow, pulmonary hypertension, and finally, congestive heart failure. The VOGM produces a large shunt, which can decrease diastolic pressure and may reverse flow within the aorta. Along with increased ventricular pressure, blood flow within the coronary arteries may be reduced resulting in myocardial ischemia and renal hypoperfusion. Ischemic brain injury can result because of diversion of blood flow via the fistula, and cerebral edema can result from increased venous pressure and impaired cerebrospinal fluid absorption. Because of extensive shunting, the choroid form of VOGM tends to present with high-output cardiac failure, thus is more difficult to treat and has higher morbidity and mortality. The mural type, which has less arteriovenous shunting, tends to present with developmental delay, hydrocephalus and seizures, is easier to treat and has a better prognosis.

Imaging Findings

Prenatal ultrasound (US) diagnosis is more common in recent years and is useful to plan delivery at an institution where immediate endovascular palliative or definitive treatment can be provided if the newborn has high-output cardiac failure. Prenatal US can be used to diagnose VOGM in the third trimester. Both pre- and postnatal US reveal a "cystic-appearing" lesion posterior to the third ventricle at the tentorial incisura. Doppler evaluation shows turbulent, pulsatile flow within the lesion, differentiating it from other midline congenital cystic structures (Fig. 106.1). High resistance in the middle cerebral arteries occurs secondary to vascular steal. Hydrocephalus and cardiac dysfunction may also be identified on US. After birth, it is helpful to assess the aorta for direction of flow. Postnatal US will show a mildly echogenic varix with turbulent flow on Doppler that drains into the straight sinus or persistent falcine sinus. Ultrasound can be used to establish a baseline appearance for frequent monitoring after treatment, including documenting and quantifying postembolization flow. On unenhanced CT, VOGMs are isoattenuated to mildly hyperattenuated.

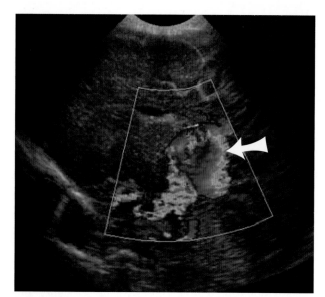

Figure 106.1. Sagittal midline Doppler US image in a 1-day-old female with cardiac failure demonstrates vascular flow within a well-defined cystic mass (arrow) posterior to the third ventricle consistent with VOGM.

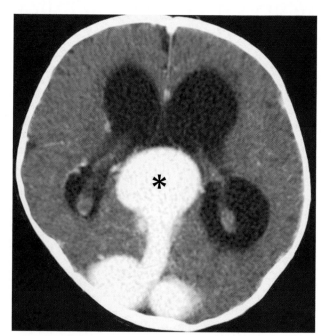

Figure 106.2. Contrast-enhanced CT image in a 2-week-old female with in utero ventriculomegaly demonstrates an enlarged midline vein of Galen (asterisk) draining into a distended straight sinus with hydrocephalus.

Calcification may be present in older individuals or those with adjacent thrombosed aneurysms. Thrombosed aneurysms may be of mixed attenuation. Additional findings include hydrocephalus, evidence of ischemia, parenchymal calcification, atrophy, and rarely, hemorrhage. After administration of IV contrast, VOGMs demonstrate strong enhancement of feeding arteries and the draining varix (Fig. 106.2). CT angiography can be useful to noninvasively map the lesion and establish a baseline for follow-up of subsequent hydrocephalus. As with prenatal US, fetal MRI can diagnose VOGM in the third trimester. Both pre- and postnatal MRI show a well-defined, hypointense, midline mass at the tentorial incisura (dorsal to the third ventricle and beneath the splenium of the corpus callosum), with associated pulsation artifact in the phase-encoding direction. Because of thrombus within the lesion, the signal may vary widely depending on the age of the blood products. Acute thrombosis is isointense on T1-weighted and hypointense on T2-weighted images, whereas in subacute thrombosis, the signal is hyperintense on both T1- and T2-weighed sequences. Diffusion-weighted sequences are helpful to reveal areas of acute ischemia and infarction. Changes of chronic ischemia and gliosis can be challenging to distinguish from the normally unmyelinated T2 hyperintense white matter in infants. MR angiography is useful to map the vascular anomaly (Figs. 106.3 and 106.4).

Imaging Strategy

Prenatal lesions are initially evaluated with antenatal US followed by MR(Fig. 106.5). Postnatal imaging may include Doppler US, CT with CTA, and/or MR with MR angiography, all of which are able to diagnose the lesion.

CT is useful for infants unable to undergo MRI. MRI with MR angiography is the study of choice to delineate the vascular anatomy along with the status of brain and ventricles. High-resolution midline sagittal images are useful to show the relationship between VOGM and the cerebral

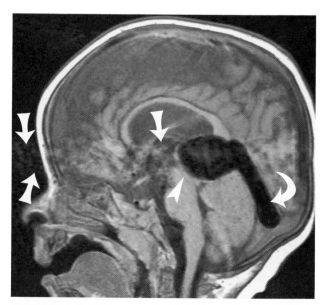

Figure 106.3. Sagittal noncontrast T1 MR image in a 4-week-old female with heart failure demonstrates a well-defined midline cystic VOGM posterior to the third ventricle and beneath the corpus callosum. Pulsation artifact is present indicating a vascular lesion (arrows), there is mass effect on the midbrain/cerebral aqueduct (arrowhead), and the draining straight sinus is distended (curved arrow).

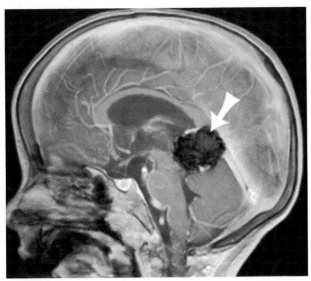

Figure 106.4. Sagittal contrast-enhanced T1-weighted MR image with fat suppression in a 6-month-old female status postembolization at age 1 month shows low signal intensity and lack of enhancement in the embolized VOGM (arrow).

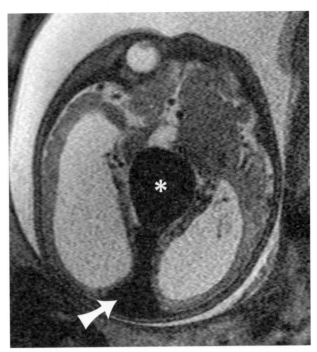

Figure 106.5. Axial single-shot fast T2 MR image in a 36-week fetus with ventriculomegaly shows a low signal intensity midline well-defined cystic mass located posterior to the third ventricle (asterisk). An enlarged midline draining straight sinus is present (arrow) in addition to ventriculomegaly.

aqueduct. Catheter angiography is not indicated for diagnosis, but is usually performed as the initial step in an embolization procedure.

Related Physics

Cranial US with Doppler can provide valuable information about anatomy and flow characteristics in newborns with VOGM. Proper sampling of a signal must obey Niquist theorem, which states that sampling frequency must be at least twice that of the signal's frequency. For Doppler US this means that twice the pulse repetition frequency (PRF) is equal to the maximum detectable Doppler shift. This affects sampling of both high- and low-flow states. In VOGM, venous flow velocities can be quite high related to arteriovenous communication. Smaller veins will show slower flow. In order to sample both ends of the spectrum one must set the PRF to match the sampled velocities (i.e., low PRF for low-flow states and high PRF for high-flow states). When a low PRF is used with high-flow, velocity aliasing will occur by exceeding the Niquist limit. When high PRF is used in low-flow environments, flow will not be detected related to decreased sensitivity to low-flow velocities. On spectral Doppler aliasing will appear as peak arterial flows in opposite direction as a result of "wrapping around" baseline. Color Doppler (red and blue map encoding red toward and blue away from the transducer) will color aliasing blood as high-velocity above or below baseline with colors yellow or green, repectively. Power Doppler is more sensitive but less specific to flow and without directional information it will not reflect the effects of aliasing. The term "bit depth" is used to portray varying shades of gray or colors. Bit depth is binary where the number of shades displayed is equal to 2^n where n is

the number of bits. In Color Doppler, if one wishes to display eight shades of red for color flow one would need 3-bit data (or 2^3). Most systems can display 256 shades of red or blue and use 8-bit processing.

Differential Diagnosis

The differential diagnosis of VOGM is relatively straightforward including congenital midline cysts and rarely teratomas/dermoids. However, the differential is quickly narrowed to include only VOGM once the presence of flow within the lesion is established. In older children and adults presenting with VOGM, one must determine if the venous enlargement is secondary to obstructed venous outflow, known as vein of Galen aneurysmal dilatation (VGAD).

Common Variants

Other venous anomalies associated with vein of Galen malformations include absence of the straight sinus, a persistent falcine sinus, and a persistent occipital sinus. Commonly associated cardiovascular conditions include aortic coarctation and secundum atrial septal defects.

Clinical Issues

Management of patients with VOGM can be difficult. Some authors have suggested use of a 21-point scale to assess patients based on cardiac, cerebral, hepatic, respiratory, and renal function. A score of < 8, usually does not warrant treatment because of an extremely poor prognosis. A score between 8 and 12 is an indication for emergent embolization. Scores > 12 are an indication for medical management until the child is older. The overall goal of VOGM treatment is to first control high-output cardiac failure, either medically if possible or with catheter embolization. Children initially treated successfully with diuretics, inotropes, and other cardiovascular agents may undergo embolization of the malformation at 5 to 6 months of age. Unfortunately, few children are controlled with medical therapy alone. More often, newborns are unstable even with medical management and must undergo catheter embolization sooner rather than later. The goal of initial embolization therapy is sufficient lesion occlusion to decrease flow through the malformation enough to prevent high-output cardiac failure and improve coronary and renal perfusion. Children with persistent heart failure require repeated embolization. Endovascular treatment using microcatheter systems and agents such as liquid adhesives (N-butyl-cyanoacrylate) or platinum microcoils are performed to occlude the fistula on the arterial side. Although some groups have used the transvenous route, some worry that occlusion on this side may severely hinder deep venous drainage and/or cause perforation of the venous aneurysms. The direct venous puncture route via a surgically created burr hole may be considered when there is bilateral severe stenosis or complete occlusion of the transverse sinuses preventing routine venous access.

Key Points

- Two types of VOGM: choroidal (90%) and mural, which have two different clinical presentations.
- Consider in the differential diagnosis of neonates presenting with congestive heart failure.
- Diagnosed on cross-sectional imaging as a defined cystic mass with internal flow posterior to the third ventricle.

Further Reading

Hoang, S, Choudhri O, Edwards M, Guzman, R. Vein of Galen malformation. *Neurosurgery Focus.* 2009;27(5):1–6.

Illner, A. Vein of Galen malfomation. In: Osborn AG, Blazer SI, Salzman KL, et al. *Diagnostic Imaging: Brain.* Salt Lake City, UT: Amirsys; 2005:I 5: 12–15.

Meyers PM, Halbach VD, Barkovich AJ. Anomalies of cerebral vasculature: diagnostic and endovascular considerations. In: Barkovich AJ, ed. *Pediatric Neuroimaging.* Fifth edition. Philadelphia, PA: Lippincott, Williams and Wilkins; 2012:1051–1107.

Lasjaunias PL, Chng SM, Sachet M, et al. The management of vein of Galen aneurysmal malformations. *Neurosurgery.* 2006;59(5 Suppl 3):S184–S194; discussion S3–13.

Soetaert AM, Lowe LH, Formen C. Pediatric cranial Doppler sonography in children: non-sickle cell applications. *Curr Probl Diagn Radiol.* 2009;38(5):219–227.

CHAPTER 107

Choanal Atresia

Anna Illner, MD

Definition

Choanal atresia (CA) is congenital obliteration of the posterior nasal aperture leading to lack of communication between the nasal cavity and nasopharynx.

Clinical Features

Cases are both sporadic and familial. Choanal atresia affects 1 in 5,000 to 8,000 newborns, with unilateral disease being slightly more common than bilateral. There is a 2:1 female predominance is unilateral disease. Unilateral CA is frequently isolated although more than half of patients with bilateral CA have additional anomalies. As neonates are obligate nasal breathers, bilateral choanal atresia presents in the newborn with severe respiratory distress relieved by crying. A nasogastric tube cannot be passed or is passed with great difficulty. Unilateral CA presents later in childhood with unilateral nasal obstruction and chronic rhinorrhea.

Anatomy and Physiology

The etiology of CA is unknown. The classic features include medial deviation and thickening of the posterior vomer, funneling of the choana, membranous or bony atresia plate, and medialization and thickening of the posterolateral nasal wall and pterygoid plates. Choanal atresia is most commonly bony and membranous (70 percent) with pure bony atresia comprising the rest. The four most accepted theories include: (1) persistence of the the foregut buccopharyngeal membrane; (2) persistence of the nasobuccal membrane; (3) faulty neural crest cell migration; and (4) persistent mesodermal nasochoanal adhesions.

Imaging Findings

Computed Tomography
- Atresia plates (Fig. 107.1)
- Posterior vomer thickening (> 0.34 cm in child < than 8 years of age)
- Medialization and thickening of the posterior lateral nasal wall/medial pterygoid (Fig. 107.2)
- Narrow, funnel-shaped posterior choana (< 0.34 cm in newborn) (Fig. 107.3)
- Deviation of nasal septum toward side of atresia (unilateral)

- Thickening, elevation of palatine bone (Fig. 107.4)
- Retained fluid in the nasal cavity
- Inferior turbinate hypoplasia

Imaging Strategy

Choanal atresia is diagnosed with flexible endoscopy and/or CT. Additionally, MRI is useful in the evaluation of associated intracranial abnormalities in suspected syndromic choanal atresia. Prior to CT imaging, the nose should be suctioned and a nasal decongestant applied for optimal evaluation of the choanal membrane and surrounding bony anatomy. The CT protocol should include 1- to 1.5-millimeter thick, axial images in bone algorithm obtained with the imaging plane parallel or 5 to 10 degrees cephalad to the hard palate with multiplanar reformations.

Related Physics

Although CT is the preferred modality for the diagnosis of CA, MR may be used to rule out associated anomalies in syndromic CA. With MR it is important to be knowledgeable about artifacts and their management in order to avoid

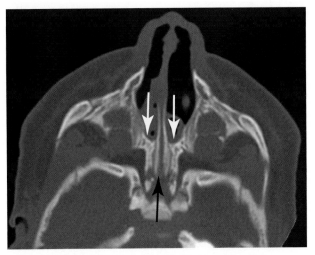

Figure 107.1. Unenhanced axial CT with bone algorithm in a 2-day-old infant with respiratory distress shows bilateral bony choanal atresia. The posterior choanae are narrow and funnel-shaped and terminate in bony atresia plates (white arrows) formed by medialized and thickened posterolateral nasal walls and thickened vomer (black arrow). Retained secretions are present proximal to the atresia plates.

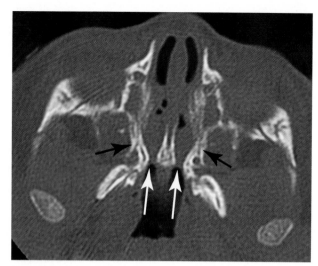

Figure 107.2. Unenhanced axial CT with bone algorithm in a 1-day-old infant with respiratory distress shows bilateral mixed bony and membranous choanal atresia. The posterior choanae are narrow and funnel-shaped with medialization and thickening of the posterolateral nasal walls (black arrows). The atresia plate (white arrows) is membranous and cannot be separated from the overlying retained secretions.

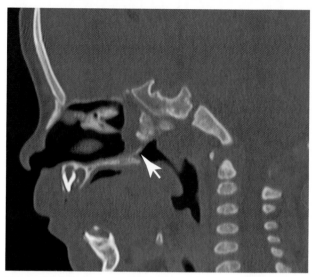

Figure 107.4. Sagittal reconstructions from unenhanced axial CT in a 4-month-old boy with chronic rhinorrhea confirms choanal atresia and shows thickening and elevation of the palatine bone (arrow).

interpretation pitfalls. Artifacts include: metal or susceptibility, field inhomogeneity, radiofrequency, k-space, motion, chemical shift, Gibb's, aliasing, partial voluming, and those related to high-speed and high field-strength imaging. This chapter will include discussion of k-space, motion, and chemical shift artifacts; the others are covered in Spinal Astrocytoma and Child Abuse (Cerebral) chapters. K-space artifact results from a spurious spike in radiofrequency (RF) frequency entering the data train. This abnormal signal strength will appear as a bright dot anywhere in k-space.

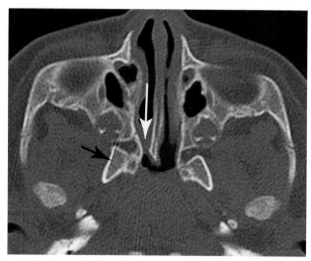

Figure 107.3. Unenhanced axial CT with bone algorithm in a 4-month-old boy with chronic rhinorrhea shows unilateral mixed bony and membranous choanal atresia. The right posterior choana is funnel-shaped (white arrow) with deviation and thickening of the posterior vomer. There is medialization and thickening of the posterolateral nasal wall and pterygoid plate (black arrow).

The x-y coordinates of the spike define the alignment and spacing of the resultant stripes that are created after Fourier transformation. For example, if the spike lies on the x-axis with y coordinate of zero, the stripes will lie vertically in an axial plane image. With regularly spaced lines, this artifact is appropriately termed "corduroy" or "stripe" artifact. K-space artifact can be corrected within the raw data by replacing the spurious signal with that from adjacent pixels. K-space artifact is used to our advantage in cardiac imaging through a process known as tagging whereby high-signal-strength pixels are injected into k-space at known spatial frequencies to purposefully create a grid pattern on the image of myocardium. The deformation of the grid pattern is analyzed to characterize cardiac motion by tracking grid line intersections. Motion artifact is a real concern in pediatric MRI. Motion in the frequency encoding direction results in blurring of the image related to misregistration. Motion in the phase direction results in ghosting, which is a repetition of the image in that direction. This occurs because the phase cycle is slower, allowing time to create a more distinct artifactual pattern. A good example of this is arterial pulsatility in the aorta. When the cardiac cycle is at a different frequency than the phase-encoding frequency, there is a replication of the aorta at different locations throughout the image, but always is the phase direction. When motion is random, one sees more of a blur without a distinct artifact. One can compensate for regular or periodic motion such as that which results from cardiac pulsation thorough ECG-triggered acquisitions. Likewise, one can compensate for respiratory motion with bellows or other devices to measure diaphragm and chest wall excursion. Each tissue has a unique Larmor frequency; fat and water differ by 220 Hertz at 1.5 T. Chemical shift artifact occurs in heterogeneous tissues containing some lipid component, whereby the lipid and nonlipid elements will separate in the frequency encoding direction resulting in two superimposed images of the structure offset by a difference of 220 Hertz at 1.5 T. This creates a dark rim along one pole of the structure and white rim along the opposite pole. One positive use of chemical shift artifact is with "in-phase" and "out-of-phase" gradient echo sequences whereby fat and soft-tissue signal can be additive or subtractive. Two images are produced, in-phase (water plus fat) and out-of-phase (water minus fat), where TE is separated by 1/220 Hertz or 4.4 milliseconds. These two images can be used to determine the fat content in a lesion.

Differential Diagnosis

- Pyriform aperture stenosis: anterior nasal cavity narrowing secondary to congenital bony overgrowth of the naso-maxillary processes
- Congenital nasolacrimal duct cyst: cyst beneath the inferior turbinate caused by an imperforate nasolacrimal duct membrane at the inferior meatus (endonasal component of dacryocystocele)
- Sincipital cephalocele: anterior skull base defect with soft tissue (meninges, brain) in the nasoethmoidal region
- Nasal glioma: heterotopic, dysplastic glial tissue within the nasal cavity (anterior skull base cephalocele that has lost its intracranial connection)

Common Variants

CHARGE syndrome (coloboma, heart defects, atresia- choanal, retardation of growth and/or development, genitourinary, and ear abnormalities/deafness) is the most common syndrome associated with CA occurring in 7 to 29 percent of cases. Additional associations include the acrocephalosyndactylies (Apert, Crouzon, Pfeiffer, Antley-Bixler), Treacher-Collins, de Lange, DiGeorge, and Down syndrome. Also, CA can be seen in association with multiple other congenital and chromosomal anomalies including cleft palate and abnormalities of chromosomes 12, 18, 22, and X.

Clinical Issues

Most cases of bilateral CA are repaired within the first few days of life. Patients with associated CHARGE syndrome or craniofacial abnormalities may have additional levels of airway obstruction requiring tracheostomy tube placement with delayed repair of CA. Unilateral CA is typically repaired after the age of 2 years. In both types of atresia, transnasal endoscopic repair with variable postoperative stenting is the preferred technique with a success rate of 85 percent. The transpalatal approach is reserved for revision operations in older children and adults given the risk of disruption of normal palate development. Patients with associated CHARGE syndrome and craniofacial abnormalities are at greater risk for postoperative complications including restenosis.

Key Points

- Unilateral CA is usually isolated.
- Bilateral CA has high association with other anomalies, particularly CHARGE syndrome.
- CT is modality for CA, MR for associated brain anomalies.
- Important to measure the size of posterior choana, thickness of the vomer and bony atresia plate (if present) and to evaluate the surrounding bony anatomy.

Further Reading

Burrow TA, Saal HM, de Alarcon A, Martin LJ, Cotton RT, Hopkin RJ. Characterization of congenital anomalies in individuals with choanal atresia. *Arch Otolaryngol Head Neck Surg.* 2009;135(6):543–547.

Corrales CE, Koltai PJ. Choanal atresia: current concepts and controversies. *Curr Opin Otolaryngol Head Neck Surg.* 2009;17:466–470.

Durmaz A, Tosun F, Yildirim N, Sahan M, Kivrakdal C, Gerek M. Transnasal endoscopic repair of choanal atresia: results of 13 cases and meta-analysis. *J Craniofacial Surg.* 2008;19(5):1270–1274.

Ibrahim AA, Magdy EA, Hassab MH. Endoscopic choanoplasty without stenting for congenital choanal atresia repair. *International J Pediatr Otolaryngol.* 2010;74:144–150.

Koch BL. Choanal atresia. In: Barkovich AJ, Moore KR, Jones BV, eds. *Diagnostic Imaging: Pediatric Neuroradiology.* Salt Lake City, UT: Amirsys; 2007:II-2-14–II-2-17.

Zuckerman JD, Zapata S, Sobol S. Single-stage choanal atresia repair in the neonate. *Arch Otolaryngol Head Neck Surg.* 2008;134(10):1090–1093.

CHAPTER 108

Otic Capsule Dysplasia

Lisa H. Lowe, MD, Zachary Bailey, MD, and Jon Phelan, MD

Definition

Otic capsule dysplasia refers to a diverse group of congenital anomalies of the bony labyrinth ranging from simple isolated malformations to complex combinations of multiple abnormal inner ear structures.

Clinical Features

Because otic capsule dysplasia involves the inner ear, it tends to present with varying degrees of sensorineural hearing loss, vertigo, and tinnitus, more so than mixed or conductive hearing loss, which are more common with middle and external ear anomalies. Early fetal insults tend to cause more severe symptoms and the degree of dysplasia tends to correlate with symptom severity. One should conduct careful search for synchronous anomalies of the middle and external ear in all children presenting with mixed or conductive hearing loss.

Anatomy and Physiology

Although the specific cause of these anomalies is not fully known, they are believed to result from a variety of insults (toxic, chromosomal, infectious, metabolic, or vascular) that disrupt normal embryologic development early in fetal life. The inner ear is composed of the membranous labyrinth contained within the bony labyrinth, which is also known as the otic capsule. Development of the inner ear and surrounding mesodermal cartilage, which gives rise to the otic capsule, begins at 3 weeks gestational age with the formation of the otic placode from ectoderm along the lateral aspect of the neural tube. The otic placode invaginates to form the otic pit during the fourth week of gestation and then closes in the fifth week to produce the otic cyst. Over the following 3 weeks, the otic cyst divides into the cochlear pouch (which gives rise to the cochlear duct and saccule) and the vestibular pouch (which give rise to the endolymphatic duct, vestibule, and semicircular canals). By the end of the eighth week, the cochlear duct has completed its growth forming a cochlea with 2-3/4 turns. Finally, during the 15th week the cartilaginous otic capsule begins to ossify forming the bony labyrinth.

Imaging Findings

Enlarged vestibular aqueduct: enlarged vestibular aqueduct syndrome has been defined as a vestibular aqueduct exceeding 1.5 millimeters at its midpoint. An easy, reliable way to quickly check the size of the vestibular aqueduct is to compare it to the adjacent superior and posterior semicircular canals, which are normally equal to or greater in size than the vestibular aqueduct (Fig. 108.1).

Cochlear aplasia (or Michel deformity): there must be complete absence of the cochlea for an imaging diagnosis of Michel deformity. Associated anomalies are frequent, including internal auditory canal hypoplasia and vestibular dysplasia. Because the cochlea never forms, the aerated middle ear often expands into the area where the cochlea would have developed. This is an important feature to distinguish cochlear aplasia from acquired cochlear nonvisualization as can occur with postmeningitic cochlear calcification, also termed calcific cochleitis or labyrinthitis obliterans (Fig. 108.2).

Mondini dysplasia: the key imaging finding of Mondini dysplasia is a cochlea with insufficient turns, typically 1.5, causing the middle and apical turns to become a single cystic chamber. In addition, the vestibule and vestibular aqueduct may often be dysplastic or enlarged (Fig. 108.3).

Imaging Strategy

The imaging strategy for children with sensorineural hearing loss and suspected otic capsular dysplasia has evolved over the years from only high-resolution CT (HRCT) to MRI as the initial imaging modality of choice. Although both modalities are able to show detailed anatomy in multiple planes, MRI has the advantages of not requiring radiation and being able to directly demonstrate the cochlear nerves. However, MRI has the disadvantages of possibly requiring sedation, it does not show the osseous structures as well as HRCT, and it may be less available in some institutions.

Temporal bone MR imaging protocols for evaluation of sensorineural hearing loss may vary between institutions, but in general include high-resolution axial and coronal T2-weighted and T1 fat-suppressed weighted sequences. Modern scanners also allow performance of isometric high-resolution heavily T2-weighted sequences that can be reconstructed in any plane and displayed using volume rendering techniques.

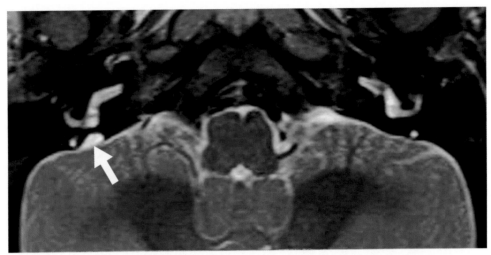

Figure 108.1. Axial T2 MR image in an 11-month-old male with sensorineural hearing loss shows an enlarged vestibular aqueduct (arrow). The normal vestibular aqueduct was noted on the left (not shown).

High-resolution CT imaging of the otic capsule has the advantage of being readily available, but requires radiation and sometimes sedation in uncooperative children. On HRCT, the temporal bone is imaged in the axial plane and reconstructed in the coronal plane at 0.5- to 1.0-millimeter slice thickness. Images are usually obtained parallel and perpendicular to the hard palate.

> **IMAGING PITFALLS:** HRCT imaging allows for visualization and measurement of the bony anatomy, but does not directly show the presence or absence of the cochlear nerve, which requires MRI. Both studies may be necessary for surgical planning, especially for possible cochlear implantation.

Related Physics

The postprocessing of CT images from children with temporal bone anomalies, if performed with care, can accentuate subtle abnormalities. Techniques include edge enhancement, noise reduction, and signal equalization. Edge enhancement is a technique that amplifies strong gradients in Hounsfield units, typically found at the edges of structures such as the tiny ossicles within the middle ear. The technique can come at the expense of increased noise in the image, which is further equilibrated using intelligent noise-reduction algorithms. Such algorithms are sensitive to Hounsfield unit gradients that appear structurally based. The noise-reduction filter will reduce randomly

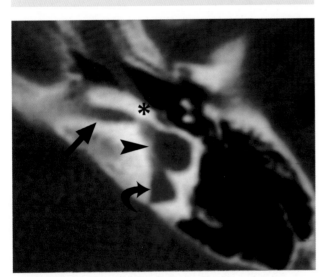

Figure 108.2. Axial noncontrast CT image of the left temporal bone in a 3-year-old female with sensorineural hearing loss resulting from complex otic capsular dysplasia demonstrates hypoplasia of the internal auditory canal (arrow), as well as dysplastic change of the vestibule (arrowhead) and semicircular canals (curved arrow). Also note cochlear aplasia (asterisk).

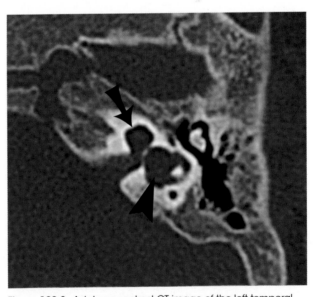

Figure 108.3. Axial noncontrast CT image of the left temporal bone in a 7-year-old female with sensorineural hearing loss resulting from otic capsular dysplasia shows a dysplastic single-cavity cochlea (arrow) and dysplastic enlargement of the vestibule (arrowhead). A normal vestibular aqueduct was seen (not shown).

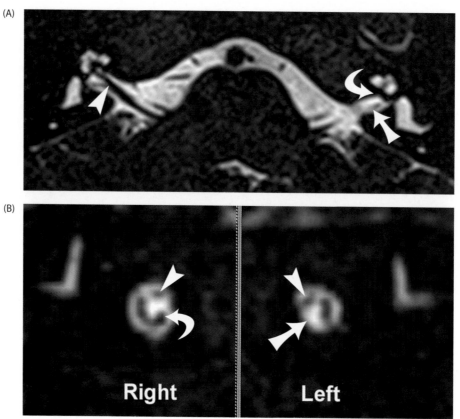

Figure 108.4. Axial T2 MR image (A) in a 4-year-old female with sensorineural hearing loss reveals a hypoplastic left internal auditory canal (arrow) with atresia of the left cochlear aperture (curved arrow), occluded by a thick bony plate, and the left eighth cranial nerve is not visualized within the internal auditory canal or at the cochlear aperture. For comparison, note the normal right eighth nerve (arrowhead) within the internal auditory canal passing through its cochlear aperture. Heavily T2-weighted MR images (B) perpendicular to the internal auditory canals demonstrate absence of the left cochlear nerve (arrow) below the seventh nerve (arrowheads). For comparison, note the right cochlear nerve within the internal auditory canal below the seventh nerve (curved arrow). Findings are consistent with left cochlear aperture and nerve aplasia.

oriented noise but will preserve the structural integrity of sharp edges. To aid in viewing the image, strong and weak signals can be averaged to a smaller dynamic range by a process known as signal equalization. This is rarely done in CT, as broadening the window width will produce a similar image. Temporal bone imaging for otic dysplasias should be performed in a head holder, with lateral padding/immobilization, high rotational speed to suppress motion, small focal-spot size, thin image thickness, small field of view and an ultra-high-resolution reconstruction kernel.

Clinical Issues

A broad array of treatment options, such as various cochlear and auditory brainstem implants are available for children with otic capsular dysplasia. All of these treatments depend upon the presence and quality of the cochlear nerve. To treat correctly, it is critical to determine if a cochlear nerve is present, which can be done with MRI (Figs. 108.4A

and B). Detailed anatomic assessment will avert complications related to abnormal facial nerve paths and potential cerebrospinal fluid (CSF) gushers secondary to stapes and anomalies of the lateral end of internal auditory canal. Often HRCT is needed in addition to MRI to fully evaluate the bony landmarks in order to avoid intraoperative injury.

Key Points

- Otic capsular dysplasia encompasses a variety of inner ear malformations.
- The type of otic capsular dysplasia depends on timing of embryologic insult.
- Otic capsular dysplasia presents with sensorineural hearing loss.
- MRI is able to definitively determine the cochlear nerve status prior to surgery.
- CT will better define the osseous anatomy.

Further Reading

Benton C, Bellet PS. Imaging of congenital anomalies of the temporal bone. *Neuroimaging Clin. N. Am.* 2000;*10*(1):35–53.

Dewan K, Wippold FJ Jr, Lieu JE. Enlarged vestibular aqueduct in pediatric SNHL. *Otolaryngol. Head Neck Surg.* 2009;*140*(4):552–558.

McClay JE, Booth TN, Parry DA, et al. Evaluation of pediatric sensorineural hearing loss with magnetic resonance imaging. *Arch. Otolaryngol. Head Neck Surg.* 2008;*134*(9):945–952.

Ozgen B, Oguz KK, Atas A, et al. Complete labyrinthine aplasia: clinical and radiological findings with review of the literature. *AJNR Am J Neuroradiol.* 2009;*30*:774–780.

CHAPTER 109

Branchial Cleft Cysts

Avrum N. Pollock, MD, FRCPC

Definition

Branchial cleft cysts (BCCs) are vestigial remnants of incomplete obliteration of the branchial apparatus in the neck or are the result of buried epithelial cells.

Clinical Features

A BCC will most often present as a mass, which tends to be recurrent, and which enlarges within days of onset of an upper respiratory tract infection (URTI). The lesion is often successfully treated symptomatically with a course of antibiotics, with resultant temporary resolution on physical examination and imaging. There is, however, a high incidence of recurrence with enlargement following the next URTI.

Anatomy and Physiology

Branchial cleft cysts are classified according to their proposed cleft or pouch of origin and are designated as either first, second, third or fourth BCCs. It should be noted that first BCCs are further divided into two types. Type I (Fig. 109.1) is thought to be caused by duplication of the membranous external auditory canal (EAC), and type II (Fig. 109.2) is a fistulous tract extending from the floor of the EAC to the submandibular area. Characteristically BCCs are found within, superficial, or deep to the parotid gland and may have direct connection with the external auditory canal. Ninety-five percent of all branchial cleft anomalies arise from the remnant of the second branchial cleft apparatus. The most common location for a second BCC (Fig. 109.3) is within the submandibular space with resultant posteromedial displacement of carotid sheath (CS), posterolateral displacement of the sternocleidomastoid muscle (SCM), and anterior displacement of the submandibular gland. The third BCC is either identified in the same region as the second BCC (rarely) or is located anywhere along the course of the third branchial cleft; along the anterior edge of the SCM in the mid to lower neck and in the posterior cervical space (posterior triangle) when it occurs in the upper cervical region (Fig. 109.4).

The fourth BCC is a misnomer, in that it is really a fourth branchial anomaly arising from a branchial pouch and not a cleft, and most commonly appears as a sinus tract from the inferior tip of the (left) piriform sinus to the ipsilateral anterior thyroid bed (Fig. 109.5).

Although sporadically described in the literature as having some malignant potential if not excised, BCCs are felt to have a very low malignant potential.

Imaging Findings

A BCC appears as a simple cyst on all imaging modalities. Lack of internal flow on Doppler ultrasound (US) confirms the cystic nature. CT shows a well-defined, fluid attenuation mass with variable enhancement of the capsule. MR shows a lesion that is hypointense on T1 and hyperintense on T2, however the lesion may be hyperintense on T1 because of internal hemorrhage or protein. The cyst can have variable appearance on imaging if there is prior hemorrhage or infection. Internal debris may be seen on US.

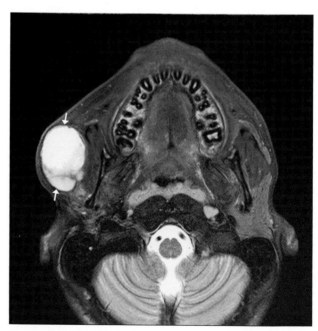

Figure 109.1. Axial fat-saturated T2 MR image of the facial region in a child with pain and swelling demonstrates a cystic lesion involving the right parotid gland (arrows) consistent with first BCC.

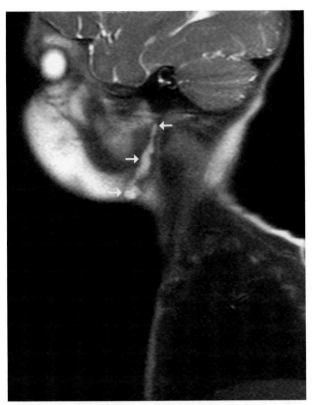

Figure 109.2. Sagittal HASTE image of the right neck in a patient with neck swelling shows a cystic lesion that extends cephalad to level of the external auditory canal (arrows) consistent with first BCC, type II.

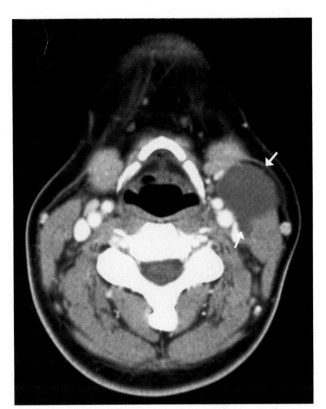

Figure 109.3. Axial contrast-enhanced CT of the neck in a child with neck swelling shows a low-attenuation lesion in the left neck, interposed between submandibular gland and the SCM muscle (arrow) consistent with second BCC.

IMAGING PITFALLS: MR can reflect the true cystic nature of these lesions. The common use of dental braces can lead to magnetic field distortion and hence limit the diagnostic quality of MRI, which is not an issue with CT limited to the neck region. In addition non-spin-echo T1-weighted techniques using gradient echo (e.g., MPRAGE/SPGR) can make the contents of the cyst appear spuriously bright, thereby falsely suggesting that the lesion may be solid, when in fact it is cystic on the standard spin-echo T1-weighted sequences. This phenomenon increases with increasing field strength.

Imaging Strategy

Ultrasound is helpful as the initial study to elucidate the cystic nature of BCC, but may lack the ability to assess the full extent of the lesion as in many cases there is deeper extension toward the trachea. Given its superior soft-tissue contrast and lack of ionizing radiation, MRI is the definitive imaging study for complete assessment of lesion characteristics and extent.

Related Physics

In order to reduce time, MR imaging for BCC can be optimized through a technique known as parallel imaging. In

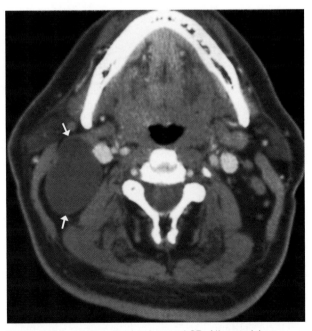

Figure 109.4. Axial contrast-enhanced CT of the neck in a child with neck mass demonstrates a low-attenuation lesion in the posterior right neck, deep to the SCM muscle (arrows) consistent with third BCC.

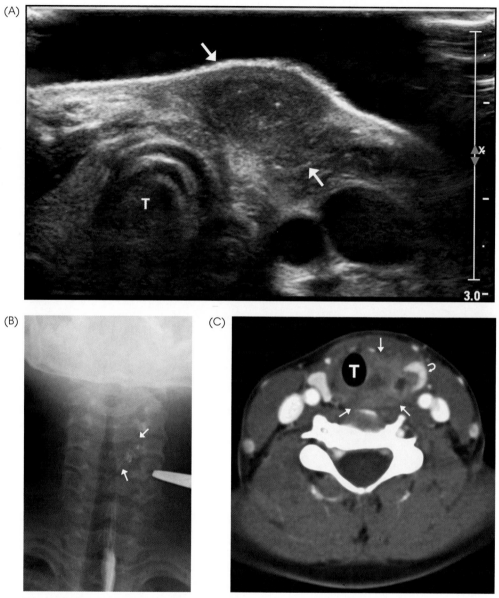

Figure 109.5. Transverse US image (A) of the left neck at the level the thyroid gland in a child with recurrent neck infection and drainage shows a mixed echogenicity lesion (arrows), which extends deep in the neck toward the level of the trachea (T). Frontal image from barium swallow (B) in the same child confirms a contrast-filled track coursing to the ipsilateral piriform sinus (arrows) consistent with fourth BCC. Axial contrast-enhanced CT (C) from a patient with recurrent neck infection and swelling shows a mixed attenuation area (arrows) deep to the left lobe of the thyroid (curved arrow) with associated mass effect on the adjacent trachea (T) consistent with fourth BCC.

general this occurs at the expense of image quality (i.e., decreased signal to noise ratio (SNR). Parallel imaging can be implemented in the image or frequency domain (k-space) and requires placement of a multi-array coil where the coil elements can be operated separately in paired sets. For parallel imaging in the image domain, the general principle is to reduce the number of phase-encoding steps and therefore time. Each coil produces a low-quality image and, when combined with the low-quality image from the other coils, produces one image of reasonable quality. For parallel imaging in the frequency domain, each coil set fills a unique fraction of k-space simultaneously, resulting in

full population of k-space in a fraction of the time taken for a single coil. The operator has the choice of several "parallel factors," with the ability to increase acquisition speeds by factors of two (at the same time reducing SNR by a factor of two). This technology will be limited by the availability of multi-element array coils and high-speed hardware and software to process highly parallel data. The most common artifact encountered with the phase method results from undersampling, which results in a band of signal through the center of the image secondary to aliasing; this is most easily rectified by opening the field of view (FOV) to 100 percent.

Differential Diagnosis

- Infected/necrotic lymph node
- Intraparotid cyst, tumor, lymph node pathology, or venolymphatic malformation
- Cystic thyroid nodule

Clinical Issues

The BCC is usually completely surgically excised with no need for further follow-up. The exception is the fourth branchial anomaly with its associated fistula that can be very difficult to completely excise, given the communication with the adjacent piriform sinus. A fourth BCC may require additional CT/MRI, barium swallow, or fistulogram for presurgical planning to ensure complete excision.

Key Points

- Present as recurrent neck mass post-URTI
- Variable imaging appearances related to internal contents
- Congenital anomalies of branchial apparatus
- Ninety-five % arise from the remnant of the second branchial cleft apparatus
- Surgically treatable
- Low malignant potential

Further Reading

Bauer PW, Lusk RP. Neck masses. In: Bluestone CR, Stool, Alper CM, Arjmand EM, Casselbrant ML, Dohar JE, Yellon RF, eds. *Pediatric Otolaryngology*. Philadelphia, PA: Saunders; 2003:1629–166

Becker M.. Oral cavity and oropharynx. In: Mafee MF, Valvassori GE, Becker M, eds. *Imaging of the Head and Neck*. New York, NY: Thieme; 2005a:720–723.

Becker M.. Other infrahyoid neck lesions. In: Mafee MF, Valvassori GE, Becker M, eds. *Imaging of the Head and Neck*. New York, NY: Thieme; 2005b:834–837.

Hudgins PA, Cure J. Pediatric and trans-spatial lesions. In: Harnsberger HR, ed. *Diagnositic Imaging Head and Neck*. Salt Lake City, UT: Amirysys; 2004:Part IV,Section 1,2–21.

Mafee MF. Salivary glands. In: Mafee MF, Valvassori GE, Becker M, eds. *Imaging of the Head and Neck*. New York, NY: Thieme; 2005:638–639.

Mafee MF. Nasopharynx. In: Mafee MF, Valvassori GE, Becker M, eds. *Imaging of the Head and Neck*. New York, NY: Thieme; 2005:560–561.

Nour SG, Lewin JS. Parapharyngeal and masticator spaces. In: Mafee MF, Valvassori GE, Becker M, eds. *Imaging of the Head and Neck*. New York, NY: Thieme; 2005:613–615.

Som PM, Smoker WRK, Reidenberg JS, Bergemann AD, Hudgins PA, Laitman J. Embryology and anatomy of the neck. In: Som PM, Curtin HD, eds. *Head and Neck Imaging*. St. Louis, MO: Elsevier Mosby; 2011:2217–2124.

Som PM, Smoker WRK, Curtin HD, Reidenberg JS, Laitman J. Congenital lesions of the neck. In: Som PM, Curtin HD, eds. *Head and Neck Imaging*. St. Louis, MO: Elsevier Mosby; 2011:2235–2252.

CHAPTER 110

Orbital Cellulitis

Alexia M. Egloff, MD

Definition

Orbital cellulitis is an inflammatory condition affecting the orbit, most often secondary to bacterial infection of the paranasal sinuses or face.

Clinical Features

Orbital cellulitis is the most common disorder affecting the orbit in children, representing 60 percent of orbital pathology. It is usually unilateral and can involve the preseptal and postseptal soft tissues (see anatomy and physiology section). *Preseptal cellulitis*, an inflammation superficial to the orbital septum, is characterized by eyelid swelling and erythema. When the inflammation extends behind the orbital septum, it is called *postseptal orbital cellulitis*. In addition to the eyelid swelling, there is associated proptosis and impaired function of the extraocular muscles. Increased postseptal pressure by a subperiosteal or orbital abscess can result in worsening proptosis with progressive visual loss and ophthalmoplegia.

Anatomy and Physiology

Orbital cellulitis is usually bacterial in origin and secondary to other inflammatory processes of the face, most commonly sinusitis. It can also be seen after trauma or secondary to foreign bodies, or septicemia. Fungal or granulomatous infection is also possible in immunocompromised patients. The pre- and postseptal spaces are separated by the orbital septum. The septum is formed by a thin sheet of fibrous tissue and attaches to the rim of the bony orbit. The postseptal area can be further divided into extraconal and intraconal regions by the extraocular muscles (Fig. 110.1). Preseptal cellulitis results from untreated sinusitis with local spread of the inflammation to the eyelid. Postseptal cellulitis almost always arises from direct extension of the ethmoid sinusitis through the porous lamina papyracea. Alternatively, the increased sinus pressure can be transmitted to the orbital veins resulting in leakage of inflammatory elements into the orbit. Infection rarely spreads posteriorly beyond the tendinous ring at the apex of the orbit.

Imaging Findings

Preseptal cellulitis
- Eyelid and facial swelling with increased attenuation of fatty tissues and fat plane obliteration (Fig. 110.2)

Postseptal cellulitis
- Swelling of the extraconal and intraconal soft tissues
- Increased attenuation of the intraconal fat
- Inflammation of adjacent lacrimal gland
- Thickening and displacement of extraocular muscles

Subperiosteal phlegmon
- Hypodense, rim-enhancing, lentiform collection along the wall of the orbit, most commonly involving the lamina papyracea with postseptal cellulitis (Fig. 110.3)
- Displaces the adjacent extraocular muscle and can cause thickening and increase in attenuation
- Adjacent sinusitis

Orbital abscess
- Rim-enhancing fluid collection with adjacent cellulitis.
- Intra- or extraconal processes can involve the extraocular muscles

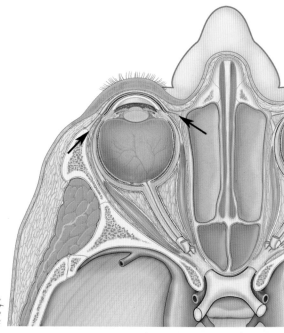

Figure 110.1. Normal orbital anatomy. Orbital septum (arrow) divides disease processes into preseptal (anterior to septum) and postseptal (posterior to septum).

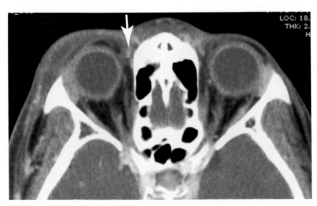

Figure 110.2. Axial contrast-enhanced CT image in a 13-year-old patient with eye swelling shows moderate thickening of right preseptal soft tissues (arrow), with no postseptal involvement consistent with preseptal cellulitis.

Ophthalmic vein and cavernous sinus thrombosis

- Engorgement of the superior ophthalmic vein
- Hypodense, heterogeneous, convex cavernous sinus with meningeal enhancement (Fig. 110.4)
- MRI demonstrates expanded cavernous sinus without normal internal enhancement

Imaging Strategy

When postseptal orbital cellulitis is a concern, contrast-enhanced CT should be performed. Thin axial images are obtained and coronal reformats are performed. Soft tissue and bone windows should be reviewed before rendering a diagnosis. The cavernous sinus and anterior frontal regions must be assessed for intracranial complications. When intracranial complications are suspected and for better evaluation of the orbital apex, MRI is performed.

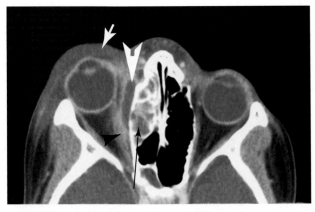

Figure 110.3. Axial contrast-enhanced CT image in an 11-year-old patient with right orbital cellulitis, pain, and proptosis shows preseptal soft-tissue thickening and increased fat attenuation (white arrow), proptosis, and a subperiosteal collection (white arrowhead) outside the lamina papyracea. Note opacification of the ipsilateral paranasal sinuses (black arrow). Fat stranding of postseptal, extraconal fat is noted with lateral displacement and thickening of medial rectus muscle (black arrowhead) consistent with postseptal cellulitis.

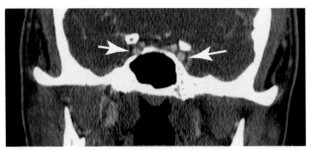

Figure 110.4. Coronal contrast-enhanced CT image in a teen with persistent neurological deficits and ptosis demonstrates incomplete contrast enhancement of the cavernous sinuses (arrows) suggestive of thrombosis.

IMAGING PITFALLS: Contrast-enhanced CT is the initial imaging modality for orbital cellulitis and is insensitive to orbital apex pathology or intracranial extension; MRI must be performed if such complications are suspected.

Related Physics

The main modality used for investigation of orbital infection is CT. There are several choices for technique for head and orbit imaging with CT. One must first decide between axial and helical (spiral) mode. The second choice is between fixed and auto-mAs. Finally one must decide if gantry angulation will be necessary. Axial mode, although slower, is less prone to artifact especially where the object of interest has considerable changes in shape and size in the z-axis, such as the head and orbits. In helical mode, as the shape changes in the z-axis, a "swirl" develops at the periphery of the curved surface related to partial volume averaging as the table moves. On some newer-generation scanners, axial mode is no longer available, so that several parameters can be adjusted to reduce this unwanted artifact. Suggestions would include lowering the pitch to 1 and narrowing the X-ray beam width (collimation). It is also advantageous to scan in helical mode to support full-resolution multiplanar reconstruction, eliminating the need for direct imaging in the axial and coronal plane. Lowest dose is imperative for CT orbits, and this can be best accomplished by choosing fixed mAs technique. Auto-mAs is not as desirable for orbital imaging as there are very few dimension differences in the left-right and anterior-posterior direction, so that the choice of mAs by the scanner may in fact be unnecessarily high. Gantry angulation would not be necessary with orbital imaging as angulation is usually used to avoid the orbits. Finally, image reconstruction should be performed both in the axial and coronal planes using both soft-tissue kernel for orbital and brain mass/abscess and high-frequency kernel to rule out bone erosion.

Differential Diagnosis

- Orbital pseudotumor (Fig. 110.5): an inflammatory process of unknown etiology, it can involve the lacrimal gland, intraconal fat, sclera, and extraocular muscles. It

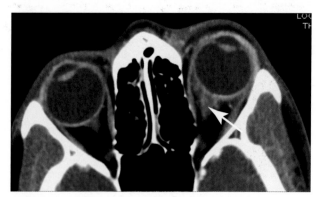

Figure 110.5. Axial contrast-enhanced CT image in a 14-year-old patient with 3 weeks of progressive swelling, pain, and proptosis demonstrates thickening of the left sclera with enhancement and surrounding preseptal and intraconal fat stranding (arrow) caused by orbital pseudotumor.

can look similar to orbital cellulitis and presents with pain, without associated fever or leukocytosis.

■ Sarcoidosis: an enhancing intra- and extraconal mass, associated with sinonasal granulomas. Associated with vasculitis and gomerulonephritis. No abscess is present.

■ Orbital rhabdomyosarcoma: this must be differentiated from cellulitis with abscess and is a an enhancing soft-tissue mass presenting with unilateral, rapidly progressive proptosis. When large, the lesion can show necrosis and hemorrhage, osseous involvement, and extension into paranasal sinuses.

Clinical Issues

If not properly treated, postseptal involvement of the orbital structures can result in optic nerve ischemia, optic neuritis, vascular thrombosis and intracranial spread with complications including empyema, meningitis, or cerebritis.

Key Points

■ Orbital cellulitis is the most common orbital pathology in pediatrics.
■ It can be preseptal or postseptal.
■ Most commonly it is secondary to sinus infection.
■ It can present with subperiosteal collection or orbital abscess.
■ Ophthalmic vein thrombosis, cavernous sinus thrombosis, and intracranial complications can occur.

Further Reading

Chung EM, Smirniotopoulos JG, Specht CS, Schroeder JW, Cube R. From the archives of the AFIP. Pediatric orbit tumors and tumorlike lesions: nonosseous lesions of the extraocular orbit. *Radiographics.* 2007;27(6):1777–1799.

Reid, JR. Complications of pediatric paranasal sinusitis. *Pediatr Radiol.* 2004;34(12):933–942.

Som PM. Orbit: embryology, anatomy, and pathology. In: Curtin HD, ed. *Head and Neck Imaging.* Fourth edition. St. Louis, MO: Mosby;579–580.

CHAPTER 111

Retinoblastoma

Janet R. Reid, MD, FRCPC

Definition

Retinoblastoma is a malignant childhood neoplasm whose origin is the immature retina of the eye.

Clinical Features

Retinoblastoma is the most common intraocular tumor of childhood with an incidence of 1 in 15,000 to 20,000. There is no gender or ethnic predominance and the most common presentation is a child under 2 years with leukocoria, or "white reflex" replacing the normal red reflex on ophthalmoscopic evaluation. Strabismus is also common. Less common presentations include heterochromia, pain, glaucoma, and ocular inflammation.

There are two forms of retinoblastoma: heritable and nonheritable. The heritable form presents on average 1 year earlier than the sporadic form. Nonheritable tumors are always unilateral. Sixty percent of retinoblastoma cases are unilateral (always sporadic) and 40 percent are bilateral (in which three-quarters of these are sporadic). The heritable form is transmitted with an autosomal dominant pattern and is related to a mutation or deletion of the RB1 tumor suppressor gene on the long arm of chromosome 13. New theories have emerged that implicate aneuploidy and chromosome instability in the pathogenesis of this disease. Patients with retinoblastoma have an increased incidence of secondary tumors including osteogenic sarcoma, melanoma, and various sarcomas as well as intracranial neuroblastomas. Radiation accelerates the formation of secondary tumors, 30 percent within the field and 9 percent outside the field of radiation. For this reason it is very important to avoid diagnostic studies that use ionizing radiation in patients with possible retinoblastoma.

Anatomy and Physiology

Normal retinal anatomy is illustrated in Figure 111.1. Retinoblastoma originates in the precursors of cone cells in the developing sensory retina. Retinoblastoma cells have a large nuclear to cytoplasmic ratio and grow rapidly with numerous mitoses, lack of intercellular matrix, and large areas of necrosis between cells. Chunks of calcification are common. More differentiated tumors may contain Flexner-Wintersteiner rosettes, which refers to a tubular array of mature cells representing primitive photoreceptors. Homer-Wright rosettes may also form in more primitive tumors.

The tumors may grow into the vitreous humor (endophytic), or through the retina and choroid (exophytic). Exophytic tumors may invade the ciliary vessels, Bruch's membrane, and extend into the orbit or along the optic nerve (postlaminar invasion). A rare infiltrative form may cause diffuse retinal thickening that can encase the globe. Metastatic spread can occur by direct local invasion of brain, or through hematogenous or lymphatic dissemination. The tumor may metastasize to lungs, bone, brain, and almost any other organ in the body.

Imaging Findings

The most common imaging finding is a nodular retina-based mass with dense calcification and areas of cystic degeneration or necrosis. The presence of calcification strongly favors the diagnosis of retinoblastoma. Exophytic tumors extending through the choroid will often cause retinal detachment with subretinal hemorrhage. Extension through the globe or along the optic nerve will be evident on MRI. Although CT is not recommended because of increased susceptibility to radiation in these patients, the tumor will be soft tissue in density with scattered or diffuse hyperdense chunky calcification with enhancement following contrast administration. On MRI the soft-tissue tumor is intermediate in signal intensity on T1 (slightly brighter than vitreous; Fig. 111.2) and dark on T2 (owing to high nuclear-to-cytoplasmic ratio; Fig. 111.3) with calcification seen as foci of bright signal on T1 and dark signal on T2. There is often intense enhancement after gadolinium. Postlaminar spread (through the optic disk) is confirmed as enhancement on high-resolution images of the orbit (Fig. 111.4). High-resolution ultrasound will show a solid mass with scattered calcification with posterior acoustic shadowing in 75 percent (Fig. 111.5). Fine calcification may be difficult to detect. Echogenic foci within the vitreous may represent hemorrhage or tumor seeding.

Imaging Strategy

Indications for imaging include leukocoria and/or positive family history for retinoblastoma. In those with

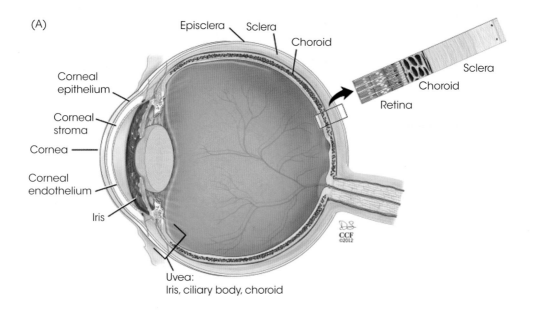

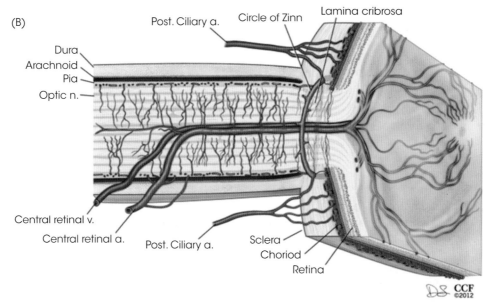

Figure 111.1. Normal anatomy of the orbit, retina and optic nerve. (A) Retinoblastoma can invade the vitreous and uvea or spread outward through the uvea and sclera, or (B) through the lamina cribrosa (postlaminar) along the optic nerve.

sonographic unilateral tumor, brain and orbital imaging are recommended to evaluate for bilateral disease and to rule out associated pineoblastoma (trilateral retinoblastoma) or pituitary germ cell tumor (quadilateral retinoblastoma with bilateral retinoblastoma and synchronous pineal and pituitary tumors). Although CT is the most sensitive modality to detect calcification, it is strongly discouraged because ionizing radiation leads to increased incidence of RB1 allelic mutations causing secondary malignancies. Recommended imaging strategy includes brain and high-resolution orbital MRI with gadolinium.

Related Physics

It is important to have a strong foundation in the biologic effects of ionizing radiation. This is particularly important when planning the imaging workup of patients with retinoblastoma. The response of cells to ionizing radiation has been described according to the Laws of Bergonie and Tribondeau, which state that radiosensitivity increases in cells that are younger, less-differentiated and faster-replicating as well as younger organisms. The rules almost perfectly encapsulate the paradox of imaging children in that if cured there is a long lifespan ahead of them; if harmed their lives are cut short. With too little radiation we

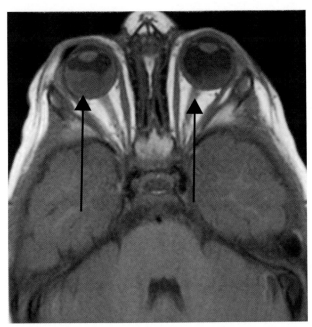

Figure 111.2. Axial noncontrast T1 MR image in a 12-month-old female with bilateral retinoblastoma shows bilateral posterior lesions of soft-tissue signal intensity (arrows).

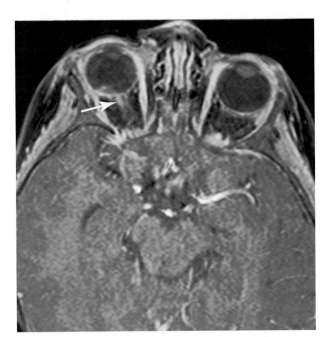

Figure 111.4. Axial contrast-enhanced T1 image of the orbits with fat suppression in a 15-month-old female with retinoblastoma shows diffuse enhancement of the small lesion of the right eye as well as enhancement of the deeper layers of the retina, sclera, and the optic nerve consistent with postlaminar invasion (arrow).

might miss a life-threatening disease that could be cured at its early stage; with too much radiation we might promote that same cancer. Radiosensitivity varies by cell type: neural and other highly differentiating tissues are radioresistant; cells that are rapidly dividing such as hair, skin, and mucosa are radiosensitive. Within any cell type, sensitivity will vary

by phase cell division; cells with greater mitoses are more radiosensitive whereas those in more dormant phases are relatively resistant. Cells can be damaged through direct injury to DNA, or indirectly through free radical formation

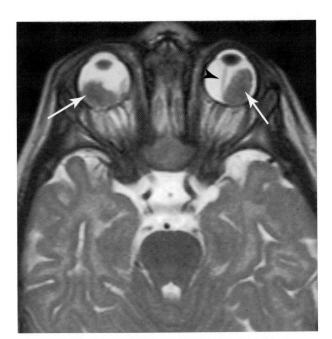

Figure 111.3. Axial T2 MR image with fat suppression in an 8-month-old male with bilateral leukocoria and family history of retinoblastoma shows bilateral posterior tumors of low signal intensity because of calcification and high nuclear-cytoplasmic ratio (arrows). Linear structure represents associated retinal detachment (arrowhead).

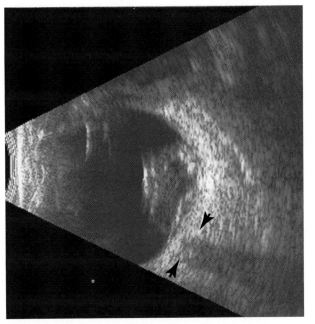

Figure 111.5. Sagittal high-resolution ultrasound image in a 15-month-old child with leukocoria shows the echogenic intraocular mass originating from the retina with a focus of posterior acoustic shadowing consistent with calcification (arrow).

in intracellular fluid resulting in disruption of DNA bonds. Most radiobiology information has been gleaned from in vitro cell experiments that have followed cell survival after exposure to various doses of radiation. In these experiments cells of a specific type were exposed to varying amounts of radiation and percent survival was determined at a fixed time postirradiation. A typical endpoint was the dose at which 50 percent of the cells in a population died within 30 days known as the LD 50/30.

Differential Diagnosis

Differential diagnosis of leukocoria includes a number of entities that rarely, if ever, calcify:

- Persistent hyperplastic primary vitreous
- Coat's disease
- Norrie's disease
- Toxocara canis infection
- Retinopathy of prematurity
- Retinal astrocytic hamartoma
- Retinocytoma is the benign equivalent and has smooth borders

Common Variants

Retinoblastoma may be bilateral, multifocal, exophytic, or diffusely infiltrative. Trilateral retinoblastoma refers to bilateral orbital tumors and pineoblastoma. Quadrilateral retinoblastoma is trilateral disease plus a germ cell tumor of the pituitary.

Clinical Issues

Retinoblastoma is often treated with enucleation. Bilateral disease and some unilateral disease may be treated with cryoablation or thermoablation to preserve vision. Other strategies include brachytherapy, chemotherapy, and external beam irradiation. Children with familial disease must be followed for life for second tumors (with an incidence as high as 38 percent). Localized disease has a cure rate of 95 percent. Disease that is metastatic at presentation has a high mortality rate.

Key Points

- Retinoblastoma is a nodular calcified orbital tumor in early childhood (calcification is rare in any other lesion of the orbit in children).
- Rarer familial form is autosomal dominant and bilateral and presents at younger age.
- CT and radiation are contraindicated.
- MRI of the orbits and brain is indicated for associated disease in pineal and pituitary.
- Retinoblastoma spreads locally along optic nerve and to lungs, bone, and brain.

Further Reading

Chung EM, Specht CS, Schroeder JW. Pediatric orbit tumors and tumorlike lesions: neuroepithelial lesions of the ocular globe and optic nerve. *Radiographics.* 2007; *27*:1159–1186.

Kleinerman RA. Radiation-sensitive genetically susceptible pediatric sub-populations. *Pediatric Radiology.* 2009;*39*:S27–S31.

Lohmann D. Retinoblastoma. In: Ahmad SI, ed. *Diseases of DNA Repair.* Vol *685*. :Springer Science and Business Media; 2010:220–227.

Mastrangelo D et al. Retinoblastoma epidemiology: does the evidence matter? *European Journal of Cancer.* 2007;*43*:1596–1603.

Ng AK, Kenney LB, Gilbert ES, Travis LB. Secondary malignancies across the age spectrum. *Seminars in Radiation Oncology.* 2010; *20*:67–78.

CHAPTER 112

Juvenile Nasopharyngeal Angiofibroma

Bhairav N. Patel, MD

Definition

Juvenile nasopharyngeal angiofibroma or simply juvenile angiofibroma (JNA) is the most common benign pediatric nasopharyngeal tumor. These tumors most likely originate from the fibrovascular stroma of the nasal wall adjacent to the sphenopalatine foramen. Although these tumors are benign, they are highly vascular and locally invasive.

Clinical Features

Juvenile angiofibroma is rare, accounting for only 0.5 percent of all head and neck tumors and occurs primarily in males between the ages of 10 to 25 years. Rare cases of JNA in females and older males have been reported. The most common presenting symptoms are unilateral nasal obstruction and/or recurrent epistaxis with less common presentations including blood-tinged sputum, nasal discharge, and serous otitis media (secondary to Eustachian tube obstruction within the nasopharynx). Extension of the tumor may cause additional symptoms including facial swelling, proptosis, sinusitis, and headache.

Anatomy and Physiology

The etiology of JNA is unknown, however growth factors, androgens, and chromosomal alterations are all believed to play a role in development. The lesion appears to originate in fibrovascular stroma of the nasal wall adjacent to the sphenopalatine foramen and contains both fibroblastic and vascular components. Often at presentation JNAs have grown to involve the posterior nasal cavity via the sphenopalatine foramen and subsequently the nasopharynx. From the pterygopalatine fossa the tumor can extend into the infratemporal fossa via the pterygomaxillary fissure into the orbit via the inferior orbital fissure, into the oral cavity via the greater and lesser palatine foramina, and intracranially via the foramen rotundum into the parasellar region and vidian canal (to the region of foramen lacerum). Involvement of smaller and inconsistent foramina originating from the pterygopalatine fossa, such as the palatovaginal canal, can also occur. Juvenile angiofibromas can also grow directly into structures such as the maxillary antrum, sphenoid sinus, and pterygoid fossa by direct osseous erosion.

Imaging Findings

- "Antral bowing" sign (anterior bowing of the posterior maxillary wall on facial radiographs)
- Mass centered in the region of the sphenopalatine foramen on CT or MR (Fig 112.1)
- Mass extends into numerous additional anatomic regions via various foramina connected to the pterygopalatine fossa and into sinuses via direct trans-osseous extension (Fig 112.2)
- Enlarged internal or external carotid artery branches, particularly the internal maxillary and ascending pharyngeal arteries on CTA or MRA
- Intermediate to low T1 signal, moderate to high T2 signal on MRI
- Avid contrast enhancement (Fig 112.3) (Fig 112.4)
- Intratumoral flow voids can be (but are not always) present on MR spin echo sequences

Angiography is typically performed as part of preoperative embolization and demonstrates a hypervascular mass fed by enlarged vessels, usually from branches of the internal maxillary and ascending pharyngeal arteries (Fig. 112.5). Importantly, blood supply from the internal carotid artery can occur through the branches of the inferolateral trunk, such as the arteries of the vidian canal and foramen rotundum.

> **IMAGING PITFALLS:** If typical hypervascularity is not present and/or lymphadenopathy is present, alternative diagnoses should be considered.
>
> One should alert the interventional radiologist if enlarged vessels are identified coursing through skull base foramina or if there is variant supply of the ophthalmic artery to avoid complications during embolization.

Imaging Strategy

A child with a known nasopharyngeal mass and/or suspected JNA based on clinical presentation should have either a contrast-enhanced CT or MRI with and without contrast of the face and neck, though both may be performed as they may provide complementary information: CT would best evaluate for osseous destruction and MRI would best

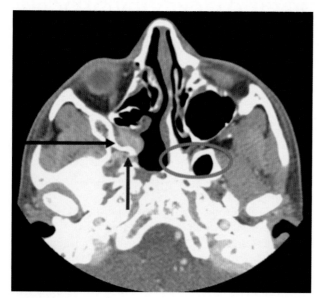

Figure 112.1. Axial contrast-enhanced CT in a teen with epistaxis demonstrates a hypervascular mass centered in the right pterygopalatine fossa (black arrow) with involvement of the sphenopalatine fossa (white arrowhead). Normal fat-filled left pterygopalatine fossa and sphenopalatine foramen (red disk).

evaluate for perineural, foraminal, and intracranial extension. A standard helically acquired contrast-enhanced CT neck with sagittal and coronal reformats can be performed. MRI should include T1 sequences without fat saturation, in axial and/or coronal plane to demonstrate replacement of fat within the pterygopalatine fossa, infratemporal fossa, retromaxillary fat pad, etc. Axial T2 with fat saturation or STIR (coronal plane can also be performed) will evaluate tumor margins and flow voids. Postcontrast axial and coronal T1 with fat saturation will best evaluate tumor margins and vascularity. Standard CT and MRI of the neck should include the skull base, orbits, and cavernous sinuses, though if significant involvement of these structures is present additional focused sequences should also be performed. Diagnostic angiography is usually performed for preoperative embolization.

Related Physics

The typical patient with JNA may have had several imaging studies by the time a diagnosis is made. Many undergo angiography to map or embolize the feeding arteries preoperatively so that it is important for the radiologist to have a good knowledge of the risks of ionizing radiation. A deterministic radiation effect occurs at the site of irradiation and is one that is directly proportional to the dose received. Deterministic effects, in order of escalating dose, include erythema, epilation, cataracts, and sterility. Although the onset of these is predictable with dose, the timing of the onset is highly variable. Erythema is the first in a progression of skin injuries and occurs when entrance

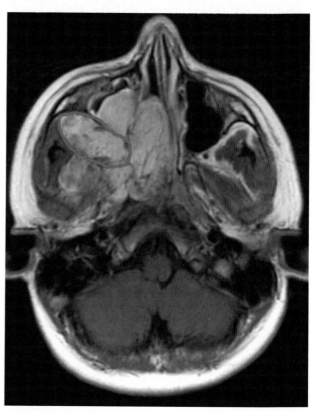

Figure 112.2. Axial contrast-enhanced T1 MR image in a 12-year-old male with right-sided epistaxis demonstrates a large JNA centered in the right pterygopalatine fossa extending into multiple regions including the infratemporal fossa through the pterygomaxillary fissure (red disk).

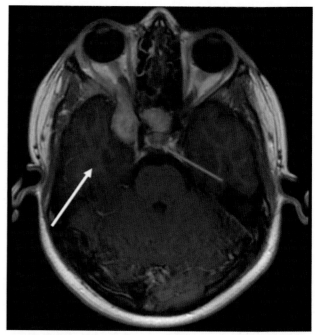

Figure 112.3. Axial contrast-enhanced T1 MR image in a 10-year-old with right-sided nasal obstruction and epistaxis demonstrates extension of JNA into the right parasellar region (white arrow). There is also extension into the sphenoid sinus (red arrow).

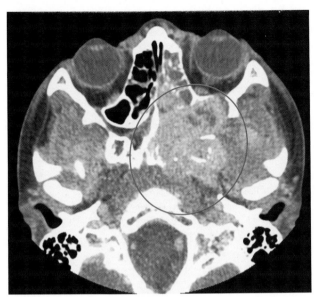

Figure 112.4. Axial contrast-enhanced CT image in a 13-year-old male with left-sided epistaxis demonstrates a large JNA eroding the left pterygoid plates with extension into the pterygoid fossa (red disk).

skin exposure exceeds 15 gray (Gy). At higher skin doses, permanent erythema may be induced, and at even higher doses one may encounter desquamation, which might require plastic surgical correction. Epilation overlaps with

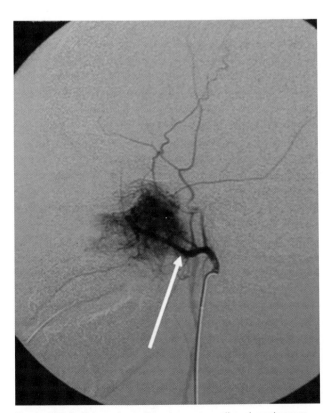

Figure 112.5. External carotid artery conventional angiogram with selective injection of the internal maxillary artery (IMA) in a 14-year-old male with epistaxis shows an enlarged IMA feeding the hypervascular JNA.

erythema and may be temporary or permanent according to dose. Temporary epilation is seen at 2 to 5 Gy; permanent epilation is seen at 7 Gy. Cataracts will form after a single exposure of 2 Gy or multiple exposures totaling 5 Gy. Recent information suggests that cataracts may form at even lower doses. All interventional radiologists should use eye protection during interventional fluoroscopy. Although not a consideration for JNA, temporary sterility results from direct irradiation of the gonads with a threshold of 2.5 Gy in males and 1.5 Gy in females with permanent sterility at 5.0 Gy and 6.0 Gy, respectively.

Differential Diagnosis

Other masses found in the nasopharynx/ptyergopalatine fossa region include the following:

- Rhabdomyosarcoma
- Nasopharyngeal carcinoma
- Hemangioma
- Venous, lymphatic, or venolymphatic malformation
- Schwannoma or neurofibroma

Common Variants

Rarely JNA can occur outside the usual location centered in the pterygopalatine fossa or sphenopalatine foramen, such as in the nasal vestibule, pterygoid musculature, or maxillary antrum. Lipomatous JNAs have also been reported. In addition, there have been rare (less than 10) reported cases of malignant transformation of JNA.

Clinical Issues

Most patients undergo preoperative embolization immediately prior to surgery to decrease vascularity and reduce intraoperative bleeding. Treatment is complete surgical resection. Often multiple surgeries are planned to achieve complete excision because of the extensive vascularity that can result in operative blood loss. For small tumors, an endoscopic endonasal approach is preferred. Craniotomy is typically performed if intracranial extension is present. Tumors felt to be inoperable because of size and involvement of critical structures are treated with radiation and antiandrogen therapy. Postoperative imaging is performed to evaluate for residual JNA and to evaluate for operative complications which, depending on the surgical techniques, can include hemorrhage, vascular injury (branches of the external carotid artery or internal carotid artery), venous thrombosis (including cavernous sinus), and standard complications of craniotomy (such as extraaxial hemorrhage). Unfortunately, JNA can have a high incidence of recurrence (up to 50 percent), especially if the skull base is involved. Depending on the extent and location of residual tumor, treatment options may include observation by serial imaging (CT or MRI), re-resection, or radiation.

Key Points

- Juvenile nasopharyngeal angiofibroma is a rare benign vascular tumor classically presenting in adolescent males with nasal obstruction and epistaxis.
- Typical location is centered in the sphenopalatine foramen or pterygopalatine fossa.
- Life-threatening hemorrhage can occur if these tumors are biopsied or partially resected.
- Pre-operative embolization is often required to reduce intraoperative hemorrhage.
- There is a high incidence of recurrence, especially if there is skull base involvement.

Further Reading

Curtin H, Rabinov J, Som P. *Central skull base: embryology, anatomy, and pathology.* In: Som P, Curtin H, eds. *Head and Neck Imaging.* Volume 2. Fourth edition. St. Louis, MO: Mosby; 2003:927.

Kania RE, Sauvaget E, Guichard JP, Chapot R, Huy PT, Herman P. Early postoperative CT scanning for juvenile nasopharyngeal angiofibroma: detection of residual disease. *Am J Neuroradiol.* 2005;*26*(1):82–88.

Momeni AK, Roberts CC, Chew FS. Imaging of chronic and exotic sinonasal disease: review. *Am J Roentgenol.* 2007;*189*(6 Suppl):S35–S45.

Robson C. Imaging of head and neck neoplasms in children. *Pediatr Radiol.* 2010;*40*:499–509.

Robson C, Hudgins P. Pediatric airway disease. In: Som P, Curtin H, eds. *Head and Neck Imaging.* Volume 2. Fourth edition. St. Louis, MO: Mosby; 2003:1579–1581.

Systemic Disease

CHAPTER 113

Sickle Cell Disease

Neha S. Kwatra, MD

Definition

Sickle cell disease (SCD), also known as sickle cell anemia or sickle cell disorder, is an autosomal recessive single-gene disorder. It is a type of hemolytic anemia characterized by the presence of sickle hemoglobin (HbS) in erythrocytes.

Clinical Features

Approximately 0.2 percent of the African-American population is affected by SCD. Most infants with SCD are healthy when born and develop symptoms later in infancy or childhood after a normal drop in fetal hemoglobin (HbF). In the United States, SCD is now identified by routine neonatal screening. Afflicted children not identified through screening commonly present in infancy or early childhood with painful dactylitis, pneumococcal sepsis or meningitis, severe anemia, splenic sequestration, acute chest syndrome, jaundice, or splenomegaly. Older children usually present with recurring abdominal or musculoskeletal pain, acute chest syndrome, aplastic crisis, splenic sequestration, cholelithiasis, and anemia. Chronic manifestations of SCD also include functional asplenia, cardiomegaly, proteinuria, delayed growth and sexual maturation, restrictive lung disease, pulmonary hypertension, avascular necrosis, proliferative retinopathy, leg ulcers, and transfusional hemosiderosis. Sickle cell trait with one abnormal and one normal gene often remains asymptomatic throughout life with implications mostly for genetic counseling.

Anatomy and Physiology

The genetic abnormality in sickle cell disease is the substitution of the amino acid valine for glutamic acid at the sixth position of the beta-globin chain of hemoglobin. Hemoglobin S that is formed as a result of this mutation undergoes polymerization when in a deoxygenated state. This distorts the shape of the red blood cells, which in turn decreases their pliability when passing through the microcirculation. Sickle hemoglobin also affects the erythrocyte cell membrane causing oxidative injury, cell dehydration, and increased adherence to endothelial cells. This in turn can cause excessive hemolysis leading to episodic vascular occlusion and tissue ischemia. Sickle cell disease affects practically every organ system with both acute and chronic involvement (Fig. 113.1).

Imaging Findings

Cardiopulmonary

The lung is commonly involved and manifestations include pneumonia and acute chest syndrome (ACS). Pneumonia is most frequently caused by *Streptococcus pneumoniae* and *Hemophilus influenzae*. Acute chest syndrome is new pulmonary consolidation and some permutation of fever, chest pain, and respiratory symptoms. The pathogenesis of ACS is largely ill-understood. Infection, fat embolism, and pulmonary vaso-occlusion with in situ thrombosis have been variably postulated as etiologies. The second major cause of hospitalization and the principal cause of death in SCD is ACS. The radiographic finding essential for the diagnosis of ACS is segmental, lobar, or multifocal air space disease with or without pleural effusions. Middle and lower lobes are more commonly affected. However, in about 30 to 60 percent cases the radiographs may initially not reveal any abnormality (Fig. 113.2). Pulmonary fibrosis is a chronic complication of SCD in 4 percent of patients. A fine reticular pattern is seen radiographically. CT findings include septal thickening, traction bronchiectasis, and architectural distortion in a patchy distribution, though predominantly involving the lung bases. Cardiomegaly with pulmonary plethora are related to chronic anemia and hyperdynamic circulation.

Musculoskeletal

Intramedullary hyperplasia presents as diploic space widening, thinning of cortical bone with hair-on-end appearance in the skull, trabecular prominence in both long and flat bones, biconcave vertebrae, and osteopenia. Infarction of bones characteristically occurs in the medullary cavity and the epiphysis. Infarction initially appears as an ill-defined radiolucency and then as arc-like subchondral and intramedullary lucent regions with intermixed sclerotic areas. A peripheral rim of sclerosis is often noted with medullary bone infarcts. Because MR imaging is very sensitive an infarct initially appears bright on T2-weighted and inversion recovery images. Later it becomes low in signal intensity on all MR pulse sequences because of fibrosis and sclerosis. Epiphyseal osteonecrosis frequently involves humeral and femoral heads. Initially there is no radiographic abnormality, although MR images reveal regions of high signal intensity because of bone marrow edema

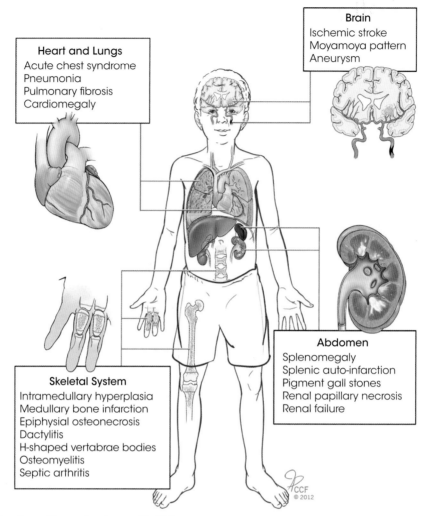

Brain
Ischemic stroke
Moyamoya pattern
Aneurysm

Heart and Lungs
Acute chest syndrome
Pneumonia
Pulmonary fibrosis
Cardiomegaly

Abdomen
Splenomegaly
Splenic auto-infarction
Pigment gall stones
Renal papillary necrosis
Renal failure

Skeletal System
Intramedullary hyperplasia
Medullary bone infarction
Epiphysial osteonecrosis
Dactylitis
H-shaped vertabrae bodies
Osteomyelitis
Septic arthritis

Figure 113.1. Illustration for multiorgan involvement in SCD.

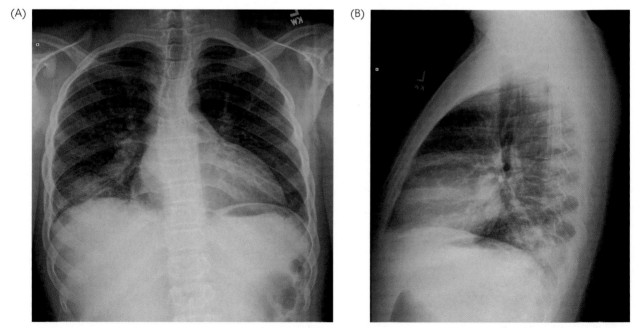

(A)   (B)

Figure 113.2. Frontal (A) and lateral (B) chest radiographs in a 16-year-old male with sickle cell disease with fever and chest pain reveals right lower lobe consolidation, which is compatible with either ACS or pneumonia. Also note cardiomegaly and vertebral end plate changes at multiple levels.

(A)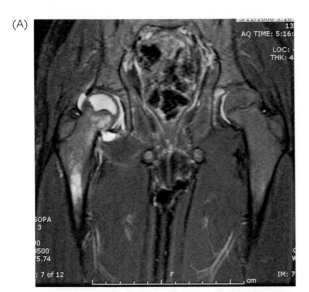

(B)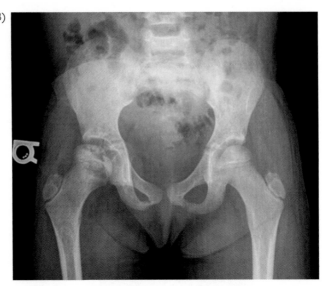

Figure 113.3. Coronal T2-weighted MR image of the pelvis (A) in a 7-year-old female patient with SCD and right hip pain shows increased signal intensity in the right femoral epiphysis and metaphysis consistent with edema representing early ischemia. Radiograph of the pelvis (B) taken 2 years later reveals sequelae to bilateral femoral epiphyseal osteonecrosis with right femoral epiphyseal flattening and subchondral lucencies with areas of sclerosis. There is also coxa magna. Left femoral epiphysis is also slightly flattened.

on T2-weighted or inversion recovery images. The "double line" sign may be seen, which consists of a hyperintense inner border and hypointense outer rim. Later, radiographic changes become apparent and include lucency and sclerosis within the epiphysis or crescent-shaped subchondral lucencies. Ultimately collapse, fragmentation, joint space narrowing, and osteophytosis develop (Fig. 113.3). In the spine, microvascular end plate occlusion and infarction results in "H-shaped" or "Lincoln log" vertebral deformity seen in about 10 percent of patients and is quite characteristic of SCD. Dactylitis or hand-foot syndrome is usually seen in children younger than 4 years old. Periostitis with cortical thinning and overall moth-eaten appearance is typical. Osteomyelitis is most common in the diaphyses of the femur, tibia, and humerus. The most commonly encountered organism is Salmonella followed by *Staphylococcus aureus*. Radiographic findings are often delayed and nonspecific, including periostitis, osteopenia, and sclerosis. On MR imaging, areas of high marrow signal with ill-defined margins are seen on T2-weighted images with corresponding enhancement following gadolinium. A sequestrum appears as a central area of low signal. Communication of soft-tissue fluid collections with intramedullary fluid collections through cortical breaks can also be established by MRI (Fig. 113.4). Septic arthritis is less common than osteomyelitis and MR findings include perisynovial edema, synovial enhancement, and joint effusion.

Cerebrovascular

Ischemic stroke from occlusive vasculopathy is a major complication. Both "silent" and clinical infarcts are best detected with MRI. Infarcts in patients with SCD are usually seen in the deep white matter or in the frontal and parietal periventricular white matter. Infarction can be identified as early as 6 hours after the initial insult on diffusion-weighted imaging. Distal ICA and proximal ACA and MCA most commonly show stenotic lesions on MRA (Fig. 113.5). Transcranial Doppler (TCD) is a noninvasive technique used to predict risk for stroke. Time-averaged mean of the maximum velocity of greater than 200 centimeters/second is associated with high risk for stroke; 170 to 200 centimeters/second is in the conditional range with a moderate risk for stroke (Fig. 113.6).

Moyamoya pattern can be seen in approximately 35 percent of SCD patients on angiography. Aneurysms are common, often multiple, and involve the vertebrobasilar system.

Miscellaneous

Splenic autoinfarction results from chronic sludging of red cells whereby the spleen becomes progressively smaller and later may calcify. Uptake of Tc-99m sulfur colloid decreases and finally may completely disappear. A rarer complication is sequestration syndrome with splenomegaly. Both are rare after 8 years of age and are becoming rarer with good maintenance therapy. Fifty percent of patients with SCD have large kidneys on imaging, however progressive renal failure is associated with renal atrophy. The kidneys may be echogenic on ultrasound. Papillary necrosis is also a known complication. Hepatobiliary complications include cholelithiasis (from pigment stones), bile sludging, and hepatitis. Head and neck involvement includes labyrinthine hemorrhage, labyrinthitis ossificans, lacrimal gland swelling, orbital wall infarction, subperiosteal hemorrhage, extramedullary hematopoiesis in paranasal sinuses, maxillofacial bone infarction, osteomyelitis, marrow hyperplasia, and lymphadenopathy.

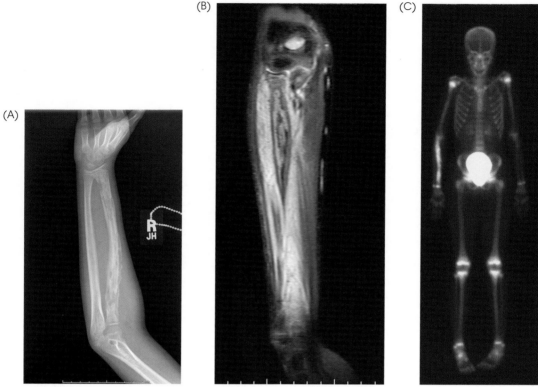

Figure 113.4. Frontal radiograph of the right forearm (A) in a 10-year-old female with SCD and pain, swelling, and fever reveals mixed lucent and sclerotic areas and extensive periosteal reaction and cortical destruction involving the radius. Coronal T1-weighted postgadolinium MR image of the forearm (B) reveals extensive abnormal signal involving the visualized proximal radius with surrounding abnormal enhancing soft tissue. Anterior bone scan image (C) reveals heterogeneously increased tracer uptake in the radius. Differential considerations are osteomyelitis and extensive infarction. Bone biopsy confirmed osteomyelitis resulting from Salmonella.

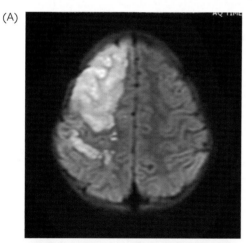

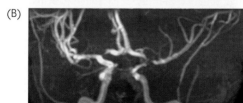

Figure113.5. Axial diffusion-weighted image (A) in a 4-year-old patient with SCD reveals acute infarction in right MCA/ACA territory. Frontal maximum intensity projection (MIP) from MRA (B) in a 10-year-old female patient with SCD cerebral vasculopathy reveals near complete occlusion of the left distal ICA and origins of left ACA/MCA with marked narrowing of the right A1 segment.

Imaging Strategy

The most common presentations for sickle cell disease include acute chest syndrome, bone pain from osteomyelitis/infarction and cerebrovascular events. Chest disease should be evaluated with chest radiography. Bone disease should undergo radiography and MRI, where T1, T2, and short tau inversion recovery sequences are helpful for evaluation of marrow. Cerebrovascular disease requires MRI and MRA. Ongoing monitoring should include TCD to predict risk for cerebrovascular disease and abdominal ultrasound to screen for gallstones and monitor spleen size. The use of gadolinium in MRI is controversial, although the American College of Radiology does not recommend withholding gadolinium in SCD.

Related Physics

A CT scan may be ordered to better elucidate pathology in ACS. As the scan is performed through air-filled lung, lower-dose scanning can be performed. mAs and kVp can be lowered to 20 to 40 mAs and 80 kVp by using a soft-tissue algorithm to help minimize quantum noise. Another promising method is partial rotation scanning. In this technique the X-ray tube is active through less than 360 degrees of rotation (from the 1 to the 11 o'clock position on a clockwise rotation) and "turned off" between 11 and 1 o'clock, with

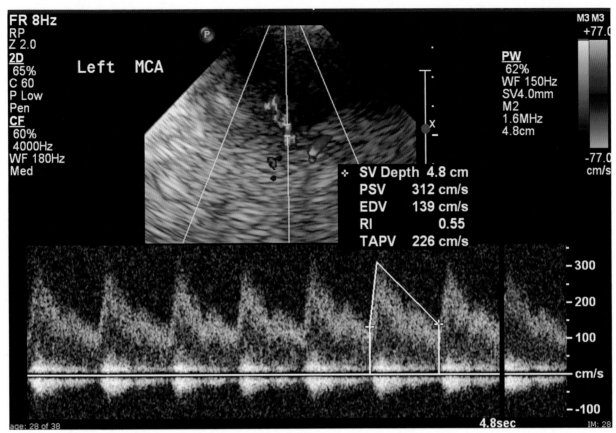

Figure 113.6. Transcranial Doppler in a 6-year-old sickle cell patient for routine screening shows a time-averaged mean of maximum velocity (TAMMX) over 200 centimeters/second in the left MCA, indicating high risk for stroke.

the overall effect of globally reducing dose by 25 percent and more significantly reducing the skin-entry dose at the anterior chest. Images are measured on bone windows from 2-D multiplanar and 3-D volume-rendered reconstructions.

Differential Diagnosis

Anemia:
- Acute hemolytic anemias

Abdominal pain:
- Appendicitis
- Cholecystitis
- Pneumonia
- Urinary tract infection

Bone pain:
- Osteomyelitis
- Acute rheumatic fever

Central nervous system signs:
- Meningitis
- Stroke

Moyamoya:
- Neurofibromatosis
- Trisomy 21
- Tuberous sclerosis
- Fibromuscular dysplasia
- Cranial irradiation

- Tuberculous meningitis
- Grave's disease

Small foci of increased T2 signal intensity on brain MRI:
- Migraine
- Hemophilia
- Vasculitides

Common Variants

Heterozygous individuals with asymptomatic sickle cell trait may develop medullary carcinoma, an infiltrative renal tumor with necrosis, calyceal dilation, and regional lymph nodal enlargement.

Other variants include homozygous and compound heterozygous individuals (e.g., Hb SC, sickle B-thalassemia) with symptomatic disease.

Clinical Issues

All patients with SCD should receive regular complete medical evaluations including monitoring of growth and development to identify early signs of chronic organ damage. Round-the-clock availability of clinical resources for management of acute complications is imperative. Severe manifestations of SCD may require maintenance chronic blood transfusions, an approach which considerably reduces the risk of recurrent stroke as well as decreasing the incidence vaso-occlusive crises, ACS, and admissions for febrile illness. In addition, chronic transfusions can avert progression to chronic organ damage and also reverse some preexisting organ dysfunction. Other more specific therapy, such as hydroxyurea, or stem cell transplantation can also be used.

Key Points

- Is an autosomal recessive hemolytic anemia with homozygous and heterozygous forms
- There is multiorgan involvement related to anemia, vasoocclusion, and infection
- Acute chest syndrome is the single important cause for mortality in SCD.
- Osteomyelitis and infarction cannot be reliably differentiated by imaging.
- MRI most sensitive for avascular necrosis. Radiographs are usually normal initially.
- Transcranial Doppler predicts risk for stroke.

Further Reading

Blitman NM, Berkenblit RG, Rozenblit AM, Levin TL. Renal medullary carcinoma: CT and MRI features. *AJR.* 2005;*185*:268–272.

Bulas D. Screening children for sickle cell vasculopathy: guidelines for transcranial Doppler evaluation. *Pediatr Radiol.* 2005;*35*(3):235–241. Epub Feb 10, 2005.

Ejindu VC, Hine AL, Mashayekhi M, Shorvon PJ, Misra RR. Musculoskeletal manifestations of sickle cell disease. *Radiographics.* 2007;*27*(4):1005–1021.

Leong CS, Stark P. Thoracic manifestations of sickle cell disease. *J Thorac Imaging.* 1998;*13*(2):128–134.

Lonergan GJ, Cline DB, Abbondanzo SL. Sickle cell anemia. *Radiographics.* 2001;*21*(4):971–994.

Section on Hematology/Oncology Committee on Genetics; American Academy of Pediatrics. Health supervision for children with sickle cell disease. *Pediatrics.* 2002;*109*(3): 526–535.

CHAPTER 114

Cystic Fibrosis

Alexis B. Rothenberg, MD, Catherine Kier, MD, FAAP, and Jeffrey C. Hellinger, MD, FAC

Definition

Cystic fibrosis (CF) is an autosomal recessive inherited disorder that is caused by defective epithelial cell chloride channel regulation and secondary abnormal exocrine gland function, affecting multiple organs and sweat glands systemically.

Clinical Features

The prevalence of CF is approximately 60,000 people worldwide. In the United States, it has an incidence of 1 in 4,000 births, most commonly occurring in Caucasians (1 in 2,500 births). Less commonly, CF occurs in African-American, Hispanic, and Asian populations, respectively. Approximately 70 percent of CF patients present within the first 12 months of life with a mean age of 6 months; 80 percent present by 4 years and 90 percent by 12 years of age, with manifestations of disease continuing during adulthood. This trend will likely change as CF newborn screening universally expands and CF is diagnosed earlier, before symptoms arise.

Although CF is a multisystemic disorder, respiratory and gastrointestinal manifestations are most prevalent. Gastrointestinal (GI) symptoms predominate in neonates and infants; lower respiratory symptoms are more common in young children and adolescents, progressing through adulthood. In the majority of cases, demise results from chronic end-stage lung disease. Upper respiratory (nasosinus) and urogenital systems are also commonly affected, however symptoms are typically less debilitating and can be more readily managed. In most patients, the chloride level in sweat is abnormally elevated.

Intestinal tract, pancreatic, and hepatobiliary abnormalities account for most GI symptoms. If not detected during prenatal ultrasound or newborn screening, neonates may present with meconium ileus, which occurs in 15 to 20 percent of CF patients. Symptoms include abdominal distention, bilious vomiting, and delayed passage of meconium, related to meconium obstructing the ileum, with or without in-utero perforation. Less commonly, intestinal obstruction in a CF neonate may result from intestinal atresia or malrotation with midgut volvulus.

Beyond the neonatal period, in addition to abdominal distention, infants more often present with increased stool frequency, steatorrhea, flatulence, and/or failure to thrive, related to insufficient pancreatic enzymes and secondary bowel malabsorption (pancreatic insufficiency [PI] phenotype). However, PI may also occur in the neonatal period. Approximately 60 percent of neonates screened for CF may have insufficient enzymes; this increases to 85 to 90 percent for CF patients during childhood. Pancreatic insufficiency presents lifetime challenges for nutrition, growth, and energy capacity and predisposes patients to secondary disorders related to depletion of fat-soluble vitamins.

Malnutrition contributes to and is further exacerbated by CF-related diabetes (CFRD), which commonly manifests by young adulthood in approximately 15 to 30 percent of CF patients; clinically, patients with CFRD have features of both type 1 and type 2 diabetes. Pancreatic disease in young children and older patients less commonly may manifest as recurrent pancreatitis (pancreatic sufficiency [PS] phenotype).

Additional intestinal disease in the young child, adolescent, and adult may include gastroesophageal reflux, peptic ulcer disease, obstructive ileocecal fecal impaction (*Distal Intestinal Obstruction Syndrome*, DIOS), appendiceal disease (acute appendicitis, mucopyoceles, and intussusception), rectal prolapse, and fibrosing colonopathy.

Hepatobiliary disease may occur as early as the first year of life, but is more common beginning in the young child, enduring through adulthood, with a prevalence of approximately 15 to 20 percent of CF patients. Presenting features include jaundice, acholic stools, abdominal pain (e.g., biliary colic), and/or elevated hepatic enzymes, related to obstructive intra- or extrahepatic cholestasis, with infectious and/or inflammatory cholangitis; cholelithiasis, with or without acute or chonic cholecystitis; and choledocholithiasis with or without cholangitis. Presentation of cholestasis in the neonate with CF may simulate biliary atresia. Patients are at increased risk for biliary cirrhosis and cholangiocarcinoma; cirrhosis may lead to portal hypertension with CF patients then presenting with hepatosplenomegaly, variceal bleeding, and hypersplenism. Hepatic disease may also be complicated by steatosis.

Pulmonary symptoms of cough, sputum (mucoid versus purulent), and/or wheezing, related to infectious and inflammatory bronchiolitis, bronchitis, and/or pneumonia, may not manifest until the first few months of life; these symptoms become more prevalent in mid to late infancy, childhood, and adolescence. Recurrent infections and inflammation progress to chronic respiratory disease, which may manifest as a chronic cough, chronic wheezing, shortness of breath, dyspnea on exertion, tachypnea, hypoxia, digital clubbing, right heart failure, and hemoptysis. Right heart failure may result in hepatic congestion, leading or contributing to hepatic dysfunction, including cirrhosis.

Additional Clinical Features

- Fevers and/or craniofacial pain and tenderness, secondary to acute or chronic sinusitis. Chronic sinusitis is more common, often associated with mass (e.g., nasal polyps, mucoceles, and mucopyoceles).
- The majority of males with CF are infertile secondary to obstructive azoospermia; females may have delayed secondary sexual development, amenorrhea, or both, related to malabsorption and nutritional deficiencies. Males may also have hydroceles and undescended testes.
- The sweat chloride test is the most readily diagnostic tool for CF (positive: >60 mmol/L, intermediate: 40 to 60mmol/L intermediate, negative: < 40mmol/L). Neonatal screening is achieved by measuring the level of immunoreactive trypsinogen in dried blood; elevated levels should be followed by sweat chloride or genetic testing.

Anatomy and Physiology

The CF gene is located on the long arm of chromosome 7. It encodes the Cystic Fibrosis Transmembrane Conductance Regulator (CFTR), a single exocrine gland apical epithelial cell membrane protein, which functions as a chloride channel to control: (1) the concentrations (i.e., osmolality) of sodium and chloride (e.g., bronchioles) or bicarbonate (e.g., pancreas); (2) the balance of cellular fluid; and (3) the degree of extracellular surface fluid. In sweat glands, a defective CFTR transport channel impairs chloride reabsorption, leading to the high content of sodium chloride in sweat. In visceral and nasosinus exocrine glands, abnormal transport causes intracellular anion retention (e.g., decreased chloride secretion) and secondary reabsorption of sodium and water (to maintain ionic and osmotic balance). The hydration decreases within the secretions and along the epithelial cellular surfaces; exocrine gland secretions become thick and viscous, obstructing ducts and organ lumens (Fig. 114.1).

Thick respiratory secretions along with abnormal ciliary motility result in endobronchial impaction and decreased clearance of bacteria and other foreign material; this leads to lower respiratory infections with neutrophil-mediated inflammation. The inflammatory response damages airways and increases endobronchial viscosity and mucous plugging, and eventually promotes colonization with distinctive bacterial flora (with *Pseudomonas aeruginosa* and *Staphylococcus aureus*). Chronic colonization along with

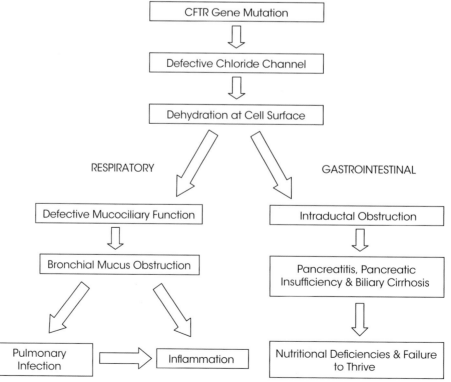

Figure 114.1. Cystic fibrosis pathophysiology: respiratory & gastrointestinal disease.

repeated episodes of infection and inflammation occur in a perpetual, worsening cycle, with ultimate complications of chronic bronchiectasis, end-stage parenchymal disease, and cor pulmonale (pulmonary hypertension with right heart dysfunction). Abnormal gas exchange leads to recruitment of systemic arteries (e.g., bronchial arteries, thyrocervical branches, and phrenic arteries); hemoptysis commonly occurs in this case, related to high-pressure systemic collateral arteries directly supplying abnormal (lower-pressure) lung. Spontaneous pneumothoraces can occur when a cystic bleb ruptures.

In the gastrointestinal system, low bicarbonate in pancreatic secretions results in impaired pancreatic enzyme function. Inspissated pancreatic secretions cause intraluminal ductal obstruction and dilatation with acinar tissue inflammation and eventual fibrosis, cyst formation, and fatty replacement, leading to pancreatic enzyme insufficiency. Included in this process is reduced β–cell mass (possibly secondary to apoptosis) and reduced insulin secretion, accounting for CFRD (i.e., type 1 diabetes effect with decreased insulin). Insulin resistance contributes to the CFRD pathophysiology; etiologies include infection, cellular inflammatory mediators, steroid treatments, and liver disease (type 2 diabetes effect). Thick intestinal secretions with abnormal intestinal motility account for meconium ileus and DIOS. Cholelithiasis and choledocholithiasis result from fecal bile acid loss secondary to intestinal malabsorption; the gallbladder may be hypoplastic with an atretic cystic duct. Bile secretions plug biliary ductules, leading to ductal dilatation, inflammation, hyperplasia, and fibrosis in the portal triad; biliary stenosis and cirrhosis are the main complications.

Additional Pathophysiology

- Mucoid obstruction of the nasal sinus ostia, abnormal mucociliary clearance, inflammatory mediators, and bacterial colonization result in chronic sinus infections and inflammation and space-occupying masses.
- In males, secretions obstruct the developing vas deferens, leading to in-utero atrophy (congenital bilateral absence of the vas deferens, CBAVD) and infertility.

Imaging Findings

Respiratory

Initially airway and lungs may be normal or may have nonspecific imaging findings. As disease progresses, lower respiratory and thoracic findings in the CF patient include peribronchial thickening, linear and nodular mucus plugging, endobronchial air-fluid levels, bronchiectasis, bronchomalacia, regional air trapping, global hyperinflation, atelectasis, consolidation, linear bands, cysts, pneumothoraces, pulmonary hemorrhage, and reactive hilar lymph nodes (Figs. 114.2 and 114.3). In addition, the right heart and central pulmonary arteries may be enlarged with peripheral pruning, related to secondary pulmonary hypertension. These findings are all readily detected by both thoracic radiography and computed tomography (CT), with CT providing greater detail and sensitivity. CT angiography (CTA) may detect systemic collateral arteries (Fig. 114.4), as a source for hemoptysis. In addition, abnormal cardiopulmonary and systemic venous morphology (related to cor pulmonale) are evaluated with superior accuracy with CTA. Less commonly, MRI is applied to assess airway and parenchymal structure; T1 and T2 sequences can readily depict peribronchial thickening, mucus plugging, bronchiectasis, and parenchymal abnormalities. For its functional imaging capabilities, MRI is advantageous. Ventilation defects are depicted and quantified with MRI using hyperpolarized helium imaging techniques; pulmonary perfusion abnormalities are depicted with contrast-enhanced MR angiography; and differential pulmonary flow is quantified with phase-contrast imaging. Alternatively, ventilation and perfusion are assessed and quantified by nuclear scintigraphy. Rarely, invasive bronchoscopy may be required for endobronchial direct real-time visualization of mucosal inflammation, viscous secretions, impaction, bronchiectasis, and bronchomalacia (Fig. 114.5). More commonly bronchoscopy is performed for therapeutic lavage.

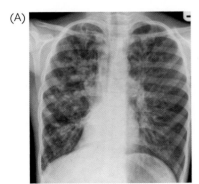 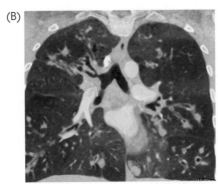 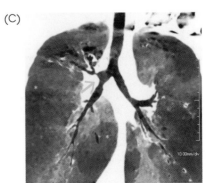

(A) (B) (C)

Figure 114.2. Frontal chest radiograph (A) and coronal CT multiplanar reformation—MPR (B) from a 17-year-old female with moderately severe CF show peribronchial thickening, bronchiectasis, and hyperinflation. Minimum intensity projection—MinIP (C) shows right upper lobe central airways bronchomalacia (arrow) with mosaic attenuation (asterisks) secondary to air trapping.

Gastrointestinal

In the fetus, meconium ileus will manifest as distended bowel loops—hyperechoic by ultrasound and T1 hyperintense by MRI; intra-abdominal calcifications would suggest in-utero perforation, although ascites would suggest secondary peritonitis. In neonates, meconium ileus manifests on abdominal radiography as a distal small bowel obstruction (Fig. 114.6); calcifications and pneumoperitoneum may be seen. A barium or water-soluble enema will reveal a microcolon with a decompressed, impacted distal ileum (Fig. 114.7). Malrotation with midgut volvulus may be demonstrated by ultrasound and/or upper gastrointestinal fluoroscopy with a small bowel follow-through (SBFT); intussusception may be detected by ultrasound and/or a contrast (barium, saline, or air) enema.

In older patients, abdominal radiographic findings of small bowel obstruction with a bubbly soft-tissue mass in the right lower quadrant (e.g., ileal-colic junction) should raise the possibility for DIOS. Fecal impaction is confirmed with SBFT or contrast (barium or water soluble iodine)

enema. Extraintestinal findings (detected by ultrasound, CT, or MRI) include pancreatic cysts, fatty replacement (lipomatous pseudohypertrophy) of the pancreas, cholelithiasis, choledocholithiasis, microgallbladder, biliary ductal stenosis and dilatation (beading; sclerosing cholangitis), hepatic steatosis, and cirrhosis (focal biliary fibrosis or multilobular biliary types) with or without portal hypertension (Fig. 114.8).

Imaging Strategy

Respiratory

The current recommendation from the Cystic Fibrosis Foundation (CFF) is to perform chest radiographs every 2 to 4 years for medically stable patients and yearly for those with declining medical status or frequent respiratory infections. Multiple systems (e.g., the Brasfield; Chrispin-Norman; NIH; Weatherly scores) can be used to grade radiographic findings for the severity of disease. During an acute exacerbation, however, chest radiographic findings may not be significantly different from those at baseline. Although there are no current recommendations from the CFF regarding the routine use of CT, with its greater sensitivity CT is useful during the early disease course to establish a baseline; during exacerbations; and during surveillance of disease at 18- to 24-month intervals, particularly in those patients who have progressive worsening of disease but have stable pulmonary function tests. CT angiography should be considered when there is

(A)

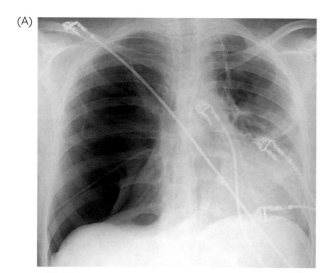

(B)

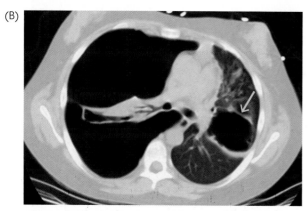

Figure 114.3. Frontal chest radiograph (A) and axial CT (B) in an 18-year-old patient with advanced CF reveal an extensive right tension pneumothorax with complete collapse of the right lung and leftward mediastinal shift with a large cyst (arrow) in the contralateral left lung, which is at risk for rupture and spontaneous pneumothorax.

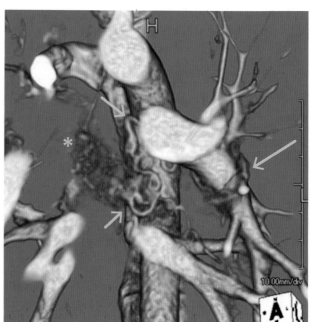

Figure 114.4. Contrast-enhanced CT with volume rendering shows abnormal bronchial artery supply to the right lung (short arrows) and left lung (long arrow) with increased right lung parenchymal vascularity (asterisks), corresponding to active pulmonary hemorrhage.

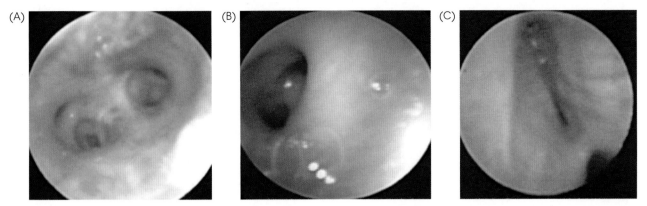

Figure114.5. Bronchoscopic images from three separate CF patients, demonstrating bronchial erythema (A); thick endobronchial viscous secretions (B); and bronchomalacia (C).

hemoptysis and transcatheter embolization is a consideration and/or when pulmonary hypertension is known or suspected and cardiopulmonary structures also require evaluation. With its lack of radiation, MRI is emerging as an important and useful modality for follow-up structural imaging of CF patients and, in select centers, ventilation-perfusion imaging. At present, however, nuclear scintigraphy remains the recommended noninvasive modality for ventilation-perfusion imaging and differential pulmonary flow quantification.

Gastrointestinal

In the postnatal patient, diagnostic evaluation of the intestinal tract, pancreas, liver, and gallbladder begins with abdominal-pelvic radiographs and ultrasound. In the neonate, if additional imaging is required for suspected low intestinal obstruction secondary to meconium ileus, a water-soluble contrast enema is performed. For an older child with GI complaints, an SBFT or contrast enema may be performed. For nonemergent hepatobiliary and pancreatic disease, MR cholangiography should be performed; CT is reserved for emergent imaging of complicated hepatobiliary and pancreatic disease.

Related Physics

One can achieve CT dose reduction in a number of ways including mAs and kVp reduction. An optimal value for mAs is usually determined from preset standards based on patient girth, weight or age, and can be held constant in conventional imaging or can be made variable using a technique referred to as "dose modulation." Radiation output can be modulated in the axial plane as the X-ray tube orbits the patient, delivering higher output to thick or bony projections and less to thin or air-filled projections. Radiation output can also be modulated along the long axis of the body by using information from a plan view. This is generally referred to as "Z-axis modulation." Each of the previously described modulations can be used separately or together. Dose modulation techniques offer a reasonable

approach to managing dose delivery in pediatric radiology where patient size varies so widely.

Differential Diagnosis

Failure to thrive:
- Increased metabolic demand
- Inadequate intake
- Malabsorption syndromes

Infectious and inflammatory etiologies of chronic sinus disease, bronchiolitis, bronchitis, and bronchiectasis:
- Primary cilliary dyskinesia (Kartagener's syndrome)
- Immunocompromised states (leading to recurrent pneumonias)

Intestinal obstruction and/or abnormal stools:
- Inflammatory bowel disease
- Celiac disease

Common Variants

More than 1,500 CFTR mutations have been identified, accounting for variable presentations. The most common is the ΔF508 mutation (90 percent of CF patients) in which there is deletion of phenylalanine at position 508 of the protein. The majority of patients with this genotype convey the PI phenotype. Patients with non- ΔF508 mutations often have residual CFTR transmembrane protein function and typically have a greater association with the PS phenotype. In these patients, disease is less severe and often diagnosed at a later age (e.g., childhood); lung, intestinal, and hepatic function as well as nutritional status are better preserved, yielding an overall better prognosis. Consistent with this, in the absence of screening, between 5 and 10 percent of patients may not be diagnosed until after 10 years of age as they may present with mild pulmonary disease, chronic pancreatitis and a normal or borderline sweat test.

Clinical Issues

Life expectancy for CF patients continues to increase as a result of frequent monitoring of patients, early

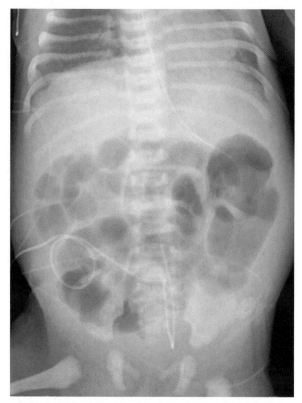

Figure 114.6. Frontal abdominal radiograph in a 2-day-old male with failure to pass meconium and progressive abdominal distention reveals multiple dilated small bowel loops with absence of rectal air.

interventions, and advances in treatment; the expected life expectancy for an infant born with CF today is estimated to be greater than 50 years of age. For respiratory care, aggressive chest physiotherapy (to clear endobronchial secretions), antibiotics (to treat infections), and antiinflammatory agents are core management strategies. In addition to manual external percussion and mechanical physiotherapy techniques (e.g., airway oscillators, high-frequency vest compression), airway clearance is also augmented by the use of beta-agonists, inhaled hypertonic saline and mucolytics (e.g., recombinant human DNase). Endovascular small particle embolization is indicated for recurrent hemoptysis, refractory to medical management (Fig. 114.9). Young adults often require lung transplantation to extend their life span in the setting of severe lung disease. Surgical management may also be indicated for treatment of recurrent pneumothoraces, hemoptysis refractory to endovascular embolization, nasal polyps, and sinusitis. For gastrointestinal disease, medical management of nutrition and growth includes a high-calorie diet with high-protein and normal-to high-lipid content, administration of pancreatic enzymes, and treatment of CFRD (e.g., insulin, diet). Oral glucose tolerance testing is recommended annually in children age 10 years and older to screen for CFRD. Fecal impaction may be treated by laxatives, pharmacologic enemas, or contrast enemas (e.g., barium, water-soluble iodine). Surgical intervention may be required for meconium ileus, malrotation, volvulus, intussusception, and rectal prolapse.

(A)

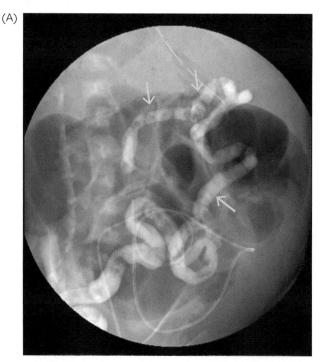

(B)

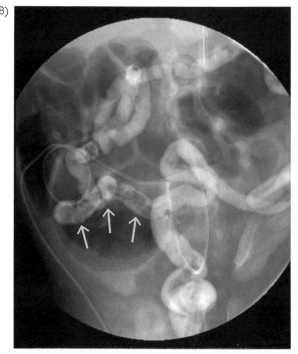

Figure 114.7. Water-soluble enema images demonstrate microcolon (arrows) with impacted meconium (arrows) in a decompressed terminal ileum consistent with meconium ileus.

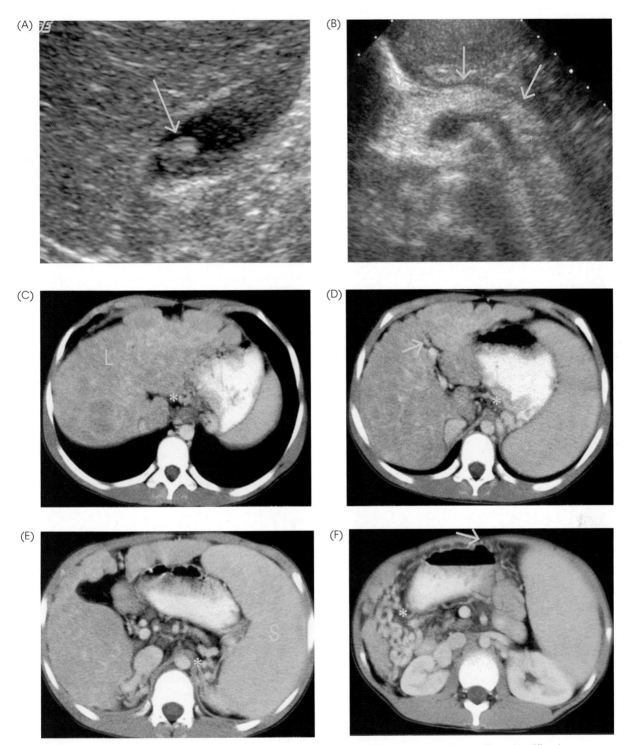

Figure 114.8. Ultrasound (A, B) from a 10-year-old with CF shows cholelithiasis (arrowon image A) and a diffusely hyperechoic pancreas (arrows on image B) consistent with fatty replacement. Contrast-enhanced abdominal CT images (C, D, E, F) in another 10-year-old patient with CF reveal macronodular cirrhosis with portal hypertension, splenomegaly, gastroesophageal, perigastric, perisplenic and mesenteric varices (asterisks on images C, D, E, F); and a recannalized periumbilical vein (arrows on images D and F). Liver (L). Spleen (S).

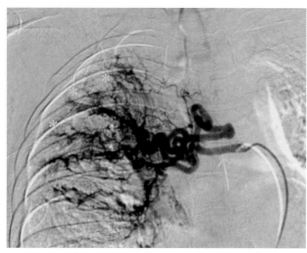

Figure 114.9. Pre-embolization catheter angiogram shows the abnormal bronchial artery supply to the right lung (short arrows) and the left lung (long arrow) with increased right lung parenchymal vascularity (asterisks), corresponding to active pulmonary hemorrhage.

Key Points

- CF is an autosomal recessive multisystemic disease, caused by CFTR mutations (most commonly ΔF508).
- Meconium ileus in the neonate is indicative of CF until proven otherwise.
- Chest radiography is most commonly used to follow progression of lung disease.
- CT has greater sensitivity and is currently considered most reliable for detection of early disease and acute exacerbations, but may also be considered for surveillance.

- MRI with structural and ventilation-perfusion imaging is advantageous for follow-up of the pediatric CF patient.
- Common pulmonary findings include peribronchial thickening, mucus plugging, bronchiectasis, regional air trapping, global hyperinflation, linear bands, and parenchymal cysts.
- Common radiologic gastrointestinal findings include small bowel obstruction, fatty replacement of the pancreas, cholelithiasis, steatosis, and cirrhosis.

Further Reading

Mogayzel PJ, Flume PA. Update in cystic fibrosis 2009. *Am J Respir Crit Care Med.* 2010;*181*:539–544.

Nathan BM, Laguna T, Moran A. Recent trends in cystic fibrosis-related diabetes. *Curr Opin Endocrinol Diabetes Obesity.* 2010;*17*(4):335–341.

Noone PG, Knowles MR. "CFTR-opathies": disease phenotypes associated with cystic fibrosis transmembrane regulator gene mutations. *Respir Res.* 2001;*2*(6): 328–332.

O'Sullivan BP, Freedman SP. Cystic fibrosis. *Lancet.* 2009;*373*: 1891–1904.

Puderbach M, Eichinger M. The role of advanced imaging techniques in cystic fibrosis follow-up: is there a place for MRI? *Pediatr Radiol.* 2010;*40*:844–849.

Ratjen FA. Cystic fibrosis: pathogenesis and future treatment strategies. *Respir Care.* 2009;*54*(5):595–602.

Robertson MB, Choe KA, Joseph PM. Review of the abdominal manifestations of cystic fibrosis in the adult patient. *Radiographics.* 2006;*26*:679–690.

Robinson TE. Imaging of the chest in cystic fibrosis. *Clin Chest Med.* 2007;*28*:405–421.

CHAPTER 115

Child Abuse: Musculoskeletal

Stephen Done, MD

Definition

The World Health Organization has defined child abuse in the following terms:

> "Child abuse, sometimes referred to as child abuse and neglect, includes all forms of physical and emotional ill-treatment, sexual abuse, neglect, and exploitation that results in actual or potential harm to the child's health, development or dignity."

Within this broad definition, five subtypes can be distinguished: physical abuse; sexual abuse; neglect and negligent treatment; emotional abuse; and exploitation.

Clinical Features

Nonaccidental trauma (NAT) is a significant cause of morbidity and mortality in America and the rest of the world. In America its incidence exceeds the combined prevalence of the common childhood problems, asthma and diabetes mellitus. The consequences are severe with death or significant disability in many cases. Neglect is most common (63 percent) followed by physical abuse (19 percent), sexual abuse (10 percent), and emotional abuse (8 percent). Most children suffering physical abuse are under 3 years of age.

Anatomy and Physiology

Fractures have been reported in almost every bone in the appendicular and axial skeleton, including the sternum, spinous processes, and digits in infants. Skeletal injury is found in 11 to 55 percent of physically abused children, making recognition of skeletal injury an important issue. Abuse fractures are common in nonambulatory infants in whom fractures of any kind are unusual except under extraordinary circumstances such as a fall from a height or an automobile accident.

Many fractures in NAT are a result of traction or torsional forces, jerking or shaking, and may be the result of using the limb as a handle for shaking the infant (Fig. 115.1). Fractures may result from squeezing the chest between the fingers while shaking the child; these types of maneuvers result in specific types of fracture patterns that are considered highly specific for abusive injuries. Knowledge of forces applied to bones and the resultant fractures is key to understanding the fractures of abuse. It is important to correlate the fractures with the clinical history. One must be aware of the acuity of the fracture in order to assist in timing and dating of the injury, because fractures in various states of healing are also considered moderately specific for NAT. If the history given is of an acute injury but the fracture is already in a state of healing, then the fracture must be viewed with suspicion.

Imaging Findings

Most fractures of abuse are occult without associated bruising or swelling. Long bone fractures are often spiral or bending types of injuries. Skull fractures are often linear, but may be complex and diastatic. Rib fractures are considered by experts in the field to be highly specific for abuse injury; rib fractures are rare in any other form of childhood trauma including birth trauma and automobile injury. They are seldom associated with other significant internal injury or bruising and may be multiple and occult. Acute rib fractures may be obscure on plain radiographs and may only be detected on follow-up examinations because of callus formation (Fig. 115.2). They may even be difficult to find at autopsy, requiring stripping of the periosteum to positively identify. These have been shown by Kleinman and Schlesinger in an infant rabbit model to be caused by violent compression of the chest. Rib fractures are usually posteromedial, paraspinal and may be accompanied by lateral or anterolateral fractures as well. Brewer and Feldman showed that these rarely occur with CPR even in unskilled hands. In a large study of birth injuries in Holland, van Rijn showed that posterolateral rib fractures in infants are rarely associated with birth trauma. The lesion considered by most authors to be most specific for NAT is the classic metaphyseal lesion (CML). Previously called "corner" or "bucket-handle" fractures because of their resemblance to the handle of a bucket resting upon its rim, these were originally recognized by John Caffey in his earliest descriptions of the "Shaken Baby Syndrome" and clarified by Fred Silverman who brought worldwide awareness to this problem (Fig. 115.3). Elegant studies done by Kleinman and Blackbourne demonstrated their pathophysiology and showed these to be fractures through the primary spongiosa. Their appearance, whether resembling the handle of

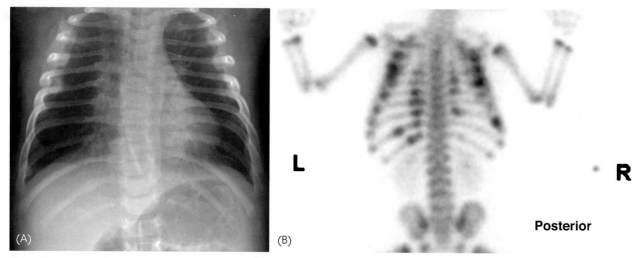

(A)   (B)

L   R

Posterior

Figure115.2. (A) Frontal chest radiograph in a 6-month-old with irritability shows multiple right-sided healing rib fractures posteromedially adjacent to the spine at the costovertebral junction. Anterolateral and anterior fractures are also present bilaterally. (B) Posterior view from a radionuclide bone scan shows multiple bilateral rib fractures at almost every level.

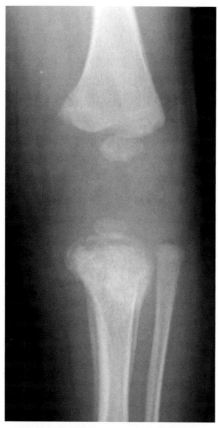

Figure 115.3. Frontal radiograph of the left knee in a child with irritability from NAT shows classic metaphyseal lesion or bucket-handle fracture in the proximal tibia associated with a single layer of perioseal new bone formation. There is a CML of the distal femur without periosteal new bone formation.

a bucket or a corner of metaphysis, is dependent upon the angle of the X-ray beam to the fracture.

Most fractures in children result from accidents and they are usually easily predictable by patterns of presentation and mechanisms of injury. Recognition of patterns of fractures that are highly specific for abusive injury is vitally important. Although long bone fractures and linear skull fractures are of low specificity, any fracture in a nonambulatory infant without adequate cause, or with obvious delay in seeking medical attention, must be viewed with suspicion as to its origin and mechanism (Fig. 115.4). Such delay may present as a diastatic skull fracture or a long bone fracture already in a state of healing when first viewed.

Imaging Strategy

Because the majority of physical abuse occurs in infants and children less than 2 years of age where physical examination may be nonspecific, a directed approach at imaging is not fruitful. Many fractures discovered in infants who are abused are asymptomatic and manifest neither pain, swelling, nor bruising at the site of the fracture. Therefore a complete radiographic skeletal survey is required to adequately evaluate for occult fractures. Nuclear medicine bone scan is more sensitive in the detection of acute rib fractures and skull fractures and is the test of choice in children over age 2 years. Head CT is also part of the routine workup of NAT.

Related Physics

Nuclear medicine bone scan with single photon emission computed tomography (SPECT) is highly sensitive in the detection of high metabolic bone activity present in occult fractures. Single photon emission computed tomography (SPECT) cameras can be used in a variety of modes of operation that include single and multiheaded units, rotational arc

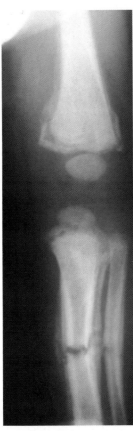

Figure 115.4. Frontal radiograph of the left knee in a child with leg swelling following NAT shows healing CML with diffuse PNBF. There is a new acute tranverse fracture through the new bone of the tibia and an associated fibular fracture.

acquisition, continuous motion acquisition, step-and-shoot, and noncircular orbits. Gamma cameras may be single-, dual-, or tripleheaded. The advantage of more than one head is that counts can be more efficiently captured, thereby reducing imaging time. Gamma cameras may remain stationary, however by rotating these around the patient's long axis ("rotational arc" acquisition), cross-sectional images can be reconstructed. Continuous motion refers to a slow linear motion over the anterior surface of the patient to collect counts over a large volume such as in whole body bone scan. When higher counts are needed than can be acquired with continuous motion, the camera can be positioned over a specific anatomic region until adequate counts are achieved before being moved to the next location ("step-and-shoot" acquisition). More recently, noncircular orbits have been created to more closely follow the patient contour. This technique has the advantage of more efficient capture of counts while reducing image artifacts.

Differential Diagnosis

Classic metaphyseal lesion:

- Spondylometaphyseal dysplasia: corner fracture type (Sutcliffe)

- Menke's kinky hair syndrome (a rare disorder of copper metabolism)
- Adenosine deaminase deficiency with severe combined immune deficiency (SCID)

Fragile bones or increased risk of fracture:

- Prematurity (inadequate calcium stores)
- Osteogenesis imperfecta
- Osteoporosis (from disuse, neurologic impairment, scurvy, or drugs such as steroids)
- Osteomalacia (rickets or resulting from trace metal deficiency such as copper in severely malnourished infants or infants on hyperalimentation for short gut or liver problems)

Although infants and children with rickets are at greater risk for fractures, these are unusual in nonambulatory infants and where the bones appear normal on radiographs.

Clinical Issues

Some fractures are seen incidentally, especially rib fractures, making it necessary for all radiologists to carefully examine the bones on all infant radiographs as the radiologist may be the first to suspect NAT.

Key Points

- The radiologist is required by law to report suspected cases of abuse and is protected by the same law for doing so.
- The role of the radiologist is to detect fractures, associated injuries, determine severity and cause but not to determine guilt.
- Nonambulatory infants require complete skeletal survey.
- Older children require a directed examination.
- Classic metaphyseal lesion and posteromedial rib fractures are specific but not most common.

Further Reading

Barsness, KA, Cha E-S, Bensard DD, Calkins CM, Partrick DA, Karrer FM, Strain JD. The positive predictive value of rib fractures as an indicator of nonaccidental trauma in children. *Journal of Trauma.* 2003;54:1107–1110.

Bilo RAC, Robben SGF, vanRijn RR. *Forensic Aspects of Paediatric Fractures.* London: Springer; 2010.

Bishop N, Sprigg A, Dalton, A. Unexplained fractures in infancy: looking for fragile bones. *Archives Diseases Childhood.* 2007;92:251–256.

Cadzow SP, Armstrong KL. Rib fractures in infants: red alert! The clinical features, investigations and child protection outcomes. *J Paediatric Child Health.* 2000;36:322–326.

Chapman T, Sugar N, Done S, Marasigan J, Wambold N, Feldman K. Fractures in infants and toddlers with rickets. *Pediatric Radiology.* 2010;40:1184–1189.

Kleinman PK, *Diagnostic Imaging of Child Abuse.* St. Louis, MO: Mosby; 1998.

Lonergan GF, Baker AM, Morey MK, Boos SC. From the archives of the AFIP: child abuse: radiologic-pathologic correlation. *Radiographics.* 2003; 23:811–845.

van Rijn RR, Bilo RAC, Robben SGF. Birth-related mid-posterior rib fractures in neonates: a report of three cases (and a possible fourth case) and a review of the literature. *Pediatric Radiology.* 2009;39:30–34.

CHAPTER 116

Child Abuse: Thoracoabdominal Trauma

Stephen Done, MD

Definition

In the older child, nonaccidental trauma to the chest or abdomen results in nonspecific patterns of injury. Thoracoabdominal nonaccidental trauma (NAT) is less common than either skeletal trauma or abusive head injury.

Clinical Features

Nonaccidental trauma is a problem known to every culture and throughout history. Traumatic injury is the leading cause of death in pediatric patients of all ages. Death from nonaccidental causes is estimated at between 2,000 and 5,000 each year in the United States. Most of the deaths and significant disability related to inflicted trauma occur as a result of head trauma (most common under the age of 2 years). Abdominal trauma is less common in the infant, usually seen in older children. Most of these children survive with less long-term morbidity than seen with abusive head trauma. In some children central nervous system (CNS) and thoracoabdominal trauma coexist, and in those cases it is usually the CNS injury that causes the most morbidity or mortality.

The child presents with abdominal pain, distention, and vomiting. There may be a delay in seeking medical care. Physical findings include tachypnea, tenderness, bruising, abdominal distention, and other evidence of injury, shock, and dehydration. Bruising is more common with thoracoabdominal injury than with either abusive head trauma or skeletal injury.

Anatomy and Physiology

Classic posterolateral rib fractures seen in the infant are the result of squeezing, shaking, and throwing the child down resulting in associated direct impact. Rib fractures are less common in the older child with direct chest trauma. Blunt injury to the chest may result in bruising, rib fractures, pneumothorax, pleural effusion, or pulmonary contusion. Rib fractures from direct trauma may be multiple and linear in distribution with overlying bruises. As in other forms of abuse they may be in various stages of healing (Fig. 116.1).

The patterns of abdominal injury are very similar to those seen in motor vehicle accidents, direct trauma by bicycle handlebars, or from falling from a height (Fig. 116.2). Liver, spleen, and kidney lacerations are most common. Also seen are liver subcapsular hematomas or hemorrhagic ascites. Kidney lacerations may result in urinoma or uriniferous ascites. Pancreatic lacerations may present as acute pancreatitis, pancreatic pseudocyst, or diffuse peritonitis, depending upon the timing of injury and severity. Pancreatitis in a child is more often caused by trauma than any other cause; NAT must always be considered. Duodenal hematoma occurs at the third portion because of compression against the spine and may result in bowel obstruction. Bowel laceration results in perforation and peritonitis with ileus. Bladder rupture is very uncommon in NAT.

Imaging Findings

Computed tomography (CT) with intravenous contrast is the study of choice for all thoracoabdominal trauma in children. Oral contrast is rarely given because of transient gastroparesis induced by abdominal pain. Rib fractures are better visualized on CT scan than radiography and should raise concern for NAT, especially in the infant (Fig. 116.3). Spine fractures will also be more conspicuous on CT. Clinically relevant pulmonary contusion, pneumothorax, or pneumomediastinum is almost always evident on radiography. A CT scan will reveal additional lesions because of its superior contrast and spatial resolution but with questionable clinical significance. CT angiography is almost as sensitive and specific as catheter angiography in detecting vascular injury. Tracheal or bronchial rupture with massive pneumomediastinum or persistent pneumothorax is rare, but well-demonstrated by multiplanar CT imaging.

Liver laceration is the most common solid organ lesion in NAT and well-demonstrated on CT (Fig. 116.4). Subcapsular hematoma will show a nonenhancing lentiform peripheral collection of lower attenuation than adjacent liver. Periportal edema is often related to fluid resuscitation. Splenic laceration and subcapsular hematoma are graded by severity of the laceration (Fig. 116.5). Pancreatic injuries include laceration and acute necrotizing pancreatitis. Pancreatic transection, peripancreatic fluid, swelling and loss of normal lobular appearance are frequently seen in abusive pancreatic injury. Renal injury may include laceration, subcapsular hematoma, poor enhancement, contusion, perfusion defects, or asymmetric nephrogram. Urinoma or vascular injuries may also occur. Duodenal

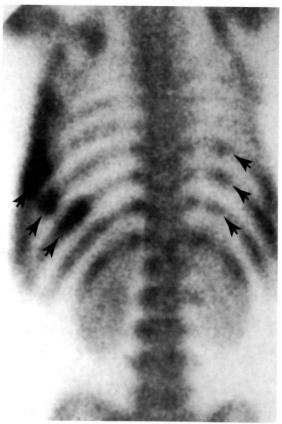

Figure 116.1. Posterior image from a radionuclide bone scan in an infant with irritability shows left posterolateral rib fractures in a linear distribution (black arrows on left). Older healing rib fractures are evident on the right with less intense uptake (arrows on right).

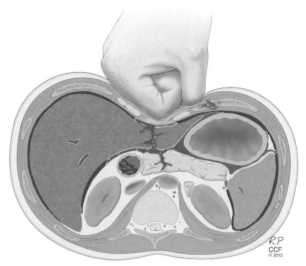

Figure 116.2. Classic abdominal injuries in NAT. Hemoperitoneum (red), liver laceration (green), pancreas laceration (orange).

hematoma appears as a mural low-attenuating mass at the second and third portion of the duodenum as it crosses the spine and is often visible on ultrasound. Intestinal laceration with perforation results in free intra-abdominal fluid and air where the fluid is usually higher in density than physiologic fluid (Fig. 116.6). Mesenteric injury results in hematoma and hemoperitoneum.

Specificity of findings increases as availability and plausibility of history decrease. Lesions specific for abusive injury are infrequent. Lacerations of solid viscera, hematoma, either subcapsular or intraparenchymal, hollow viscus injury, and mural

(A)

(B)

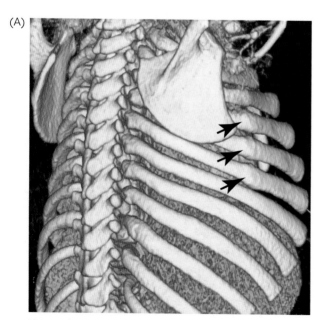
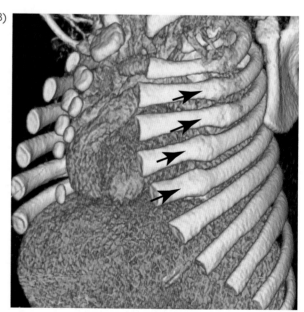

Figure 116.3. Volume-rendered chest CT in two projections in a 4-month-old with loss of consciousness shows multiple bilateral rib fractures (Arrows).

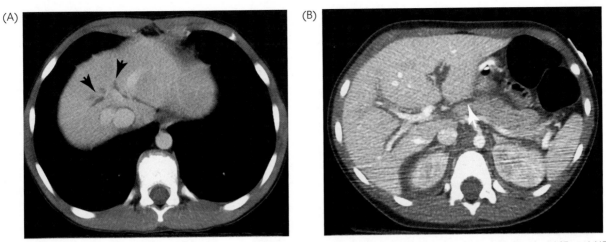

Figure116.4. (A) Axial contrast-enhanced CT of the liver in a 7-year-old child with abdominal pain and elevated AST and ALT shows a stellate liver laceration (black arrows). (B) Axial contrast-enhanced CT of the upper abdomen in a 4-year-old child with abdominal pain and elevated amylase and lipase shows pancreatic laceration (white arrow) and periportal edema.

hematoma or rupture are nonspecific and should be viewed in the context of the history and physical examination.

Imaging Strategies

A directed imaging approach is recommended. In these older children it is rarely necessary to perform a complete skeletal survey to evaluate for occult lesions. For the rare request for complete skeletal evaluation, radionuclide bone scan is preferred to radiographic skeletal survey (Fig. 116.1). The modality of choice to rule out multiple organ injury is CT scan. In some cases where the presentation may be unclear, ultrasound may be the first modality used. Upper gastrointestinal series may also be

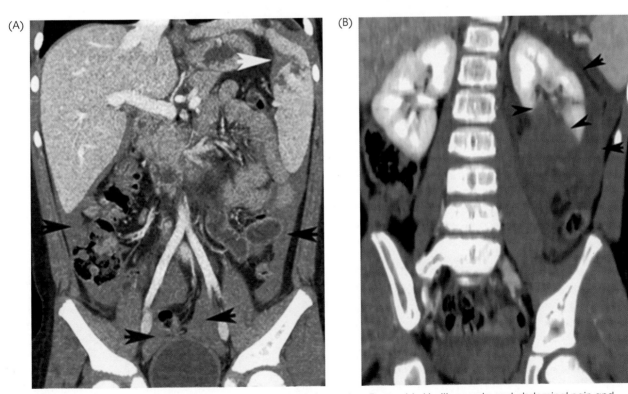

Figure 116.5. (A) Coronal contrast-enhanced CT of the abdomen in a 7-year-old girl with anemia and abdominal pain and distension shows splenic laceration (white arrow) and blood in the paracolic gutters bilaterally (black arrows). (B) Coronal contrast-enhanced CT in a 4-year-old boy with abdominal pain caused by NAT shows a left renal laceration (black arrowheads) with hematoma extending to Gerota's fascia (black arrows) and along the left psoas.

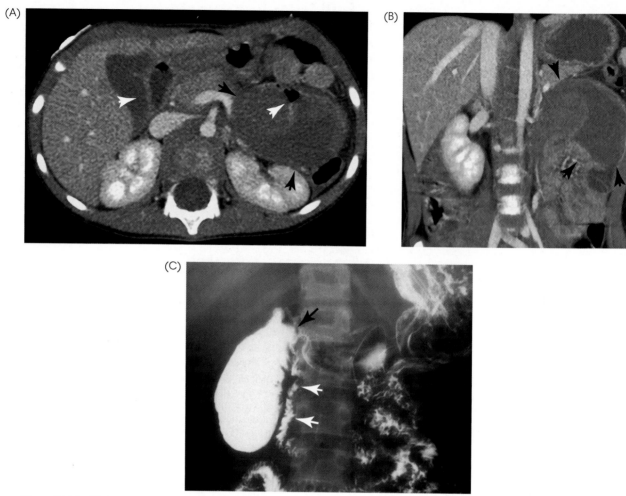

(A)

(B)

(C)

Figure 116.6. (A) Axial contrast-enhanced CT image of the abdomen in an infant with vomiting shows a large complex mass in the left upper quadrant (black arrows) compressing the duodenal lumen (white arrowhead) and proximal duodenum (white arrow) consistent with intramural duodenal hematoma. (B) Coronal reformatted image shows the complex nature of the hematoma (arrows). (C) Upper GI series from a different patient with the same symptoms shows a dilated first portion of the duodenum (black arrow) and compression of the second portion by an intramural hematoma (white arrows).

employed for the evaluation of the child who presents with vomiting. In blunt abdominal injury the presence of bruising is often a clue to the possibility of abuse.

Related Physics

Trauma imaging generates large data sets, and for practical purposes it is important that images arrive at the remote viewer fast enough so that the radiologist can render a timely report in order to guide therapy. Data compression can be performed with or without data loss, each having pros and cons. Lossless compression refers to a ratio of less than 3:1, which would be satisfactory for small data sets with few images but is rarely used in radiology because of the large number of pixels, large bit depth, and number of images per data set, especially in CT and MR. In order to effectively transfer the larger data sets with virtually no discernible image degradation, higher compression ratios such as 100:1 can be used

through lossy compression, which is the most commonly used method for imaging. This is the most common form of data compression for image storage on most pictorial archive and communication system (PACS). Modern radiology departments generate static and digital cine data sets that also can be compressed through the lossy technique. The most common image format in radiology is DICOM (Digital Imaging and Communications in Medicine) in which the ratio of DICOM to JPEG (Joint Photographic Experts Group) for a standard CT image is close to 8:1. Lossless compression looks for patterns in the data that can easily distinguish between surrounding room air and patient data and eliminates the surrounding useless data. Lossy compression works by removing pixels in an ordered fashion, dependent on the compression ratio, and further concentrating the remaining pixels through directed Fourier transformation that removes low-utility frequency according to the chosen algorithm.

Differential Diagnosis

The most frequent differential diagnosis is accidental trauma. Handlebar injuries may be identical to those seen in abusive abdominal injury. Fall from a height may be most difficult to distinguish, but here, history is important.

Clinical Issues

Abdominal injuries seldom result in death or significant morbidity and most, including liver lacerations, can be managed nonoperatively. Liver lacerations will be accompanied by elevations in AST and ALT. As is the case in accidental injury, splenic lacerations in abusive trauma seldom require surgical intervention. When there is no significant elevation in pancreatic enzymes, pancreatic injury is seldom visible on imaging studies. Operative intervention is often required with significant pancreatic injury. Pancreatic pseudocyst and chronic pancreatitis are potential sequelae of pancreatic injury. Most renal injuries are managed nonoperatively with adequate preservation of renal function. Bowel rupture and peritonitis require surgical intervention.

Long-term sequelae of abusive thoracoabdominal trauma are neither as significant nor as common as with abusive head trauma. Early recognition and intervention may have lasting impact in preventing death of the child from repeat injury.

Key Points

- Thoracoabdominal NAT is more common in the child over age 2 years.
- Mortality and morbidity are less than with head injury.

- Lesions are identical to accidental injury.
- Imaging is focused to the areas of clinical concern.
- CT scan with intravenous contrast is sensitive to solid organ and bone injury.
- Bone scan replaces radiographic survey and performed only in rare cases.

Further Reading

Hilmes MA, Hernanz-Schulman M, Greeley CS, Piercey LM, Yu C, Kan JH. CT identification of abdominal injuries in abused pre-school-age children. *Pediatric Radiology.* 2011;*41*:643–651.

Kleinman PK. *Diagnostic Imaging of Child Abuse.* St. Louis, MO: Mosby; 1998.

Lonergan GF, Baker AM, Morey MK, Boos SC. From the archives of the AFIP: child abuse: radiologic-pathologic correlation. *Radiographics.* 2003; *23*:811–845.

Mann FA, Gross JA, Blackmore CC. Imaging of blunt trauma to the pediatric torso. In: Medina LS, Applegate KE, Blackmore, CC, eds. *Evidence-Based Imaging in Pediatrics.* 2010:539–553.

Matshes EW, Lew EO. Do resuscitation-related injuries kill infants and children? *American Journal Forensic Medicine and Pathology.* 2010;*31*:178–185.

Pierce MC, Kaczor K, Aldridge S, O'Flynn J, Lorenz DJ. Bruising characteristics discriminating physical child abuse from accidental trauma. *Pediatrics.* 2010;*125*:67–74.

Trokel M, Discala C, Terrin N, Sege R. Patient and injury characteristics in abusive abdominal injuries. *Pediatric Emergency Care.* 2006;*22*:700–704.

CHAPTER 117

Child Abuse: Cerebral

Stephen Done, MD

Definition

Abusive head trauma (AHT) in infancy and childhood was first recognized by the French forensic physician Ambroise Tardieu in the nineteenth century and is a continuing problem of serious proportions and long-lasting effect. Also known today as inflicted head trauma, it was first described by John Caffey in 1974 as "whiplash shaken baby syndrome" or "shaken baby syndrome." As causal factors were further studied and doubts as to its biomechanical production arose, the term was broadened to include impact. Inasmuch as shaking, impact, and hypoxia-ischemia all have contributing effect, the terms "abusive head trauma" and "inflicted head injury" may be more appropriate because they are more inclusive of the various mechanisms of injury. The term presently preferred by the American Academy of Pediatrics is AHT, and it most frequently includes the triad of subdural hemorrhage, retinal hemorrhages, and encephalopathy.

Clinical Features

Nonaccidental trauma (NAT) is a worldwide problem. The exact incidence of AHT is difficult to clearly establish but may be as frequent as 17 per 100,000 person-years. In the United States it appears that the overall incidence of NAT may be declining but some studies report it as a leading cause of death in infancy. The most serious morbidity and mortality is a result of head trauma in its many forms. Most AHT occurs in infants under 2 years of age with peaks at 2 to 4 months and 7 to 9 months. It is more common in boys than girls. The parents, the male live-in partner, or nonbiological father are the most common assailants; there is a decreased incidence in homes with a biological father present.

The infant presents with signs of central nervous system excitation or depression, seizures, obtundation, apnea, bradycardia, poor feeding, or vomiting. There is often a delay in seeking medical attention. Physical findings such as bruising, scalp hematoma, and other evidence of injury commonly seen in accidental head injury are frequently absent in AHT.

Pathophysiology

As most cases are not witnessed, the mechanism of injury is often difficult to confirm. Biomechanical studies have shown that the act of shaking an infant results in translational and rotational forces that can cause life-threatening injury to the infant brain (Fig. 117.1). Acute subdural and subarachnoid hemorrhages and chronic subdural collections or mixed lesions may occur with shaking alone. Impact resulting from throwing the infant against a deformable object such as a bed or sofa or nondeformable surface such as the wall or floor may aggravate the injury or add skull fracture to the existing injury. Subdural hematoma or retinal hemorrhages can occur without impact and are present in the vast majority of shaken babies. Retinal hemorrhage may rarely occur with accidental injury but is never reported in the severity frequently seen with inflicted head injury.

Other injuries occurring in the infant brain include: contusion, often the result of direct blow; epidural hematoma, which may be venous or arterial and is frequently associated with skull fracture, often in the area of arteries or dural sinuses; diffuse axonal injury, probably related to hypoxia and vascular changes rather than shearing forces as once thought; and hypoxic-ischemic encephalopathy, cerebral edema, and herniation. Common histories include loss of consciousness, excessive crying that finally settled, choking or aspiration and the caregiver may admit to shaking to revive the infant or an attempt at CPR. Short falls such as rolling off a sofa or bed or falling while carrying the infant are also frequently mentioned in the history. In most cases of AHT the explanation does not fit the magnitude of the findings and severity of brain injury.

Imaging Findings

Findings on initial head CT depend upon the nature and degree of injury as well as the timing of presentation (Fig 117.2). Skull fractures are unusual, but if present may be complex or diastatic at presentation, owing to delay in seeking medical attention (Fig. 117.3). Skull fractures are better demonstrated on CT with 3-D reconstruction than any other imaging modality. Initial screening head CT often shows high-attenuation blood along the interhemispheric fissure in the parafalcine area and along the tentorium cerebelli. This subdural blood is the most commonly observed finding in AHT and may extend over the convexities of the parietal lobes depending upon the severity of the trauma (Fig. 117.4). Collections in multiple areas and of differing ages are more typical of inflicted head trauma than accidental head trauma (Fig. 117.5). The presence of both high- and

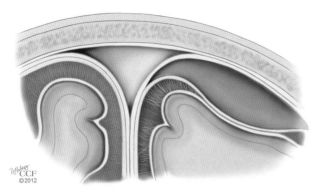

Figure 117.1. Illustration of the anatomy of the extra-axial spaces housing the vulnerable bridging cortical veins prone to hemorrhage with shaken impact trauma in child abuse.

low-attenuation extra-axial fluid does not necessarily indicate repeated trauma, however. Studies have shown that even acute subdural collections may present with mixed attenuation fluid. Intra-axial hemorrhage or contusions in the absence of skull fracture are rare in AHT and more common in accidental injury. Hypoxic ischemic encephalopathy with diffuse cerebral swelling results in obliteration of the extra-axial fluid spaces, basal cisterns and effacement of the sulcal and gyral pattern (Fig. 117.6). The cerebral hemispheres on CT become diffusely low in attenuation and stand out in stark contrast to the higher-attenuating thalami and cerebellum. The interhemispheric falx appears

relatively high in density. Brain swelling is usually apparent on CT by 12 to 48 hours.

Subarachnoid hemorrhage is much more clearly demonstrated on MRI. Additionally, MRI is superior in demonstrating chronic subdural hematoma owing to its ability to differentiate fluid with higher protein content from normal cerebrospinal fluid. Petechial hemorrhage and diffuse axonal injury are both more clearly demonstrated by MRI. Diffusion-weighted MRI shows areas of diffusion restriction in cytotoxic edema and cerebral infarction. This technique suggests that hypoxic ischemic encephalopathy is responsible for the parenchymal brain damage seen in most AHT.

Imaging Strategies

Head CT is the first imaging study obtained in the infant or child with suspected CNS injury. Its availability, ease and speed of acquisition, and sensitivity are all adequate for initial screening. Three-dimensional reconstruction increases the sensitivity for skull fractures, because some fractures may lie in the plane of imaging and be invisible on standard CT scans with bone algorithm. MRI is more sensitive to smaller collections of blood, principally subarachnoid and petechial hemorrhage. It is also more sensitive to timing and evolution of blood products (Table 117.1). Newer sequences are sensitive to diffuse axonal injury, hypoxic ischemic encephalopathy, and infarction.

(A)

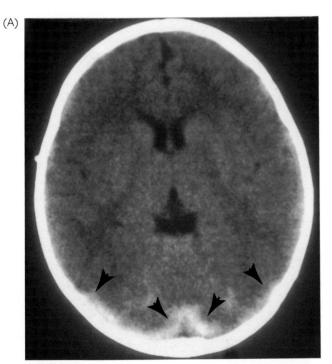

(B)

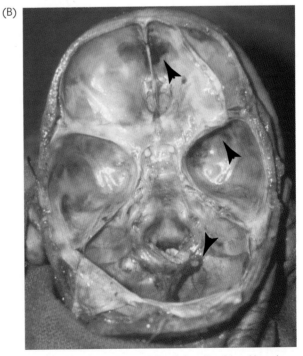

Figure 117.2. (A) Axial noncontrast head CT in a 4-month-old with loss of consciousness shows high-attenuation blood layering along the falx and tentorium cerebelli (arrowheads). (B) Autopsy specimen in the same child shows blood in the anterior, middle, and posterior fossae (black arrows).

(A)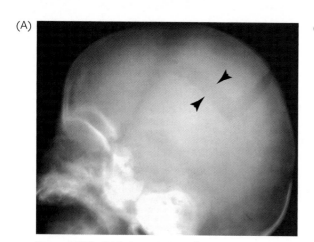

(B)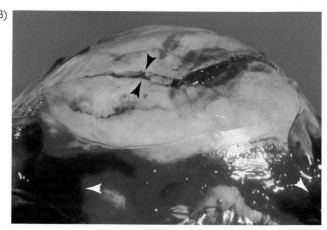

Figure 117.3. (A) Lateral skull radiograph in a 2-month-old with loss of consciousness resulting from a blow to the head shows a diastatic skull fracture (black arrows). (B) Autopsy specimen shows the diastatic fracture is mildly depressed (black arrows).

Related Physics

In child abuse cases, MRI may serve as legal evidence and therefore a high confidence level is necessary in order to avoid misinterpretation of imaging artifacts as true pathology. Artifacts can originate from a variety of sources in the imaging environment with the two most prevalent related to the patient factors or the magnet. Common MR artifacts include metal or susceptibilty, field inhomogeneity, radiofrequency, k-space, motion, chemical shift, Gibb's, aliasing, partial voluming, high-speed and high-field-strength imaging. The first three are discussed here. Susceptibility artifact is caused by local magnetic field distortions and their accelerated dephasing at that location within the image. With metal, the dephasing is almost instantaneous at the metal-tissue interface resulting in a signal void on the image. This artifact is actually used to our advantage in detecting extracellular methemoglobin related to old hemorrhage. Metal artifact can be decreased but not eliminated by using fast spin echo with short echo time (TE) in place of echo planar imaging, while increasing the bandwidth. This may lead to increased heating effects, especially with higher field strengths, so that one must pay heed to the specific absorption rates (SAR). Static field inhomogeneities cause geometric distortion in the image, most often seen as bowing at the polar ends of the magnet. As the static magnetic field, B_0, exits one end of the bore, its tendency is to wrap around and reenter the other end of the bore, which causes the lines of magnetic force to diverge from parallel. For this reason, static field inhomogeneities increase with shorter and wider bore magnets. One can overcome this through active or passive shimming. Radiofrequency (RF) artifacts may be related to spurious RF signals from support equipment in the room or signal entering the room from FM transmitters. These appear as a row of pixels in the frequency encoding direction whose signal strength is high or low relative to adjacent structures, the so-called "zipper" artifact. One can determine the source by disconnecting power to all support equipment in the MR room

and imaging a water phantom. If artifacts are still present, these must originate outside the room, meaning there is a leak in the room's RF shielding.

Differential Diagnosis

- Accidental trauma (most studies suggest that short-distance falls do not result in skull fracture or significant intracranial hemorrhage although point-of-impact small subdural hemorrhages may be seen)
- Superior sagittal sinus thrombosis (every MRI in suspected AHT should include MR venography)

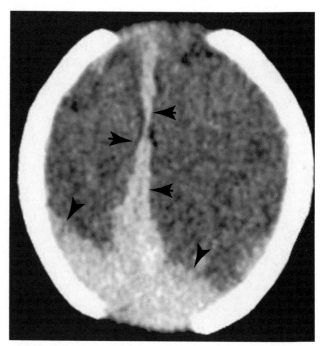

Figure 117.4. Axial noncontrast CT scan in a 3-week-old following shaking injury shows high-attenuation blood along the interhemispheric fissure (black arrows) extending over the convexities (black arrowheads).

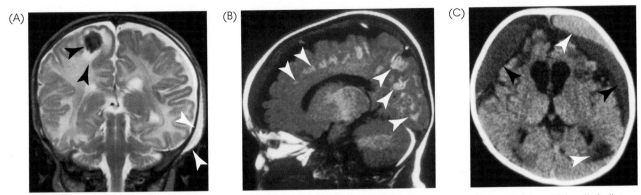

Figure 117.5. (A) Coronal fat-suppressed T2-weighted image in a child with head injury shows decreased signal intensity in the right frontal lobe (black arrowheads) consistent with hemorrhagic contusion. Left subtemporal subgaleal edema represents the site of impact (white arrowheads). (B) Parasagittal T1-weighted image in another child shows multiple foci of increased signal intensity at the gray-white interface, previously thought to represent shear injuries, but more likely caused by hypoxia (arrows). (C) Axial CT of the brain in an infant following NAT shows multiple subdural collections of differing ages—acute (white arrow), chronic (black arrows), and encephalomalacia (white arrowhead)—as long-term sequelae of repeated head trauma.

- Coagulopathies
- Glutaric aciduria type 1
- Newborn subdural hemorrhage (between 26 and 46 percent of asymptomatic normal-term newborn infants screened with MRI may have small infratentorial subdural hematomas that usually resolve by 1 to 3 months of age)
- Meningitis
- Vasculitis
- Craniotomy
- Ventriculoperitoneal shunting

Clinical Issues

Patients with AHT are in most cases younger than those with accidental head injury, usually presenting between 6 weeks to 9 months of age. Minor injuries and small hemorrhages or chronic subdural collections may be clinically inapparent and the diagnosis may be unsuspected on initial presentation. In some cases of severe or fatal AHT the infants have been seen by medical practitioners shortly before the significant event and the diagnosis of NAT has not been made. Most frequently the considerations in AHT are whether the injuries seen in an injured infant are consistent with the history given, both

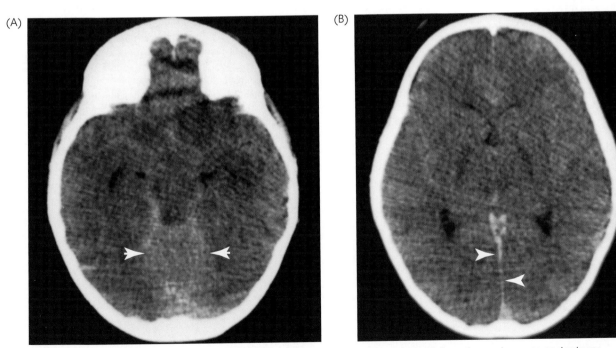

Figure 117.6. (A and B) Axial noncontrast CT images of the brain in a 6-month-old with loss of consciousness and seizures show diffuse cerebral edema including bright cerebellum and tentorium (arrowheads) and decreased attenuation in the basal ganglia and loss of normal gray-white differentiation.

Table 117.1 – Characteristics of Blood Products and Edema on CT and MRI

AGENT	TIMING	MRI T1 (SIGNAL INTENSITY)	MRI T2 (SIGNAL INTENSITY)	CT (ATTENUATION)
Oxyhemoglobin	Hyperacute (6 hours)	Iso to low	High	High
Deoxyhemoglobin	Acute (6 hrs to 3 days)	Iso to low	Low	High
Methemoglobin	Intracellular-EARLY SUBACUTE (3 days to 1–2 wks)	High	Low	High
	Extracellular- LATE SUBACUTE (1–2 wks to 4–6 wks)	High	High	Iso
Hemosiderin	Chronic (4–6 weeks)	Very low	Very low	Iso/low
Edema		Low	High	Low

in regards to the mechanism of injury and the timing. Death is almost always from hypoxia-ischemia from multifactorial processes. Mortality rates are between 11 and 33 percent. Sixty-seven percent of infants suffering AHT have neurological impairment including hemiplegia, visual or hearing impairment, microcephaly, hydrocephalus, learning disabilities, behavioral, developmental, and cognitive sequelae.

Key Points

- Exact timing of events is not always possible.
- AHT is the most common cause of death in NAT.
- Mixed attenuation extra-axial hemorrhages do not always indicate multiple events.
- Violent shaking of an infant by itself appears to be capable of causing the triad of subdural hemorrhage, retinal hemorrhages, and encephalopathy; impact does not appear to be necessary.
- Although skull fractures may occur from a short fall, fatal head injury is extremely rare.
- The province of radiology is not to determine who, but what, how, and when AHT occurred.

Further Reading

Adamsbaum C, Grabar S, Mejean N, Rey-Salmon C. Abusive head trauma: judicial admissions highlight violent and repetitive shaking. *Pediatrics*. 2010;*126*:546–555.

Christian CW, Block R. Abusive head trauma in infants and children. *Pediatrics*. 2009;*123*:1409–1411.

Cory CZ, Jones MD. Can shaking alone cause fatal brain injury? A biomechanical assessment of the Duhaime shaken baby syndrome model. *Medical Science Law*. 2003;*43*:317–333.

Couper Z, Albermani F. Mechanical response of infant brain to manually inflicted shaking. Proceedings Institution Mechanical Engineering Part H: *J Engineering in Medicine*. 2010;*224*:1–15.

Ehsani JP, Ibraham JE, Bugeja L, Cordner S. The role of epidemiology in determining if a simple short fall can cause fatal head injury in an infant. *American Journal Forensic Medicine and Pathology*. 2010;*31*:287–298.

Oehmichen M, Schleiss D, Pedal I, Saternus K-S, Gerling I, Meissner C. Shaken baby syndrome: re-examination of diffuse axonal injury as cause of death. *Acta Neuropathologica*. 2008;*116*:317–329.

Pierce MC, Bertocci G. Injury biomechanics and child abuse. *Annual Review Biomedical Engineering*. 2008;*10*:85–106.

Rooks VJ, Eaton JP, Ruess L, Petermann GW, Keck Wherley J, Pedersen RC. Prevalence and evolution of intracranial hemorrhage in asymptomatic term infants. *American Journal of Neuroradiology*. 2008;*29*:1082–1089.

Sato Y, Moritani T. Imaging of non-accidental head injury. In: Santiago-Medina L, Applegate KE, Blackmore CC, eds. *Evidence-Based Imaging in Pediatrics*. New York: Spinger; 2010:161–174.

Vinchon M, deFoort-Dhellemmes S, Desurmont M, Delestret I. Confessed abuse versus witnessed accidents in infants: comparison of clinical, radiological, and ophthalmological data in corroborated cases. *Childs Nervous System*. 2010;*26*:637–645.

CHAPTER 118

Langerhans Cell Histiocytosis

Kamaldine Oudjhane, MD and Janet R. Reid, MD, FRCPC

Definition

Langerhans cell histiocytosis (LCH), formerly known as Histiocytosis X, is characterized by the proliferation of histiocytes (Langerhans cells) of the dendritic cell system. Of historic interest, Hand Schuller Christian syndrome and Letterer-Siwe disease refer to the first individualized forms of LCH. Presently the LCH study group recommends the following stratification system: single-system LCH involving a single site (bone, skin, or lymph node); or multisystem LCH (multifocal bone or lymph nodes) characterized by two or more organs involved with/without dysfunction.

Clinical Features

The peak age for LCH is 1 to 4 years with slight predominance in males. Prevalence is two to five cases per one million children annually. Ten percent of new cases have an adverse clinical course. Single-system LCH most often involves the skeleton resulting in bone pain, local swelling, skull lump, ear discharge, proptosis, floating tooth, or pathologic limb fracture. Skin involvement results in a papular rash. Lymph node disease causes lymphadenopathy. Systemic signs are seen with multisystem disease and include fever, leukocytosis, elevated erythrocyte sedimentation rate, peripheral eosiniphilia, hepatosplenomegaly, and gastrointestinal (GI) symptoms like those of Crohn's disease. Although the lungs may be involved in single-system disease, up to 50 percent of multisystem disease has lung involvement with cough, dyspnea, chest pain, and pneumothorax. Pituitary infundibular infiltration results in diabetes insipidus. Other central nervous system (CNS) signs include ataxia, tremor, and pyramidal signs. Twenty percent of the patients with multisystem disease may be at low risk with a good prognosis if the risk organs (liver, lung, spleen) are not involved. The high-risk group (80 percent of cases) is associated with a high mortality rate, when one or more organs are involved.

Anatomy and Physiology

The Langerhans cell is a large mononuclear cell with eccentric nucleus, derived from the bone marrow stem cell CD34. Cells migrate to the epidermis and lymph nodes and may infiltrate an organ with subsequent immunologic reaction. The mechanism of lesion proliferation is thought to be lack of auto-regulation, delayed apoptosis, or an exaggerated immune reaction. It is no longer believed that LCH is a neoplasm. Biopsy may demonstrate granulomata with histiocytes, eosinophils, lymphocytes, and bone necrosis. The histiocytes house the antigens and are identified on electron microscopy (EM) as containing cytoplasmic Birbeck granules. Many surface antigen markers are used for diagnosis including CD1a and protein S100.

Imaging Findings

Bones

The skeletal system is involved in at least 60 percent of cases where "eosinophilic granuloma" is the classic form. The most commonly involved bones include skull (Figs. 118.1 and 118.2), mandible, ribs, femur (Fig. 118.3), pelvis, and spine. There is a variable radiographic appearance of LCH because of different stages of evolution. Findings include:

- Osteolytic lesion with well-defined or sclerotic borders when healing
- Skull lytic lesion with beveled edges resulting from advanced erosion of the internal table
- Associated soft-tissue mass on CT
- Abnormal marrow signal intensity on MR
- Extra-osseous and meningeal soft-tissue mass with edema
- Enhancement of active lesion
- Rat-bite-like temporal bone destruction with soft-tissue mass best demonstrated by CT
- Vertebra plana resulting from collapse of the vertebral body
- Preserved intervertebral disc spaces bordering a vertebral lesion (Fig. 118.4)
- Expansile osteolysis of rib lesions

Lungs

Chest CT is more informative than radiography and shows a reticulonodular pattern with cysts, with predilection for the upper lobes sparing the costophrenic sulci. Pneumothorax may result (Fig. 118.5). Thymic involvement is most often

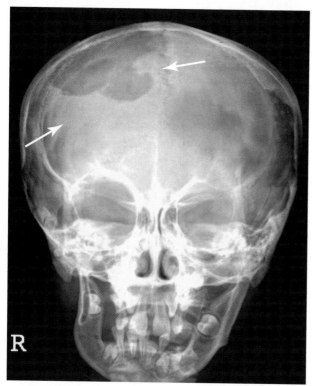

Figure 118.1. Frontal radiograph of the skull in a 6-year-old boy with fevers shows two large well-defined bone defects near the left pterion and the right parietal eminence (arrows). Notice also the remodeled left orbital rim from previously healed lesion 1 year prior.

present in infants with systemic disease resulting in medi-astinal widening, cysts, and calcifications.

Abdomen

Langerhans cell histiocytosis can infiltrate the intestines resulting in mucosal disease akin to Crohn's enteritis or colitis. Liver involvement results in focal liver lesions that

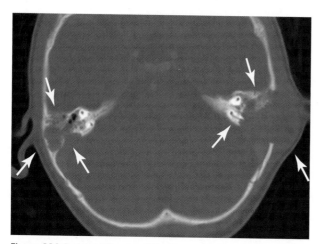

Figure 118.2. Axial CT scan of the temporal bones in a 2-year-old with acute onset of left mastoid area swelling with ear discharge shows bilateral soft-tissue masses with associated "rat bite" erosion of the mastoids (arrows). The radiographic skeletal survey also detected a fibular lesion.

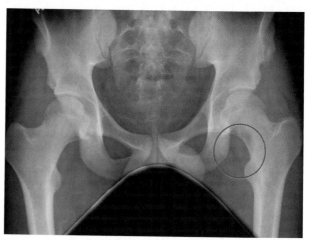

Figure 118.3. Frontal radiograph of the pelvis in a 16-year-old male with recurrent left hip pain and past history of LCH shows an osteolytic lesion (red circle) at the medial aspect of the left proximal femoral metaphysis. Bone scan showed multiple additional sites of involvement.

are heterogeneous on ultrasound (US) and hypodense on CT. Biliary infiltration will appear on CT or MRI as irregular dilatation of the intrahepatic biliary system.

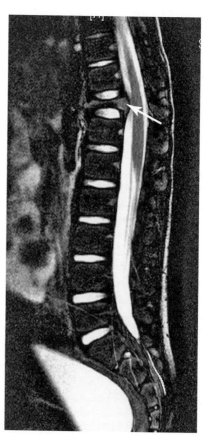

Figure 118.4. Sagittal FSE T2 MR image with fat saturation in a 6-year-old male with 1-week history of nontraumatic back pain depicts vertebra plana of the T11 vertebral body, abnormal marrow signal and retropulsion of the vertebral body into the spinal canal with effacement of the CSF space anterior to the spinal cord (arrow). Disk spaces are preserved.

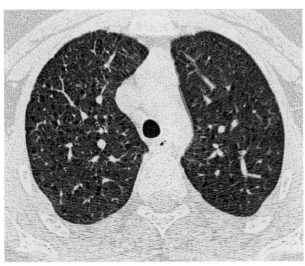

Figure 118.5. Thin-section chest CT in a 12-year-old male with liver and bone LCH and recent respiratory symptoms shows numerous air filled cysts through the lungs.

Central Nervous System

Classic CNS disease causes infiltration of the pituitary infundibulum with loss of the normal high signal intensity in the neurohypophysis on T1. The thickened infundibulum measures more than 2 millimeters and enhances avidly following intravenous gadolinium (Fig. 118.6). Langerhans cell histiocytosis of the CNS may result in tumefactive intra-axial supratentorial and infratentorial lesions, as well as meningeal and intramedullary spinal cord infiltration. Additional findings include increased free water in white matter tracts consistent with demyelination and gliosis, abnormal signal intensity in basal ganglia, parenchymal calcifications, and cerebellar atrophy.

Imaging Strategies

The imaging workup includes radiographic skeletal survey and detailed MR imaging of lesions. The false-negative rate on bone scintigraphy is up to 16 percent. Whole-body MRI with short tau inversion recovery sequences is a promising modality. To evaluate the thymus and lungs, CT is optimal. Liver disease is best assessed with US and MRI including magnetic resonance cholangiopancreatography (MRCP). Diabetes insipidus and skull lesions require brain MRI with gadolinium.

Related Physics

A standard way to evaluate bones for additional lesions in LCH is radiographic skeletal survey. It is important to understand the various photon interactions that are responsible for the production of radiation dose to the patient and the operator. These include Compton scattering and photoelectric absorption. Compton scattering is the primary mode of interaction in soft tissues at diagnostic X-ray energies. It is

(A)

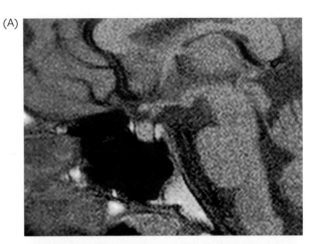

(B)

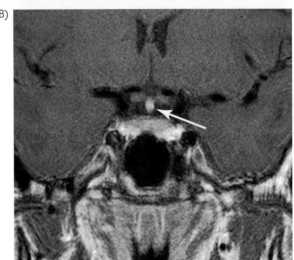

Figure 118.6. Sagittal T1 MR image (A) in a 13-year-old with diabetes insipidus and past history of multiple recurrences of osseous LCH depicts the absence of bright signal at the neurohypophysis. Coronal T1 MR image with fat saturation following IV gadolinium administration (B) shows a thickened enhancing pituitary infundibulum (arrow).

responsible for scattering of moderate energy X-rays toward the operator and all other occupants in the room especially during fluoroscopy. Compton scattering will increase with increase in body thickness so that there is very little Compton scattering when imaging a newborn. With adolescents the increase in Compton scattering can be controlled through proper collimation of the incident beam. In addition one can limit the occupational dose from Compton scattering through lead drapes and garments. Compton scattering is also related to density of tissue so that it will be lowest when imaging the chest (air) and highest when imaging the abdomen (solid organs). Photoelectric effect predominates at low energy and in tissues with a high atomic number such as bone. Unlike Compton that produces scattered photons, photoelectric absorption produces electrons that contribute directly to patient dose but not to operator dose. Photoelectric effect is the primary reason that bones are radiopaque on radiographs. This effect can be controlled by moderating the kVp whereby higher kVp will decrease the photoelectric effect (while increasing scatter). When imaging the infant versus the adolescent, the compromise becomes the balance between the deleterious effects from Compton scattering and photoelectric effect while maintaining image quality. Though not used in radiographic skeletal survey, for completeness it is important to understand the relationship between Compton scattering, photoelectric absorption, and contrast media. Contrast media work to increase image contrast, as they are designed to contain high-atomic-number atoms (iodine or barium) within their molecular structure. The iodine or barium causes photoelectric absorption and the media effectively displace tissues or fluids that would otherwise not participate in photoelectric absorption. For example, iodinated contrast replaces blood within vessels allowing us to see the vessels as radio-opaque through photoelectric effect with iodine. Likewise, ingested barium replaces and coats the esophagus, stomach and lower-GIstructures rendering them visible under X-ray imaging. A full understanding of Compton scattering and photoelectric absorption is critical to producing high-quality images with acceptable patient dose and safe radiation levels for operators.

Differential Diagnosis

A differential diagnosis can be developed based on the imaging features of the index lesion:

- Aggressive osseous lesions: osteomyelitis, leukemia, Ewing sarcoma
- Osteolysis with sclerotic edges: healing metastases, fibrous dysplasia, nonossifying fibroma, giant cell tumor, and hemangioma
- "Punched-out" skull lesion: leptomenigeal cyst, metastasis
- Rim sclerosis: fibrous dysplasia, epidermoid, meningocele
- Orbital mass: lymphoma, neuroblastoma, rhabdomyosarcoma
- Temporal bone osteolysis: mastoiditis, external ear rhabdomyosarcoma
- Vertebra plana: metastatic neuroblastoma, aneurysmal bone, tuberculosis, hemangioma, Gaucher disease, and trauma
- Extremity soft-tissue mass: granuloma or rhabdomyosarcoma
- Cervical lymphadenopathy: adenitis, reactive adenopathy, or lymphoma
- Lung disease: bronchiectasis and infection (tuberculosis)
- Liver disease: bile duct rhabdomyosarcoma, sclerosing cholangitis
- GI tract mucosal lesions: inflammatory bowel disease
- Pituitary stalk infiltration: granulomatous disease, germ cell tumor, pituitary ectopia

Clinical Variants

The very young infant may present an auto-involutive skin disease of cutaneous histiocytosis of Hashimoto-Pritzker. Letterer-Siwe is classically a multisystemic involvement in the very young patient. Hand-Schuller-Christian syndrome combines diabetes insipidus, exophthalmos, and cranial osteolysis.

Clinical Issues

The clinical presentation of LCH is polymorphous; the most common signs and symptoms are local swelling and bone pain. Single-system LCH has a high rate of spontaneous remission. Bone LCH associated with multisystem disease is treated with chemotherapy to prevent reactivation. Prognosis deteriorates with vital organ involvement. It is rare for vertebra plana to completely resolve.

Key Points

- LCH features a protean presentation and a clinical course.
- LCH includes a wide range in severity from self-healing solitary bone lesion to an acute life-threatening multisystem disease.
- Ideal imaging workup relies on radiographic skeletal survey and whole-body MRI.
- CT is helpful with skull and orbit lesions.
- Bone scan may be falsely negative in 16%.
- Top differential diagnoses for bone LCH are osteomyelitis, Ewing sarcoma, leukemia, and metastatic neuroblastoma.

Further Reading

Abla O, Egeler RM, Weitzman S. Langerhans cell histiocytosis: current concepts and treatments. Cancer Treatment Reviews. 2010;36:354–359.

Azouz ME, Saigal G, Rodriguez MM, Podda A. Langerhans cell histiocytosis: pathology, imaging and treatment of skeletal involvement. *Pediatr Radiol.* 2005;35:103–115.

Diederichs G, Hauptmann K, Schroder RJ, Kivelitz D. Case 147: Langerhans cell histiocytosis of the femur. *Radiology.* 2009;252:309–313.

Goo HW, Yang DH, Ra YS, Song JS, Im HJ, Seo JJ, et al. Whole-body MRI of Langerhans cell histiocytosis: comparison with radiography and bone scintigraphy. *Pediatr Radiol.* 2006;36:1019–1031.

Schmidt S, Eich G, Geoffray A, Hanquinet S, Waibel P, Wolf R, et al. Extraosseous Langerhans cell histiocytosis in children. *Radiographics.* 2008;28:707–726.

Weitzman S, Egeler RM. *Histolytic Disorders of Children and Adults.* Cambridge, UK: Cambridge University Press; 2005.

CHAPTER 119

Vascular Malformations

Terrence Hong, MD

Definition

Vascular malformations are collections of abnormal veins, lymphatics, arteries, capillaries or a combination of these that develop before birth and persist throughout postnatal life, growing in proportion with the patient.

Clinical Features

Vascular malformations affect 1.2 to 1.5 percent of the general population and have an equal sex distribution. Low-flow vascular malformations are more common than high-flow malformations. Depending on the type and severity of the lesion, malformations can result in disfigurement, pain, functional limitation, ischemia, cardiac failure, skeletal and joint abnormalities, limb-length discrepancy, and other complications if left untreated.

Low-Flow Vascular Malformations

Capillary malformations (CMs), also referred to as port wine stains, are the most common vascular malformation affecting the skin, appearing as red skin stains, with localized forms common on the face. In older patients, CMs may exhibit skin and subcutaneous tissue thickening.

Venous malformations (VMs) are the most common malformations seen at specialty clinics. Venous malformations are soft, compressible, nonpulsatile masses and can involve skin, mucosa, and/or deeper tissues. Most often located in the head, neck, and extremities, VMs may enlarge following compression, as well as when the patient is in a dependent position or performing Valsalva's maneuver. Lesions may also enlarge following trauma or hormonal changes, such as at puberty and during pregnancy. Intra-articular or periarticular involvement, such as in diffuse VM of the extremities, may result in secondary osteoarthritis. Intramuscular lesions may result in bone deformity, bone remodeling or skeletal hypertrophy. Intraosseous VM may result in osteopenia and increased risk of fractures. Bone involvement is often accompanied by limb undergrowth.

Lymphatic malformations (LMs) are most often located in the head and neck and may be focal or diffuse, sometimes involving multiple organ systems. They are masses with a rubbery consistency that cannot be compressed manually. Sudden enlargement may be a sign of spontaneous intralesional bleeding or infection.

High-Flow Vascular Malformations

Arteriovenous malformations (AVMs) and arteriovenous fistulae (AVF), present as masses with thrill, bruit, and sometimes, local hyperthermia. Arterial steal, hypoxia, and ischemia may lead to pain and functional impairment. In cases with large arteriovenous shunts, cardiac overload and failure may result. Other symptoms include skin bleeding or ulceration, as well as bone overgrowth resulting from increased vascularization of the cartilage growth centers. Arteriovenous fistulae and AVMs can be distinguished on imaging.

Anatomy and Physiology

Low-Flow Vascular Malformations

Capillary malformations consist of small ectatic capillaries in the dermis, which enlarge with age. Venous malformations are composed of thin-walled venous channels with flattened endothelium and a deficiency of smooth muscle cells. Venous malformations may surround normal structures, such as arteries and nerves, and can involve subcutaneous tissues, muscles, bones, and joints. Thrombi can be seen within VMs and may calcify to form phleboliths. Lymphatic malformations result from defective embryologic development of primordial lymphatic channels that did not involute over time. There are three types of LMs: macrocystic (cysts > 1 cm in diameter), microcystic (cysts <1 cm in diameter), and mixed macro-microcystic.

High-Flow Vascular Malformations

High-flow vascular malformations may result from the lack of regression of arteriovenous channels in the primitive retiform plexus during early fetal development. Arteriovenous fistulae are formed by direct connections between arteries and veins, whereas AVMs are distinguished by the presence of precapillary shunts called nidii. Both AVMs and AVFs can have multiple arteriovenous communications.

Imaging Findings

Most vascular malformations are diagnosed from history and clinical examination. Imaging of vascular malformations is usually performed to confirm the diagnosis,

(A)

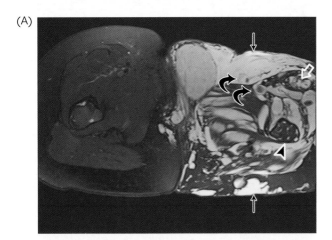

(B)

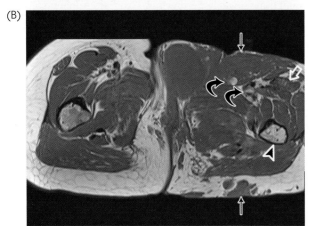

(C)

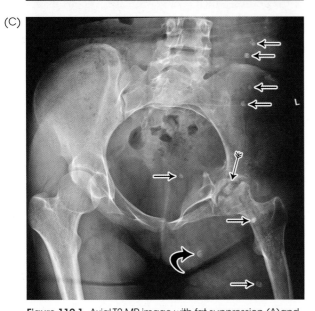

Figure 119.1. Axial T2 MR image with fat suppression (A) and axial T1 MR image (B) in a teen with venous malformation demonstrate extensive left pelvic and proximal thigh, low-flow tubular structures within the subcutaneous soft-tissue fat (arrows), muscle (arrow outline), and proximal femoral metaphysis (arrowhead). Multiple filling defects are noted in keeping with phleboliths (curved arrow). Frontal radiograph of the pelvis (C) shows multiple phleboliths (arrows), including one with MRI correlation (curved arrow), secondary left hip joint arthropathy, and left femoral head avascular necrosis (quilled arrow). Also note that the proximal left femoral is gracille compared to the contralateral side.

determine the anatomic extent of malformation, and evaluate treatment response. Ultrasound (US) and MRI are the preferred modalities for noninvasive assessment. CT does not provide tissue specificity to establish a diagnosis and should be avoided because of radiation exposure.

Low-Flow Vascular Malformations

Capillary malformations are usually confined to the dermis and are typically diagnosed clinically. Venous malformations are the only malformations that contain phleboliths, which may be seen on radiographs as rounded calcifications in a soft-tissue mass. Other radiographic features are bony hypertrophy, bowing, cortical thickening, periosteal reaction, and remodeling. Intraosseous lesions may create a lattice-like, trabecular pattern. Diffuse involvement will cause ostepenia with the risk of pathologic fracture. Secondary arthropathy may be seen with intra-articular involvement of the knee. On US, VMs will appear as hypoechoic, compressible venous lakes infiltrating subcutaneous tissue and muscle, as well as surrounding normal structures. The lesions may contain echogenic thrombi and highly echogenic phleboliths with slow flow on Doppler. On MRI, VMs appear as septated masses with ectatic, serpentine vessels, which are hyperintense on short tau inversion recovery (STIR) and on fat-saturated T2-weighted images, although signal intensity may be variable because of hemorrhage and thrombosis. Lesions are isointense to muscle on T1-weighted images and may contain fluid-fluid levels. No flow voids are seen. The lesions show marked enhancement on gadolinium-enhanced T1-weighted images. Thrombi are hyperintense on T1-weighted images and hypointense on STIR and fat-saturated T2-weighted images and phleboliths appear low in signal intensity on all sequences (Fig. 119.1). Hemarthrosis may be seen on gradient echo images because of the T2* effect of hemosiderin.

Lymphatic malformations have no characteristic radiographic features. On US, macrocystic LMs are hypoechoic, thin-walled, multilocular cystic masses without flow, except in the septae. In the case of recent hemorrhage, echogenic debris may be visible in the cysts. Microcystic lesions appear as multiple tiny, hyperechoic cysts without flow on Doppler. On MRI, macrocystic LMs are multiloculated, septated masses with low signal intensity on T1-weighted images and high signal intensity on T2-weighted images, although signal intensities may be variable because of hemorrhage or proteinaceous content (Fig. 119.2). Blood-fluid levels indicate recent bleeding or infection (Fig. 119.3A). On contrast-enhanced T1-weighted images, there is septal and marginal enhancement sparing the central channels. Diffuse enhancement could be related to superimposed infection. As lesions can be mixed venolymphatic malformations, there may be vague, ill-defined contrast enhancement throughout the lesion (Fig. 119.3B). Microcystic LMs show diffuse infiltration with intermediate signal intensity on T1-weighted images and high signal intensity on T2-weighted images. There may be lymphedema adjacent to subcutaneous fat. Lesions show decrease in size and enhancement following therapy (Fig. 119.4).

High-Flow Vascular Malformations

Arteriovenous malformation appears on US as a hypervascular lesion with both arterial and venous wave forms

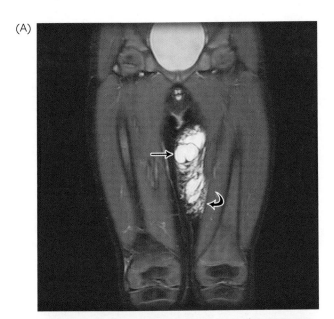

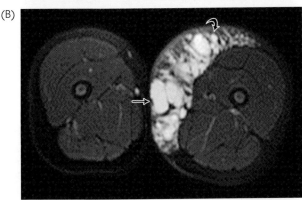

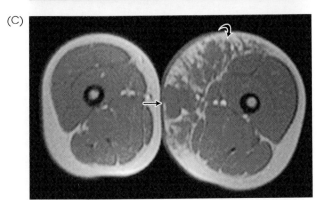

Figure 119.2. Coronal STIR (A) and axial T2 MR image with fat suppression (B) and axial T1 MR image (C) in a teen boy show macrocystic (arrow) and microcystic (curved arrow) components of a lymphatic malformation with increased left thigh girth and thickening of the superficial subcutaneous fat tissue.

on Doppler. Arteriovenous fistula shows a characteristic accentuated diastolic flow proximal to the fistula, high-velocity jet at the fistula, and pulsatile waveform in the draining vein. The hallmark of the high-flow lesion is flow voids on spin-echo sequences and absence of a parenchymal lesion. Enlarged feeding arteries and draining vessels can be displayed using MR angiography. Static information may be insufficient to assess flow dynamics. Catheter angiography is the gold standard for confirmation and assessment of high-flow vascular malformations. Arteriovenous malformation shows prominent feeding arteries, a nidus (i.e., amorphous tangle of small channels), and early-draining veins resulting from rapid shunting. Arteriovenous fistula shows direct arteriovenous connection(s) with enlarged feeding and draining veins with rapid shunting.

Imaging Strategy

Sonography and MRI are the preferred modalities for both diagnosis and monitoring of vascular malformations. Sonography may help confirm flow velocity within lesions, and MRI may be beneficial in assessing the size of the lesion and its relationship to deeper vasculature. Radiography is of limited value, but may aid in differential diagnosis (e.g., phleboliths) and alert radiologists to bone or joint involvement. Computed tomography should be avoided because of radiation exposure and inferior soft-tissue contrast compared with MRI. Because of its invasiveness, conventional angiography should only be used for high-flow vascular malformations and when therapeutic intervention is being considered.

Related Physics

Vascular malformations can be high-flow, low-flow, or mixed. These require imaging with B-mode, spectral, color, and power Doppler. B-mode will identify location and depth of involvement and characteristics such as pseudocapsule and soft-tissue component of hemangioma, phleboliths in venous malformation, or blood-fluid levels in lymphatic malformations. Once lesion location and morphology are characterized on gray scale, Doppler will significantly increase specificity in diagnosis. Spectral Doppler will differentiate between arteries and veins by characteristic waveform patterns. Once high-flow characteristics are ruled out, the low-flow lesions are further distinguished first with Color Doppler. In cases of very slow flow, Color Doppler will show signal void, which could be mistaken for absence of flow, resulting in a misdiagnosis of lymphatic malformation. Where no flow is detected on Color Doppler, power Doppler must be employed. Power is more sensitive to low-flow states at the price of sacrificing quantitative speed and directionality.

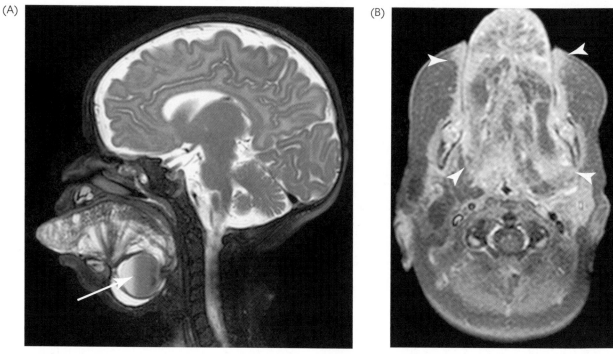

Figure 119.3. Sagittal T2 MR image with fat suppression (A) in a baby with a mass involving the tongue and floor of the mouth shows linear regions of high signal intensity and a blood-fluid level (arrow). Axial contrast-enhanced T1 MR image with fat suppression (B) shows patchy diffuse enhancement (arrowheads) in a typical venolymphatic malformation.

Differential Diagnosis

- Malignant vascular tumors: unlike tumors, AVMs are often accompanied by fat within the lesion, muscle atrophy, and rarely edema.
- Proliferative hemangioma: Doppler may be used to rule out hemangioma as VMs have limited, if any, flow.

Common Variants

- Klippel Trenaunay: low-flow malformations
- Parkes Weber: high-flow malformations
- Cobb: AVMs
- Osler-Weber Rendu: AVMs
- Blue rubber bleb nevus: venous malformations

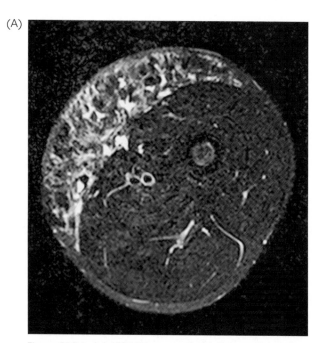

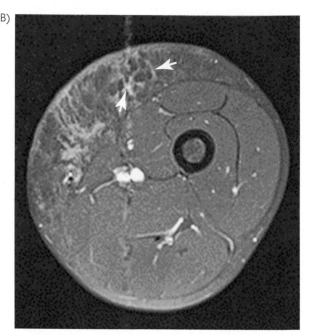

Figure 119.4. Axial T2 MR image with fat suppression (A) and axial contrast-enhanced T1 MR image with fat suppression (B) following sclerotherapy show interval shrinking of the macrocystic component and typical wall and septae pattern of enhancement (arrows).

Clinical Issues

Low-Flow Vascular Malformations

Capillary malformations are often confined to the skin and do not typically require imaging. Pulsed dye laser therapy is the treatment of choice. Venous malformations rarely regress spontaneously and may be associated with pain, functional limitation, decrease in range of motion, and disfigurement or deformity. Involvement of the brain is typically asymptomatic as VMs are usually comprised of atypical venous routes, as opposed to cavernomas. Thus, there is limited risk of cerebral hemorrhage. Noninvasive management of VMs in the extremities usually consists of use of compression bandages or garments. In patients with pain, functional limitation, disfigurement or bleeding, intervention may be indicated. Percutaneous sclerotherapy performed under general anesthesia with direct puncture and injection of a sclerosant (e.g., alcohol, sodium tetradecyl) under US and fluoroscopic guidance is the treatment of choice. Surgical resection is a good option for focal localized VM but is considered a second option for diffuse lesions because of their infiltrative nature and the risk of bleeding during surgical resection. Lymphatic malformation involvement of the mouth and tongue is associated with swelling, bleeding, and airway obstruction. Lymphatic malformation in the extremities may result in diffuse or localized swelling, accompanied by soft-tissue and skeletal overgrowth. Pelvic involvement can lead to bladder obstruction, constipation, and infection. Sudden enlargement of LM may suggest bleeding, inflammation, or infection. Microcystic lesions have a high risk of recurrence following resection; thus, conservative management is advised in mild cases. Treatment options for LM include surgery, sclerotherapy, or a combination of both. With diffuse, infiltrating lesions, complete resection of the lesion is usually not possible. Recurrence rates are high. Because of the need for multiple surgical interventions, and the potential for complications, sclerotherapy (e.g., doxicycline, bleomycin, ethanol, sodium tetradecyl) is a good therapeutic option.

High-Flow Vascular Malformations

Quiescent AVMs are managed conservatively, usually without intervention. However, in patients with pain, ulceration, gangrene, congestive heart failure, or severe overgrowth, treatment typically includes transarterial or percutaneous embolization performed under general anesthesia. The treatment aim is to destroy the AVM "nidus" preserving the feeding vessels. In difficult cases, such as in patients with previous intervention or unusual anatomy, US-guided, direct puncture of the feeding vessels may be performed. Treatment of AVM is limited, and currently, is not curative. Repeated catheter embolization, sometimes combined with surgery, is often necessary for lesion control. An AVF located in large vessels may result in cardiac failure early in life resulting from a decrease in peripheral resistance and associated elevations in cardiac output. Fistulae may be treated by ligation, stenting, or embolization (e.g., Coils, Amplatzer devices). Intervention may not be necessary in smaller lesions.

Key Points

- Vascular malformations are disorders of vascular morphogenesis occurring in early fetal life.
- Although not always visible early in postnatal life, vascular malformations are present from birth and grow in proportion to the patient.
- Low-flow malformations are more common than high-flow malformations.
- Males and females are equally affected.
- Complex malformations may be associated with various syndromes.

Further Reading

Dubois J, Alison M. Vascular anomalies: what a radiologist needs to know. *Pediatr Radiol.* 2010;*40*(6):895–905.

Konez O, Burrows PE. Magnetic resonance of vascular anomalies. *Magn Reson Imaging Clin N Am.* 2002;*10*(2):363–388, vii.

Lobo-Mueller E, Amaral JG, Babyn PS, John P. Extremity vascular anomalies in children: introduction, classification, and imaging. *Semin Musculoskelet Radiol.* 2009;*13*(3):210–235.

Lobo-Mueller E, Amaral JG, Babyn PS, Wang Q, John P. Complex combined vascular malformations and vascular malformation syndromes affecting the extremities in children. *Semin Musculoskelet Radiol.* 2009;*13*(3):255–276.

Odile Enjolras MW, Chapot R. *Introduction: ISSVA Classification. Color Atlas of Vascular Tumors and Vascular Malformations.* Cambridge University Press; 2007.

CHAPTER 120

Vascular Anomalies: Vascular Tumors

Terrence Hong, MD

Definition

Vascular tumors include infantile hemangiomas (IHs), congenital hemangiomas (CHs), and other tumors (Table 120.1). These are lesions that are characterized by endothelial proliferation producing a soft-tissue mass with high flow.

Clinical Features

Infantile Hemangiomas

Infantile hemangiomas are the most common tumor of infancy with distinct proliferation (9 to 12 months) and involution (5 to 7 years) phases. These tumors are more commonly seen in females, low-weight or preterm infants, as well as infants whose mothers underwent chorionic villus sampling. Usually diagnosed clinically, IHs appear as raised red skin lesions. Infantile hemangiomas are superficial, and thus, recognized early in life. Deep lesions may present relatively later and undergo a longer proliferative phase. Skeletal changes and growth discrepancies are rare.

Congenital Hemangiomas

Congenital hemangiomas are endothelial vascular tumors that affect the skin and subcutaneous tissues. These tumors undergo a prenatal growth phase, and thus, are already at maximal size at birth. They can be further divided into rapidly involuting or noninvoluting subtypes. Rapidly involuting congenital hemangiomas (RICHs) typically involute within 12 months after birth. They present with swelling and appear pink or purple with coarse telangiectasias and a thin surrounding white halo. Local hyperthermia, venous dilation, and arterial pulsations may be seen. Noninvoluting congenital hemangiomas (NICHs) do not involute over time and lesions are flat, round, and pink or purple. There is often a peripheral white halo and telangiectasis. They appear with less dramatic clinical symptoms than RICHs.

Anatomy and Physiology

Infantile Hemangiomas

Infantile hemangiomas are benign tumors that stain positive for glucose transporter 1 protein (GLUT-1) and Lewis Y antigen. Infantile hemangiomas are GLUT-1 positive during all three phases of the life cycle. During the proliferative phase, IHs undergo increased endothelial cell turnover, leading to rapid growth within the first 9 to 12

Table 120.1 – Classification of Vascular Anomalies	
VASCULAR TUMORS	**VASCULAR MALFORMATIONS**
Infantile hemangioma	*Low-flow*
Congenital hemangioma	■ Capillary malformation (CM)
Tufted angioma	■ Venous malformation (VM)
Kaposiform endothelioma	■ Lymphatic malformation (LM)
Hemangioendothelioma	
	High-flow
	■ Arteriovenous malformation (AM)
	■ Arteriovenous fistula (AVF)
	Complex combined malformations
	■ Klippel-Trenaunay syndrome
	■ Parkes-Weber syndrome

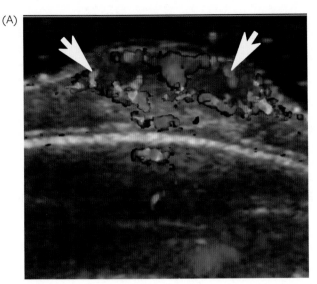

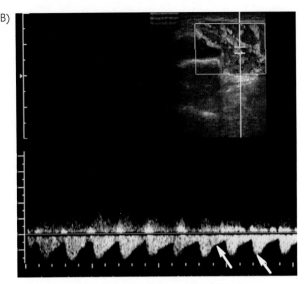

Figure 120.1. Sagittal US with color Doppler image (A) in a baby with a cheek mass noted several weeks after birth shows a soft-tissue mass containing multiple high-flow vessels (arrowheads). Transverse spectral Doppler image (B) in a 3-week-old baby with a scalp mass shows a soft-tissue mass containing multiple high-flow vessels with low-resistance pattern (arrows).

months of life. Spontaneous involution of the lesion is typically replaced with fibrofatty tissue.

Congenital Hemangiomas

Congenital hemangiomas undergo a prenatal growth phase and are fully grown at birth, unlike IHs. Furthermore, CHs are immunonegative for both GLUT-1 and Lewis Y antigen.

Imaging Findings

Infantile Hemangiomas

Infantile hemangiomas appear on ultrasound (US) as a well-circumscribed parenchymal mass often with anechoic channels with a high vessel density, high peak arterial Doppler shift, with reduction in the number of vessels during involution (Fig. 120.1A). On MRI during the proliferative phase there will be a solid, lobulated parenchymal mass that appears isointense to muscle on T1-weighted sequences and hyperintense to muscle on T2-weighted sequences. Multiple flow voids represent the high-flow vessels and there is strong enhancement after gadolinium administration (Fig. 120.1B). During the involution phase there is less gadolinium enhancement and fewer flow voids are seen resulting from reduced vascularity. Fibrofatty changes can be seen.

Congenital Hemangiomas

Rapidly involuting congenital hemangiomas appear as exophytic, hypoechoic masses with multiple, compressible vascular channels, prominent vasculature, and high flow. NICH lesions are flat hypervascular masses.

Both RICH and NICH have similar MRI characteristics: intermediate signal intensity on T1-weighted images, high signal intensity on T2-weighted fat-saturated images, and marked enhancement with intravenous gadolinium administration (Fig. 120.2A,B). Rapidly involuting congenital hemangiomas may have direct arteriovenous shunts, arterial aneurysms and thrombi. Unlike arteriovenous malformations (AVM), however, there is a soft-tissue mass.

Imaging Strategy

Ultrasound and MRI are the preferred modalities for monitoring vascular tumors as they can differentiate between different phases in the life cycle. However, many cases will require no imaging.

Doppler should be used to differentiate between different phases of the tumor life cycle and different tumor subtypes. Whenever possible, catheter angiography should be avoided because of its invasiveness and radiation exposure and is only performed in conjunction with embolization therapy.

Related Physics

Multidisciplinary clinics specializing in vascular anomalies rely on ready access to health-care information, which can include history and physical, laboratory values, biometric data, operative notes, pharmacologic data, and medical images. The Integrated Health Enterprise (IHE) embodies the goal of complete digital sharing of medical information across all specialities and platforms and is currently a work in progress both within and between institutions. Fully enacted, the IHE could greatly increase efficiency in health-care

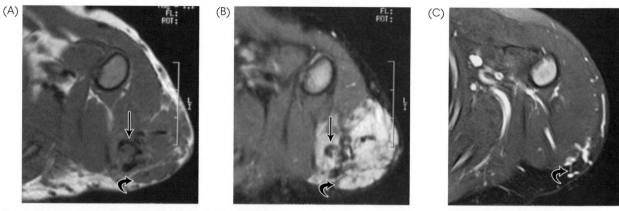

Figure 120.2. Axial T1 MR image (A) and axial T2 MR image with fat suppression (B) in a teen show a vascular tumor with high- (arrow) and low-flow (curved arrow) vascular structures involving the subcutaneous fat with a deep to the fascia component consistent with noninvoluting congenital hemangioma (NICH). Axial T2 MR image with fat suppression following treatment (C) shows almost complete interval resolution with a small residual low-flow component predominantly within the soft-tissue fat.

delivery by eliminating the need for duplicate services simply because information is not portable between institutions. One example of this is the number of times imaging studies are repeated because of lack of access to the outside images or results. Constituents within the IHE include picture archiving and communication system (PACS), hospital information systems (HIS), radiology information systems (RIS), and the electronic medical record (EMR). An industry approved language has been established to support this. The PACS is the system within the IHE for handling, moving, and storing images. The major departments that currently input into the PACS are radiology, cardiology, and obstetrics, whereas most clinical services rely on extraction of images from PACS. The HIS is where basic demographic information is stored as well as medical record numbers, insurance information, etc. One key component of IHE is that the HIS populates data downstream to the EMR and RIS without error. The RIS resides within radiology and fuses HIS and PACS information. Once a report is generated from radiology, it is sent downstream to the EMR, which collects and stores all pertinent information from other systems. At the same time this generates a signal back to the HIS to initiate billing. This loop ensures that only services rendered are billed.

Differential Diagnosis

- Venous malformations (VM) vs proliferative hemangioma: Doppler may be used to rule out hemangioma as VM has low flow
- IH vs hemangioendothelioma: unlike IH, calcifications may be present
- RICH vs AVM: RICH hemangiomas have a vascular tumor component and AVMs do not
- Fibrosarcoma, angiosarcoma, and rhabdomyosarcoma can have imaging patterns similar to deep proliferative hemangiomas

Common Variants

Patients with numerous cutaneous hemangiomas may be affected by diffuse or benign hemangiomatosis, depending on whether visceral hemangiomas are present or absent, respectively. One syndrome worth noting in pediatrics is PHACE syndrome (posterior fossa anomalies along the Dandy-Walker spectrum; multiple hemangiomas of the face, neck, and airway; arterial anomalies involving the circle of Willis; coarctation of the aorta; and eye anomalies). Some add an "S" for sternal and skin midline raphe.

Clinical Issues

Infantile Hemangiomas

For lesions near the mouth or anal-genital region, ulceration and bleeding sometimes leads to infection. Although the majority of IHs involute spontaneously, rapidly growing or "alarming" IHs may require steroid therapy, followed by sclerotherapy, embolization or surgery. NICH often undergo a combination of treatments (Fig. 120.2C).

Key Points

- Vascular tumors
- Usually diagnosed clinically, but may require imaging to assess deeper lesions
- Majority spontaneously involute
- Female predominance for IH

Further Reading

Dubois J, Alison M. Vascular anomalies: what a radiologist needs to know. *Pediatr Radiol.* 2010;*40*(6):895–905.

Dubois J, Garel L. Imaging and therapeutic approach of hemangiomas and vascular malformations in the pediatric age group. *Pediatr Radiol.* 1999;29(12):879–893.

Odile Enjolras MW, Chapot R. *Introduction: ISSVA Classification. Color Atlas of Vascular Tumors and Vascular Malformations.* Cambridge University Press; 2007.

Takahashi K, Mulliken JB, Kozakewich HP, Rogers RA, Folkman J, Ezekowitz RA. Cellular markers that distinguish the phases of hemangioma during infancy and childhood. *J Clin Invest.* 1994;93(6):2357–2364.

Index